Cardiac Surgery

Congenital Heart Disease

Color Atlas of

Cardiac Surgery

Congenital Heart Disease

James L. Monro
FRCS, Consultant Cardiac Surgeon,
Wessex Cardiac and Thoracic Centre,
Southampton General Hospital

Gerald Shore
Clinical Perfusionist, Wessex Cardiac and Thoracic Centre,
Southampton General Hospital

ACC

APPLETON-CENTURY-CROFTS/Connecticut

A Division of Prentice-Hall, Inc.

Published by Wolfe Medical Publications Ltd, 1984
Printed by Royal Smeets Offset b.v.,
Weert, Netherlands

Distributed in Continental North America by
Appleton-Century-Crofts, 25 Van Zant Street,
East Norwalk, Connecticut 06855

Library of Congress Catalog No: 82-73135
ISBN: 0-8385-1165-1

This book is one of the titles in the series of Wolfe Medical Atlases, a series which brings together probably the world's largest systematic published collection of diagnostic colour photographs.
For a full list of Atlases in the series, plus forthcoming titles and details of our surgical, dental and veterinary Atlases, please write to Wolfe Medical Publications Ltd, Wolfe House, 3 Conway Street, London W1P 6HE

Contents

To our children
Charles, Rosanne, Andrew,
Sarah and Helen

Preface

Like the previously published Coloured Atlas on aquired Heart Disease, this book of operative photographs aims to show the steps in the commoner operations performed for congenital heart disease. Explanatory diagrams have been included at the beginning of most chapters to help the understanding of the anatomy and physiology.

There are as many different ways of doing an operation as there are surgeons; however, most operations have basic set principles. Some of the rarer operations have been excluded because this book is really aimed at junior doctors starting cardiac surgery. From reading the relevant chapter they should be able to understand the various steps in each operation and hopefully be a better assistant for having done so. It is hoped that more senior surgeons will find at least some of the chapters helpful. Newly-qualified doctors, medical students and nurses will be able to refer to the appropriate chapter before watching an operation and thereby better understand what they see. Operating department nurses taking cases will find the various stages of the operations set out so that they can understand what the surgeon is doing.

The photographs in this book were taken by Mr. Gerald Shore on Kodak Ektachrome 64 ASA 19 DIN film. The camera was an Alpa Surgical Model 81 fitted with a 50mm f/1.9 Kern Macro-Switar lens and with an exposure setting of 1/60th of a second at f/22. A surgical Xenon strobe light source was used. Mr Shore is one of the perfusionists at the Wessex Cardiac and Thoracic Centre, Southampton, and has therefore been readily available to take photographs of any suitable patient. At all times the good of the patient has come first and therefore, if it would have delayed the operation unjustifiably, photography has been abandoned. This is particularly so when performing the operation under total circulatory arrest when time is pressing. Furthermore, many of the patients are very small, the exposure limited and the operation may be being performed as an emergency in the middle of the night. It has therefore taken several years to collect these photographs and, in an attempt to include only clear photographs, many series of photographs have been discarded. However, because all photographs were taken during an operation, they provide a true picture of what the operation actually looks like — unlike the line drawings, often by many different artists, in other books on operative surgery.

It is hoped that the reader will soon recognise landmarks such as the sternal retractor, which is common to so many operations. The smaller black retractor is used in infants and small children, whereas the stainless steel retractor is used in older children. This, together with the different types of cannulae used when ordinary cardiopulmonary bypass or deep hypothermia is used, enables the reader to assess the size of the patients. The orientation has been standardised, with the head of the patient at the top of the page.

We are particularly fortunate in Southampton in having a bank of antibiotic-sterilised aortic homografts for use as conduits. Particularly in the repair of persistent truncus arteriosus (Chapter 14), the Fontan procedure (Chapter 16), and correction of pulmonary atresia with ventricular septal defect (Chapter 17), these homografts are invaluable. They are the best currently available conduits but in countries where law does not permit their collection, surgeons will have to use other conduits such as pig valves mounted in Dacron tubes.

The text has been kept to a minimum so as not to detract from the atlas format that has been so effective in other books in the Wolfe series. Details of pre-operative assessment and post-operative care have been virtually excluded. Some references have been included to enable the reader to look further into the subject, and are grouped together in chapters at the end of the book.

Acknowledgements

All the photographs in this book were taken during operations performed in Southampton at the Western or General Hospitals. We are indebted to all the medical staff, operating-room nurses and technicians who have been involved. In particular we would like to thank Mr Brian Lewis (Chief Perfusionist) and Mr Charles Gilmore (Perfusionist) for standing in for Mr Shore when he unexpectedly had to take photographs. Also, we would like to thank Dr John Manners and Dr John Edwards (Consultant Anaesthetists) who have graciously made room for the photographer during those operations recorded, and Yvette Siebert for providing the beautifully prepared aortic homografts.

We would like to thank Dr Alan Johnson, Dr Neville Conway and Dr Barry Keeton for referring the patients, and the staff of the Teaching Media Department, Southampton University, for their help with developing the film.

We would like to thank Mr Duncan Larkin who drew the diagrams, our publishers for their invaluable assistance in the preparation of this book, and Mrs Julie Mintram for her secretarial help.

1: Introduction

Surgery for congenital heart disease has made dramatic advances since Gross ligated a persistent ductus arteriosus in 1938[1]. The resection of a coarctation of the aorta by Crafoord in 1945[2], the Blalock-Taussig shunt in 1945[3], pulmonary valvotomy by Brock[4] and Sellors[5] in 1948 and pulmonary artery banding by Muller and Damman in 1952[6] gave the surgeon some limited operations to treat children with congenital heart disease. However, the need to see inside a resting, empty heart to correct intracardiac lesions was essential.

Some simpler conditions were treated using moderate hypothermia and in-flow occlusion. Lewis, in 1952, successfully closed an atrial septal defect, Swan, in 1954[7], reported pulmonary valvotomy and Lewis, in 1956[8], reported aortic valvotomy using this technique.

Lillehei[9] briefly used cross-circulation with an adult for the repair of congenital defects in children, but to Gibbon[10] must go the credit of performing the first successful operation using cardiopulmonary bypass. He closed an atrial septal defect by direct suture in an 18-year-old girl on the 6 May 1953. After this, great progress was made over the next few years in the technology of cardiopulmonary bypass, and this allowed the surgeon to tackle many challenging congenital defects. In the 1960s, the oxygenators used were mainly non-disposable and, particularly in infants, the longer bypasses needed to deal with more serious conditions were not well-tolerated. Because of the disappointing results in children, there was a tendency to palliate initially and then correct at about 5 years of age.

However, with the improvement in oxygenators, post-operative care and a better understanding of the complex anatomy of some of these lesions, surgeons began to get better results when performing total correction in the first year of life[11].

The introduction of a technique of surface cooling, total circulatory arrest and bypass rewarming (Hisaka *et al*, 1967)[12] and its popularisation by Barratt-Boyes and co-workers (1971)[13] has contributed greatly to the improvement in results in infants since 1970.

The operations illustrated in this book have been performed on both infants and older children. Although each chapter sets out to illustrate the different types of operation in isolation, it is frequently necessary to perform more than one procedure at the same time in one patient. For example, a patient may need an atrial septal defect and ventricular septal defect closed, or an infant may need repair of coarctation of the aorta and banding of the pulmonary artery.

The pre-operative assessment of the patient is very important and the surgeon relies heavily on the cardiologist to provide an exact diagnosis. The surgeon must know exactly what he is going to find at operation – he should only have to confirm the diagnosis, not spend time trying to establish one. The patient must be in the best possible clinical state, and, particularly in small infants, this requires meticulous attention to treating heart failure, the acid-base state and keeping the child warm.

Before operation the child must be suitably anaesthetised and paralysed[14] and an endotracheal tube inserted. The patient is then ventilated except when on full cardiopulmonary bypass. Arterial and central venous pressure lines are inserted to help the anaesthetist monitor the patient during the operation and post-operative period. The surgeon then opens the chest; most operations are performed through a median sternotomy, as illustrated in Chapter 2. Those patients undergoing operation on cardiopulmonary bypass will require heparinisation before the insertion of arterial and venous cannulae.

If the right side of the heart is to be opened, as for the closure of an atrial or ventricular septal defect, then two venous cannulae must be inserted, one into each vena cava, and an air-tight seal achieved around it with a snugger. If the left side of the heart is being opened, as for an aortic valvotomy, then it is only necessary to insert one venous cannula into the right atrium.

Once the cannulae are in position and connected to tubing from the cardiopulmonary bypass machine, bypass can be commenced. The desaturated venous blood siphons back from the patient to a disposable bubble oxygenator. Oxygen and carbon dioxide are bubbled through the blood in the oxygenator and the fully saturated blood is defoamed and pumped back to the patient. There are many different types of cardiopulmonary bypass arrangements; the reader is referred to other descriptions[15] as this topic is outside the scope of this book.

Once bypass has been commenced, the ascending aorta can be clamped and it is usual to protect the myocardium with cold cardioplegic solution[16], which is infused directly into the ascending aorta. The heart can then be opened and the repair performed.

1
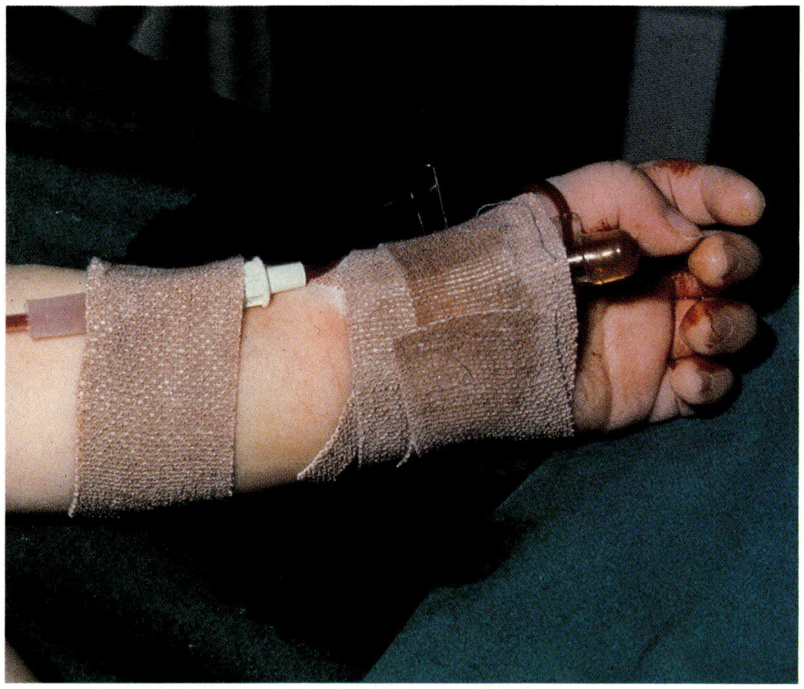

2
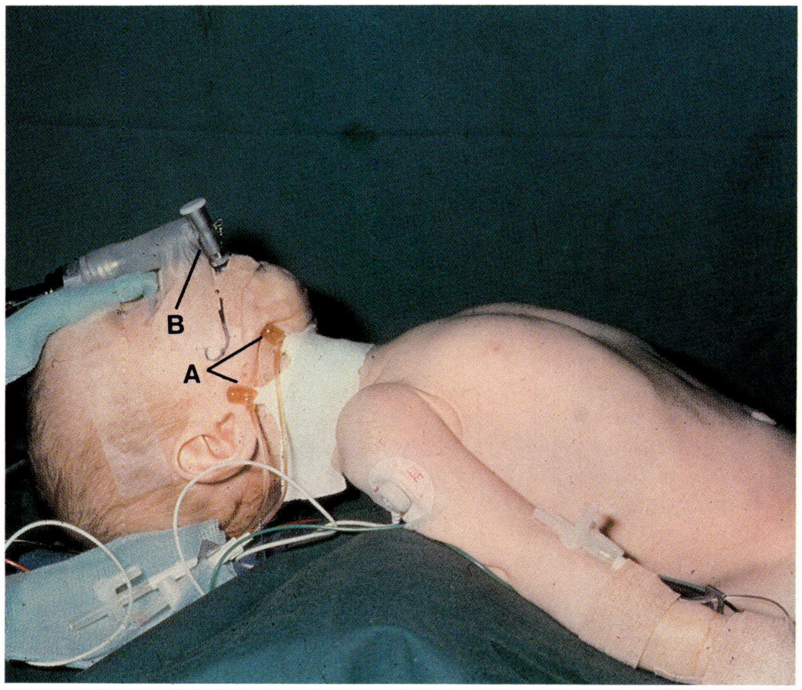

1 To monitor the arterial pressure during the operation, a cannula is inserted percutaneously into the radial artery, securely fixed and connected to a transducer and monitor giving a direct readout of the arterial pressure.

2 To monitor the venous pressure and for the administration of drugs, central venous cannulae (**A**) are inserted through the internal jugular vein. The endotracheal tube (**B**) is also shown, and it is helpful to position the child's shoulders on a pillow, to bring the chest forward for easier access.

3
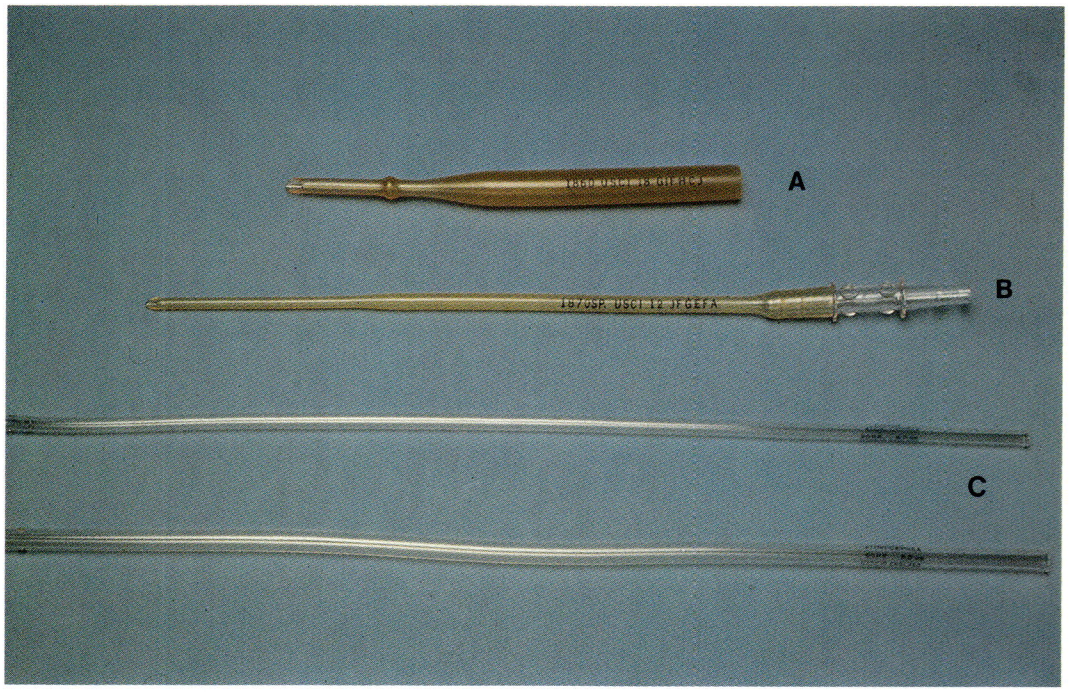

3 The arterial cannulae used in older children (**A**) and for infants (**B**) are shown together with two venous cannulae (**C**).

4

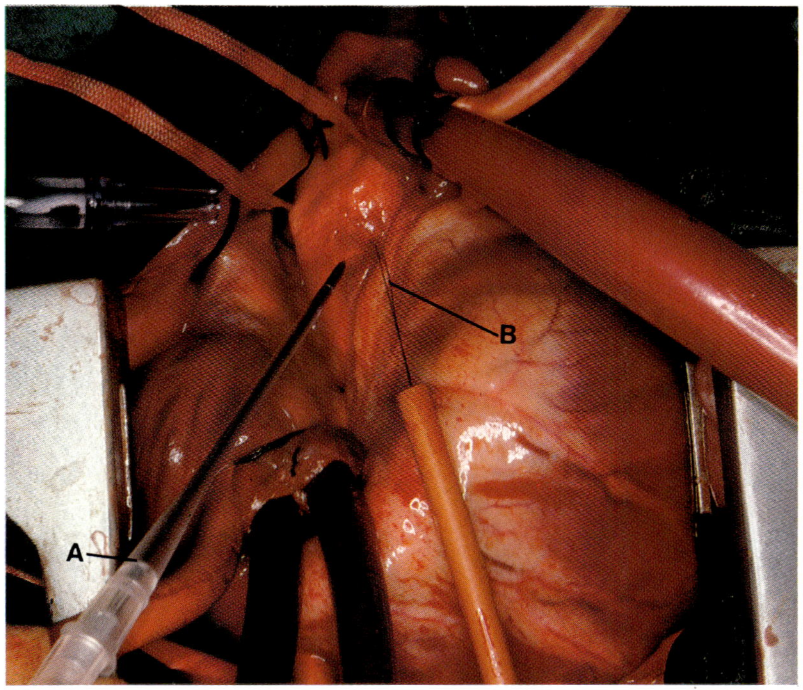

5

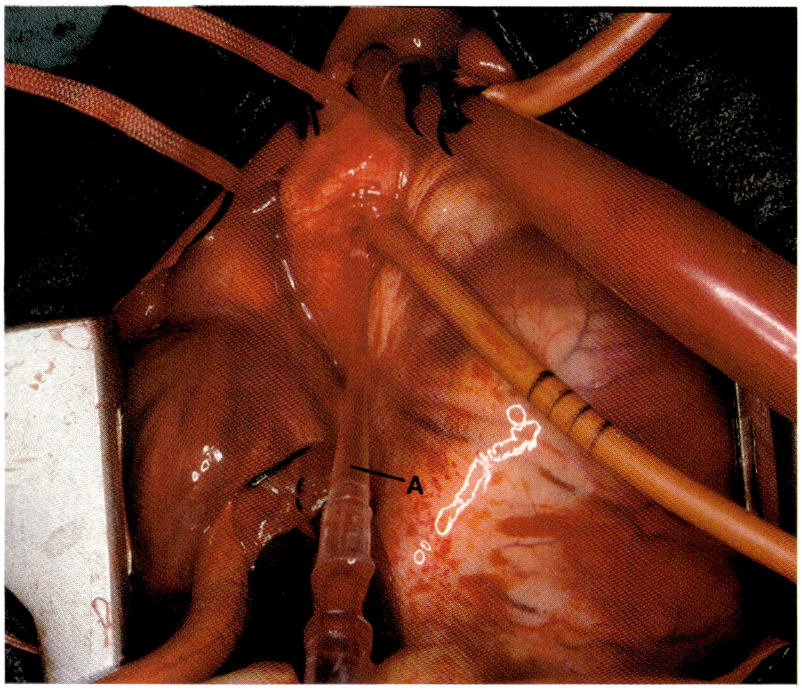

4 and 5 A small cannula (**A**) is inserted into the ascending aorta through a purse-string suture (**B**) which is snugged, and the cannula connected to drip tubing for the administration of cardioplegic solution at 4 °C.

6

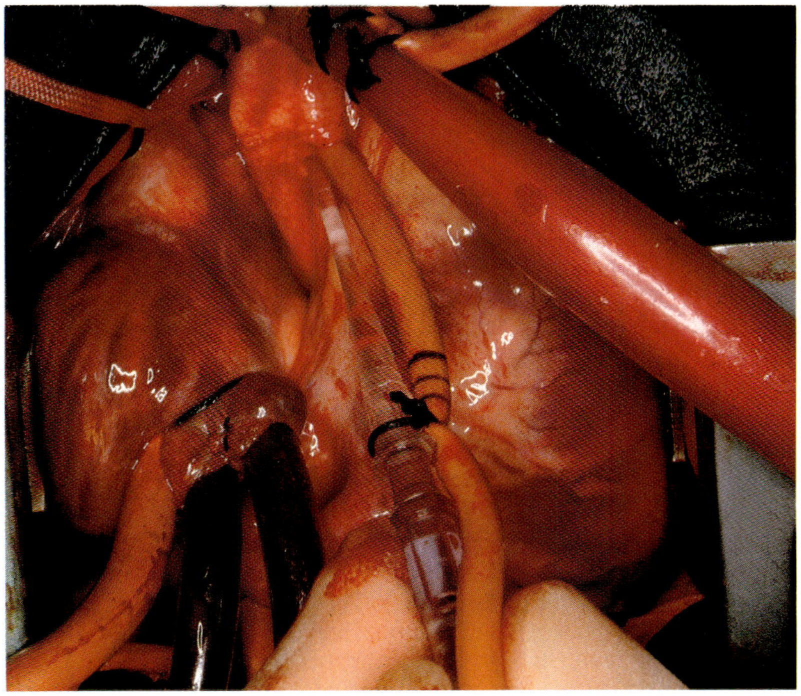

7

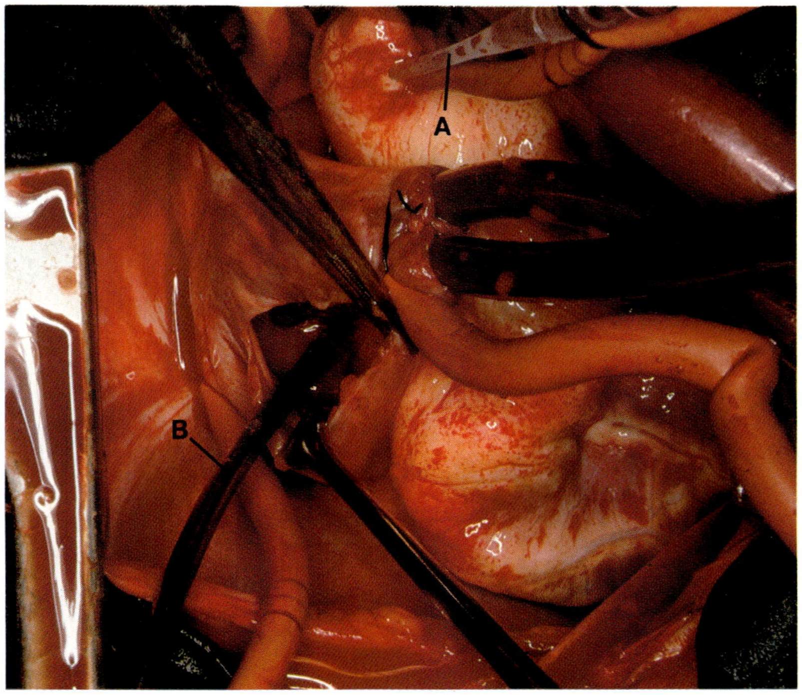

6 The cannula is tied to the rubber snugger so that it will not slip out.

7 After bypass has been started and the aorta cross-clamped, cardioplegic solution is infused through the cannula (**A**) into the ascending aorta, from where it passes through the coronary arteries, emerging from the coronary sinus in the right atrium. Here the right atrium has been opened and a sucker (**B**) removes the cardioplegic fluid.

8

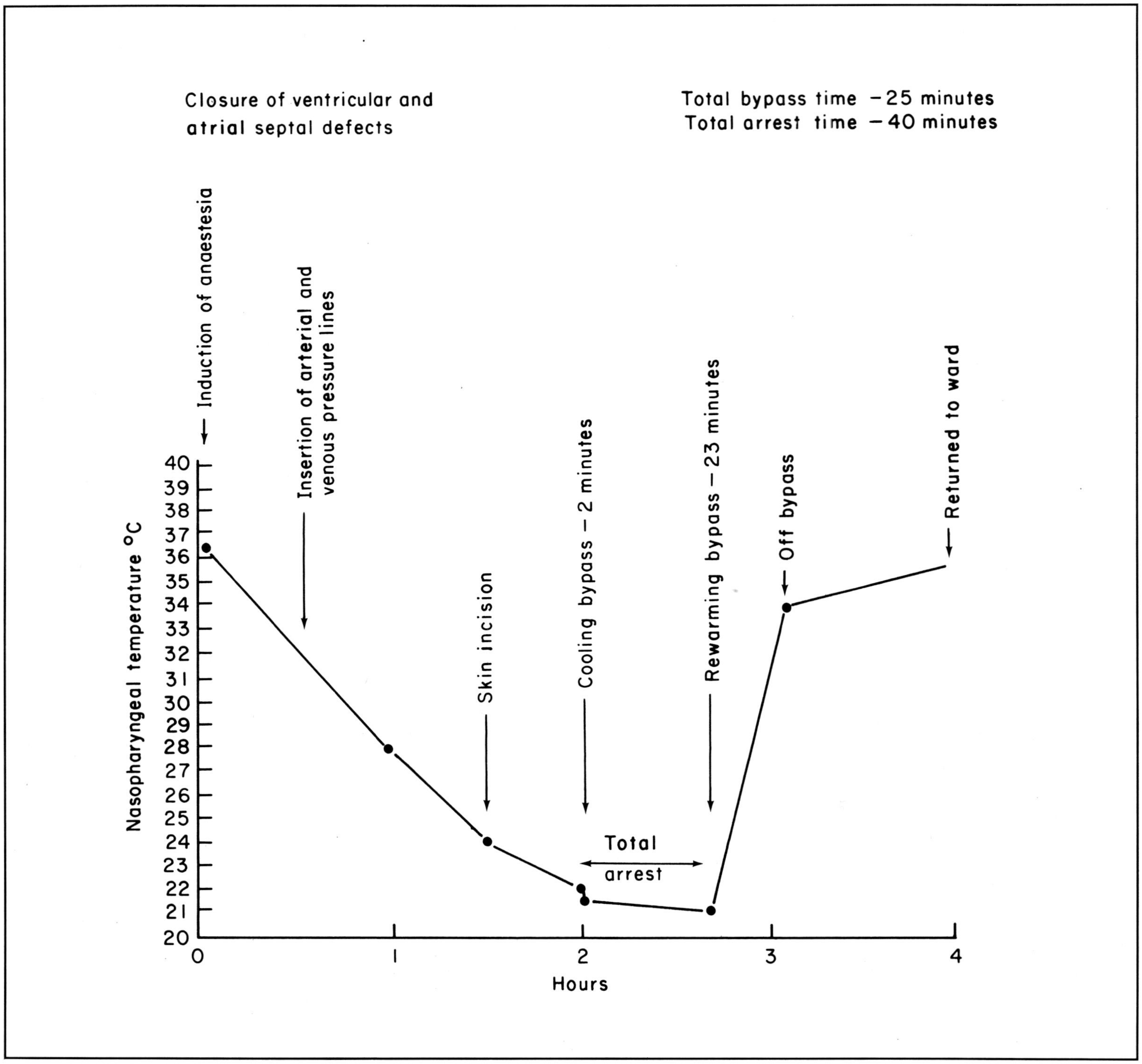

8 For many of the intricate repairs on small infants it is essential to have a still, bloodless field. This is best achieved with total circulatory arrest and it is therefore possible to remove the venous cannulae. Some surgeons prefer to use core cooling on bypass to a suitably low temperature and then stop bypass. The author's preference is for surface cooling to about 25 °C (see graph), then the chest is opened, bypass instituted and the patient cooled for a short further period on bypass. In the case illustrated, the patient needed closure of a ventricular septal defect and an atrial septal defect. As this was not expected to take very long, the patient was only cooled to 22 °C (nasopharyngeal), and the duration of total circulatory arrest was 40 minutes, which is quite safe at this temperature. However, when longer periods are needed for the correction of more complicated lesions, it is safer to cool on bypass for perhaps 5 minutes and stop at 18 °C, at which temperature it is safe to stop for at least one hour. Rewarming on bypass takes about 25 to 30 minutes and, when a nasopharyngeal temperature of 34 °C has been reached, bypass can be discontinued, the cannulae removed and the patient further slowly rewarmed on a water-blanket. Thus the total bypass time is about 30 minutes, which is considerably shorter than would be achieved with bypass alone, and the operating conditions are excellent.

The whole technique, however, is one which requires considerable experience and any prospective users are recommended to research the subject in depth [12,13,14,17].

The following pictures describe the surgical steps in using the surface cooling and total circulatory arrest technique, as used by the author.

9

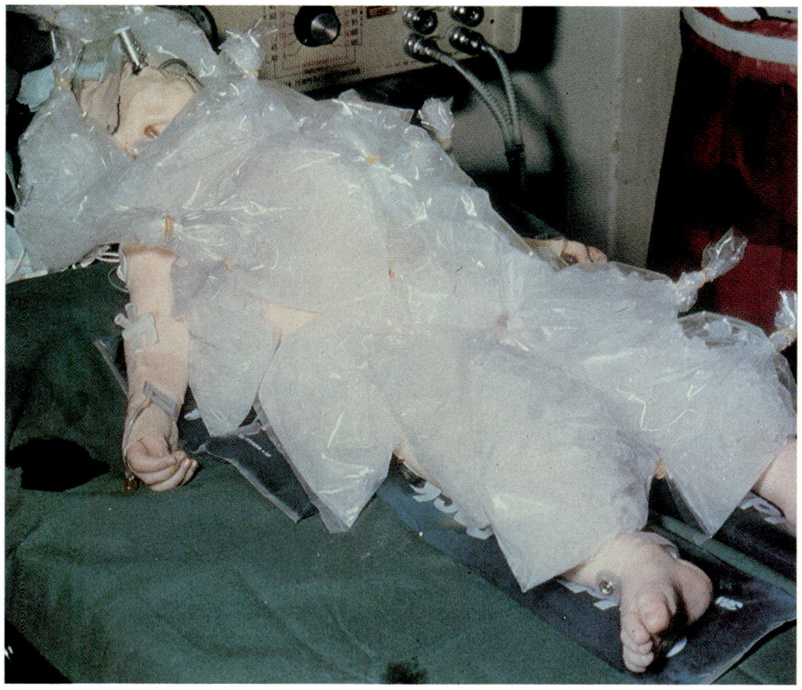

10

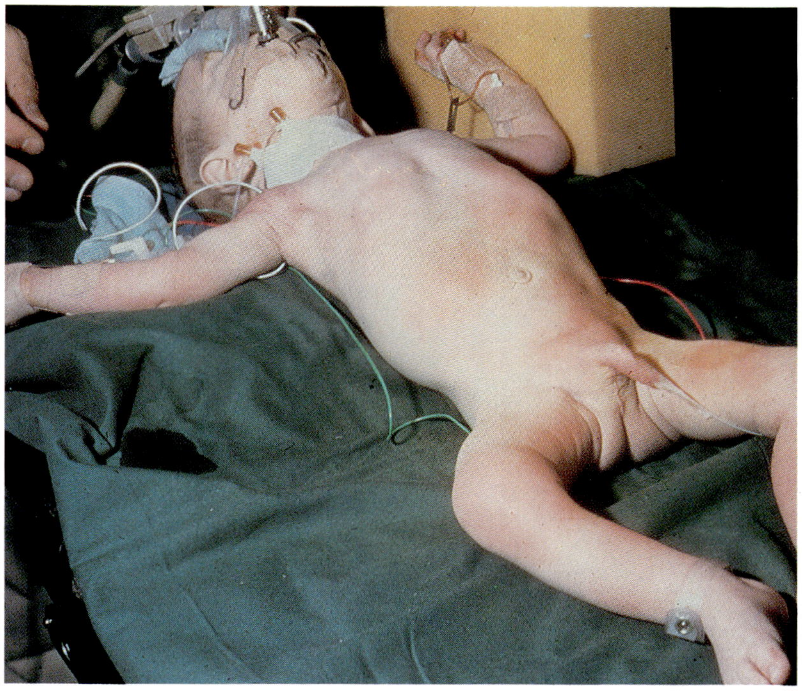

9 Once the anaesthetised patient has had the monitoring lines and a urinary catheter inserted, ice-bags are placed over the infant, who is already lying on a water-blanket.

10 When the nasopharyngeal temperature has reached a sufficiently low level, such as 25 °C, the ice is removed and the chest can be opened.

11

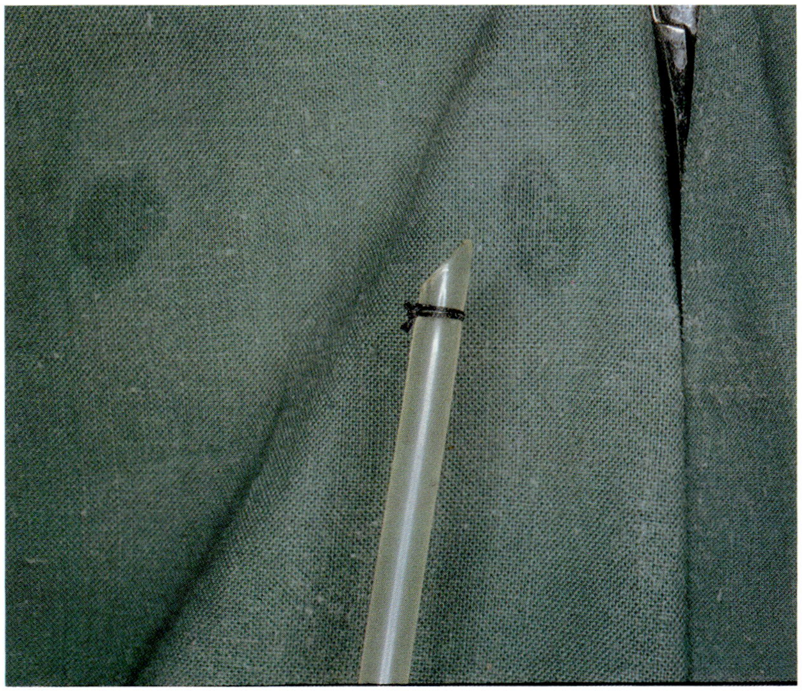

12

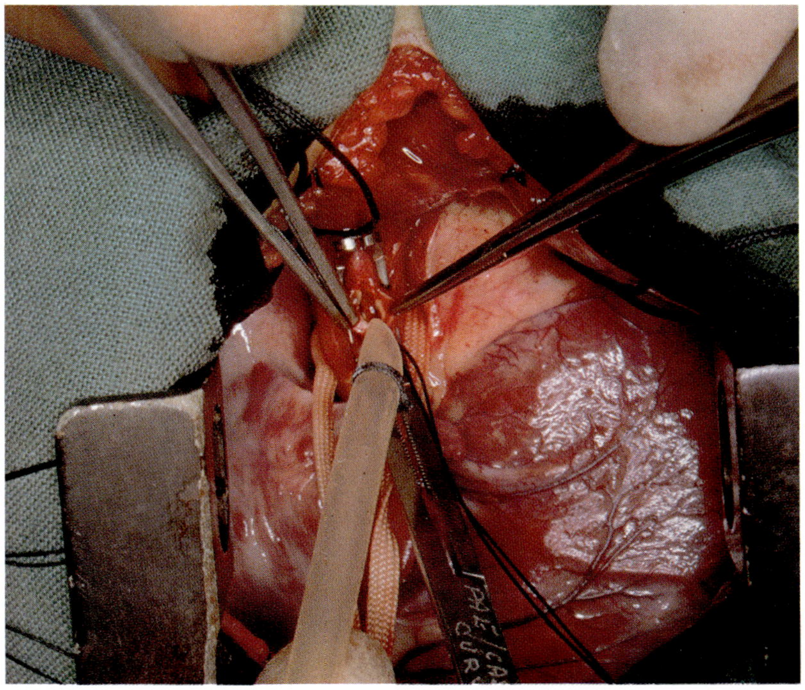

11 A tie is placed around the end of the aortic cannula to allow only the distal short end to enter the aorta. This facilitates the removal of air from the heart at the end of the operation.

12 A side-clamp has been placed on the ascending aorta, a longitudinal incision made and a purse-string suture placed. The aortic cannula is about to be inserted.

13 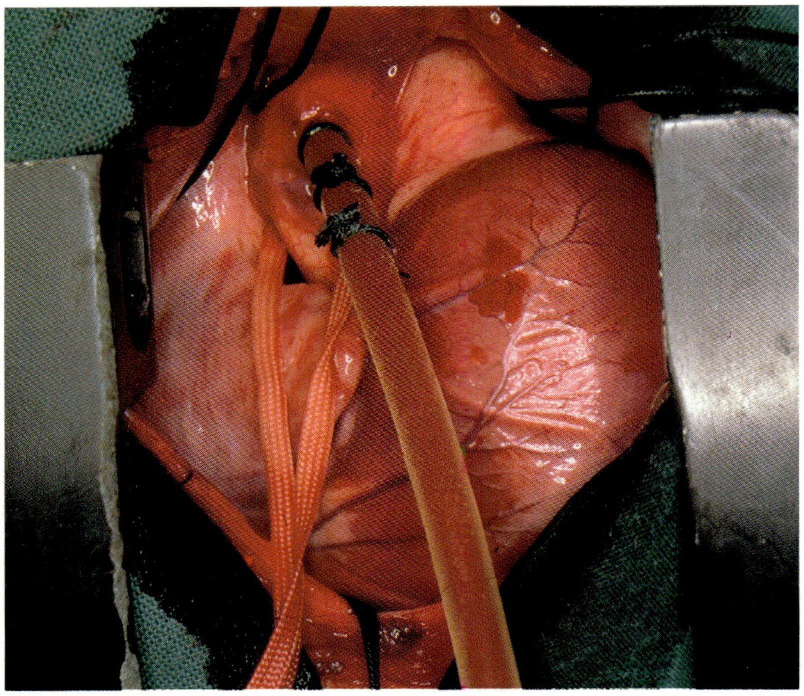

14 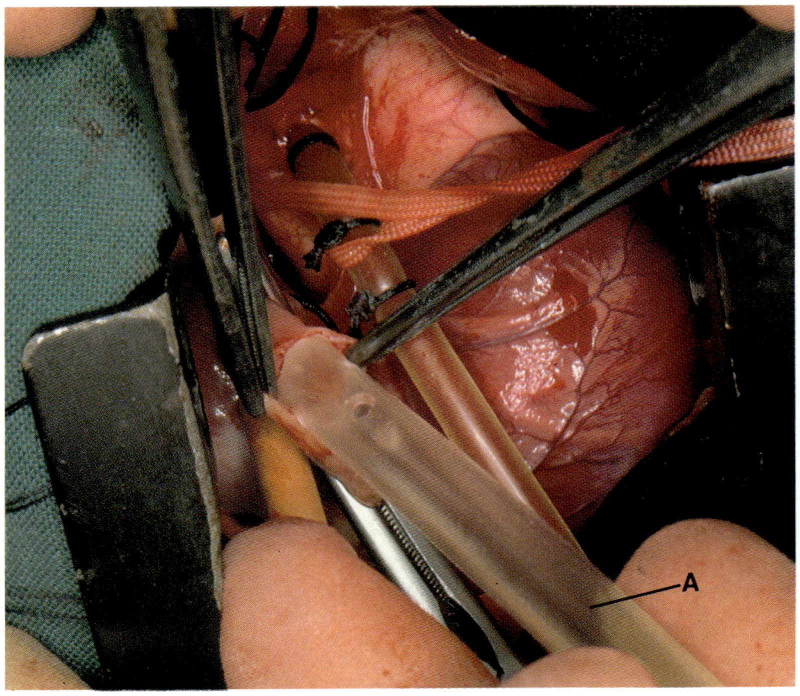

13 The aortic cannula is now in position and it is fixed in position by two silk ties which also hold the purse-string suture.

14 The single venous cannula (**A**) is now inserted into the right atrial appendage.

15 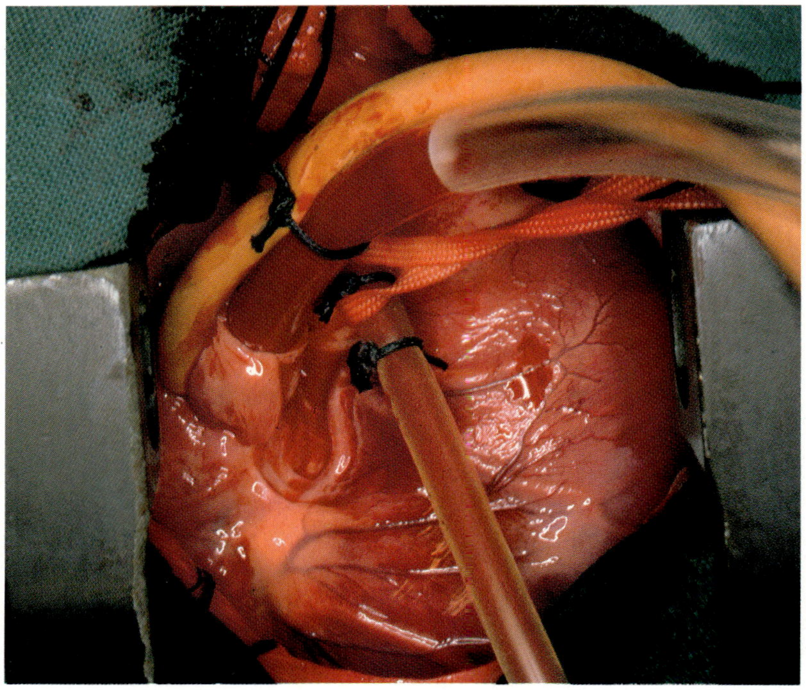

16 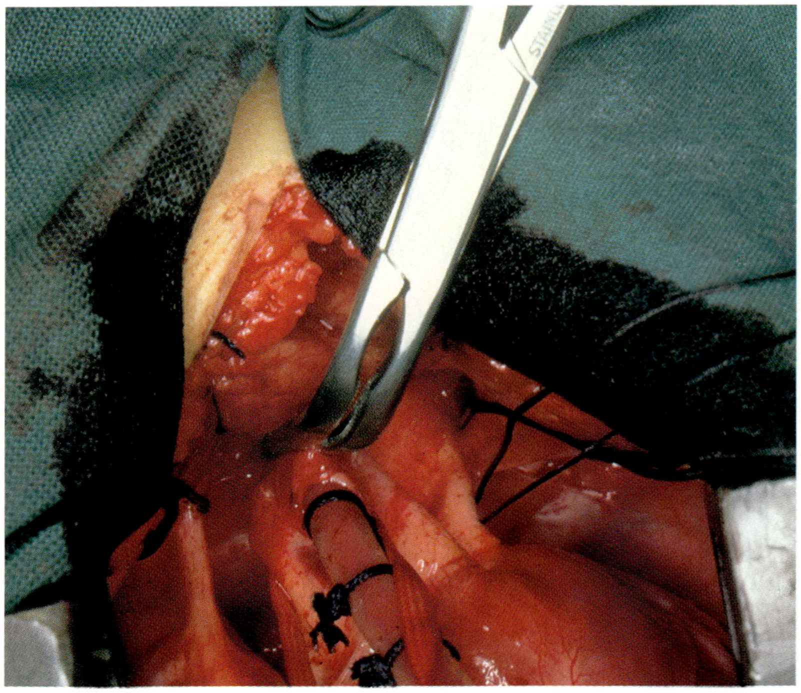

15 and 16 Bypass is begun and the patient cooled for a short period until an appropriate temperature is reached. Then the aorta is cross-clamped distal to the aortic cannula, which is possible as the cannula has only been inserted a short distance.

17

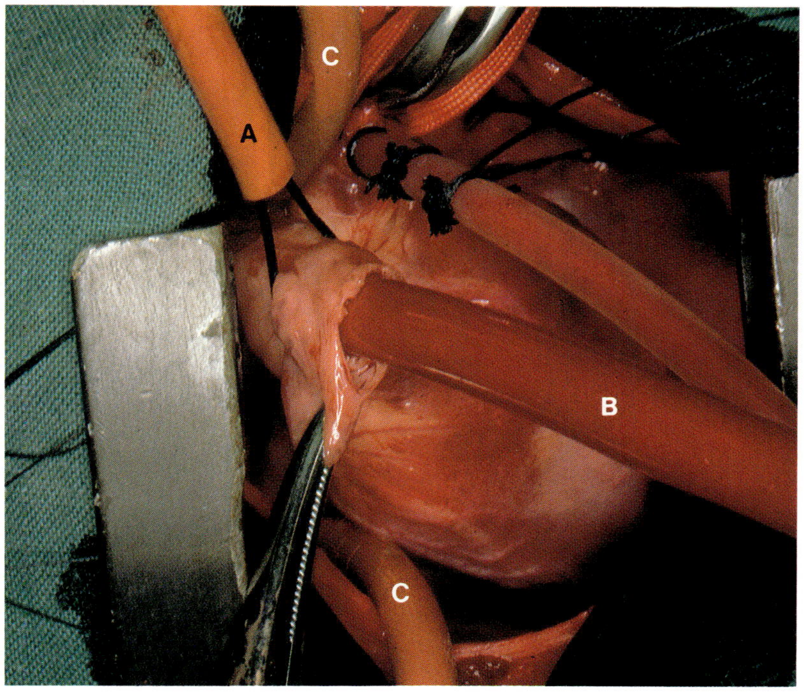

17 The snugger holding the cannula in the right atrium is released (**A**) and the cannula (**B**) removed after snugging the vena caval snares (**C**).

18

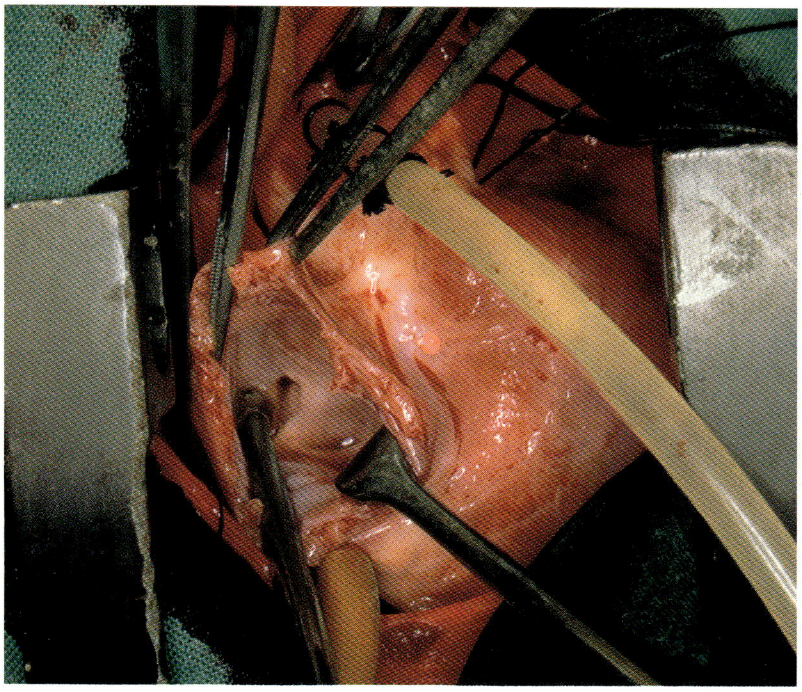

18 Cardioplegic fluid is now infused via a three-way tap into the aortic cannula and sucked from the right atrium. This rather unusual clear appearance of the aortic cannula will be seen throughout the book and indicates those patients in whom circulatory arrest was used.

19

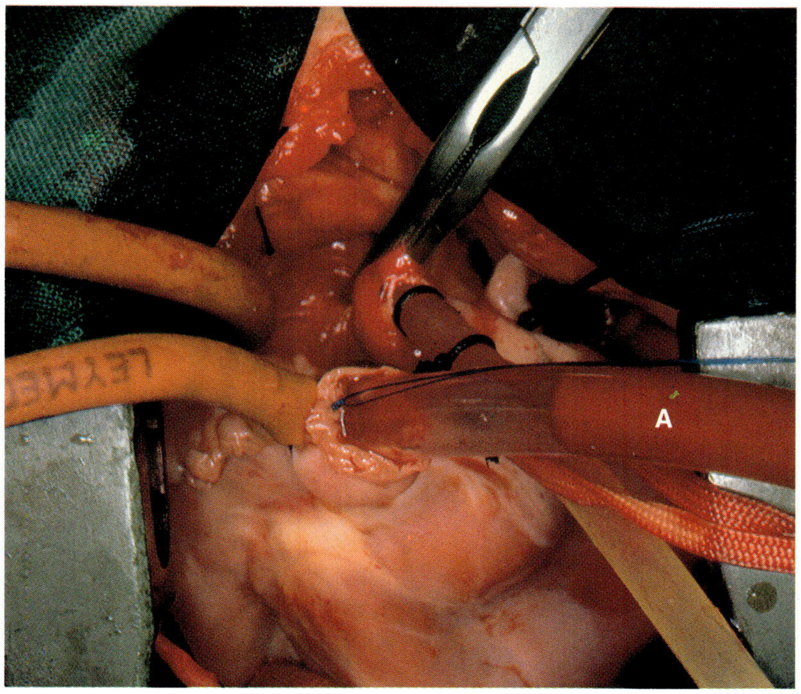

19 Once the repair is complete, the venous cannula is reinserted (**A**).

20

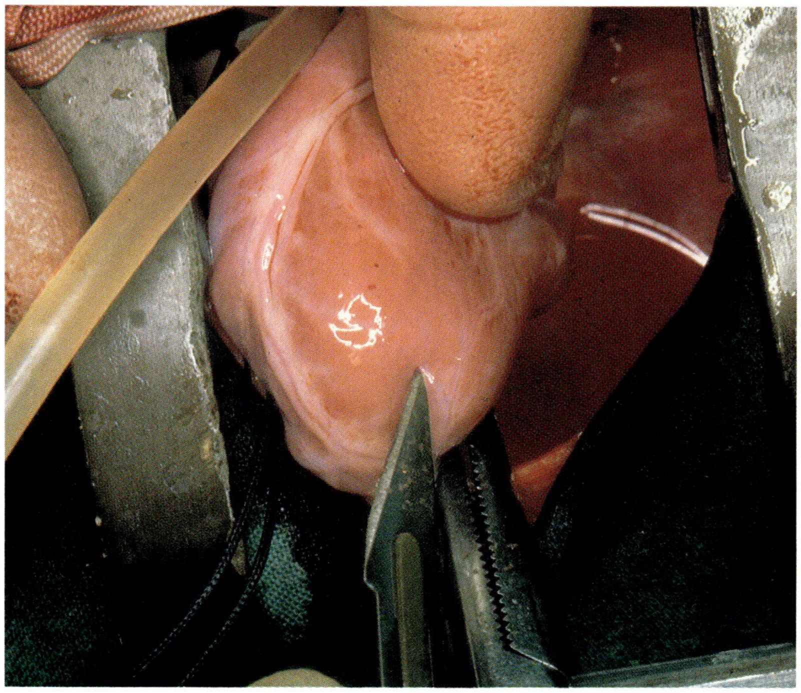

20 To remove the air from the heart, a small incision is made in the apex of the left ventricle.

21

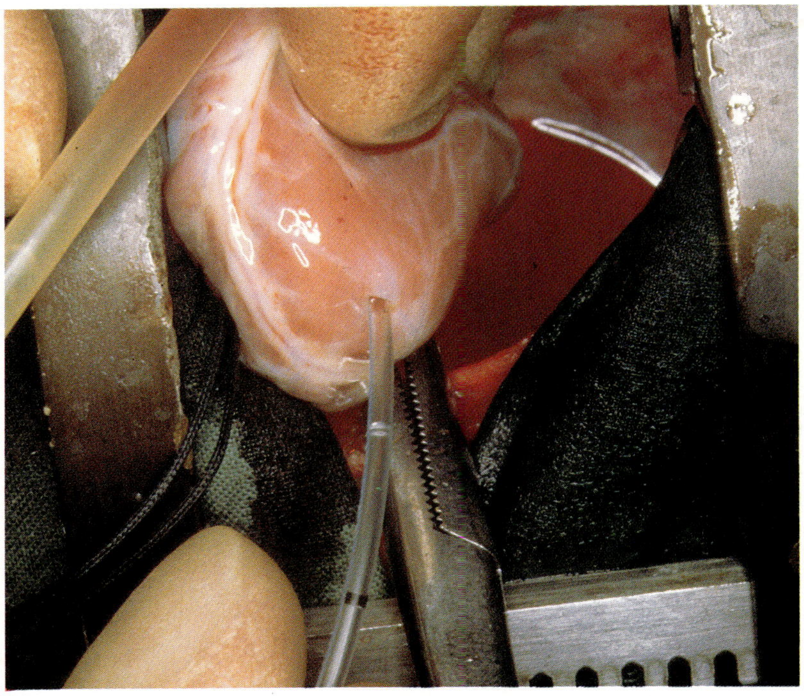

22

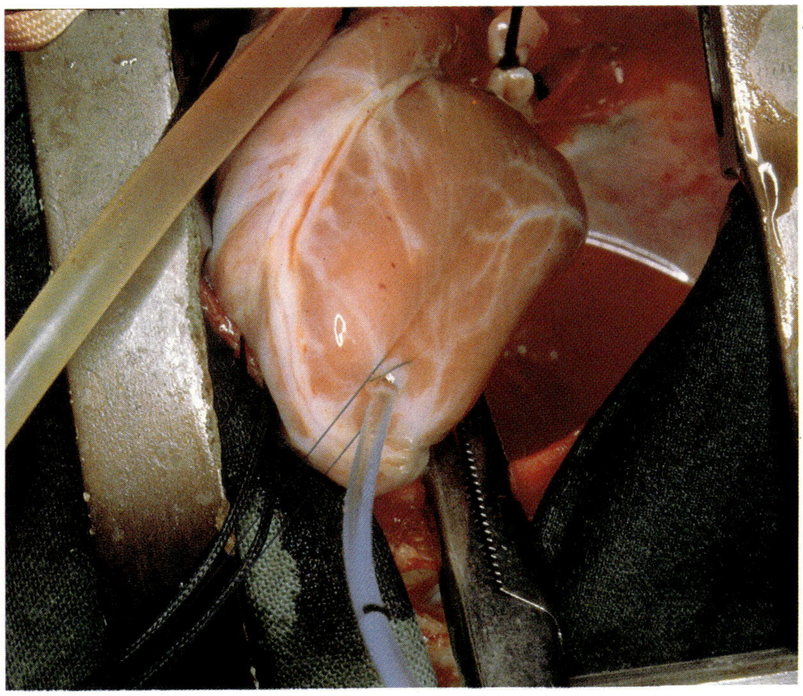

21 and 22 A fine cannula connected to a syringe of Ringer's or Hartman's solution is inserted, and a suture placed around it.

23

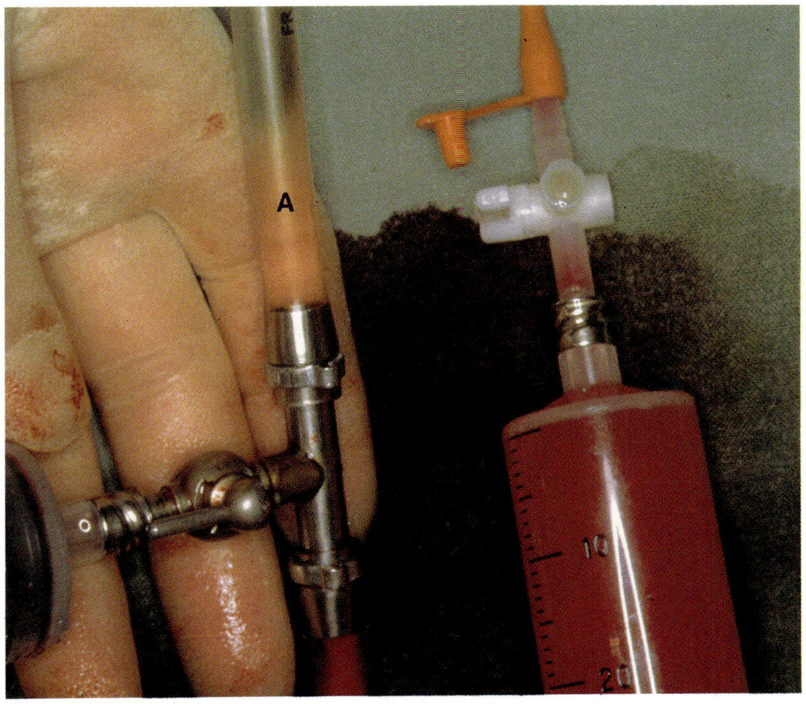

23 Then, while fluid is gently injected into the left ventricle, which has been allowed to fall back in the pericardial cavity, air and fluid are aspirated from the arterial line (**A**), until no more air is found.

24

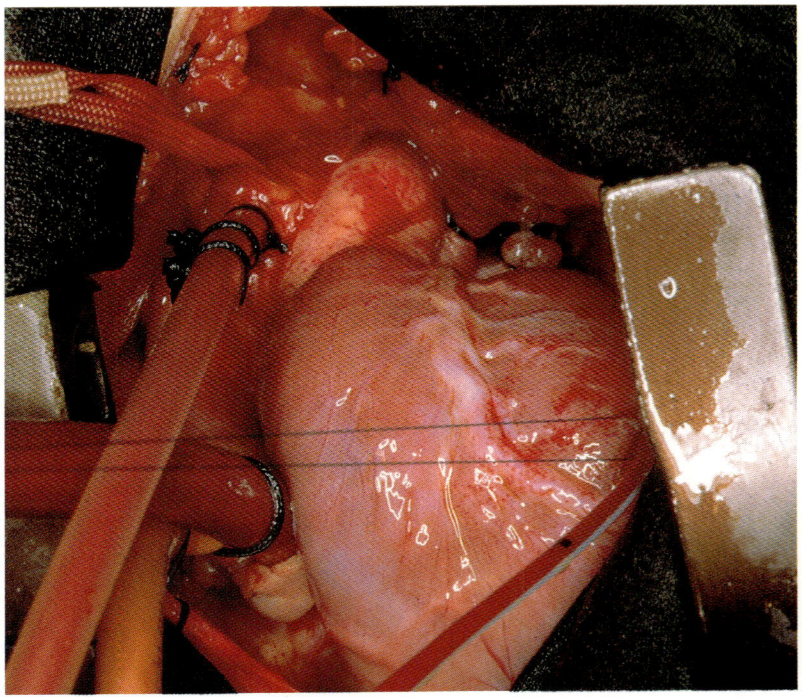

24 The aortic clamp is then released and bypass gently recommenced. To ensure removal of any further air, the ventricle is tipped up and aspirated through the same catheter a few times before removing it once the heart starts to beat. The patient is then rewarmed on bypass.

2: Median sternotomy and institution of cardiopulmonary bypass

The midline approach gives excellent exposure for all procedures requiring cardiopulmonary bypass in children. In this chapter the routine procedure for the institution of cardiopulmonary bypass will be described. Whether one or two venous cannulae are inserted depends on what operation is to be performed. Clearly, if the right atrium is to be opened (as for closure of an atrial septal defect), a cannula must be placed down each vena cava and an air-tight seal be achieved, or air will be sucked down into the venous reservoir and stop the siphon. If the right atrium does not need to be opened (as for an aortic valvotomy), one venous cannula is quite adequate. Otherwise, all procedures have the same basic steps as outlined in this chapter and if the operating team follows the same routine every time, what may otherwise be a rather tedious part of cardiac surgery can be dealt with quickly and efficiently.

1

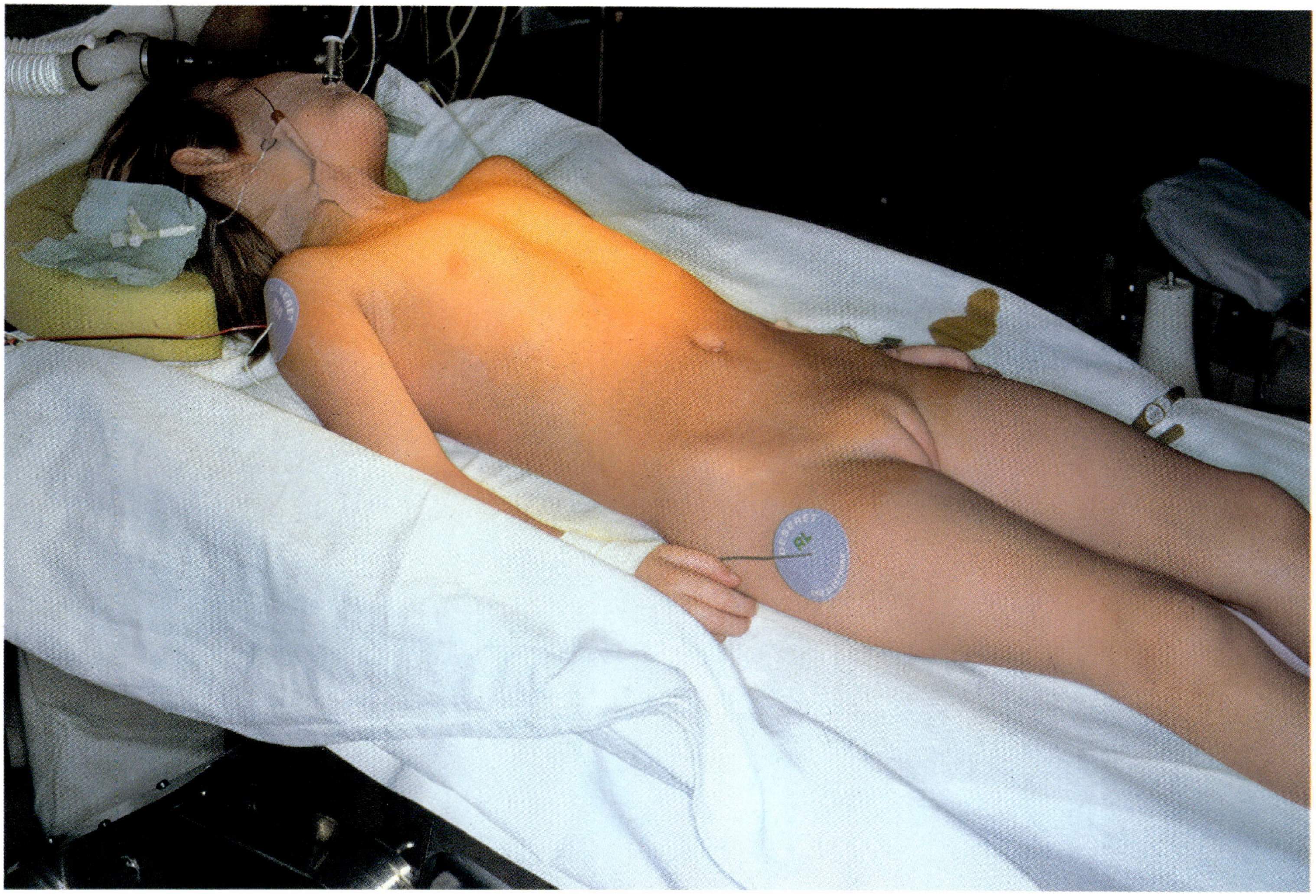

1 The anaesthetised child is placed on her back on the operating table and the skin prepared with iodine or some such antiseptic.

2

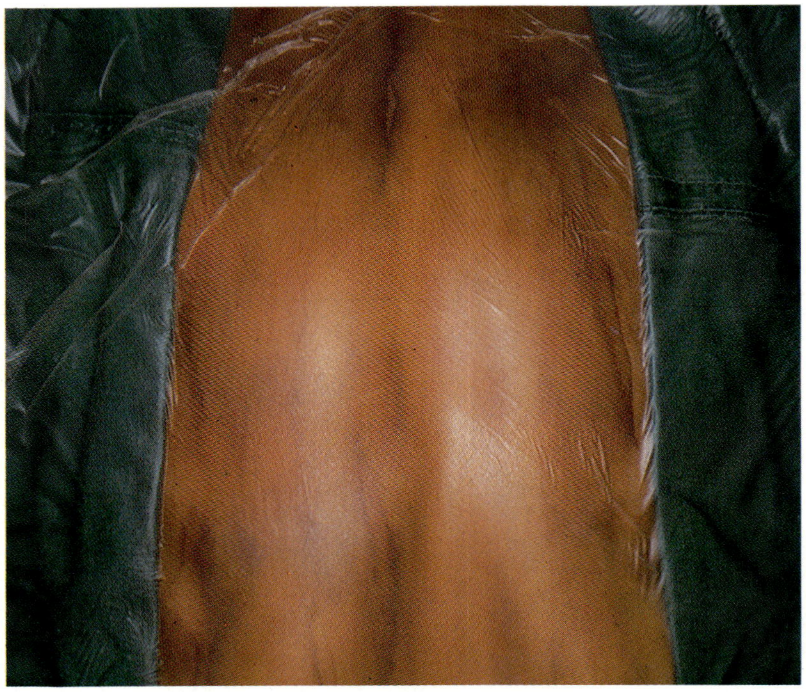

3

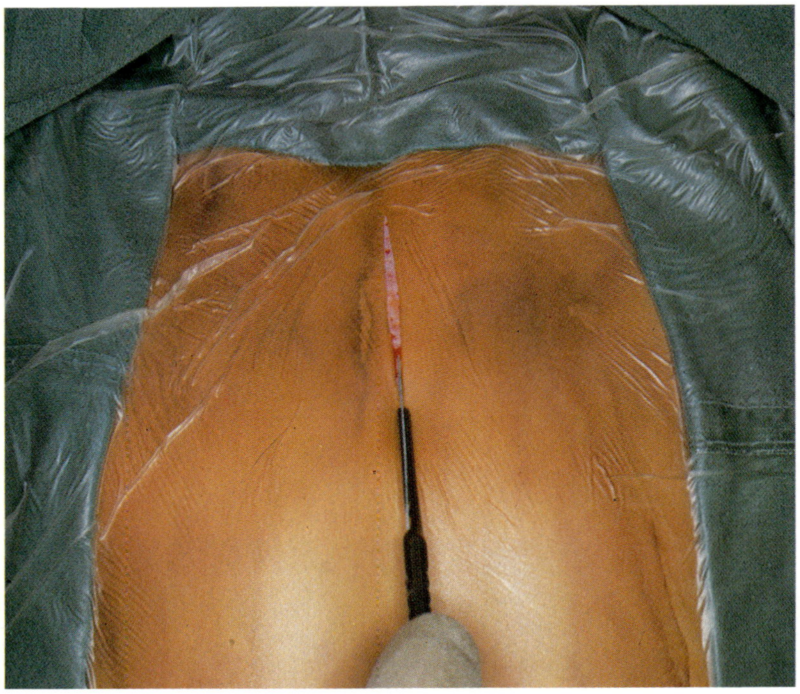

2 to 5 Drapes are placed around the chest and Steridrape applied. The knife is used to incise the skin, but the diathermy carefully used to incise the deeper layers down to the bone.

4

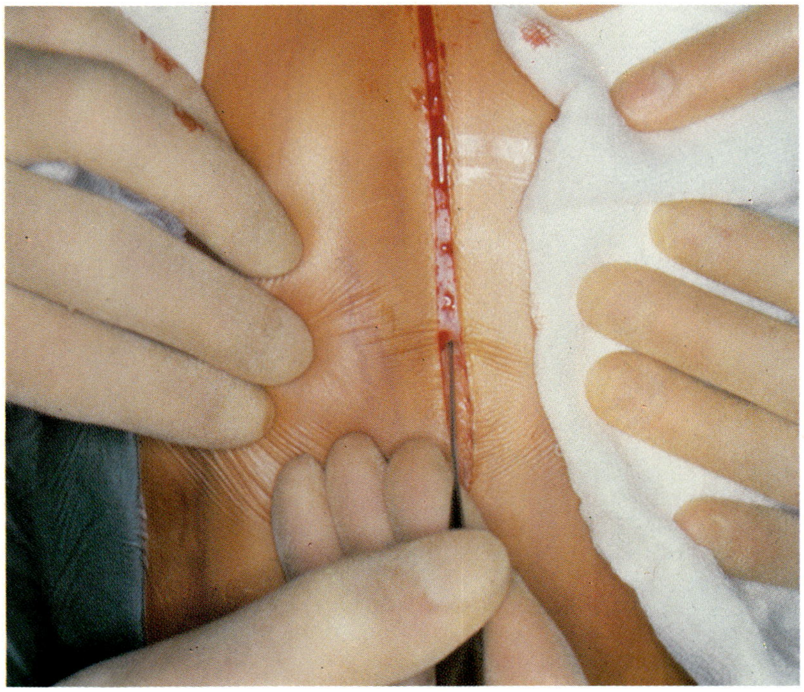

5

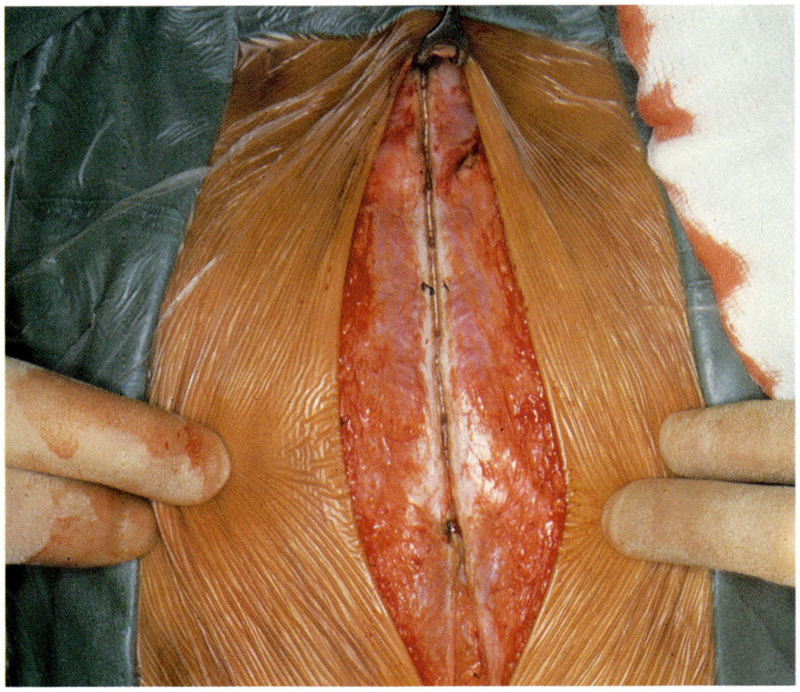

6

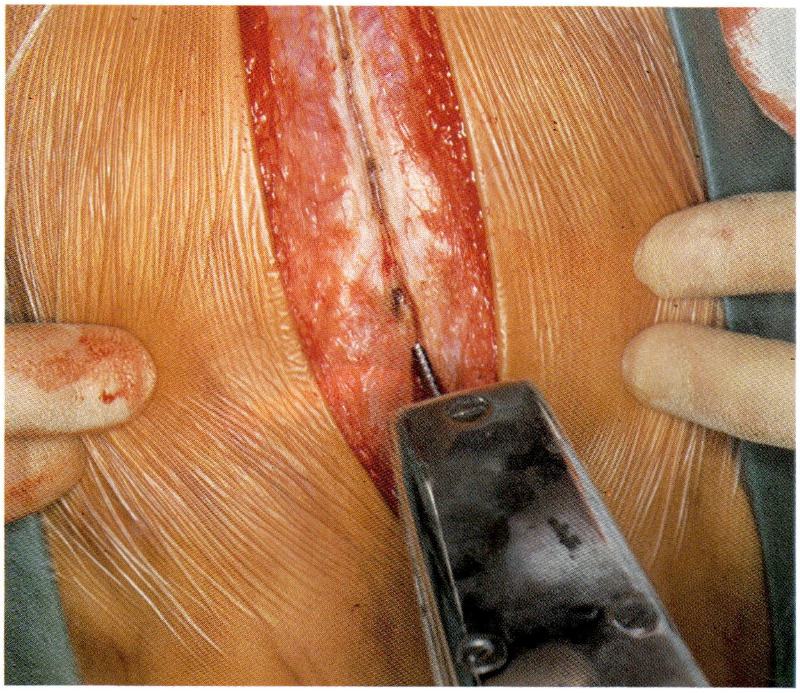

7

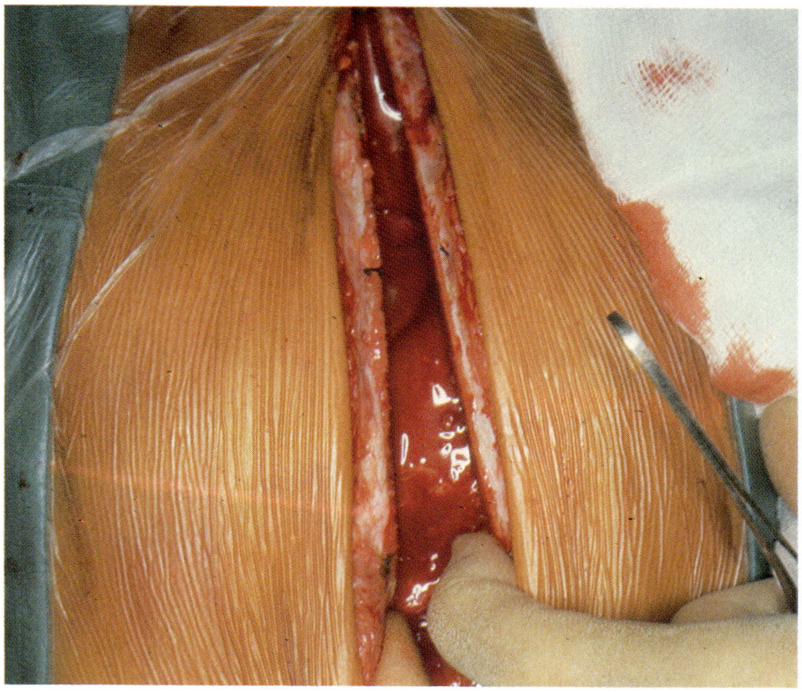

6 to 9 The sternum is then divided longitudinally with a mechanical saw, the edges of the bone diathermied and wax sparingly pressed into the cut surface of the bone to stop bleeding.

8

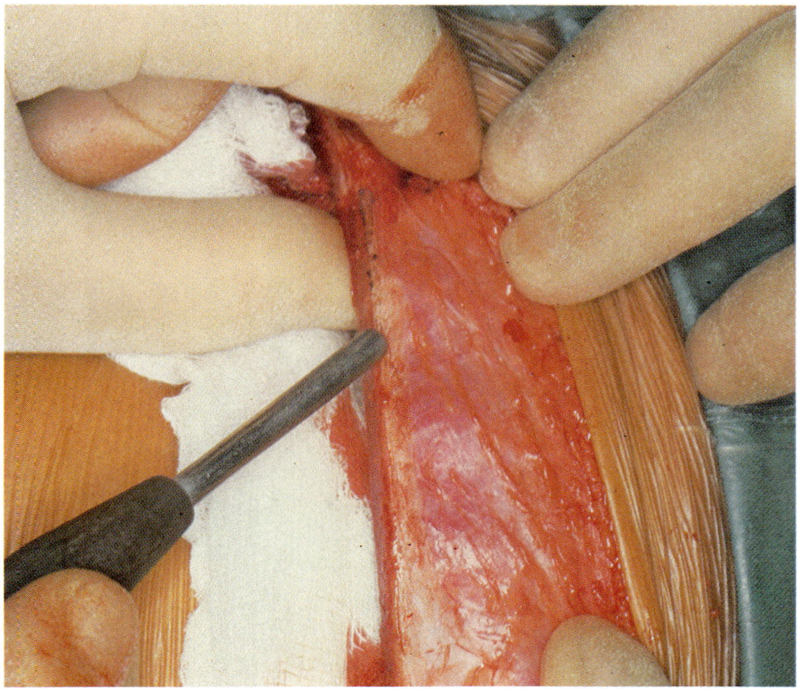

9

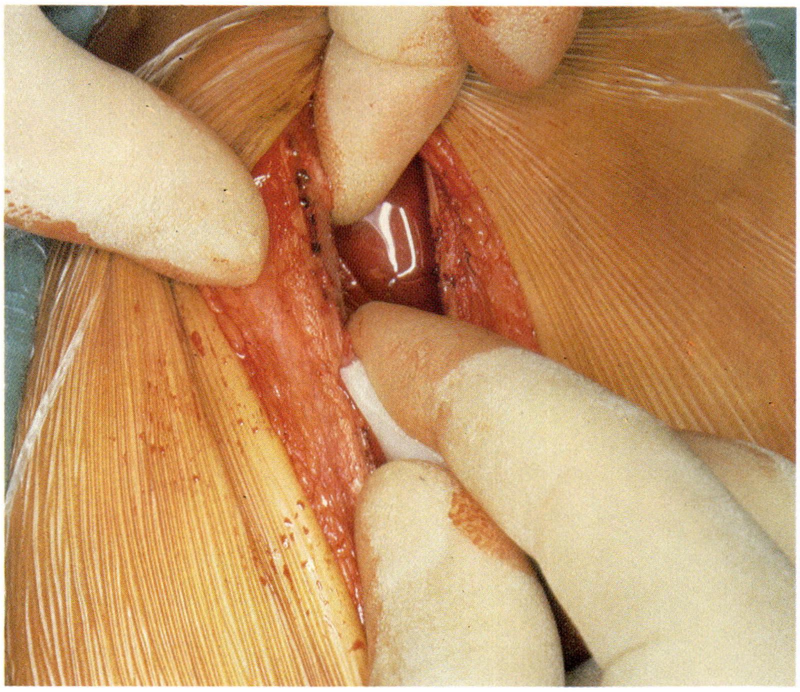

10

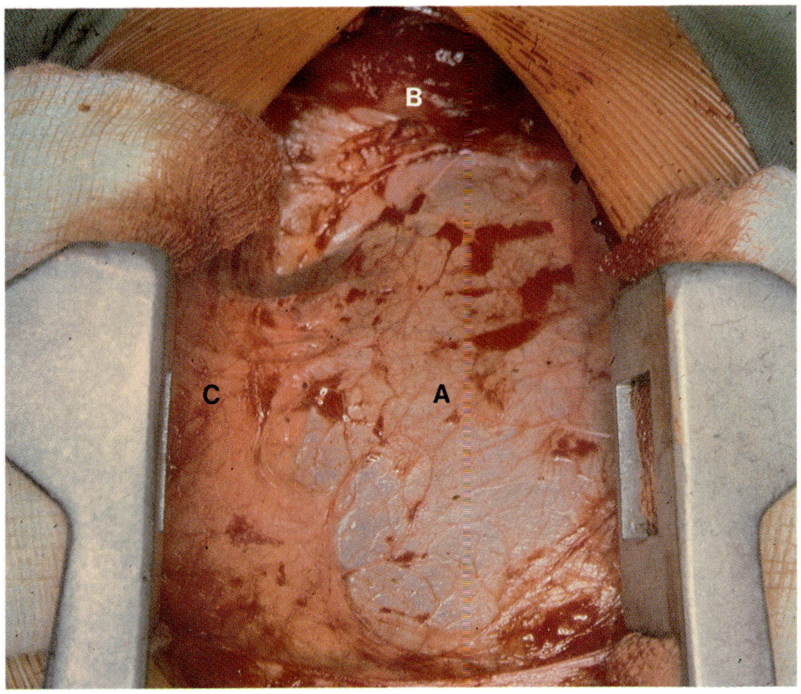

11

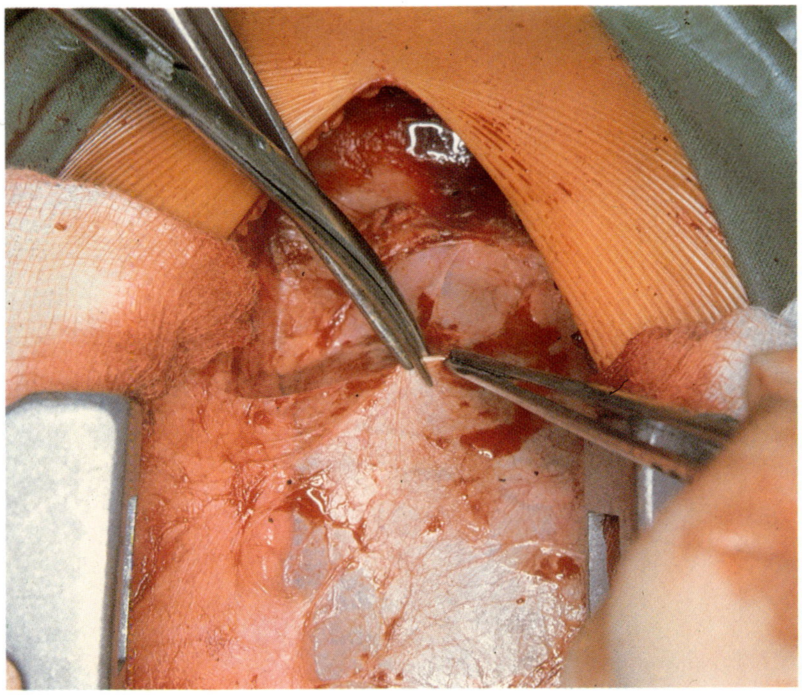

10 A swab is placed over the bone on each side and the sternal retractor inserted. The pericardium (**A**) is then exposed and it is usually necessary to dissect the thymus (**B**) upwards off it. The pleura (**C**) can be seen laterally, but it is not intentionally opened and therefore the lungs are not seen.

11 to 13 The pericardium is then incised and three stay-sutures placed in the cut edge on each side to help retraction and exposure.

12

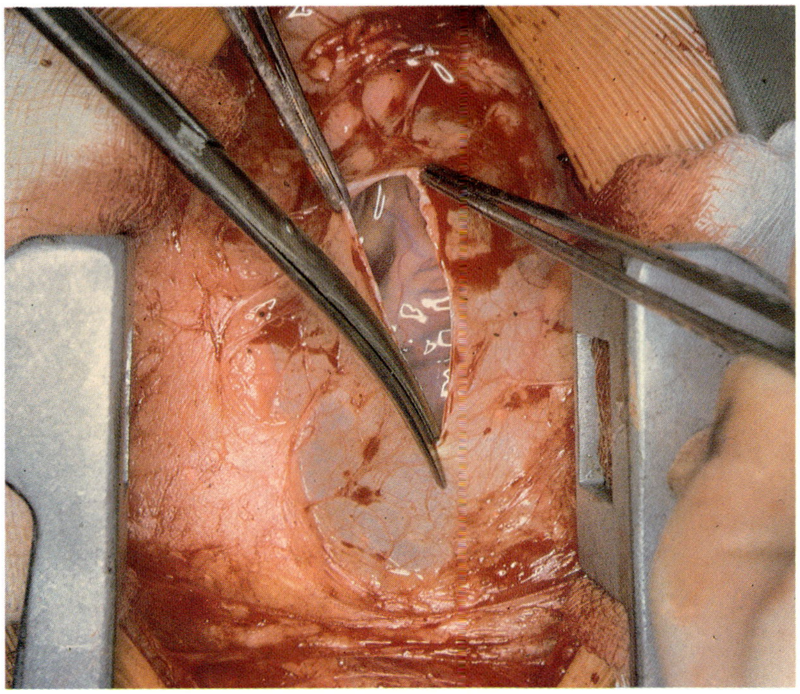

13

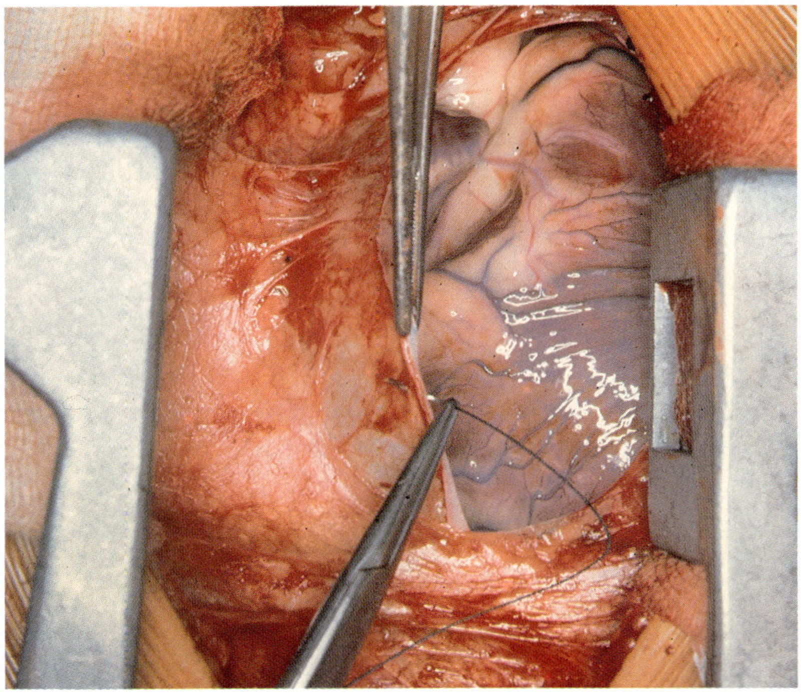

14

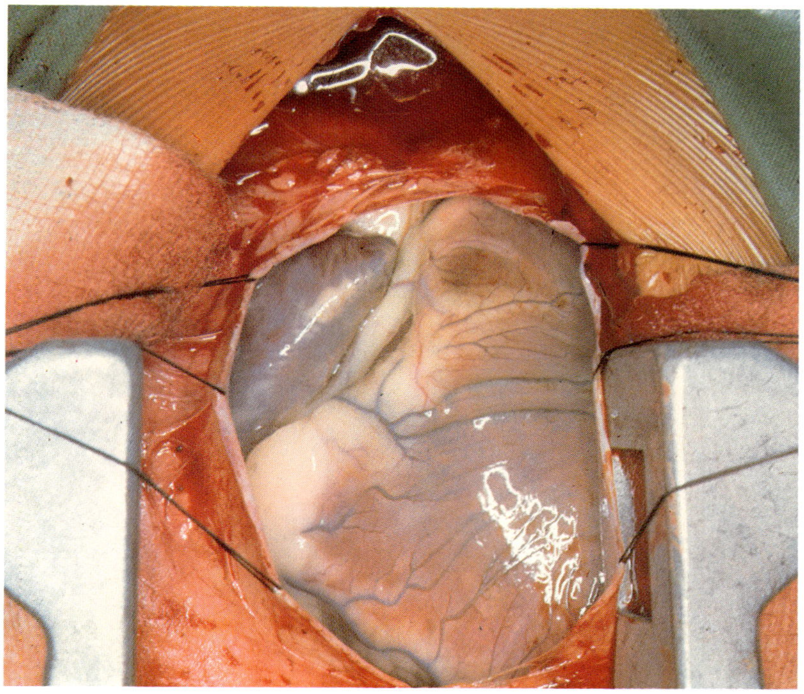

15

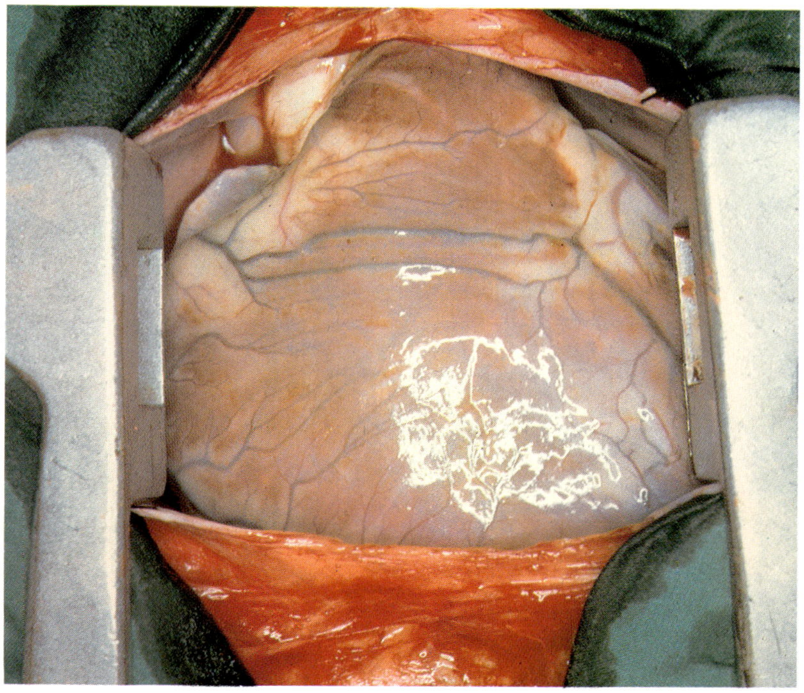

14 and 15 The retractor and swabs are then removed and side-towels placed to cover the wound edges. The stay-sutures are then pulled up and laterally and the retractor re-inserted so that the heart is then pulled forwards and a good view is obtained of the front of the heart.

16

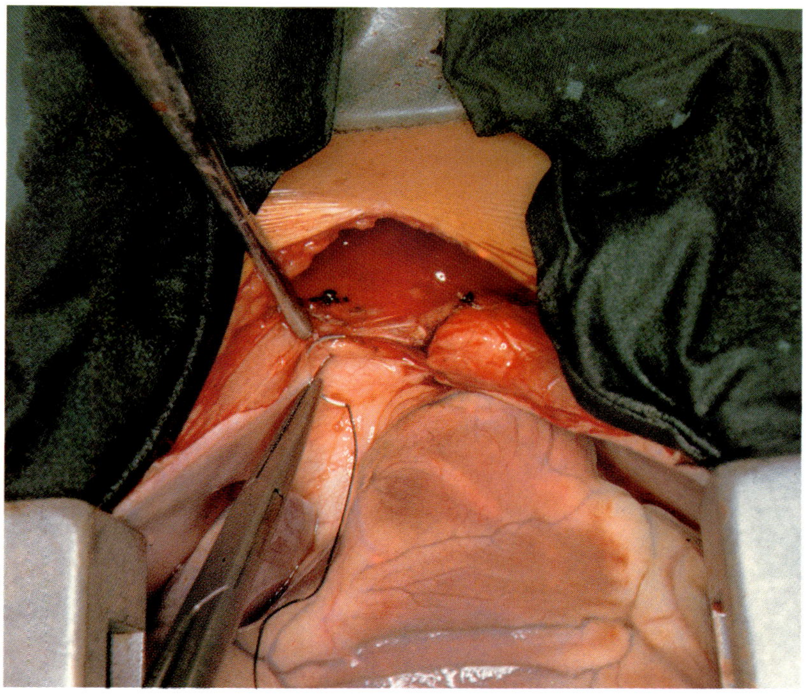

17

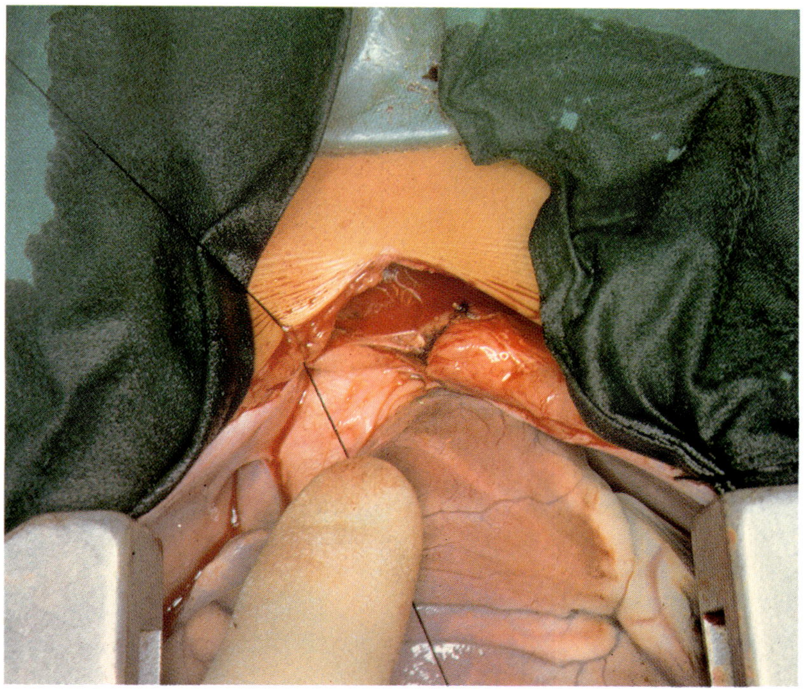

16 and 17 The exposure may be improved by placing one or two sutures at the top of the wound holding the pericardium up to the subcutaneous tissues.

18

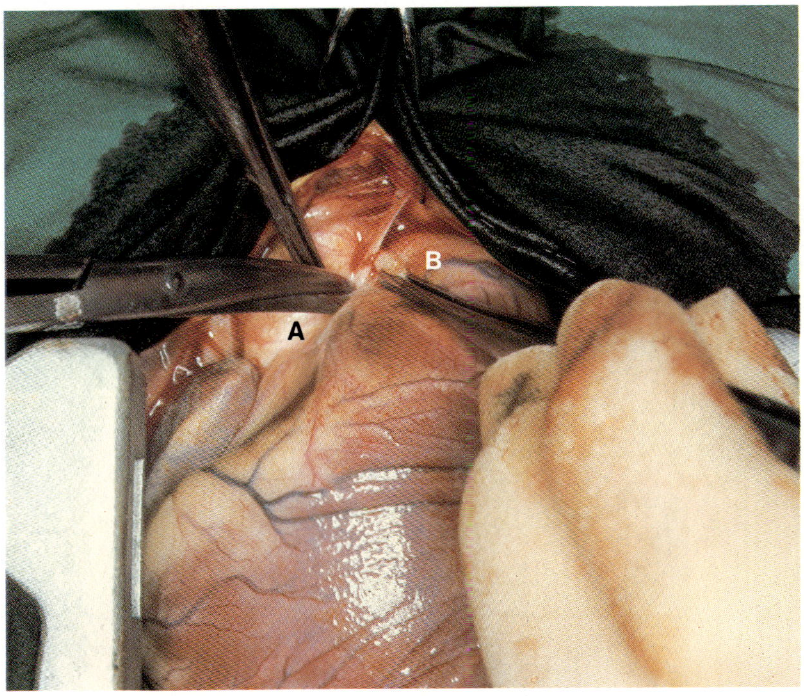

19

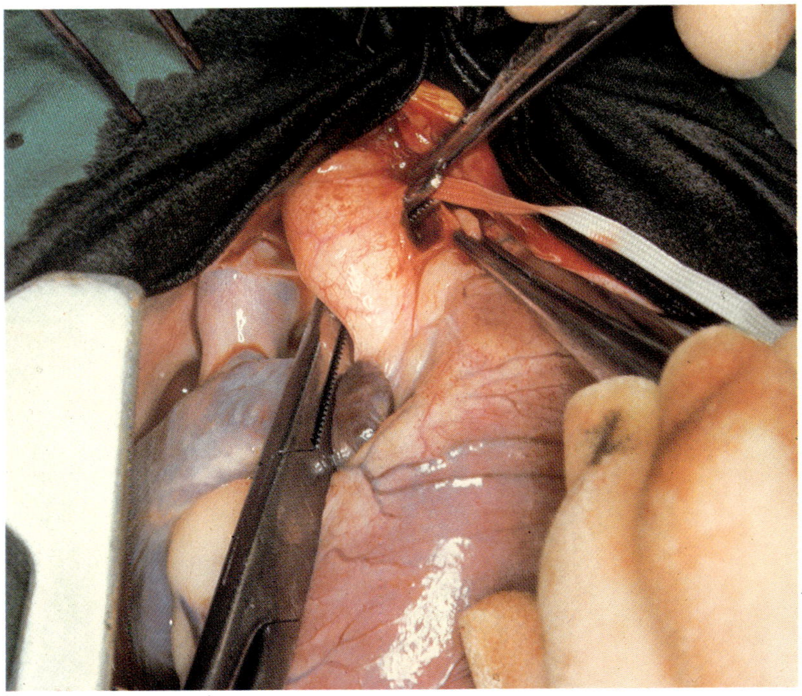

18 and 19 It is helpful to place a tape around the aorta so that it can be retracted easily once on bypass for clamping. The tissue between the aorta (**A**) and pulmonary artery, (**B**) is dissected and a curved pair of forceps passed behind the aorta to collect the tape.

20

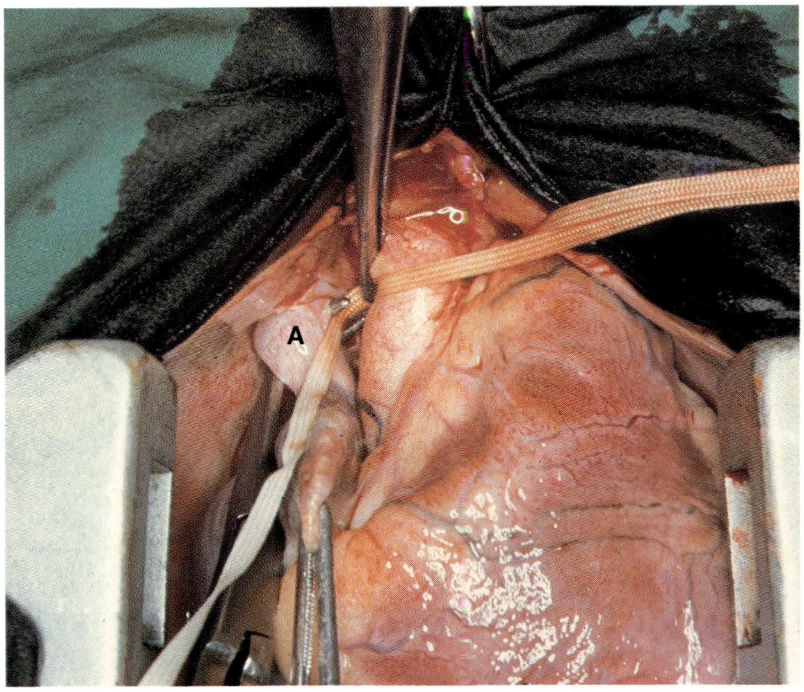

20 The aorta is retracted to the left and a tape is placed around the superior vena cava (**A**).

21

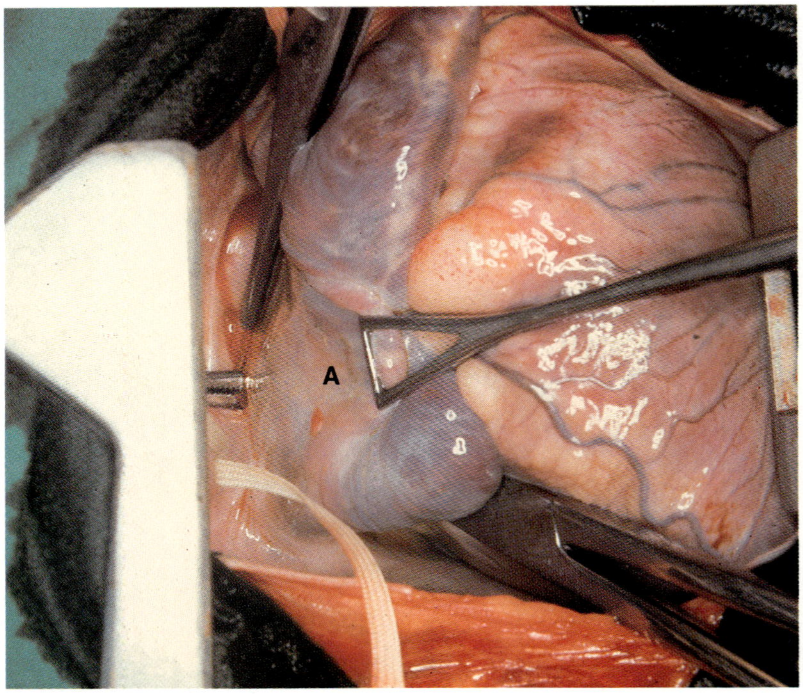

21 To facilitate passing a tape around the inferior vena cava, a Duval clamp can be placed on the right atrial wall (**A**) to retract it forwards. Again a curved clamp is placed around the inferior vena cava to collect the tape.

22

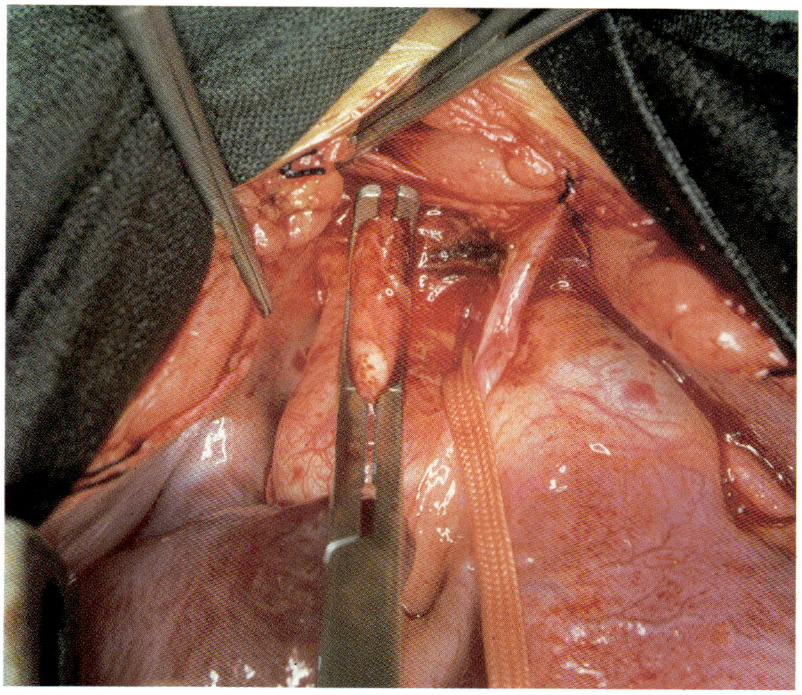

23

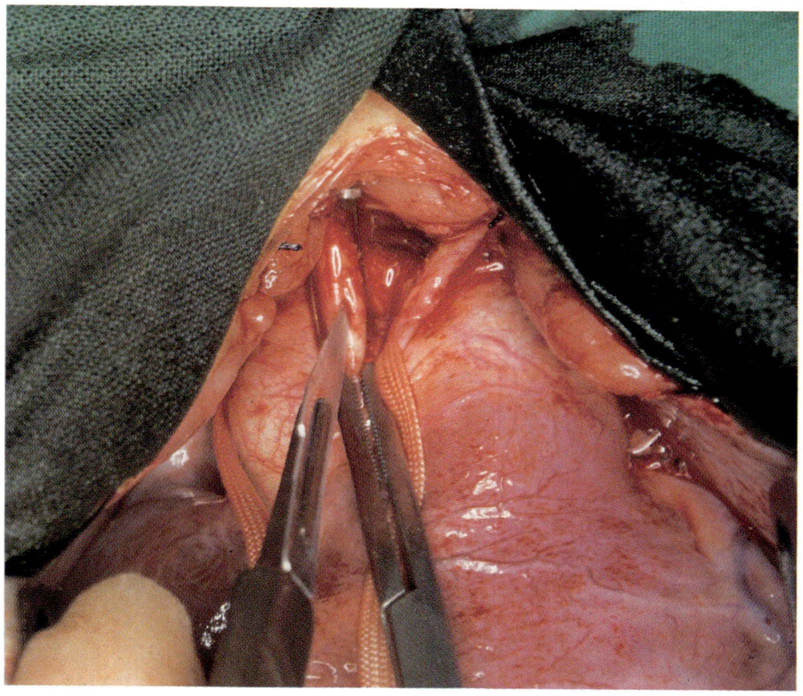

22 to 24 A side-clamp is applied on the ascending aorta and a longitudinal incision is made with a knife.

24

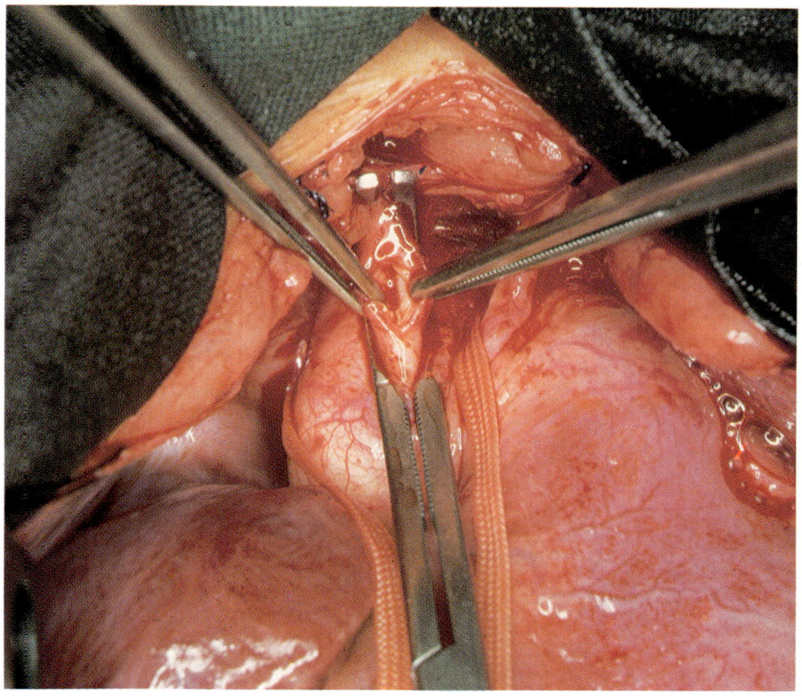

25

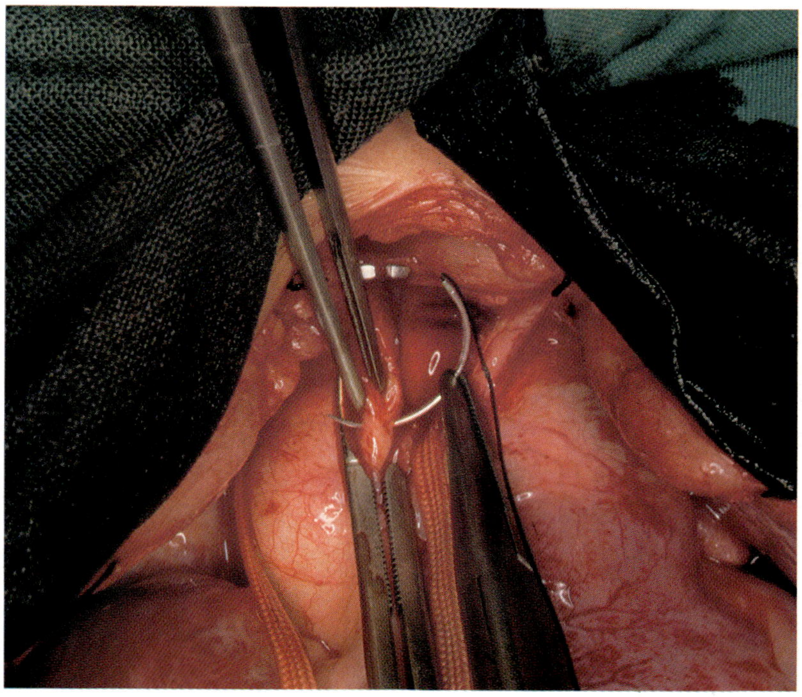

25 It is necessary to place a purse-string suture around this aortotomy to prevent leakage when the aortic cannula is inserted.

26

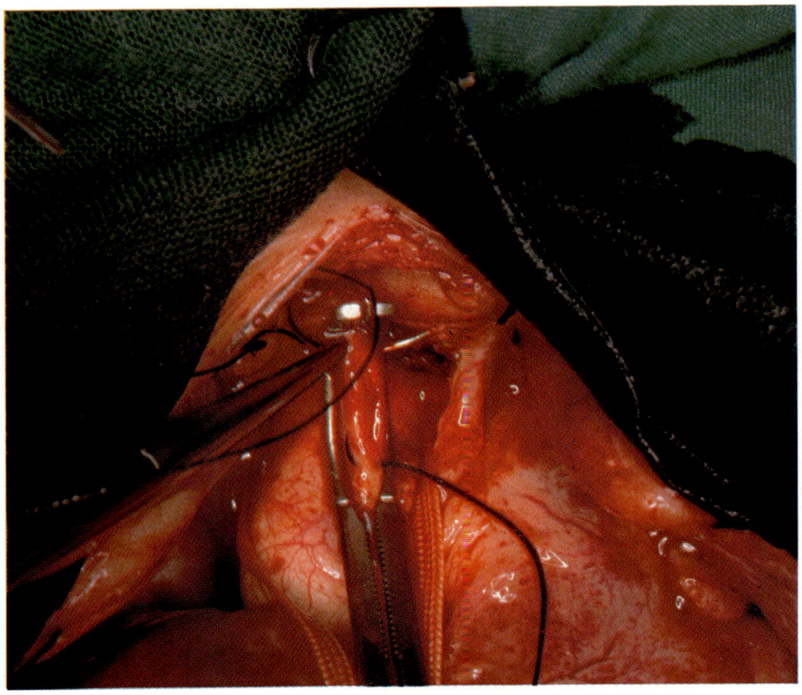

27

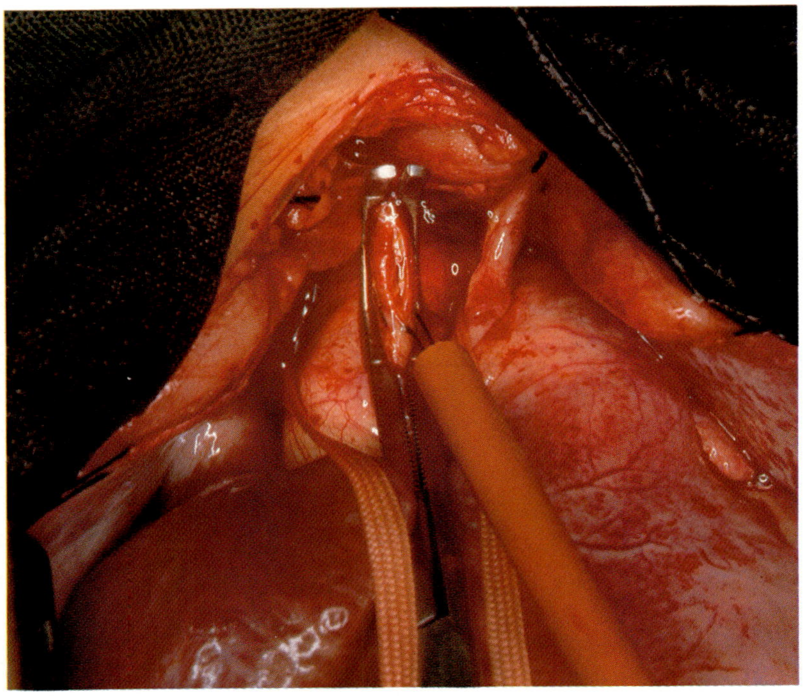

26 and 27 The remainder of the purse-string suture is inserted and the two ends of the suture pulled through a rubber snugger.

28

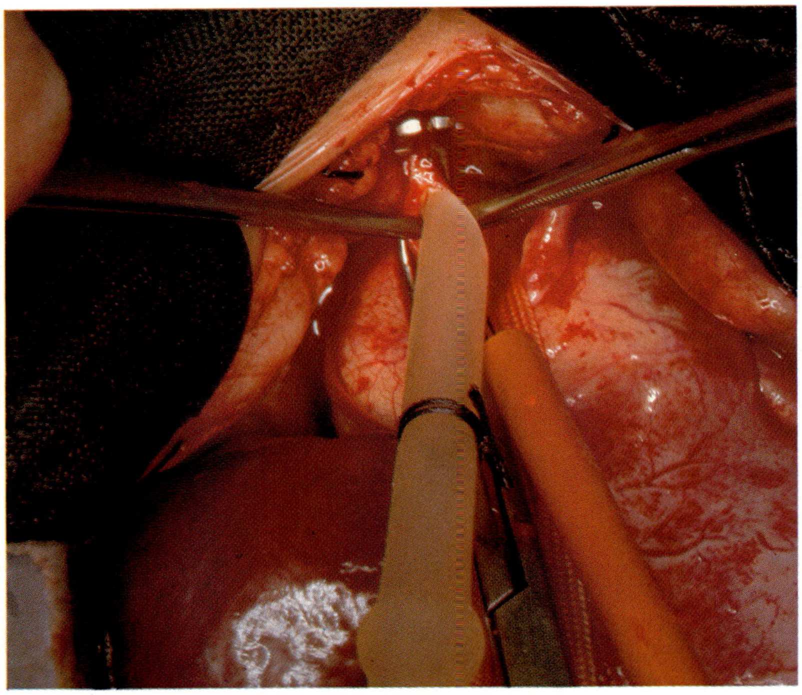

28 The aortic cannula is then ready for insertion. It is helpful to place a tie around it to prevent it going too far into the aorta. The sides of the aortotomy are held with forceps, the aortic clamp released and the cannula is inserted.

29

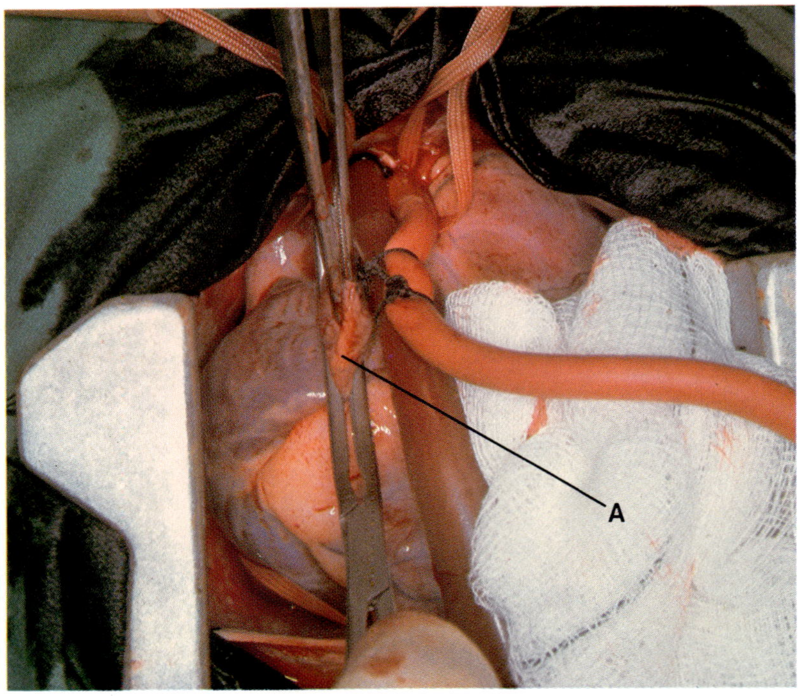

29 The purse-string suture is snugged and doubly tied to the cannula to prevent the cannula coming out of the aorta. This picture also shows the right atrial appendage (**A**) being held by forceps and a clamp being applied in preparation for the insertion of the venous cannulae.

30

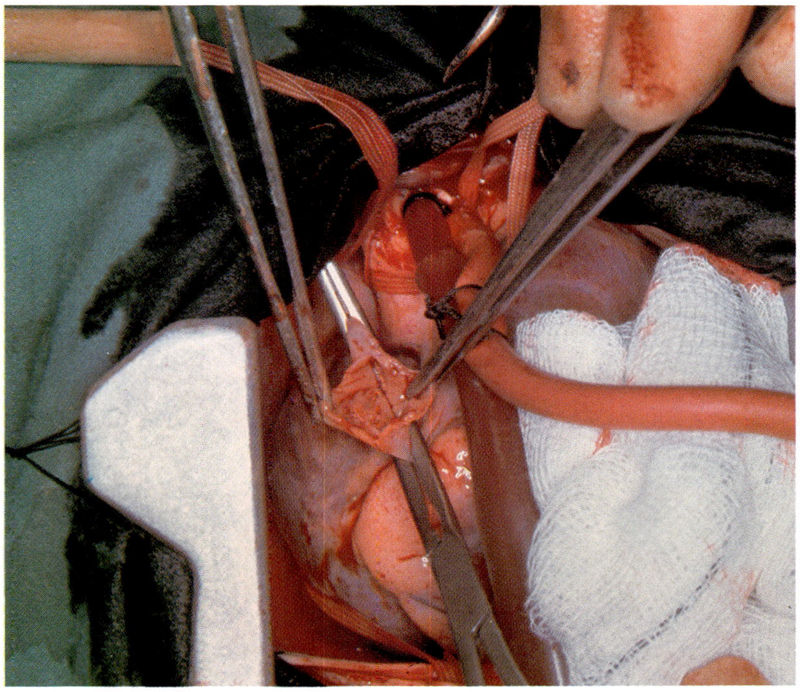

30 The tip of the atrial appendage is incised and the edges are held with forceps.

31

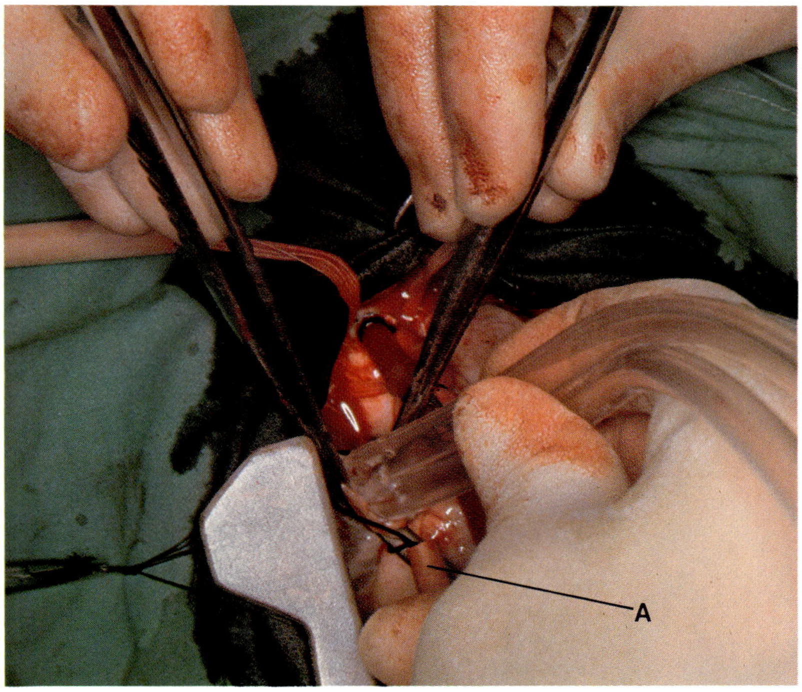

31 A tie is placed around the appendage and placed through a rubber snugger (**A**). The two tubes are ready for insertion and the edges of the atrial appendage are held with forceps. Some surgeons prefer to place only one cannula through the atrial appendage and the other directly into the atrial wall.

32

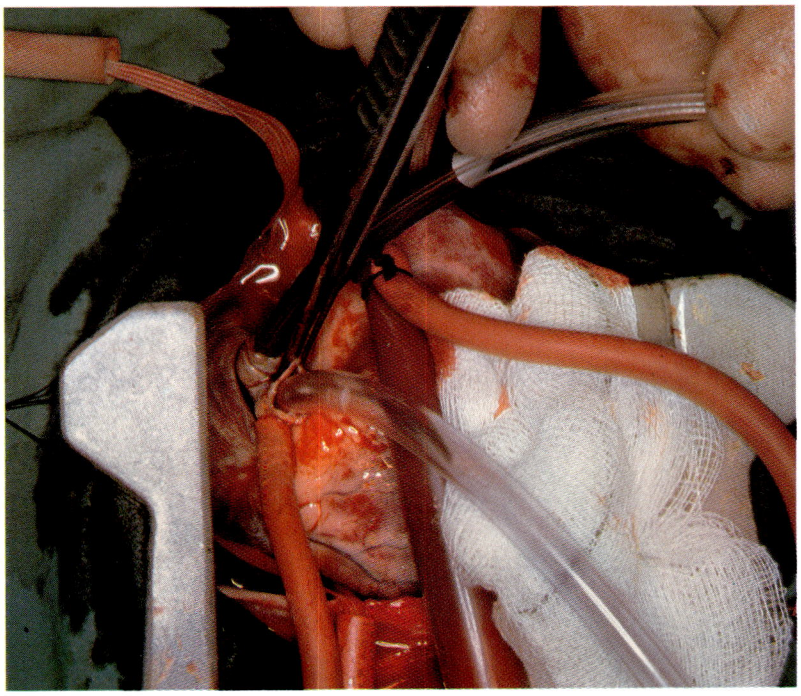

32 The atrial clamp has been removed, the tubes placed through the appendage into the right atrium and the rubber snugged.

33

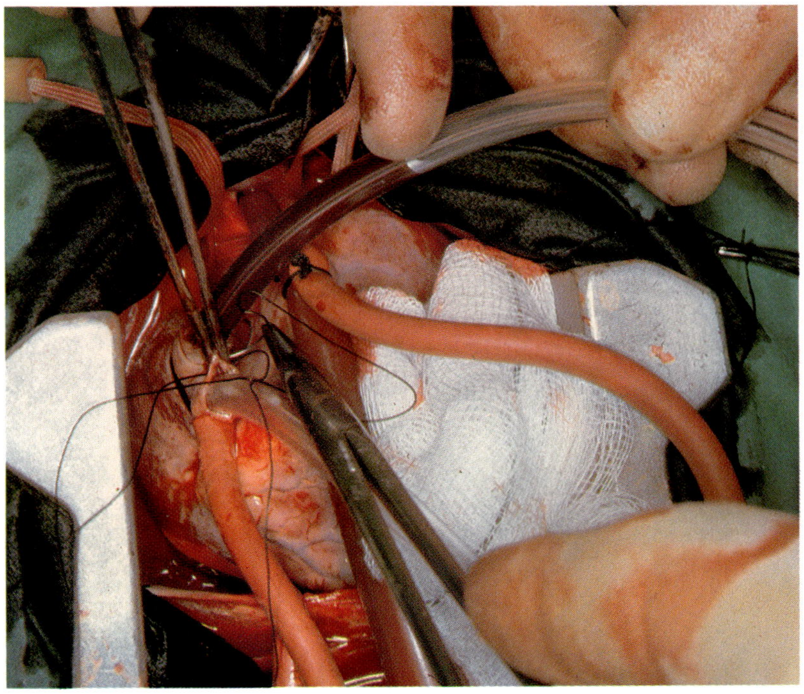

33 A suture is placed through the atrial appendage between the two cannulae to form an air-tight seal.

34

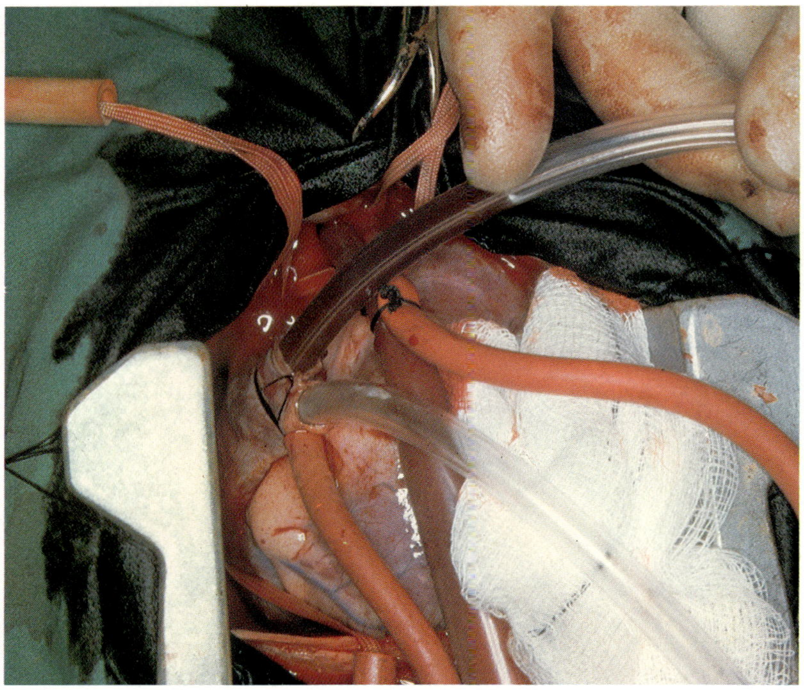

34 The venous cannulae are now in the right atrium and must be advanced carefully into their respective vena cava.

35

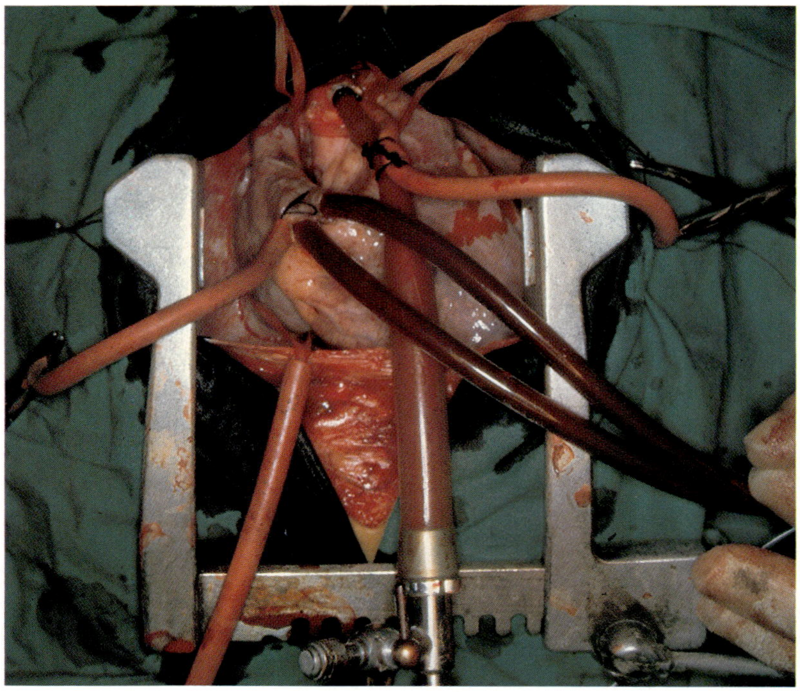

35 The arterial and venous lines have now been connected to the cardiopulmonary bypass circuit and the patient is ready for bypass to begin. It can be seen that all the air has been sucked out of the venous tubes by siphoning blood back to the cardiopulmonary bypass machine.

36

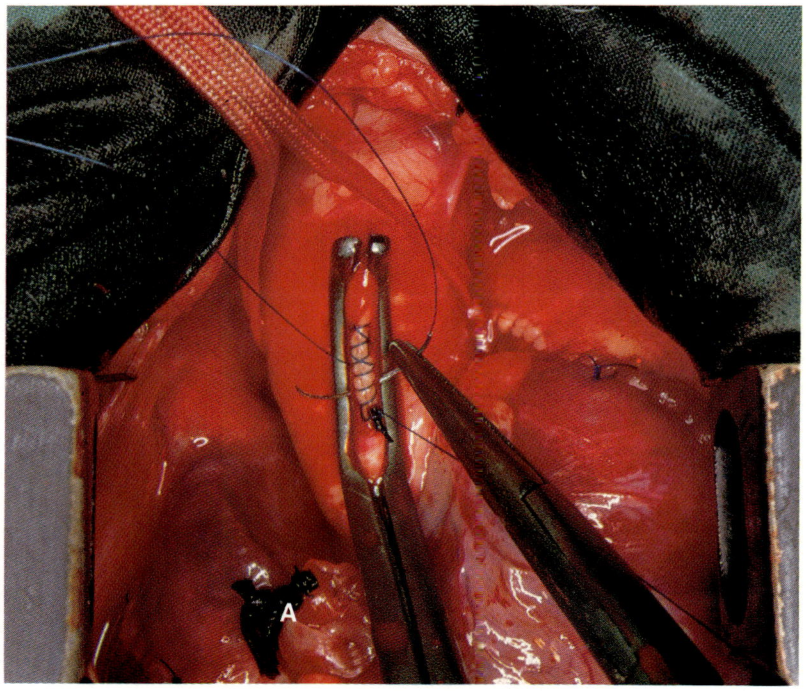

36 Once the operation has been completed and cardiopulmonary bypass stopped, the venous cannulae are removed and the right atrial appendage tied off (**A**). The aortic cannula is then removed and the aortotomy closed with a double layer of continuous Prolene. (Alternatively, the purse-string suture can be tied and the incision oversewn.)

37

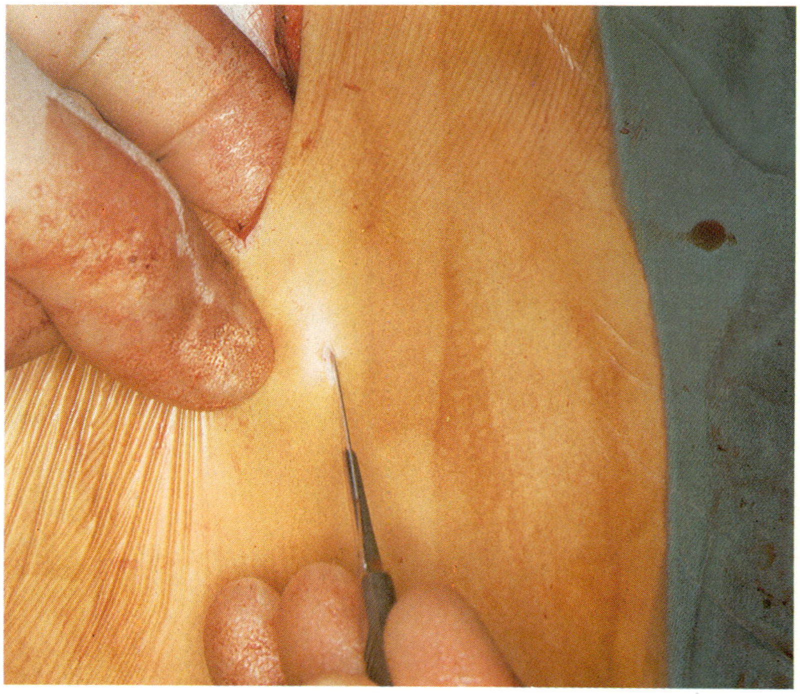

37 After removal of the arterial and venous cannulae and all the bleeding has stopped, it is necessary to insert drainage tubes to remove any further blood that accumulates after the chest is closed. A small skin incision is being made to take one of the pericardial drainage tubes.

38

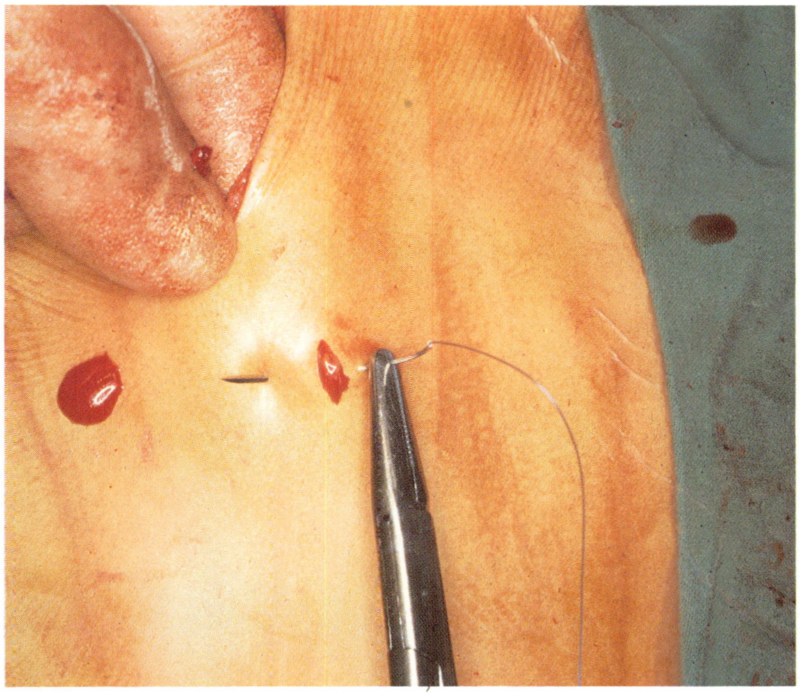

39

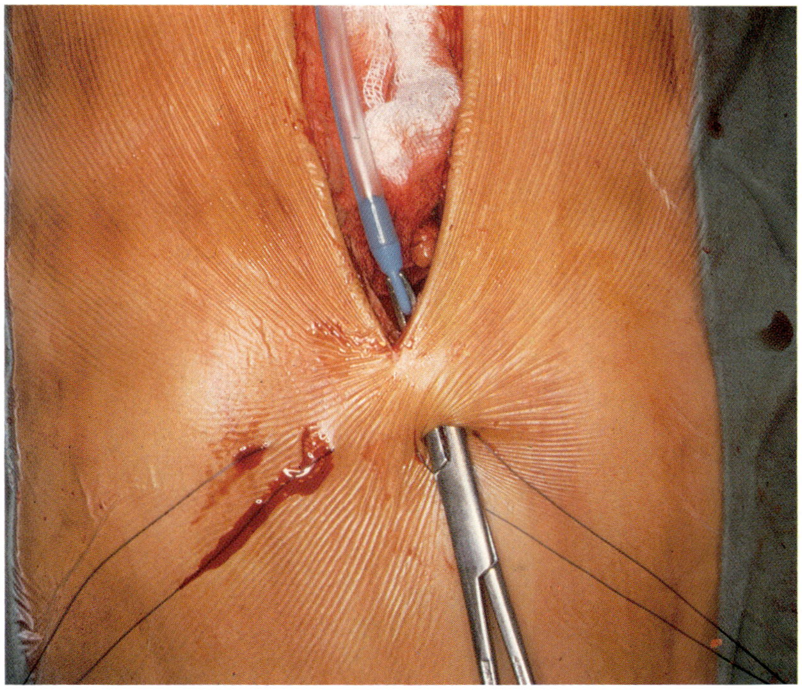

38 to 40 A suture is inserted to allow closure of the skin after the tube has been removed; the two tubes are inserted by being pulled through with a pair of forceps and tied securely in position.

40

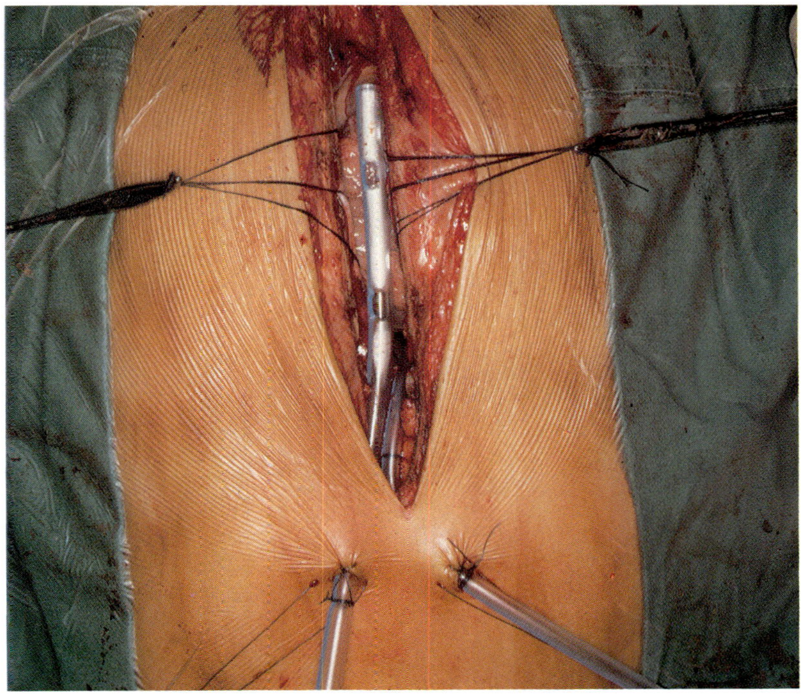

41

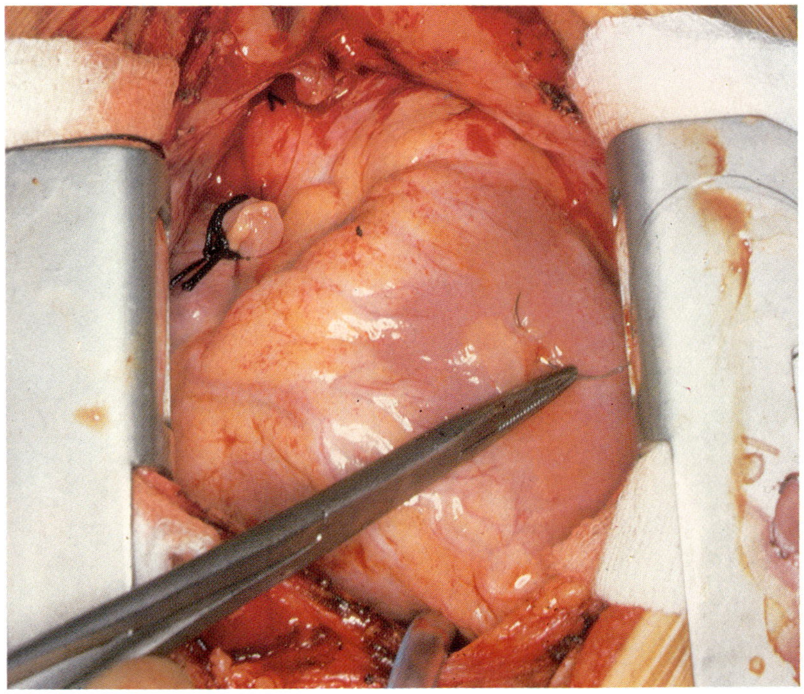

41 The sternal retractor is then reinserted and a temporary pacing wire sutured to the surface of the right ventricle.

42 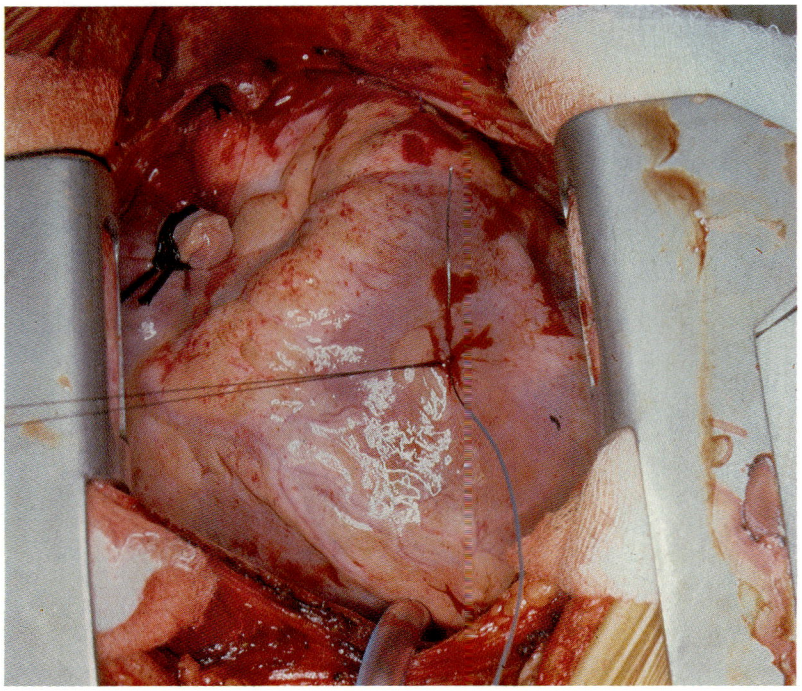

43 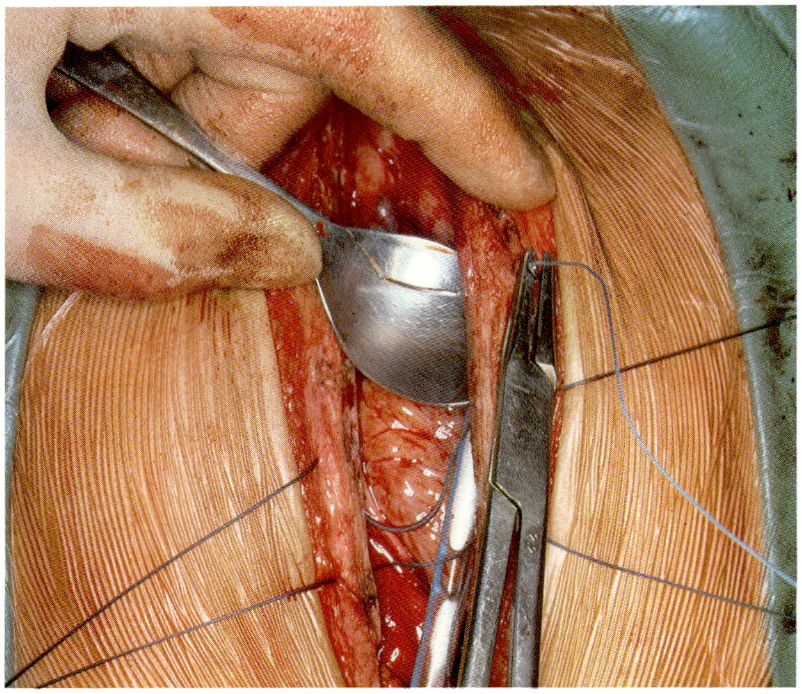

42 The pacing wire is held in position with a fine silk suture.

43 Interrupted heavy sutures are then inserted to approximate the sternal edges and the spoon protects the heart. Many surgeons prefer to use wire for sternal closure.

44 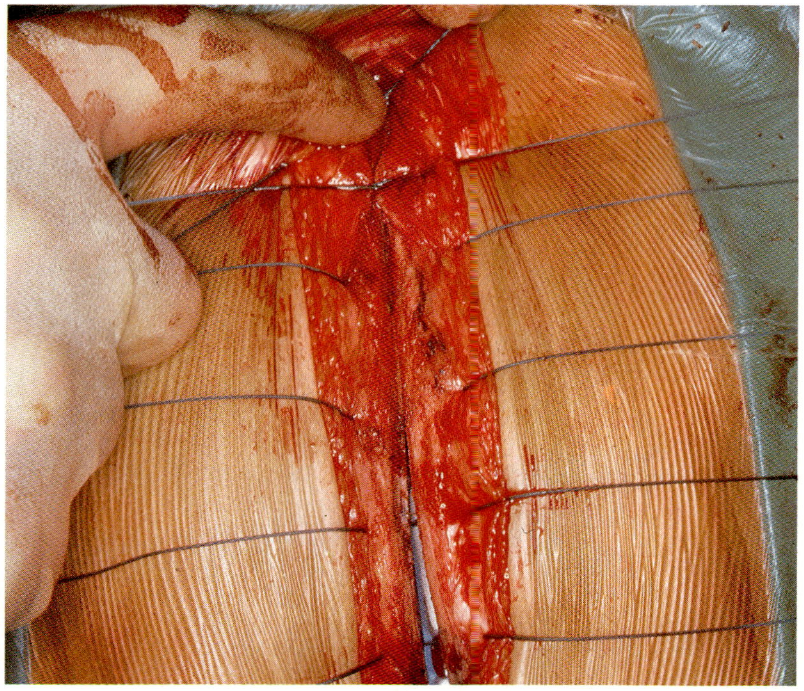

45 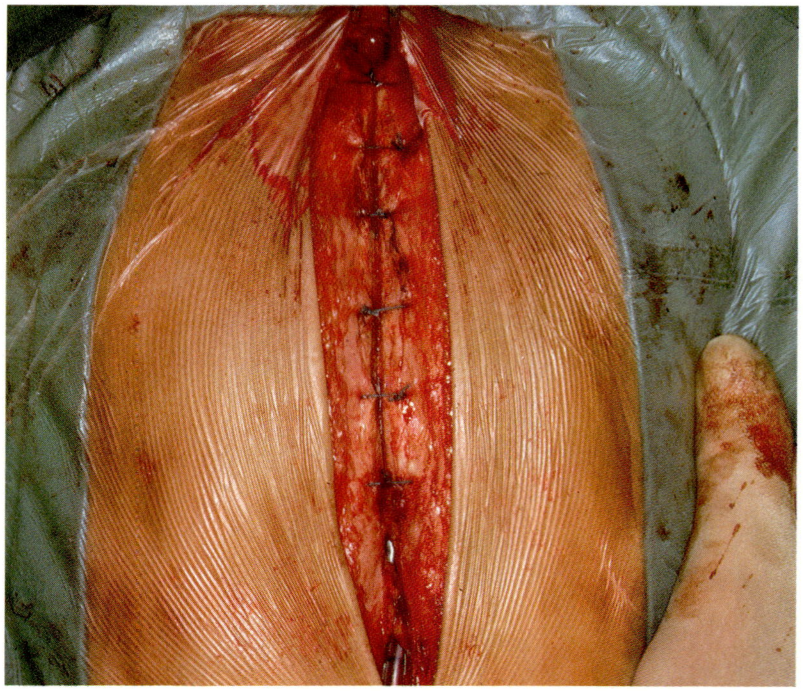

44 and 45 The sutures are then tied and cut and the sternal edges firmly approximated.

46
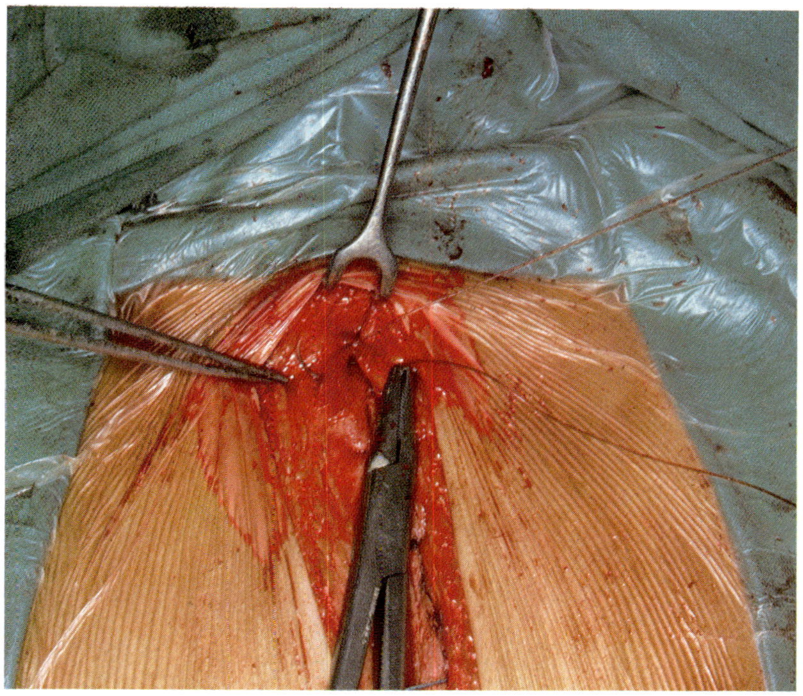

47
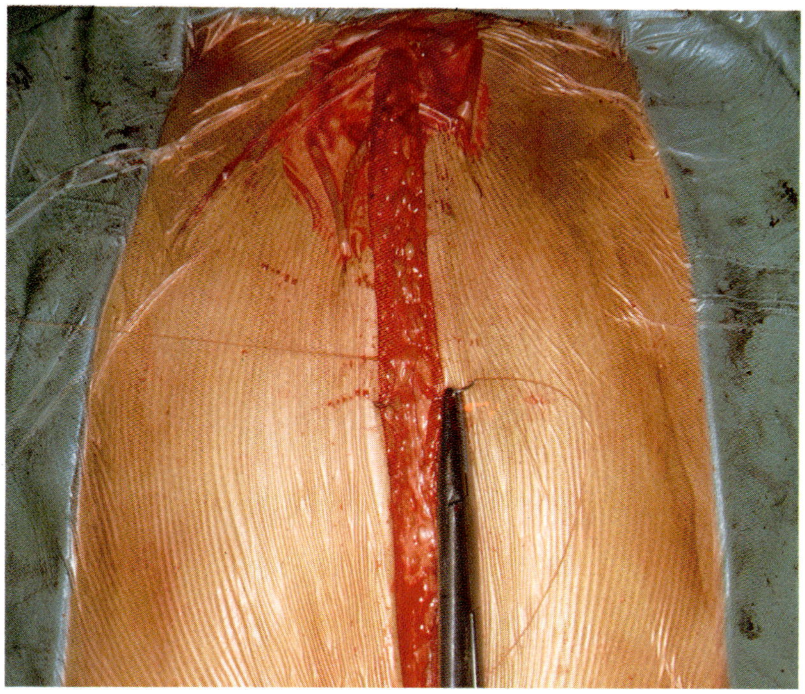

46 The deep layer is then closed with a continuous chromic cat-gut suture, taking care to bury the sternal suture knots.

47 The subcutaneous tissue is closed with continuous plain cat-gut.

48
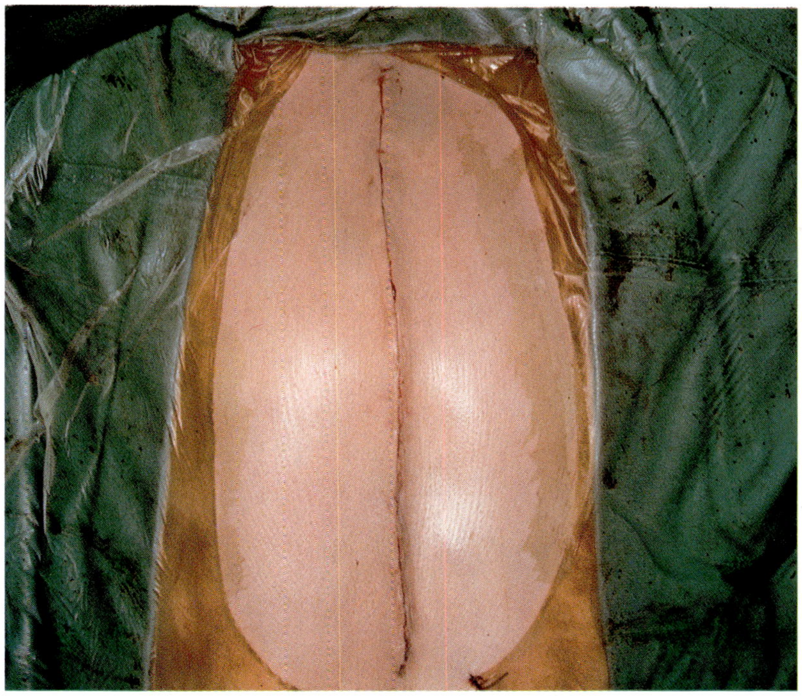

49
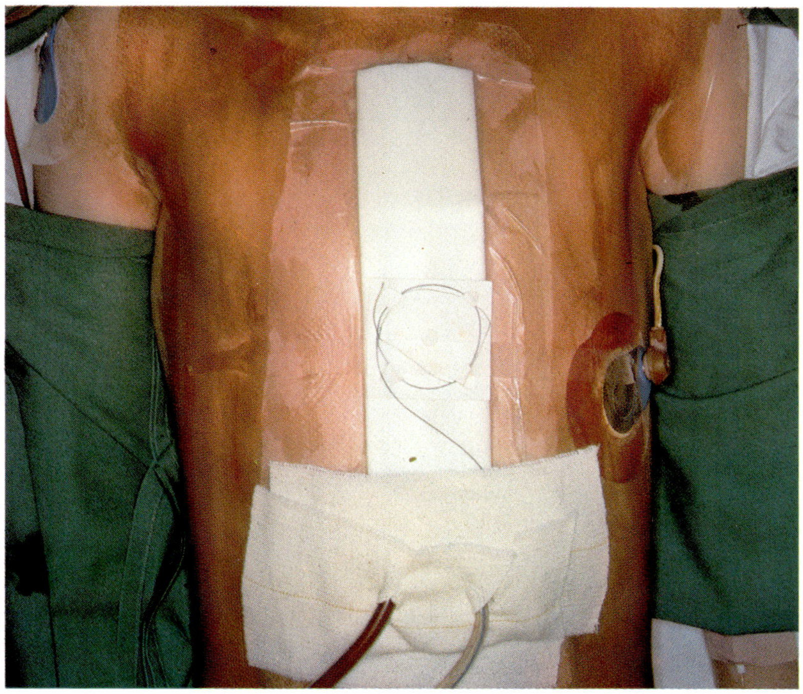

48 The skin is closed with subcuticular Dexon.

49 The dressings are applied, the drapes are removed and the patient is ready for transfer to the recovery room.

3: Thoracotomy

A left thoractomy is used for repair of coarctation of the aorta and for approaching a persistent ductus arteriosus, and it is usual to use the fourth intercostal space. A thoracotomy is also used for palliative procedures such as a Blalock-Taussig procedure, which is performed on the side opposite the aortic arch, therefore most commonly the right.

1

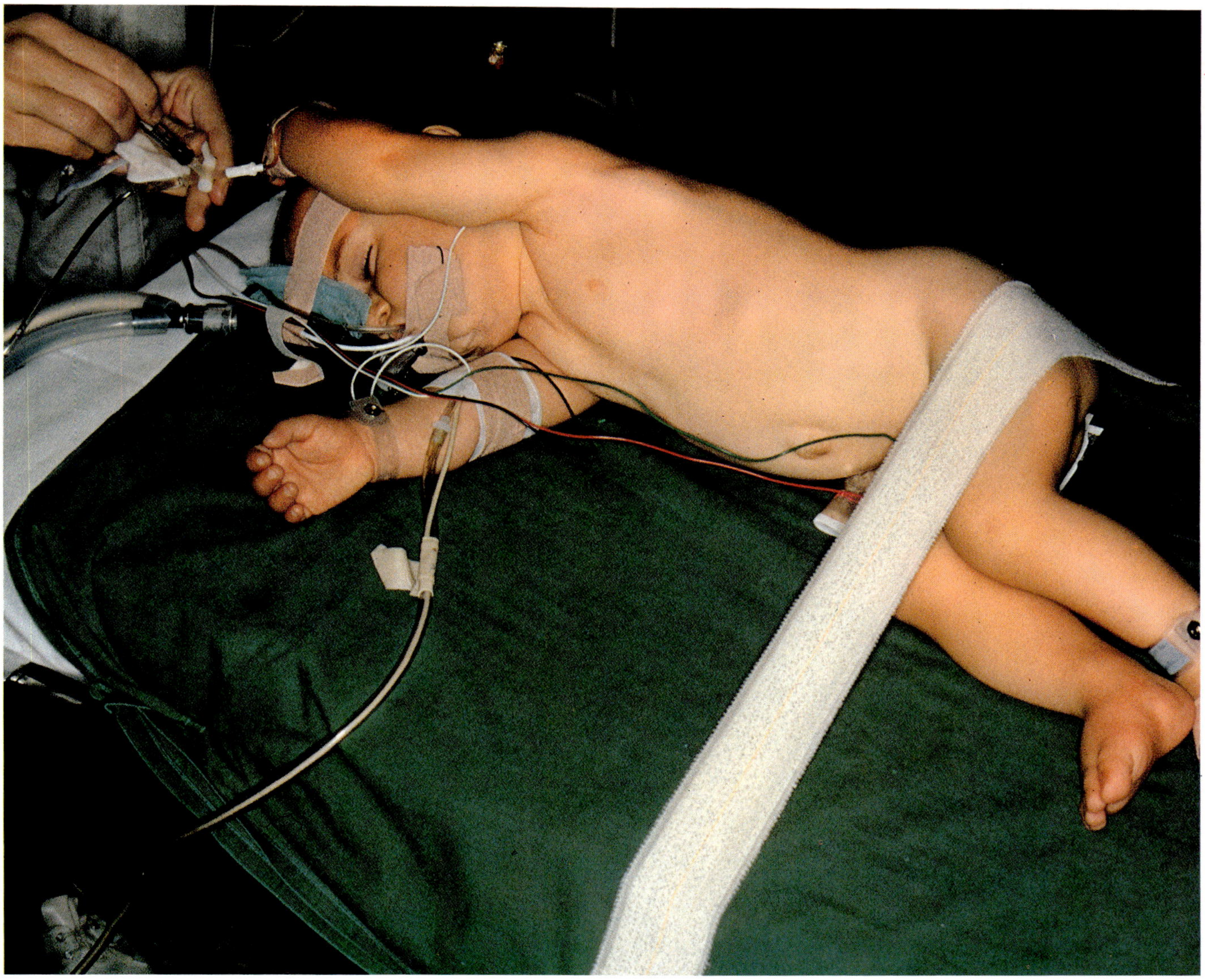

1 The patient is positioned on the operating table with the side of the chest to be operated on uppermost. The patient is held in position with firm Elastoplast over the hips. The skin is then sterilised and suitably draped.

2

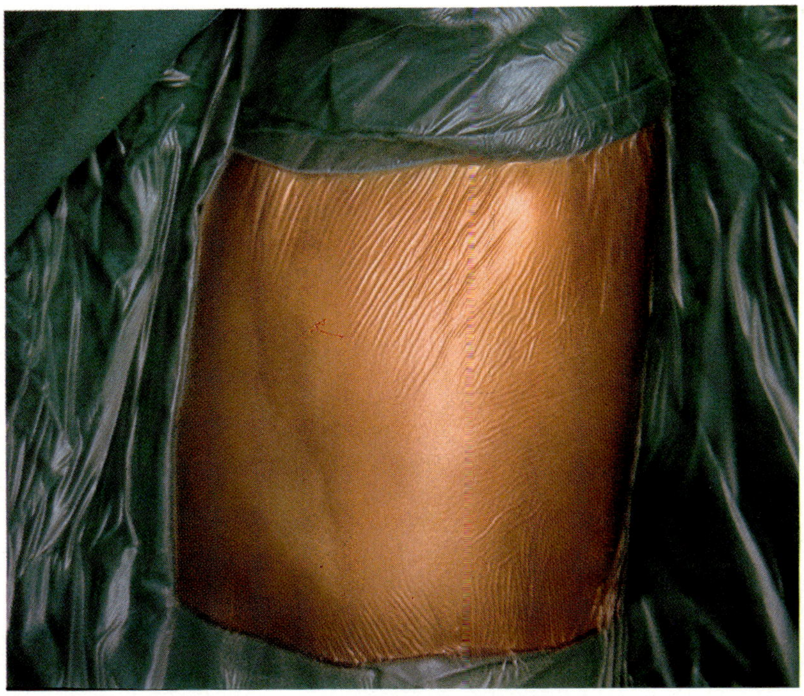

3

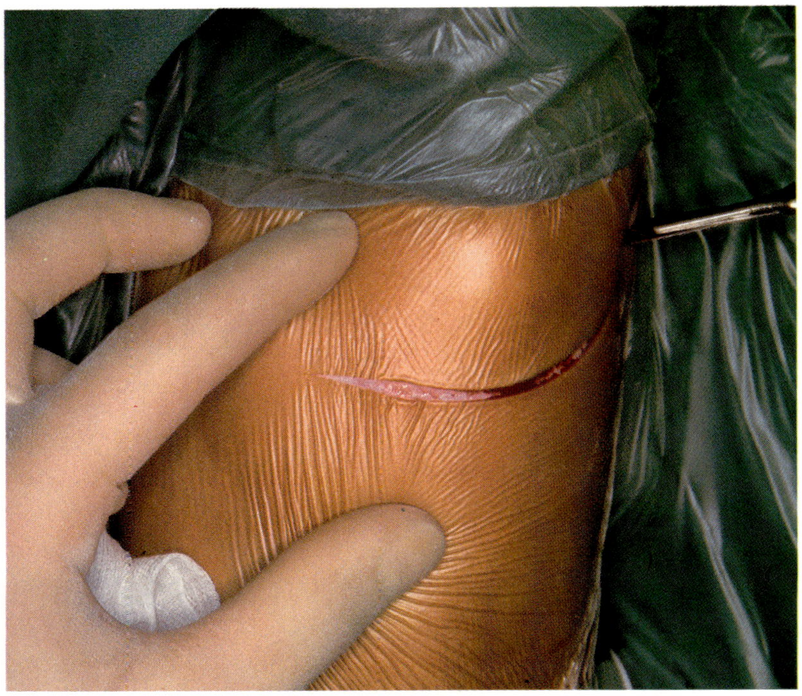

2 and 3 Steridrape has been placed over the prepared skin and surrounding towels, and the skin is incised with a knife well below the lower edge of the scapula.

4

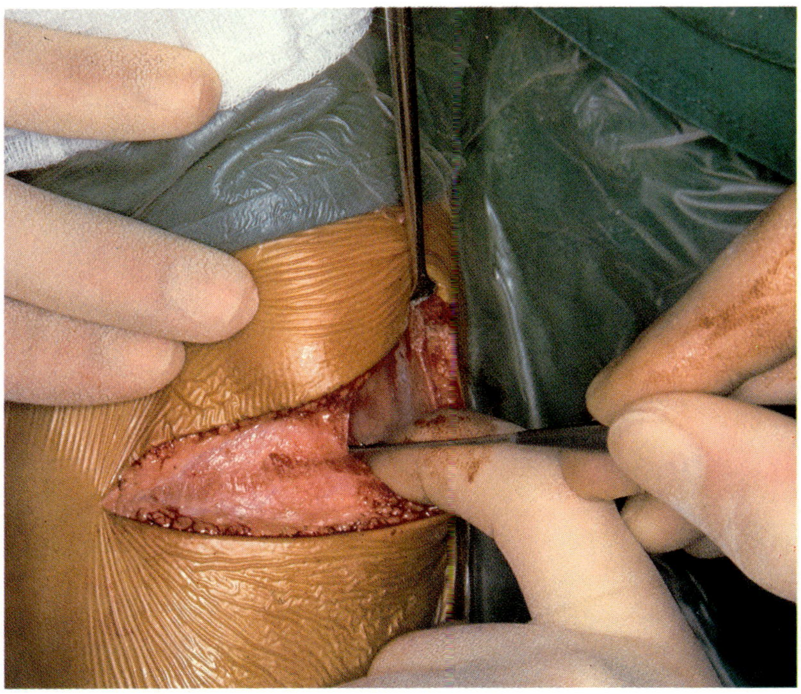

5

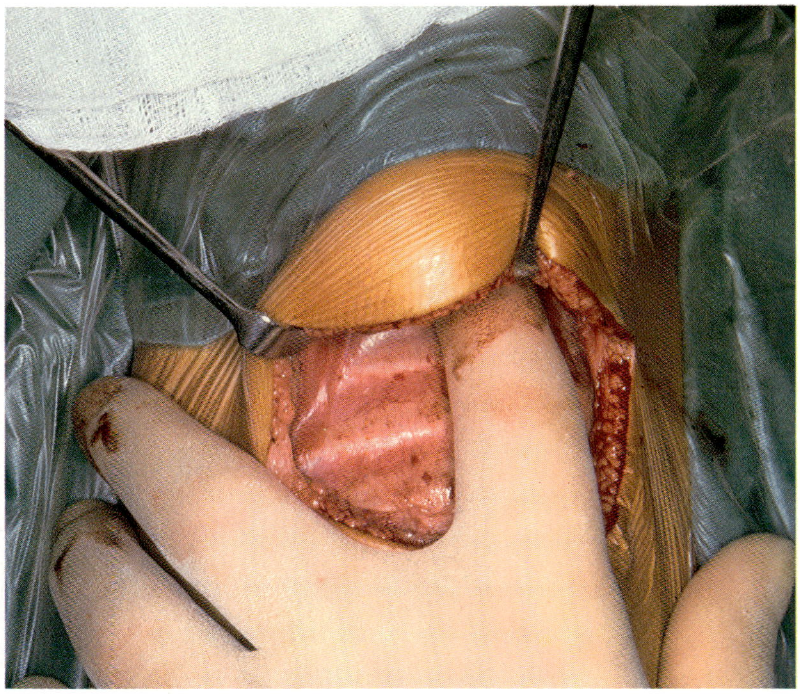

4 and 5 The muscles are incised with diathermy and the scapula retracted upwards with the upper margin of the wound. The ribs are counted from above and the fifth rib selected.

6

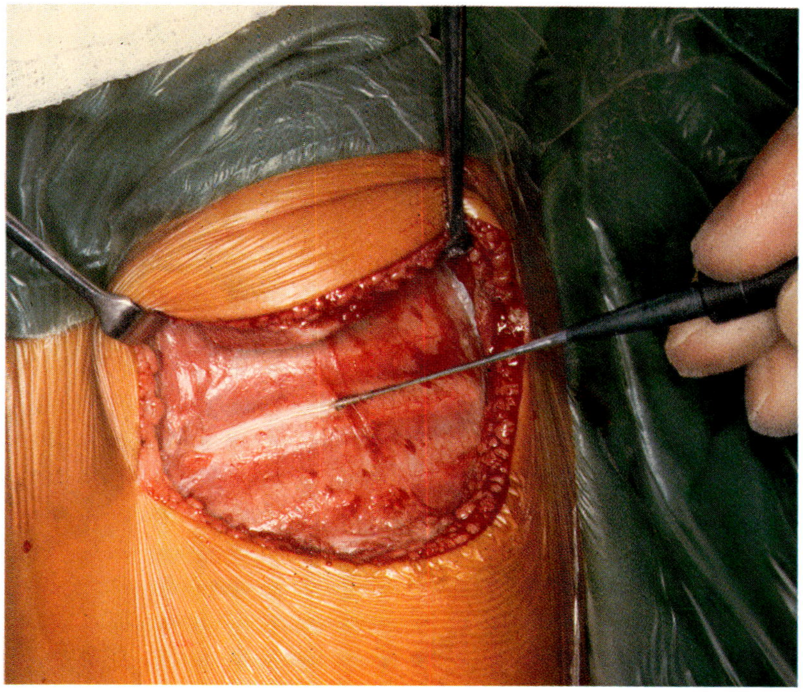

7

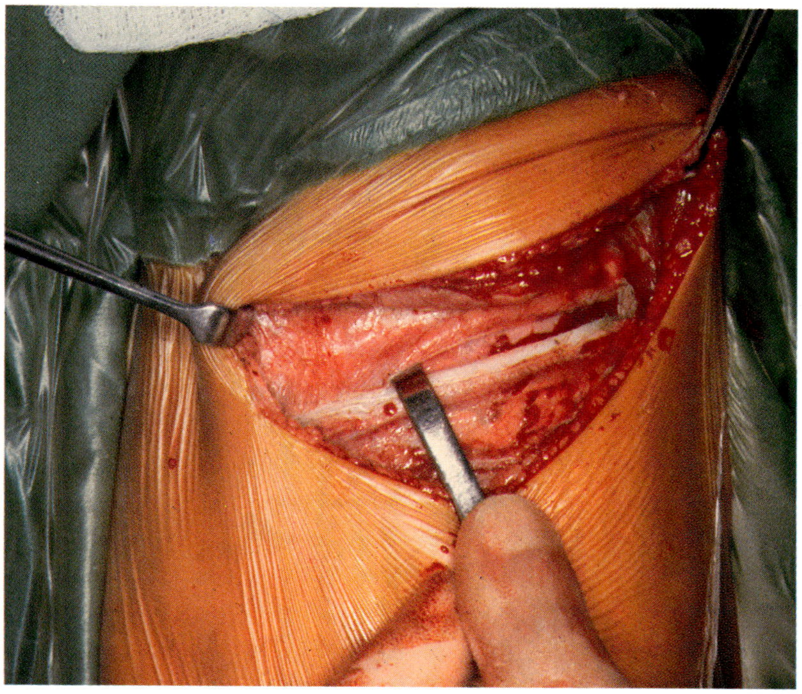

6 and 7 The periosteum of the fifth rib is incised and, using a periosteal elevator, the periosteum is scraped from the top of the rib, starting at the back.

8

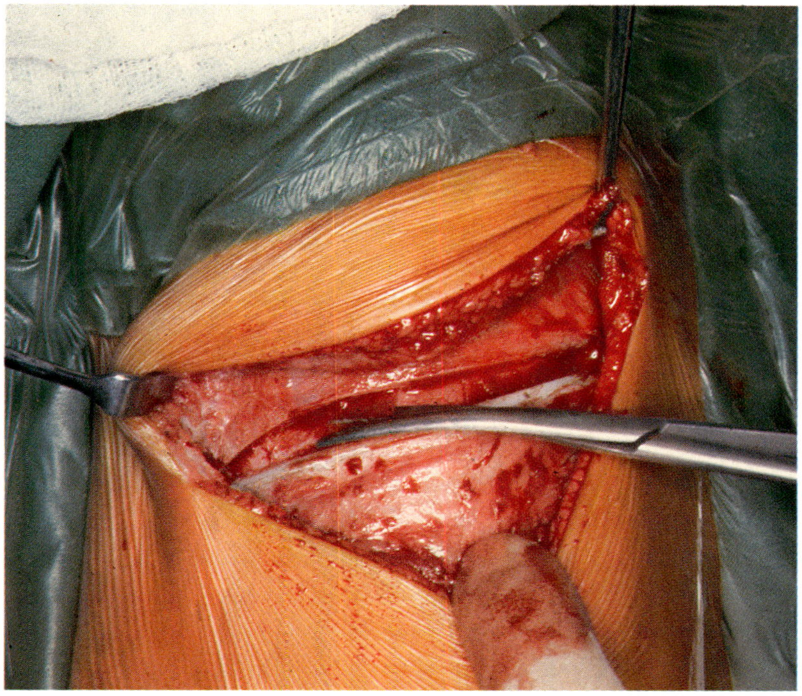

9

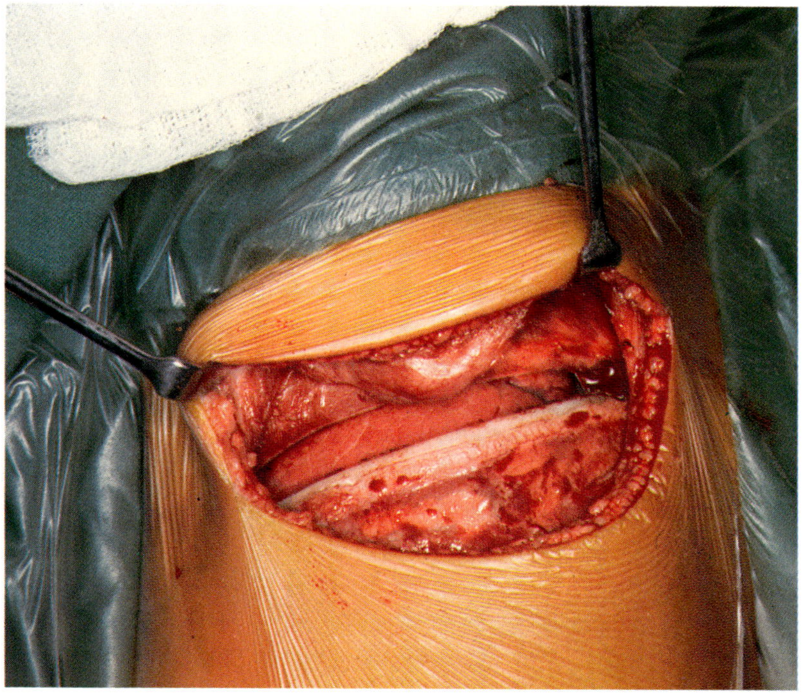

8 and 9 The pleura is incised with scissors and the expanded lung can be seen.

10

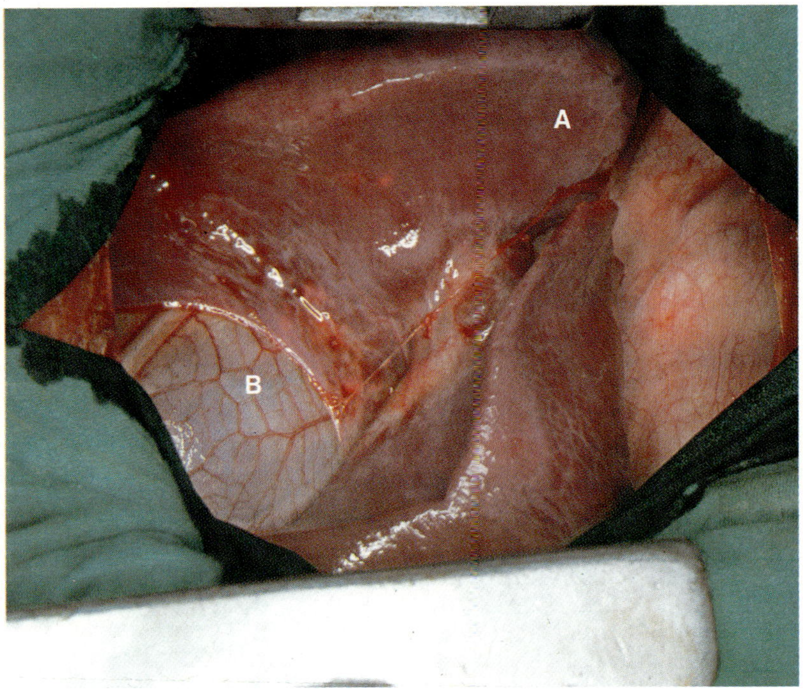

11

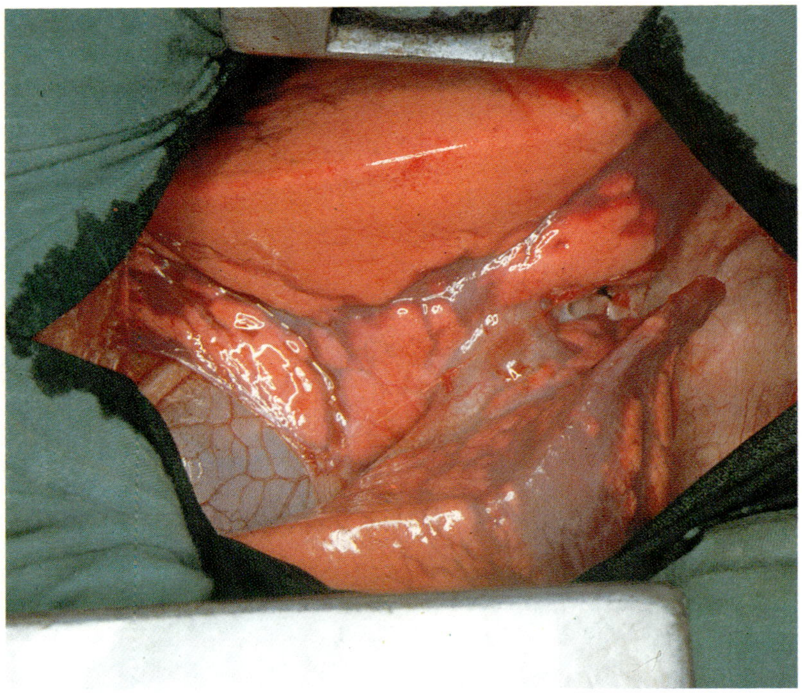

10 This picture shows the bluish, collapsed lung (**A**) ready to be retracted forwards for exposure of the aorta posteriorly. The pericardium (**B**) is seen anteriorly.

11 Once the operation is complete, the anaesthetist inflates the lung; here the lung is shown partially re-inflated.

12

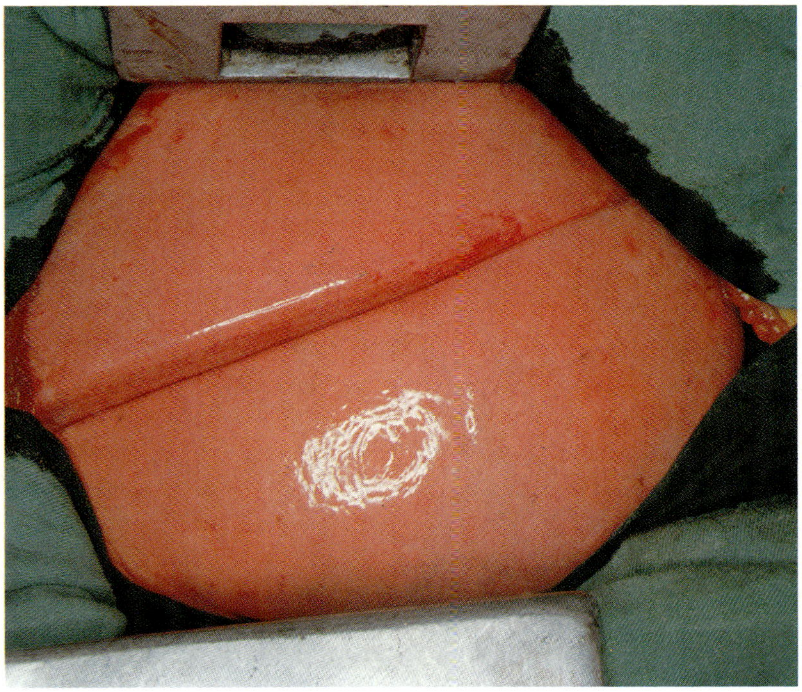

13

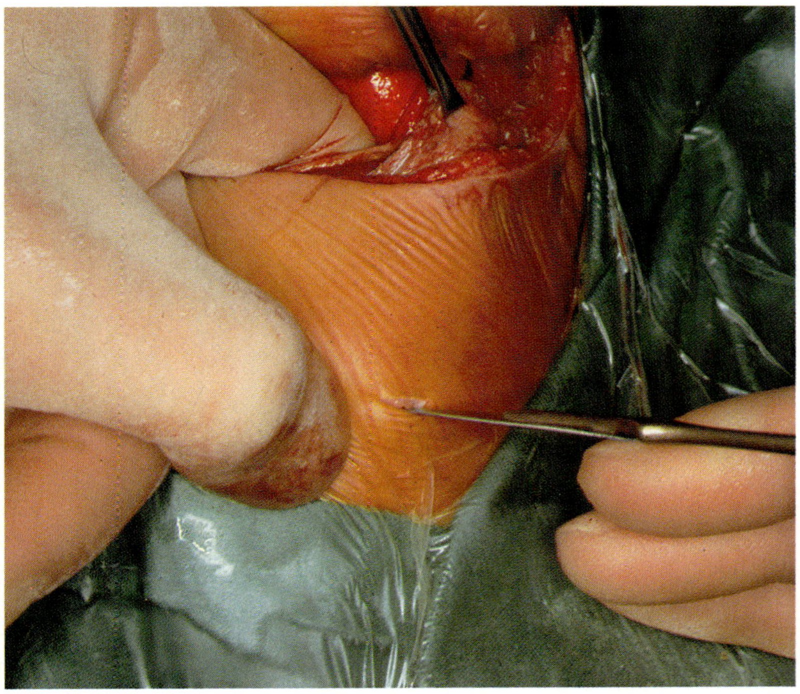

12 The lung has now been completely re-expanded and the chest can be closed.

13 It is usual to insert an intercostal drainage tube after most thoracotomies to remove air and any subsequent blood that is lost. Here a small skin incision is being made well below the incision for insertion of the drain. The muscle layer is being held up with forceps.

14
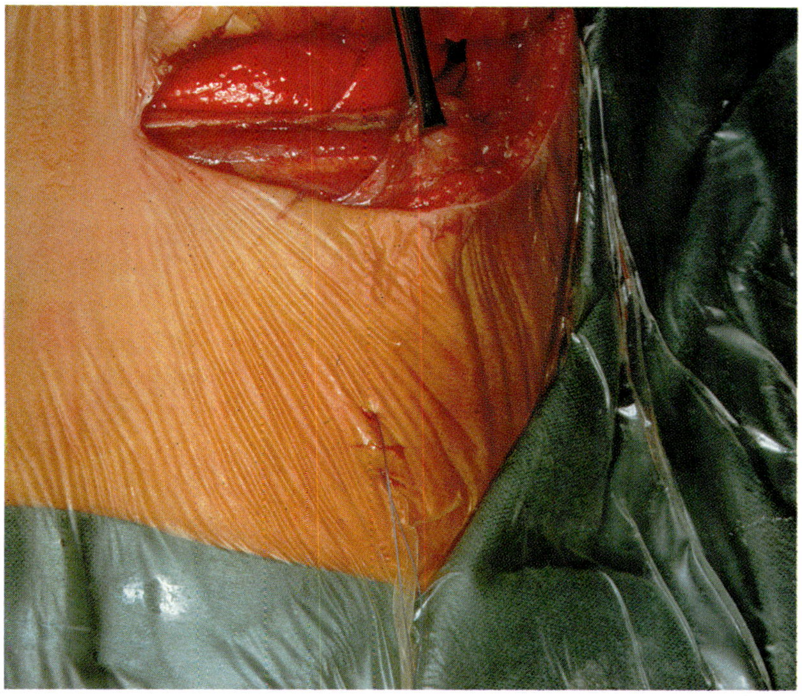

14 A stitch is placed loosely across the incision for tying when the tube is removed.

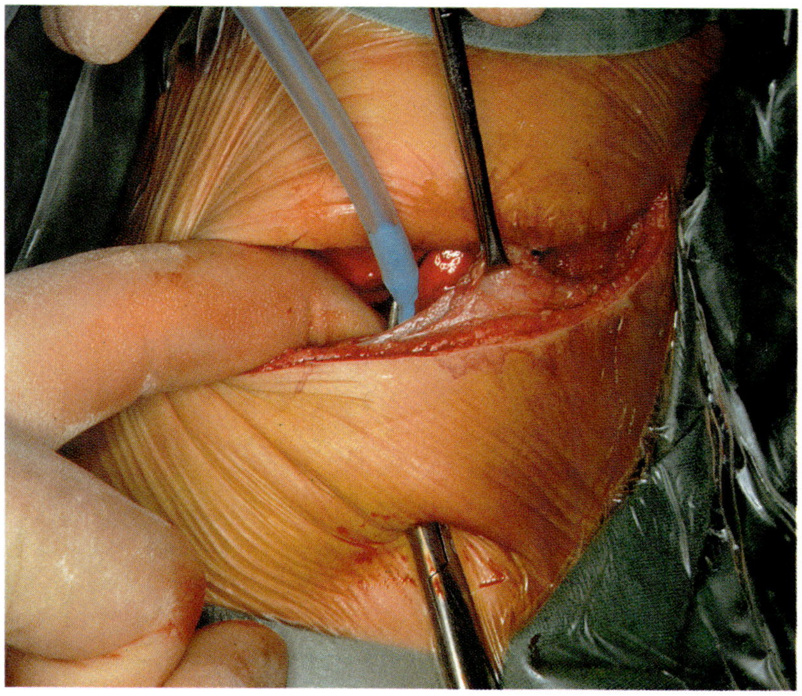
15

15 to 17 The drainage tube is then inserted by pulling through with Kelly's forceps and tied in position with another stitch.

16
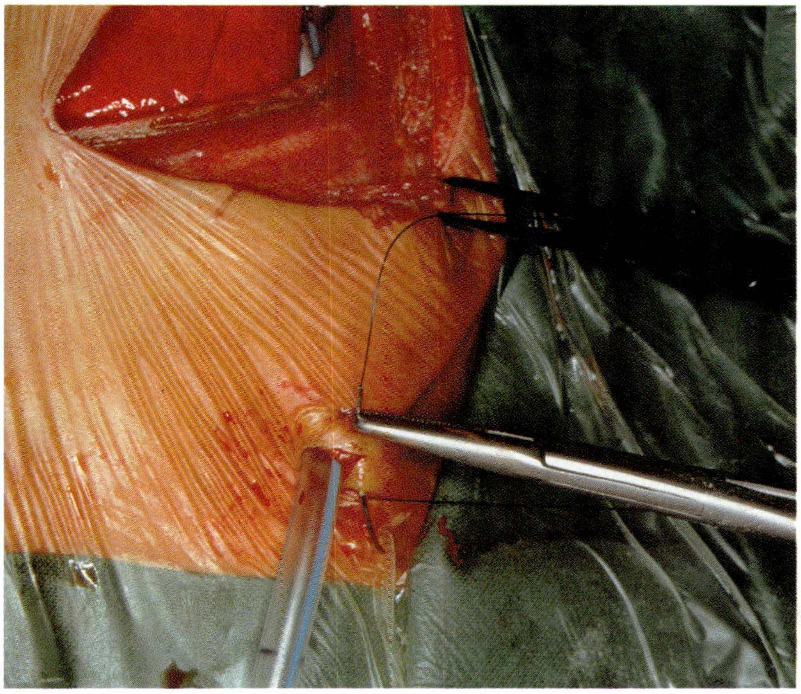

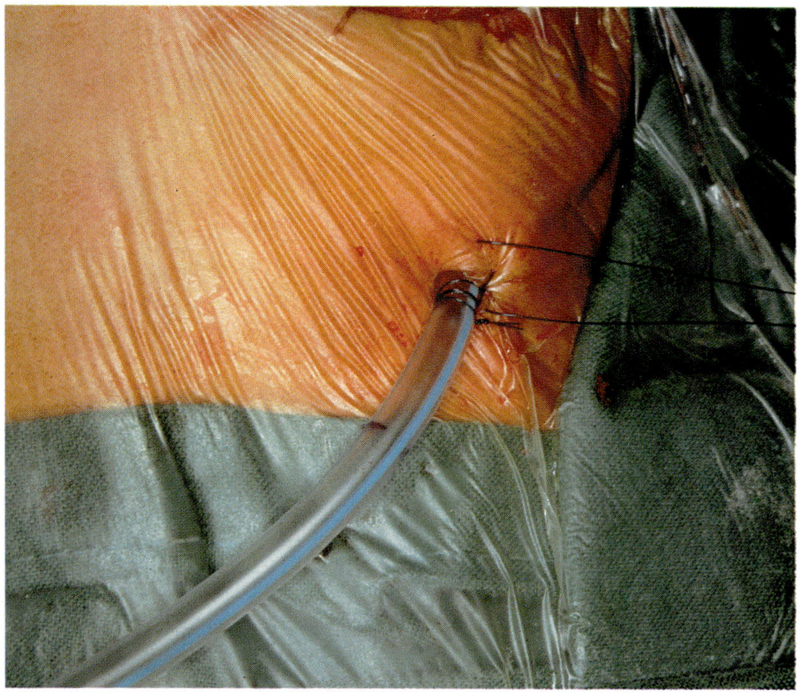
17

18
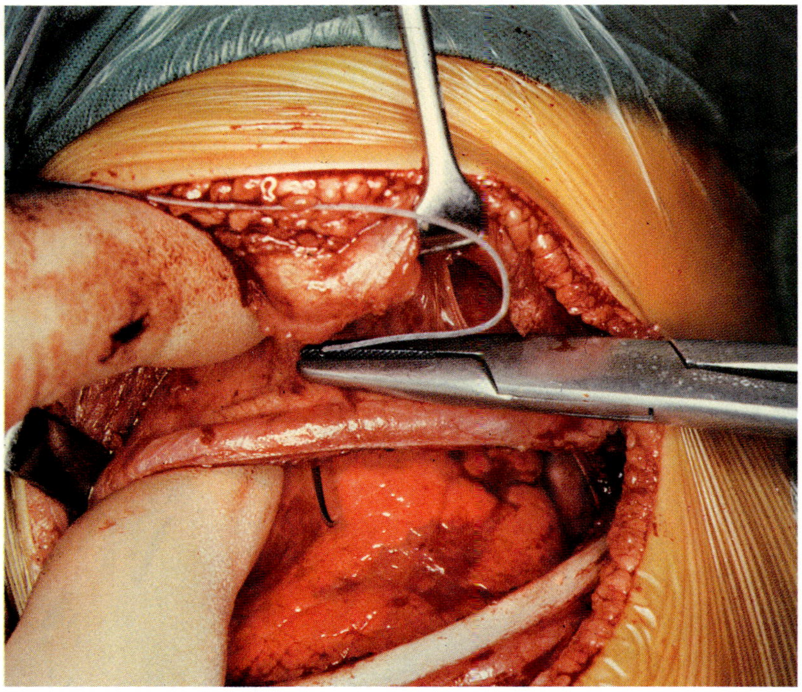
19
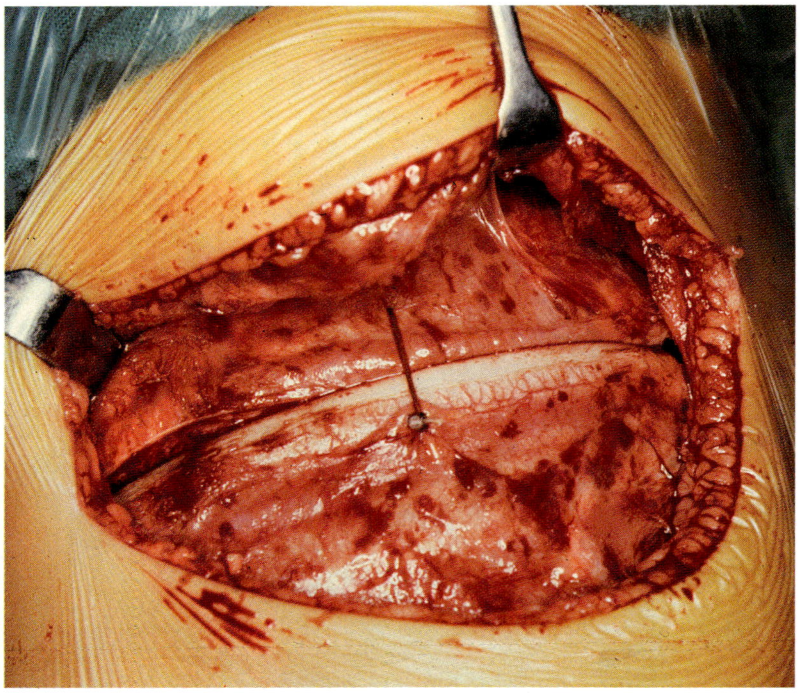

18 and 19 A chromic cat-gut suture is placed around the ribs to approximate them.

20
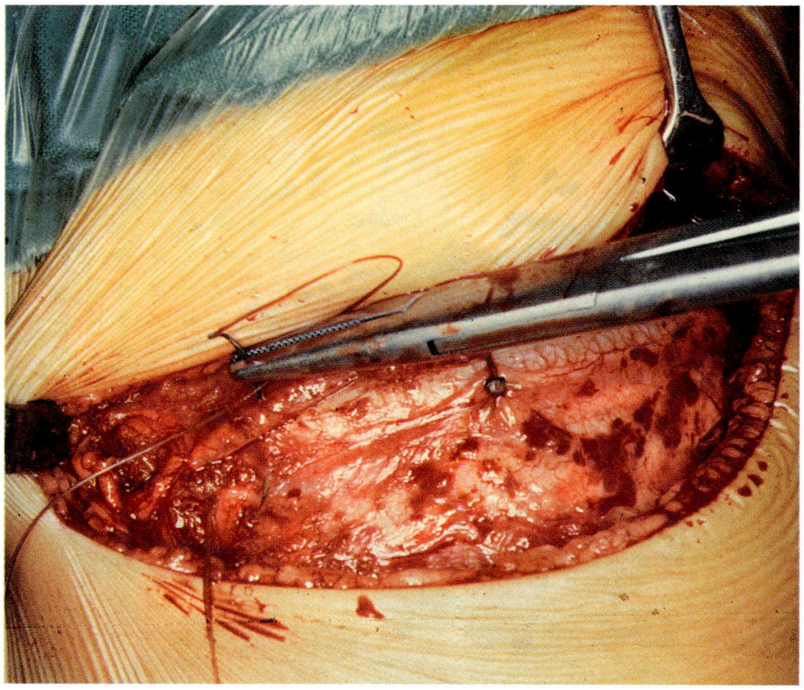
21
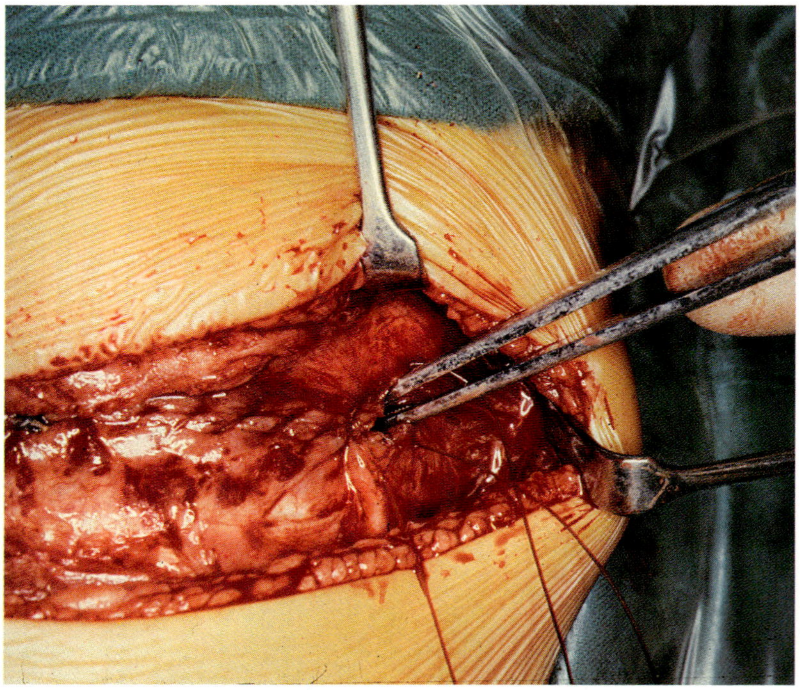

20 and 21 The upper intercostal muscle layer is sutured to the periosteum and lower intercostal muscles to seal the chest wall. If an intercostal drain has not been inserted, air is removed at this stage by holding the wound open with forceps while the anaesthetist firmly inflates the lungs to remove any air in the pleural space. The forceps are then quickly removed and the knot tied.

22

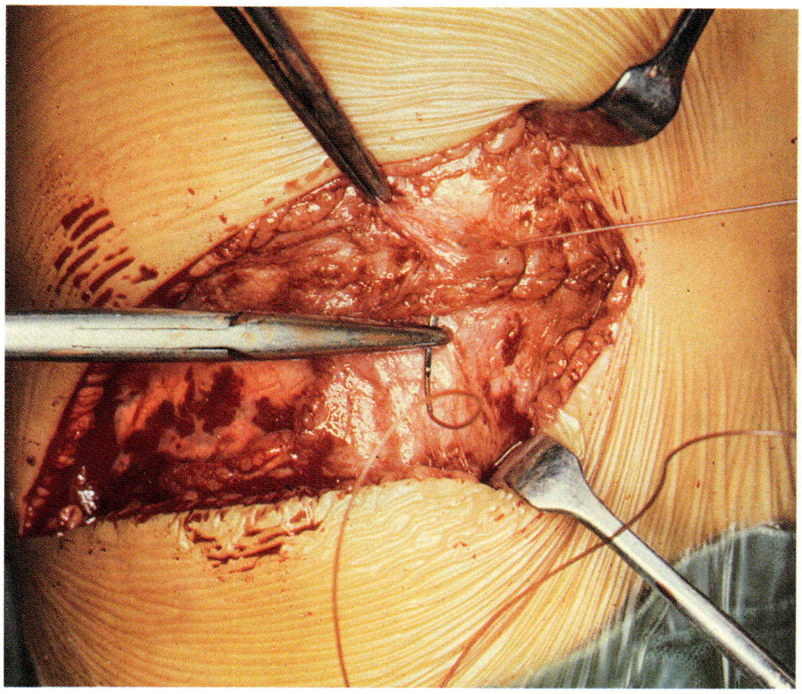

23

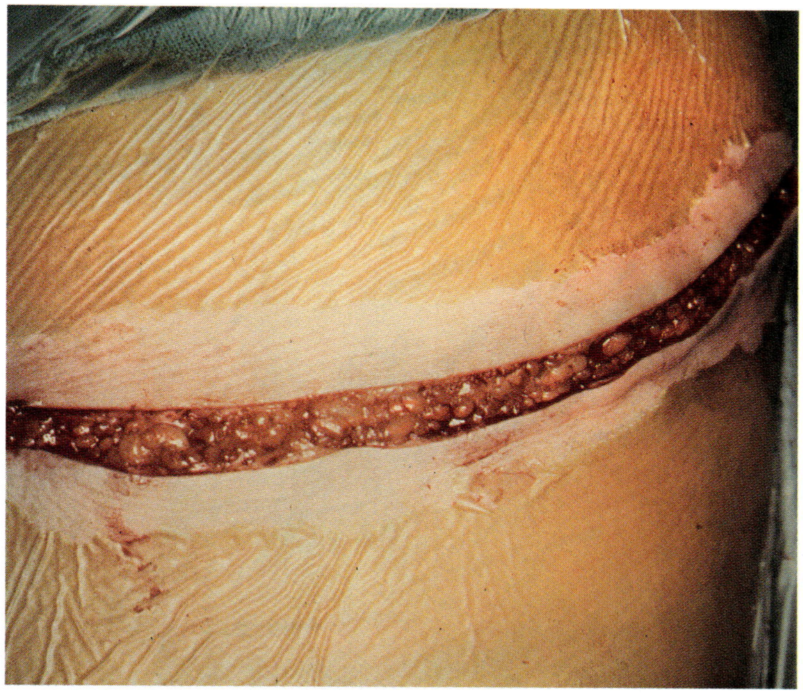

22 and 23 The muscle layers are closed with chromic cat-gut and the subcutaneous layer with plain cat-gut.

24

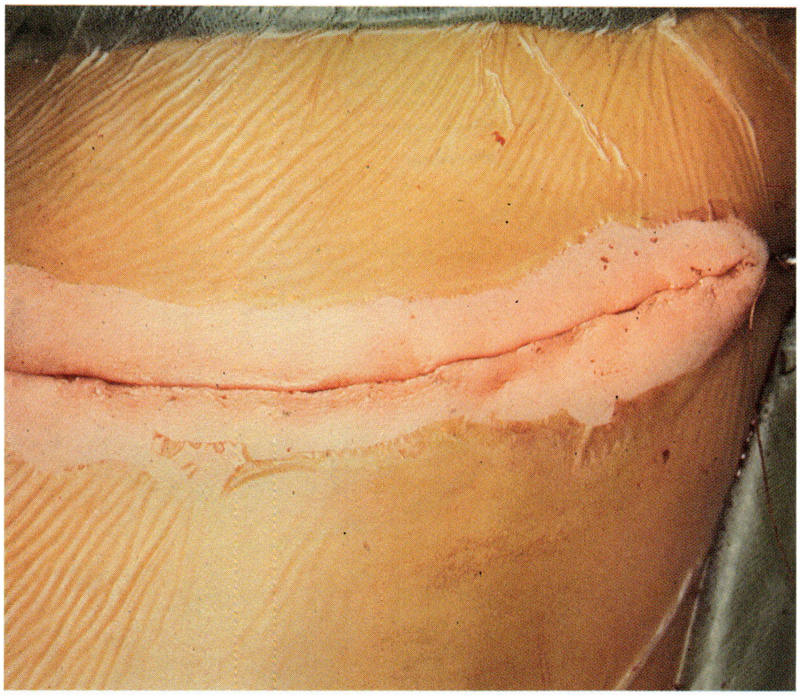

24 The skin is closed with subcuticular Dexon.

4: Closure of persistent ductus arteriosus

Closure of a persistent ductus arteriosus was first performed by Gross and Hubbard in 1938[1] and was, therefore, the first operation for congenital heart disease. The operation remains much the same today and does not require cardiopulmonary bypass. Diagram **A** demonstrates the duct (**A**) communicating between the aorta (**B**) and left pulmonary artery (**C**).

The approach is by a thoracotomy through the left fourth space (see Chapter 3) and the duct can be ligated or divided. Ligation is a quicker and simpler procedure but care must be taken not to sever the duct if the knot is tied too tightly; very rarely a recurrence has been reported after ligation. If the duct is large, it would therefore seem better to divide it; both procedures are illustrated in this chapter.

Diagram A

A – Persistent ductus arteriosus

B – Descending thoracic aorta

C – Left pulmonary artery

D – Left subclavian artery

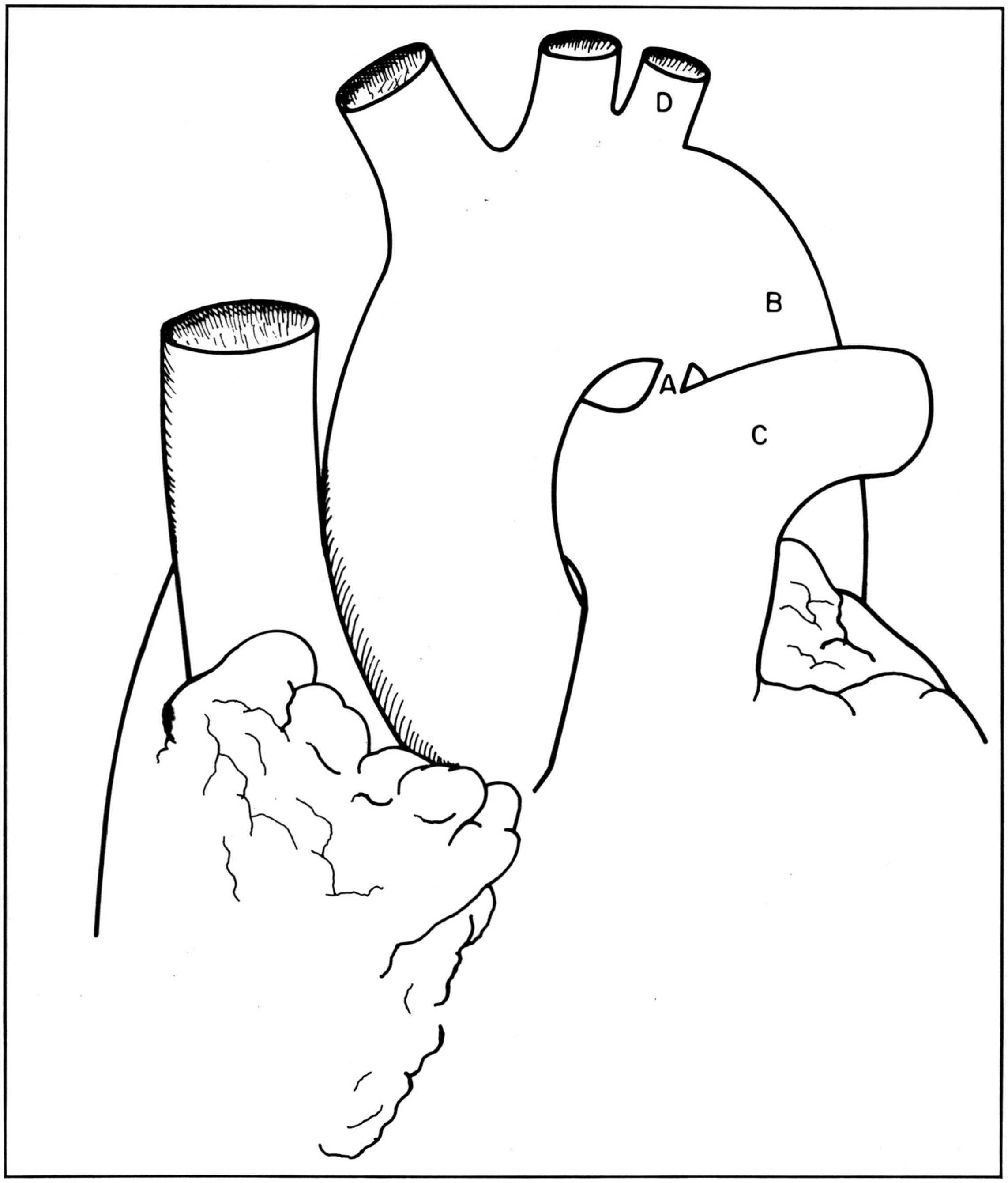

Ligation of persistent ductus arteriosus

1 The left chest has been opened and the lung retracted forward with a malleable retractor (**A**). The subclavian artery (**B**) and the descending thoracic aorta (**C**) are seen clearly, crossed by the left superior intercostal vein (**D**). The vagus nerve (**E**) can just be seen and must be safeguarded.

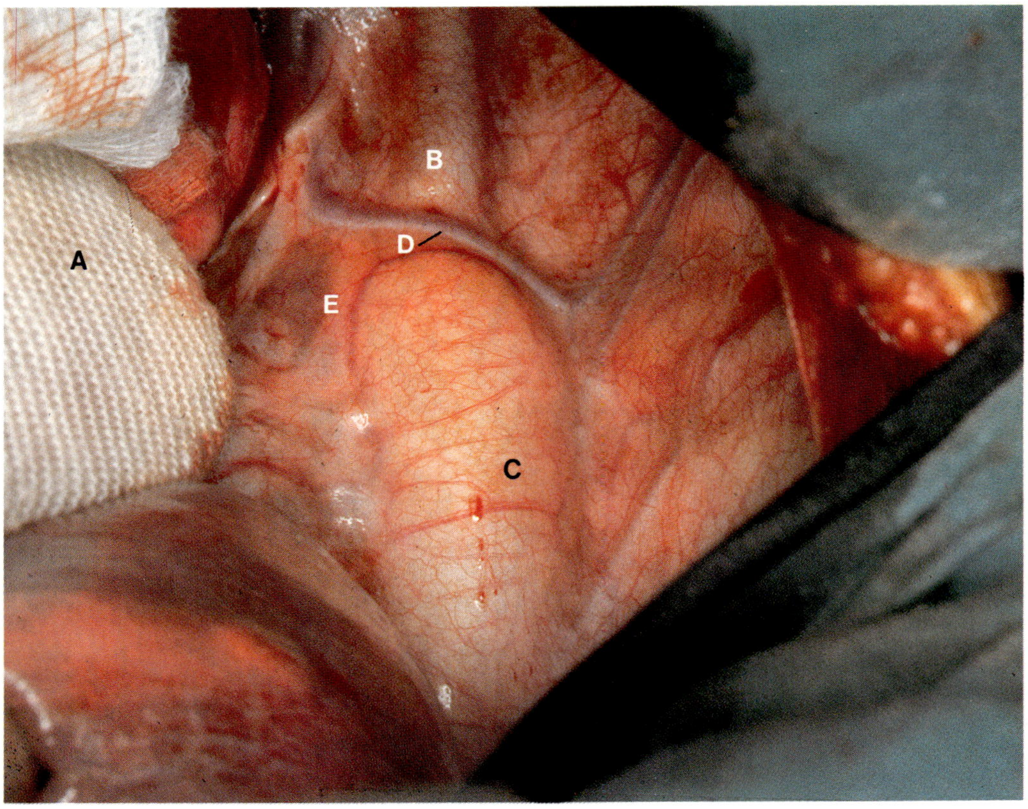

1

2

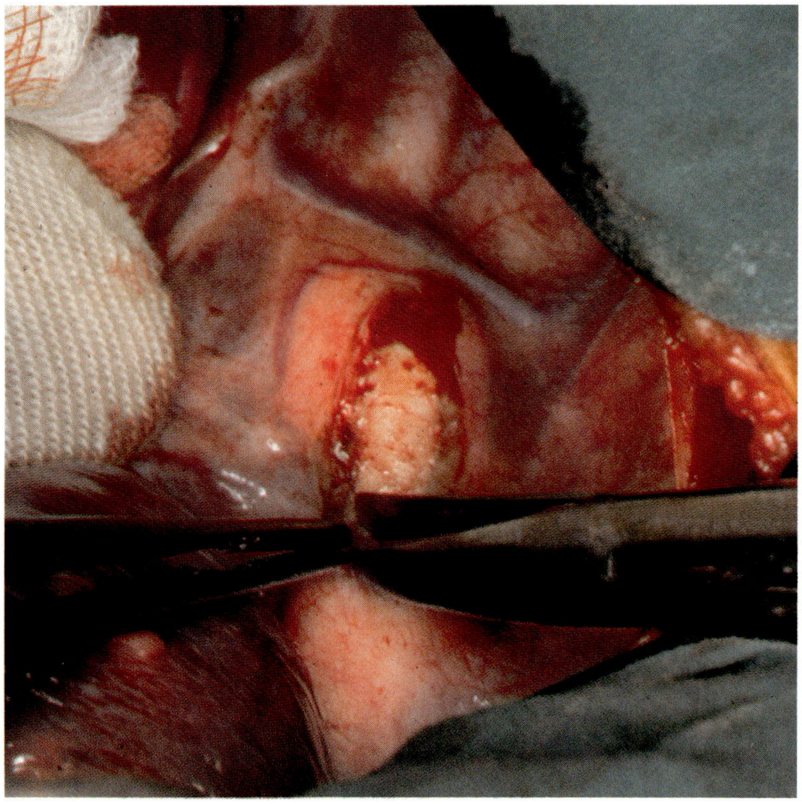

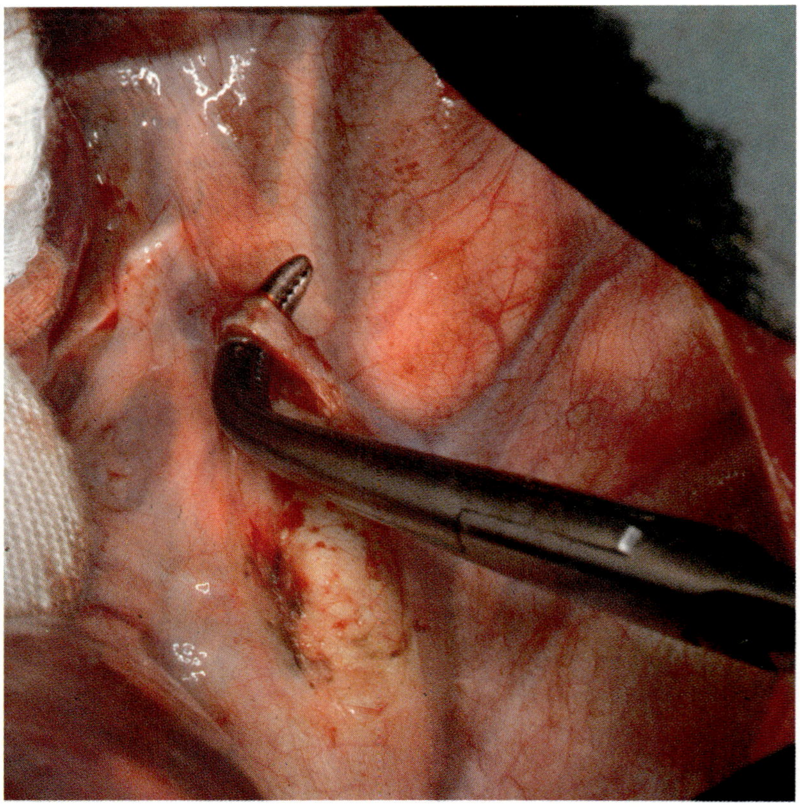

3

2 and 3 The pleura is incised vertically over the descending aorta and it is usually necessary to divide the left superior intercostal vein.

4

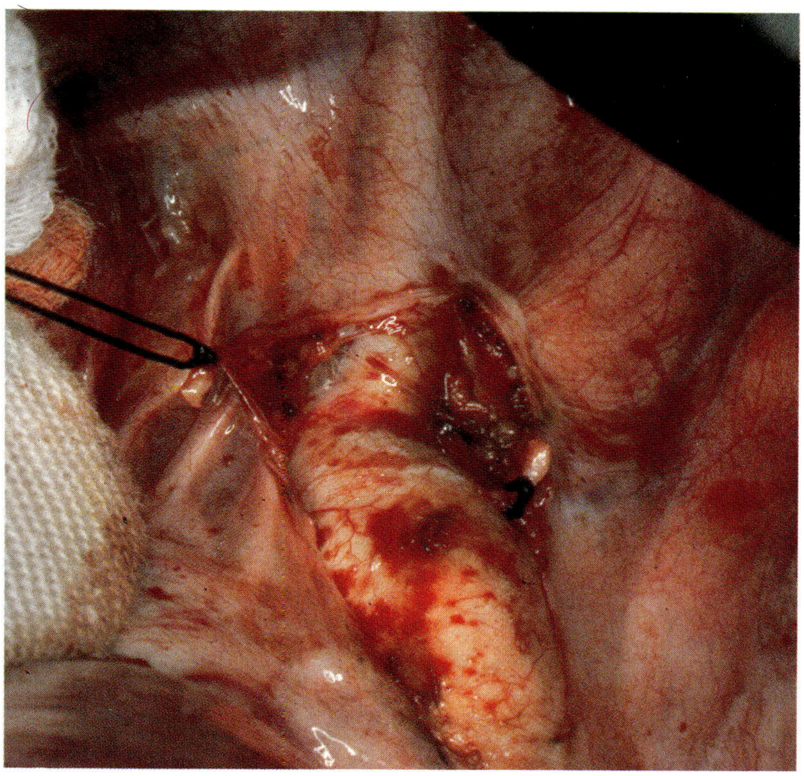

5

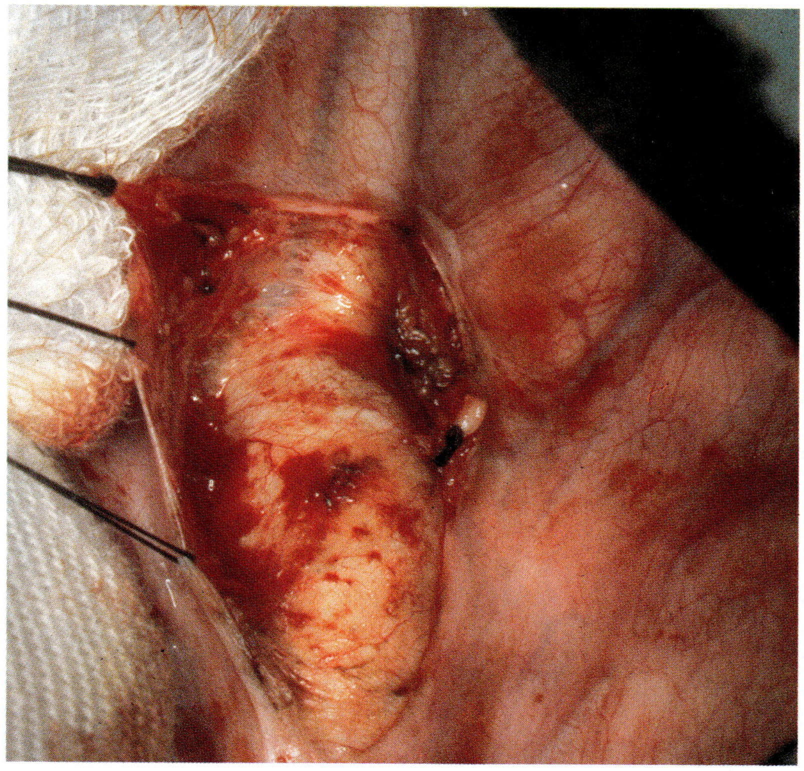

4 and 5 The anterior tie and two stay-sutures are used to retract the lung forward and can be secured anteriorly so as to free the assistant's hands.

6

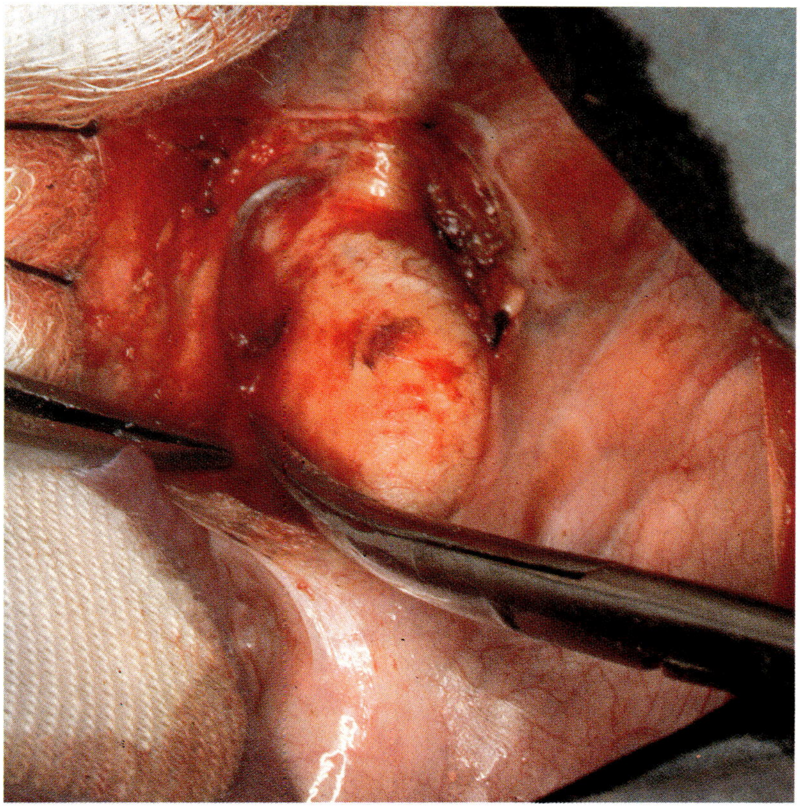

7

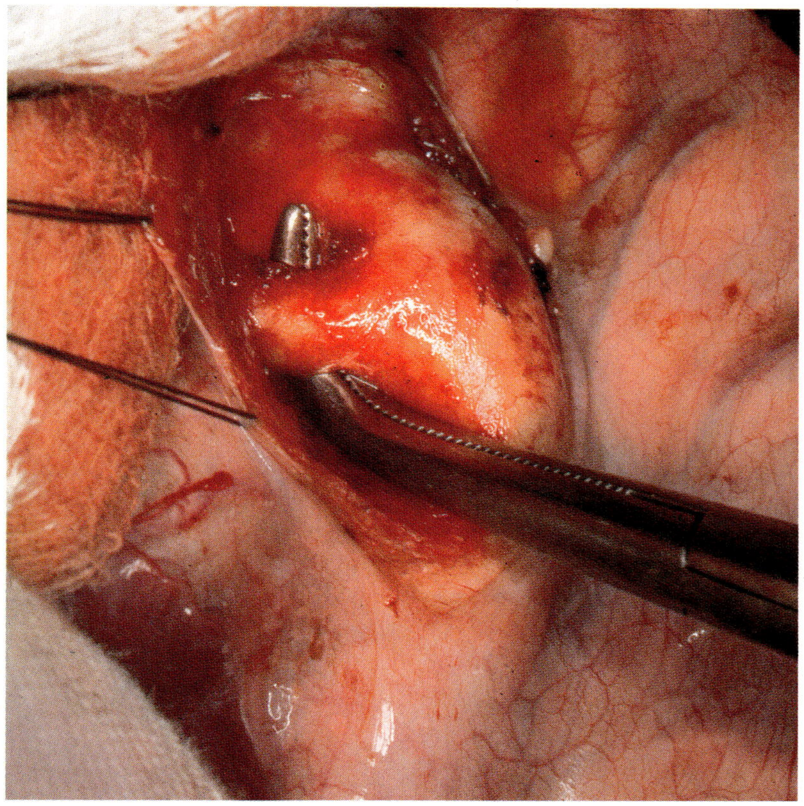

6 and 7 Careful dissection with scissors is then required to expose the fragile duct without tearing it. Dissection should be kept close to the aorta and be continued above and below the duct. Forceps can then be carefully placed around the back of the duct.

8

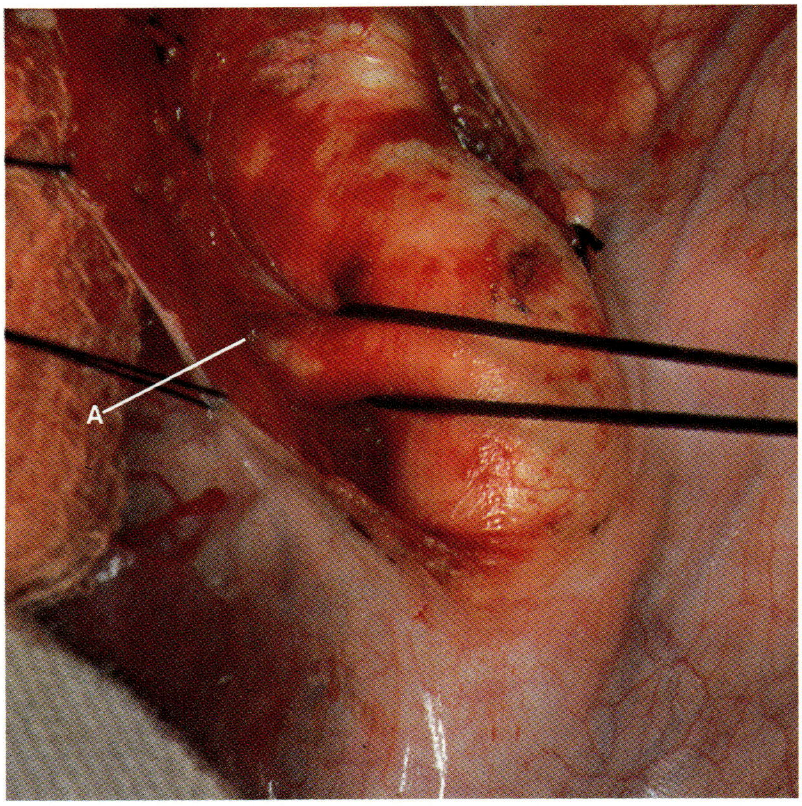

9

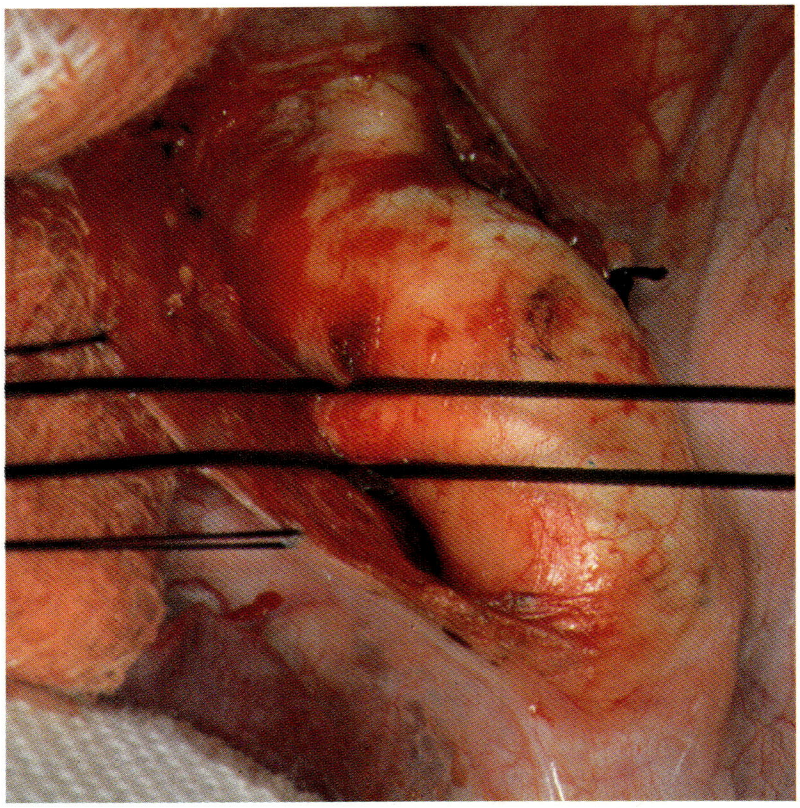

8 A '4' silk ligature is placed carefully around the duct. It is helpful to wet it so that it slides more easily. The recurrent laryngeal nerve (**A**) can be seen passing from the vagus nerve around the undersurface of the duct and must be guarded at all times.

9 to 12 A second ligature is placed around the duct and both ligatures are tied and cut.

10

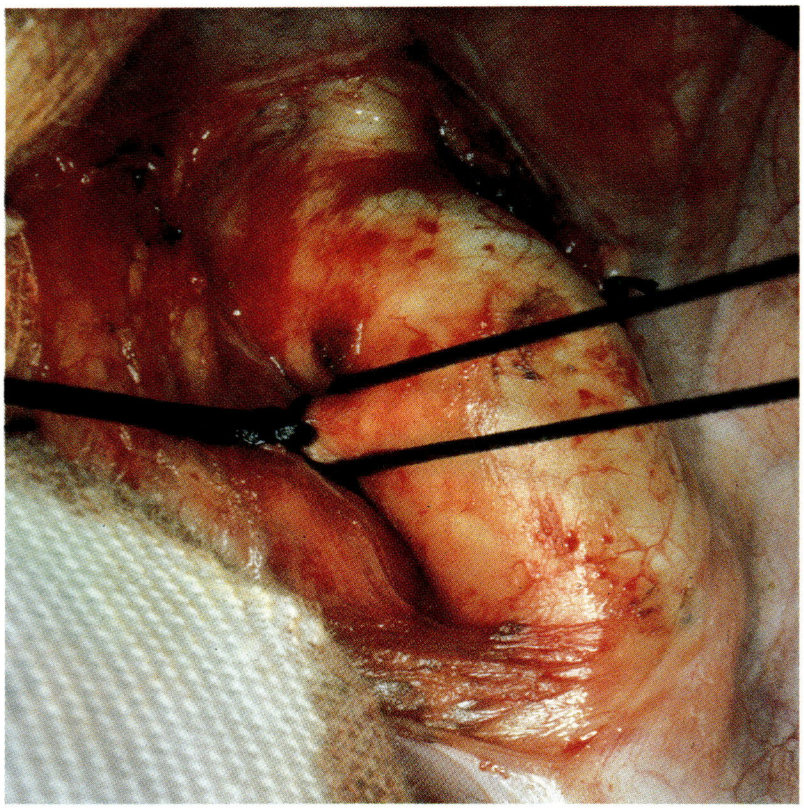

11

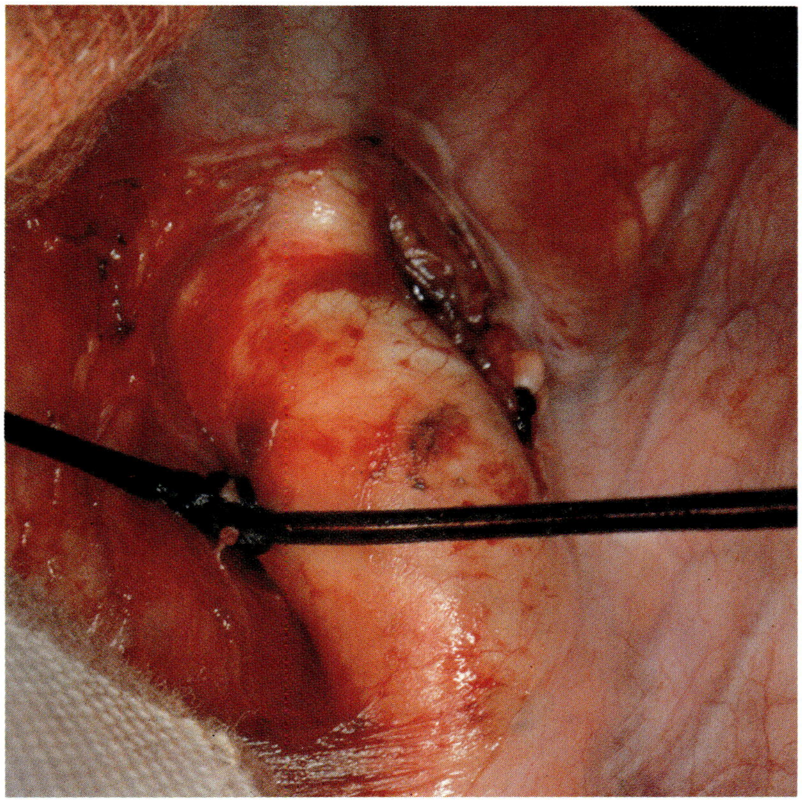

12

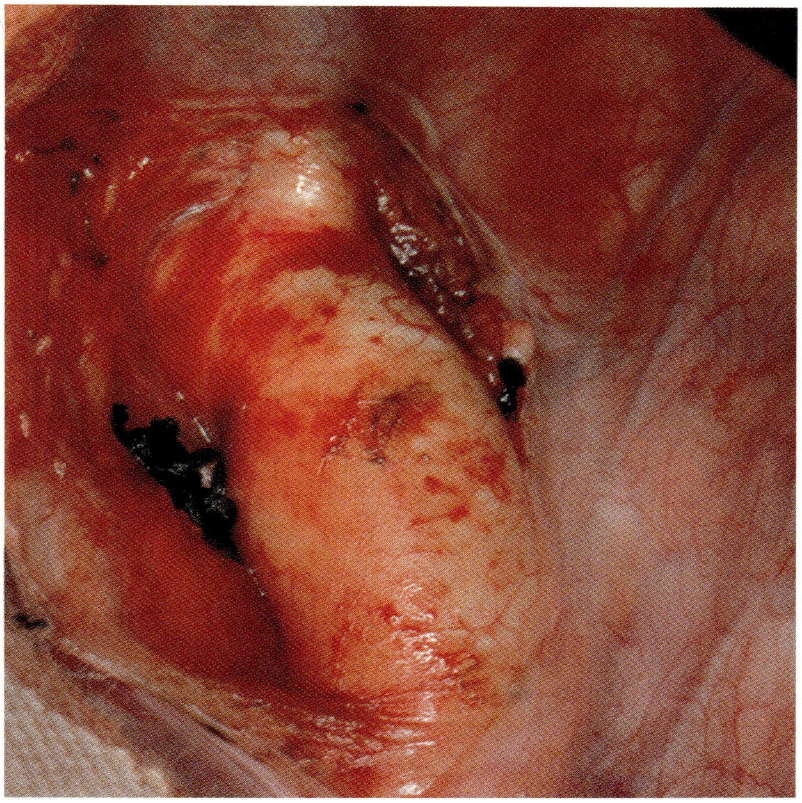

13

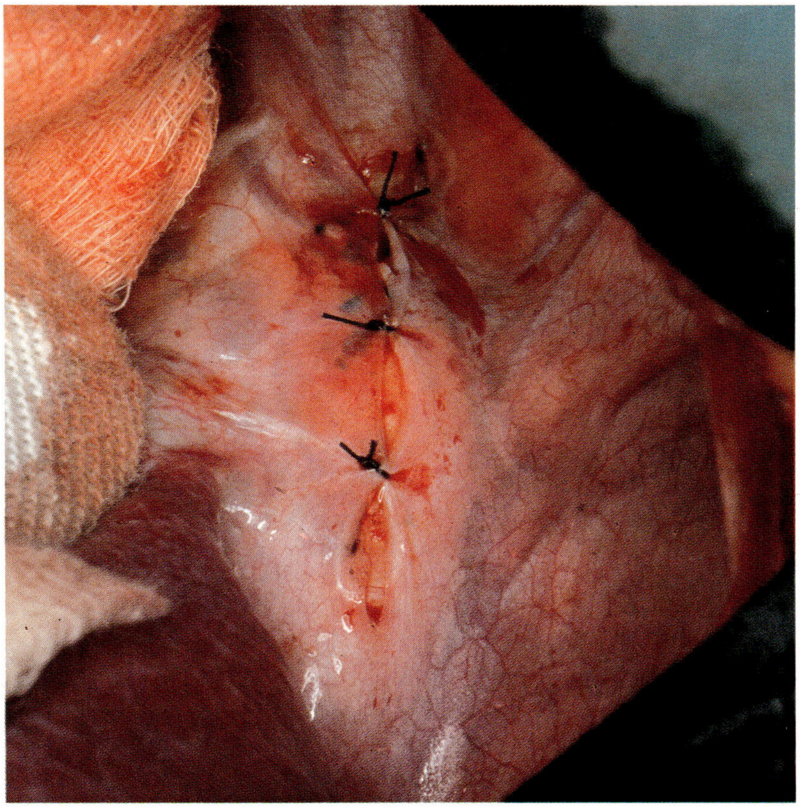

13 Finally, the pleura is approximated over the aorta with 3/0 silk or other suitable suture. The chest is closed in layers (see Chapter 3) and it is usually unnecessary to insert a drainage tube, but care must be taken to get the anaesthetist to fully expand the lung and expel all air from the pleural cavity as the intercostal muscle layer is finally closed.

Division of persistent ductus arteriosus

14

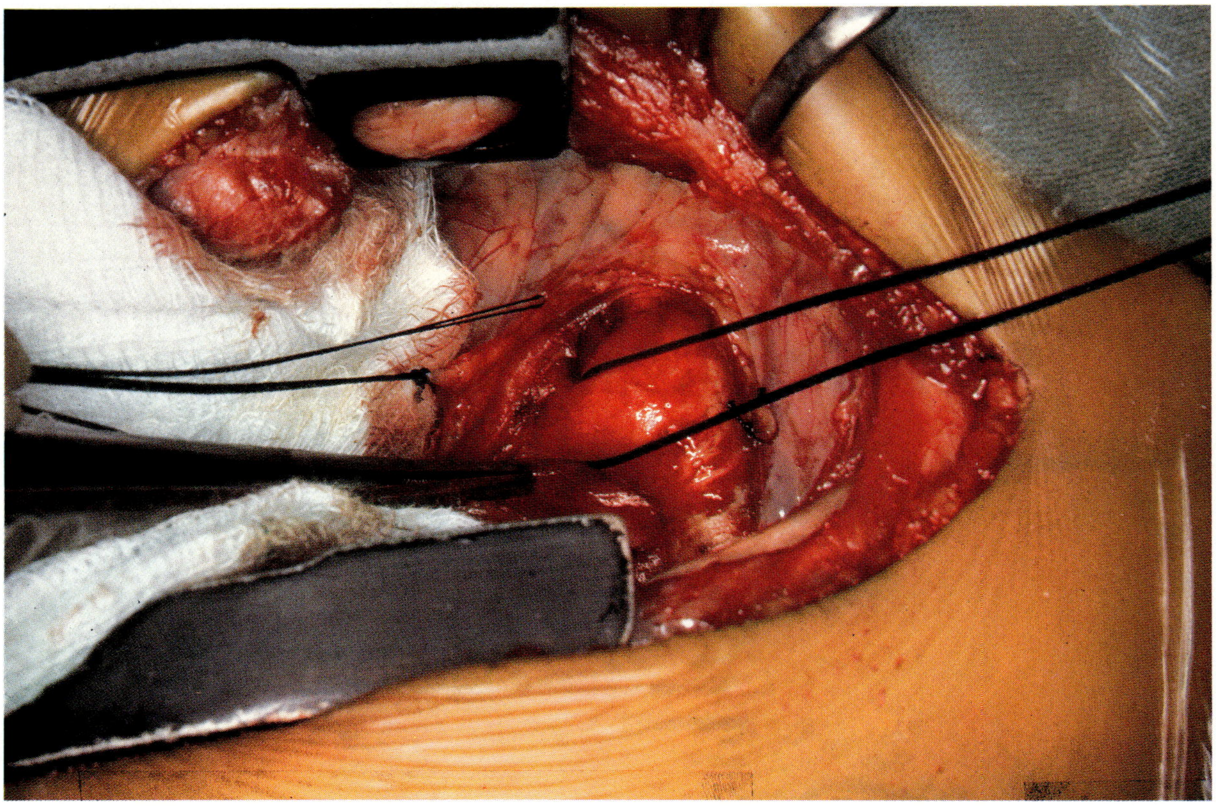

14 The duct is exposed as for ligation and a ligature is placed around it.

15

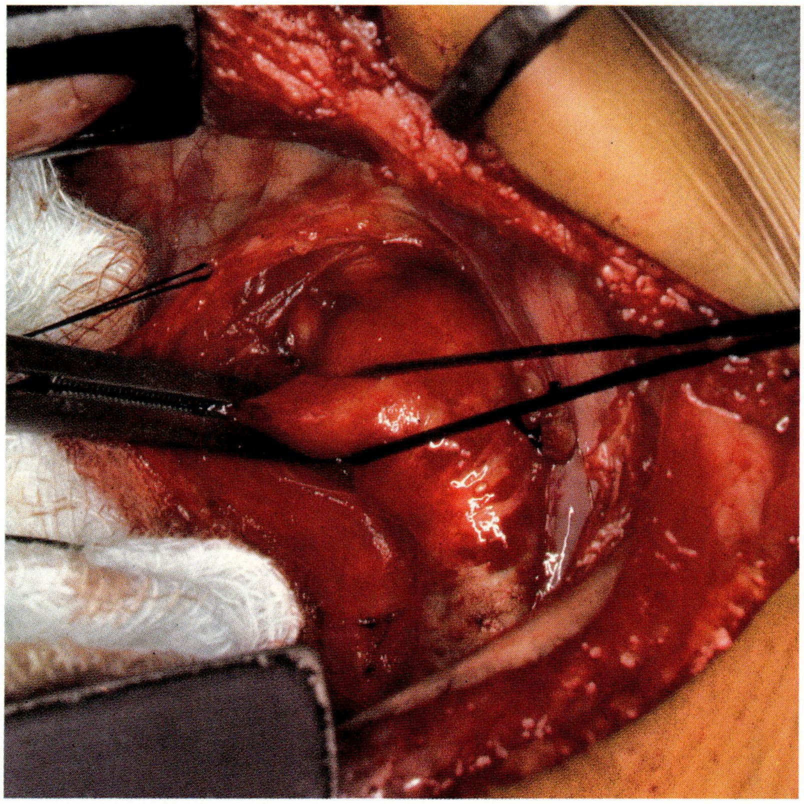

16

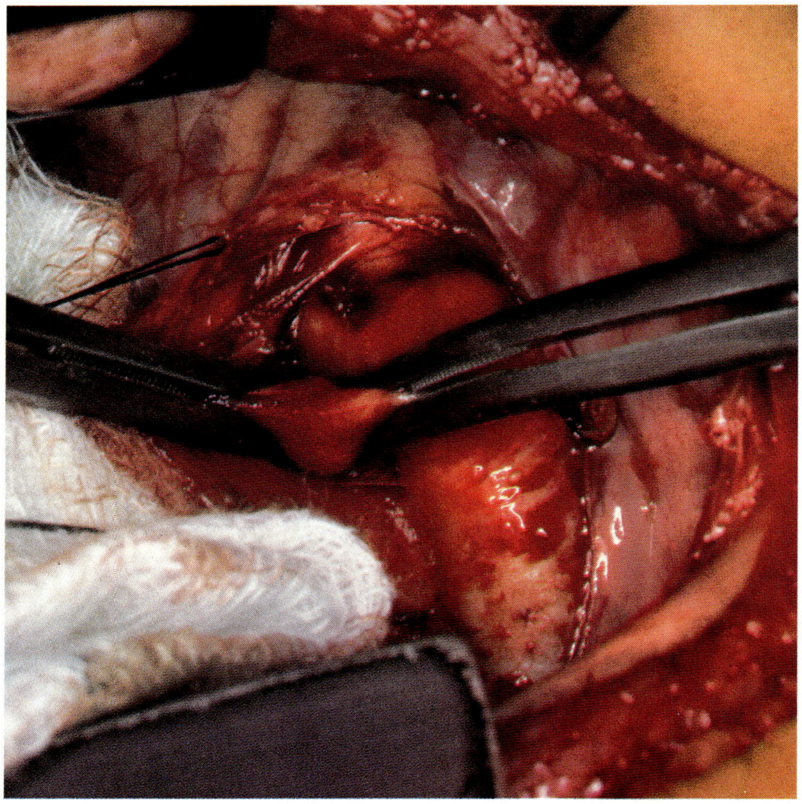

15 and 16 An arterial clamp is placed, first on the pulmonary artery end of the duct and then the aortic end, being sure to leave an adequate amount of tissue between them. The ligature is helpful in placing the clamps but is then removed.

17

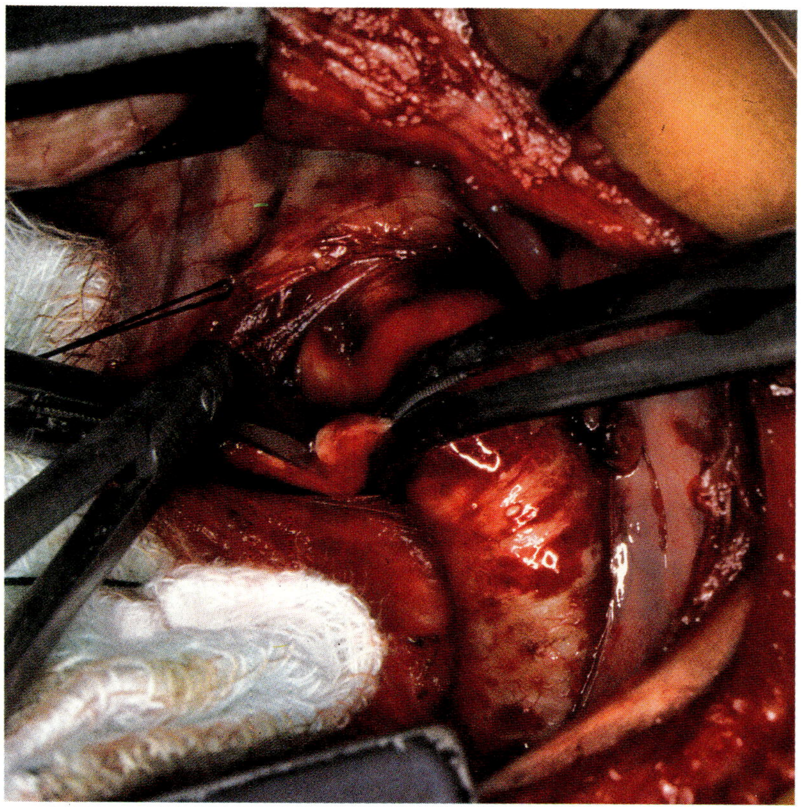

18

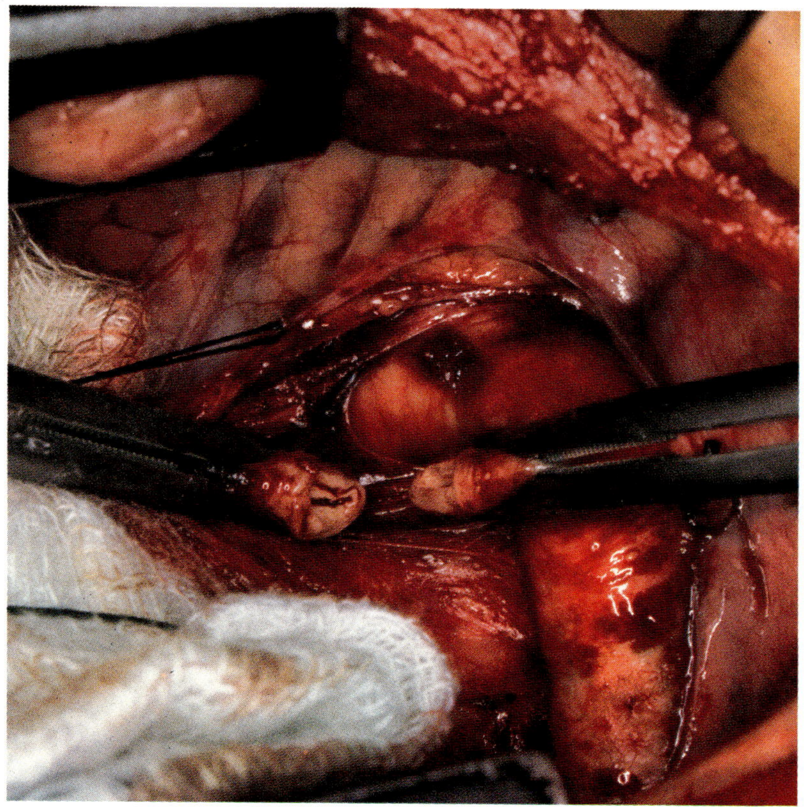

17 and 18 The duct is divided with Potts' scissors.

19

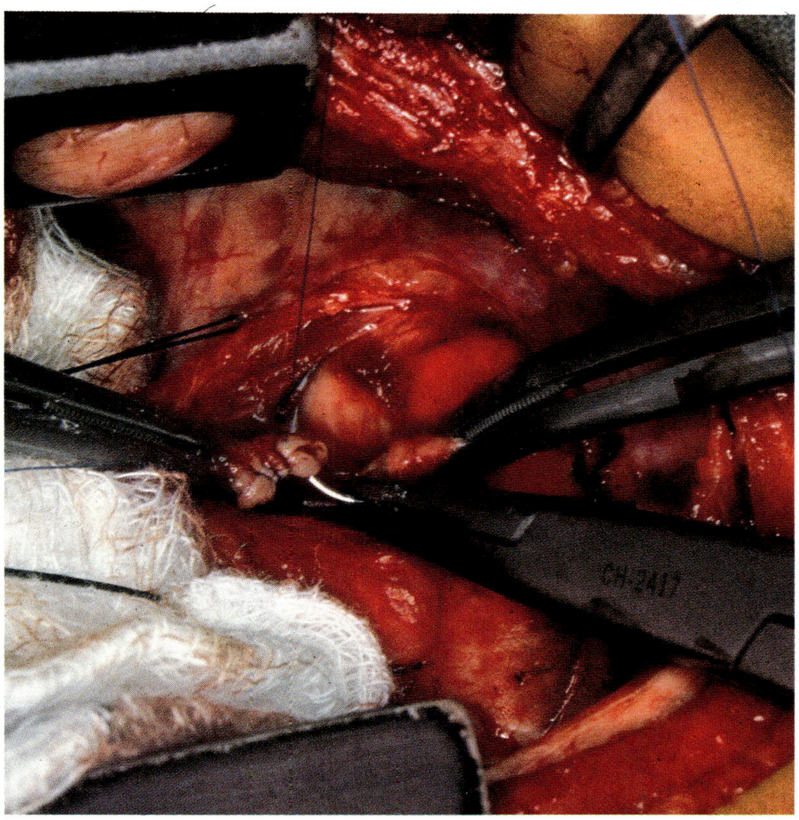

20

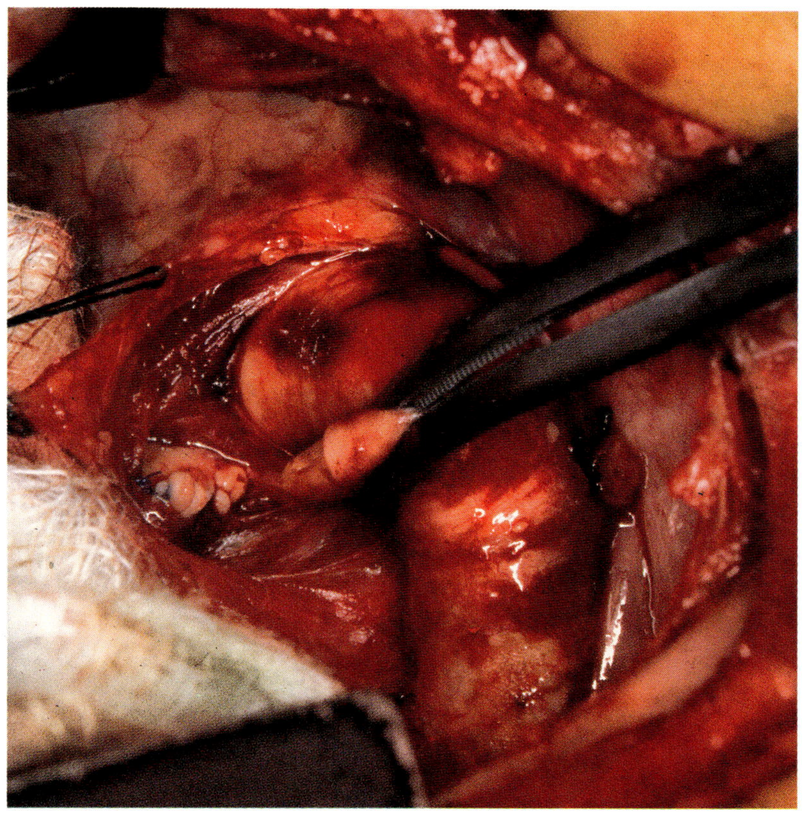

19 and 20 The pulmonary artery end is then oversewn with a double layer of continuous 5/0 Prolene and the suture cut. If there is any bleeding from the suture line, a swab can be placed over the suture line and retracted gently while the aortic end is closed.

21

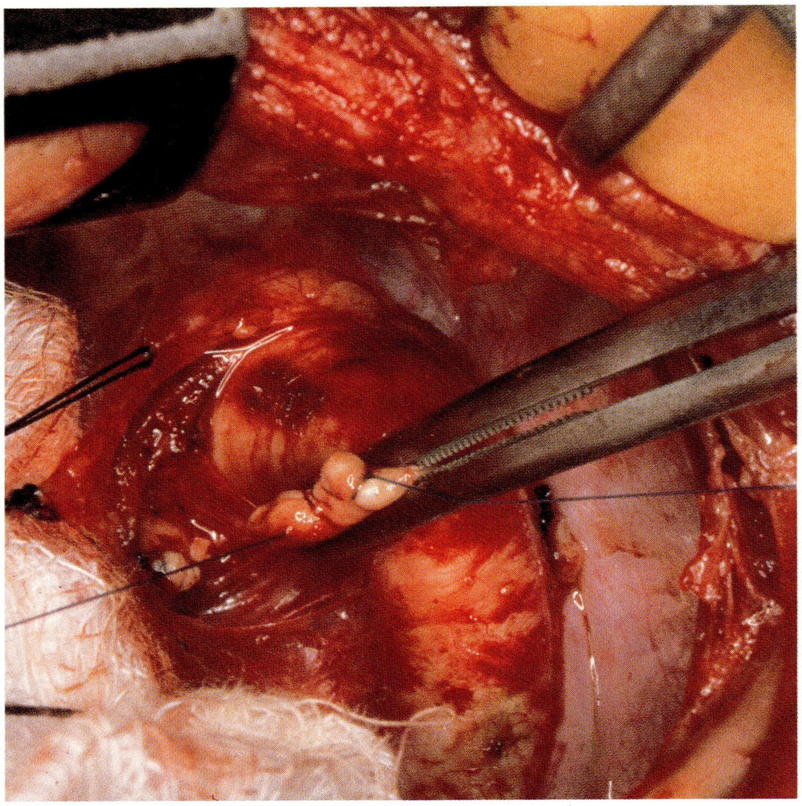

22

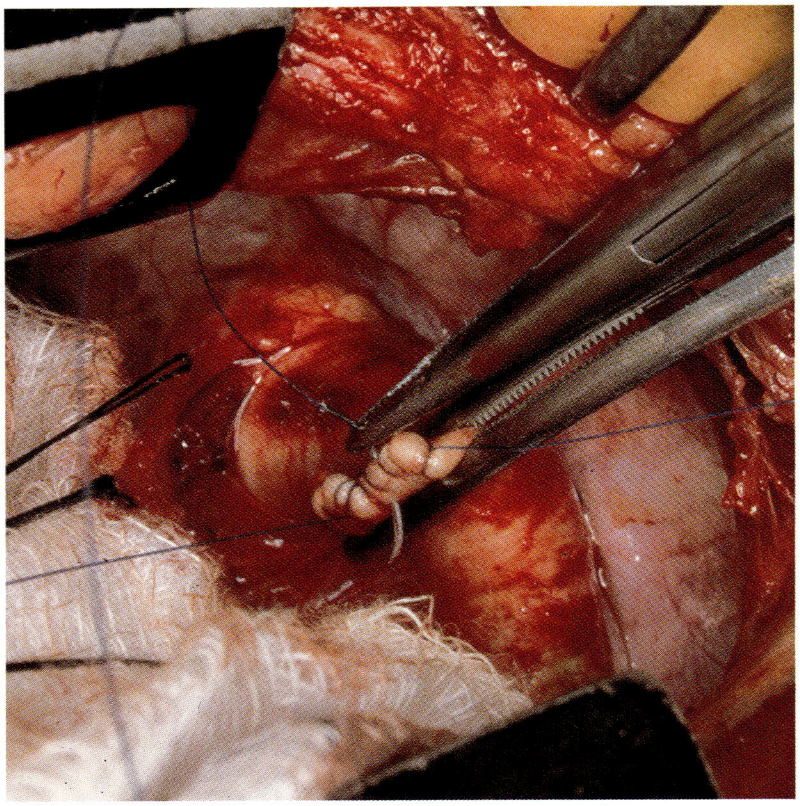

21 to 24 The aortic end is closed with a double layer of 5/0 Prolene and the clamp is removed.

23

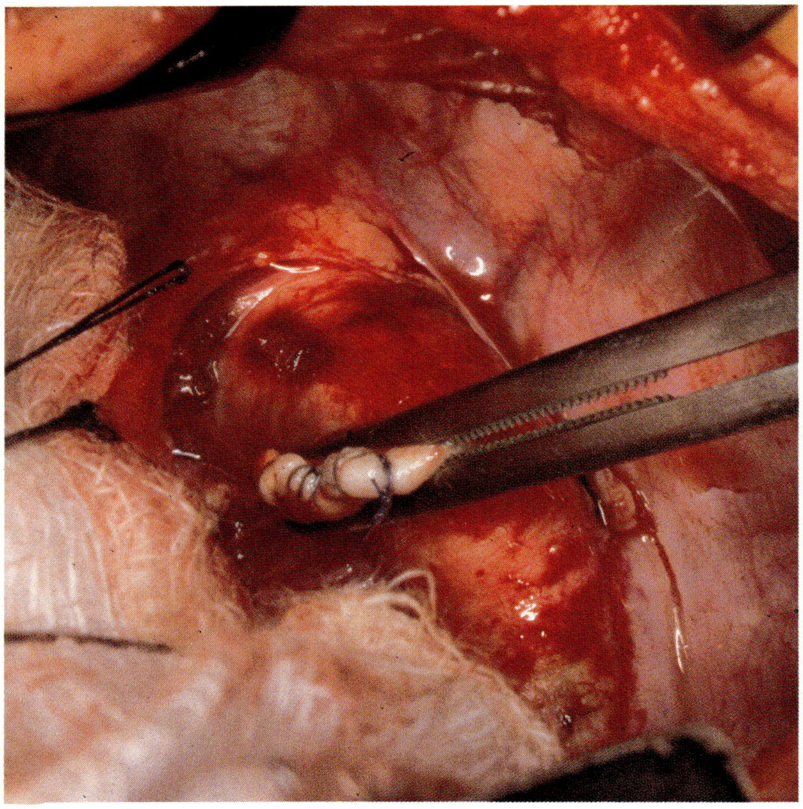

24

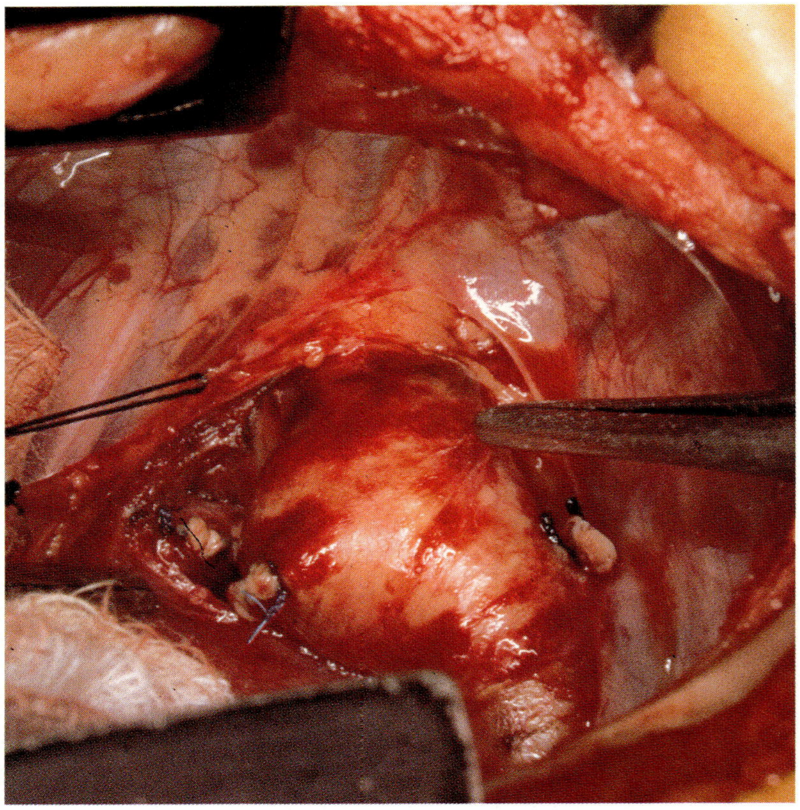

5: Repair of coarctation of the aorta

Coarctation of the aorta, as illustrated in diagram **A,** is a narrowing of the thoracic aorta just beyond the origin of the left subclavian artery (**A**). The narrowing may be localised, usually just opposite the ligamentum arteriosum (**B**), or, particularly in infants, the aorta may be narrowed over a longer segment. As the coarctation is present from early on in foetal life, blood finds its way round through collateral vessels (**C**) to the descending aorta (**D**) below the coarctation. For this reason, in severe coarctation, it is safe to clamp the aorta above and below the coarctation so that the coarctation can be resected with an end-to-end aortic anastomosis. This operation was first performed by Crafoord in 1944[1] and remains the standard form of treatment to this day.

When the coarcted segment is longer, it may be simpler to incise the narrowed segment longitudinally and insert a dacron patch. In infants, some reported series have quoted a high rate of restenosis after end-to-end anastomosis and, therefore, the use of the subclavian flap technique[2] has become popular. This technique is very useful and successful[3] and is particularly suitable when there is a long aortic isthmus (that part of the aorta between the subclavian artery and coarctation) and in the first few months of life.

When performing an end-to-end anastomosis, it is technically easier to use a continuous posterior suture line but anteriorly interrupted sutures allow for growth. It is usually unnecessary to divide any intercostal vessels, though they may need temporary occlusion during the anastomosis.

Occasionally, if the coarctation is not very severe, insufficient collaterals will have developed and prolonged aortic clamping would be unsafe. It is therefore sometimes necessary to provide a bypass to the lower part of the body, as when resecting a descending thoracic aortic aneurysm. Rarely it may be easier to place a dacron tube graft in parallel with the coarcted segment by end-to-side anastomosis rather than use cardiopulmonary bypass when the collateral circulation is inadequate.

The approach for repair of coarctation of the aorta is through the left chest in the fourth intercostal space (see Chapter 3).

Diagram A

A – Left subclavian artery

B – Ligamentum arteriosum

C – Collateral vessels (intercostal arteries)

D – Descending aorta

E – Site of coarctation

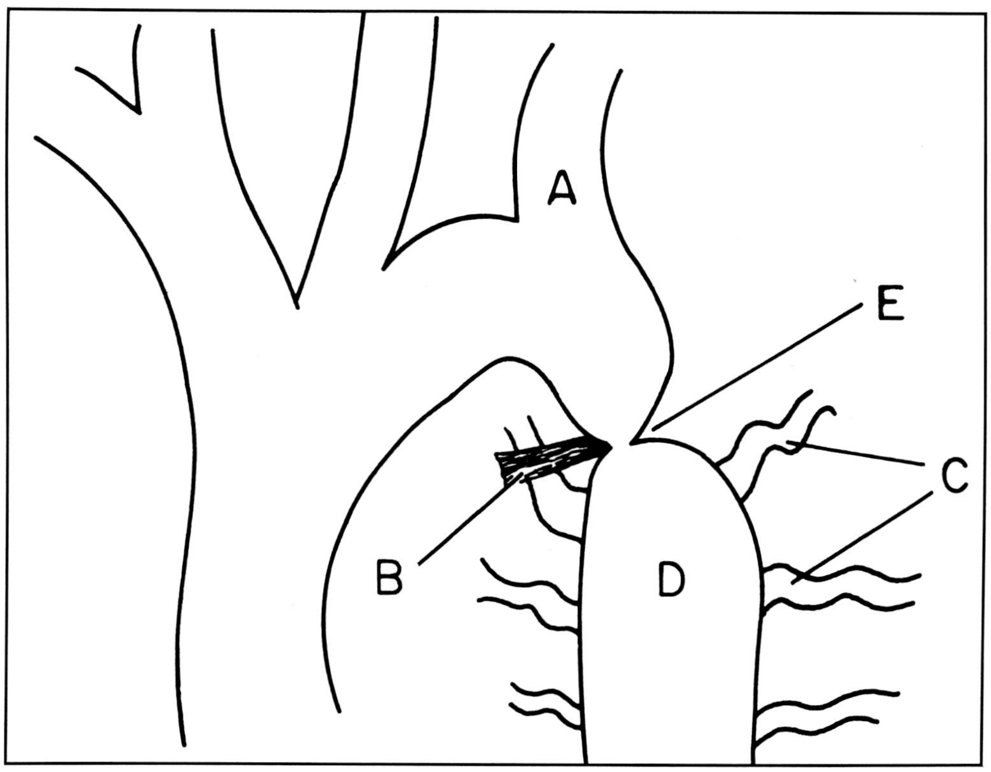

End-to-end anastamosis

1 The left chest has been opened and the lung, which is covered by a swab, retracted forwards by a cloth-covered malleable retractor (**A**). The descending thoracic aorta (**B**), left subclavian artery (**C**) and left superior intercostal vein (**D**) are clearly seen. The enlarged internal mammary artery (**E**) and an enlarged intercostal artery (**F**) are evidence of a good collateral circulation. The coarctation itself is not apparent though situated, in this case, beneath the left superior intercostal vein.

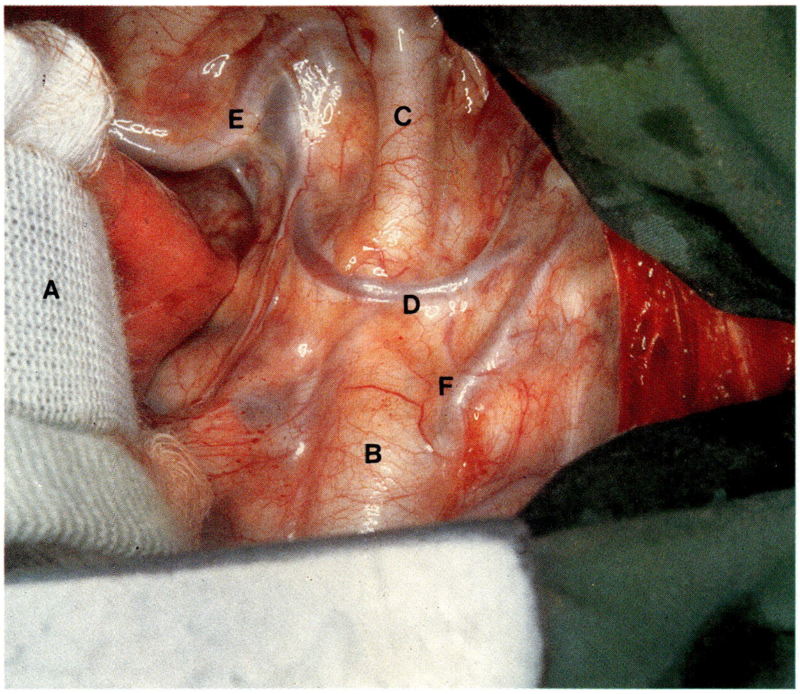

1

2

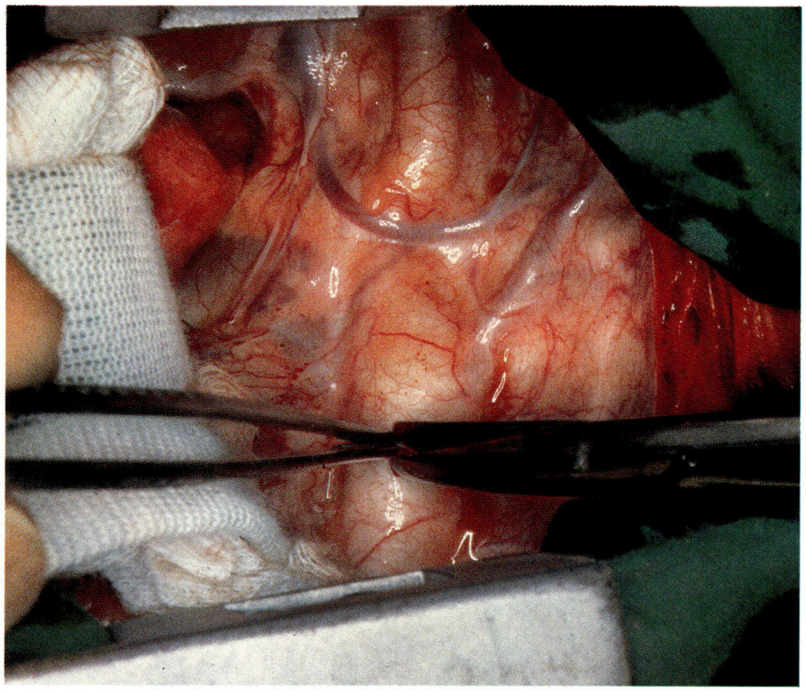

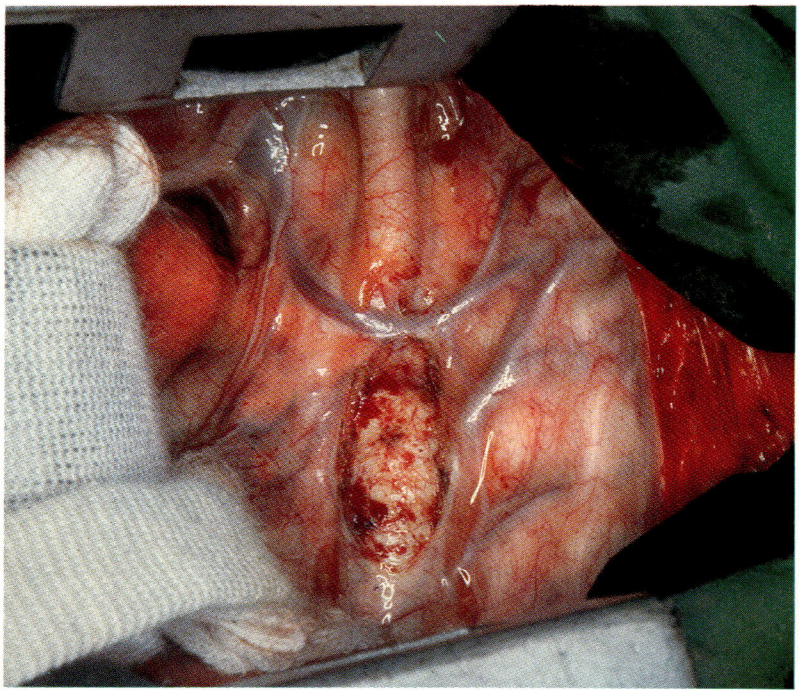

3

2 and 3 The pleura overlying the aorta is incised longitudinally to expose the aorta.

4

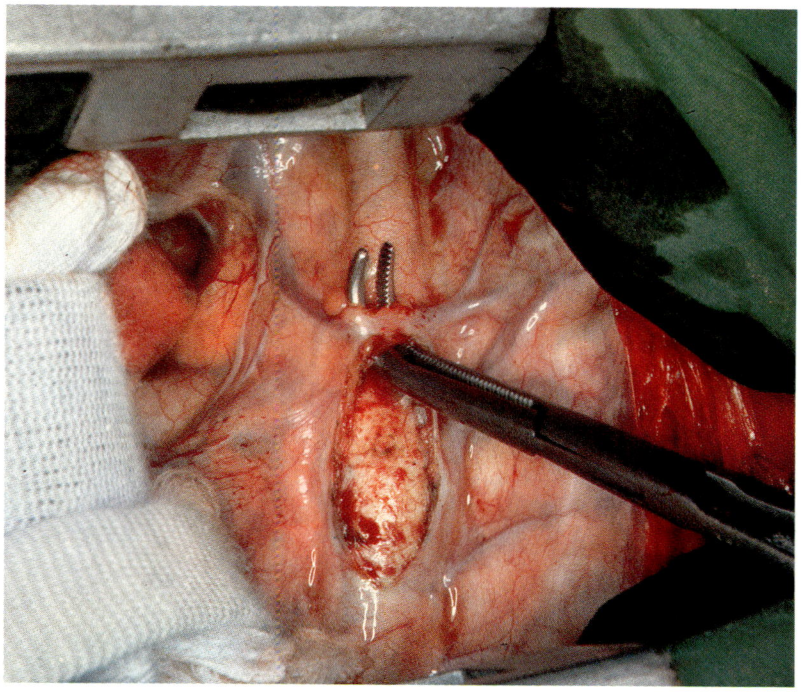

5

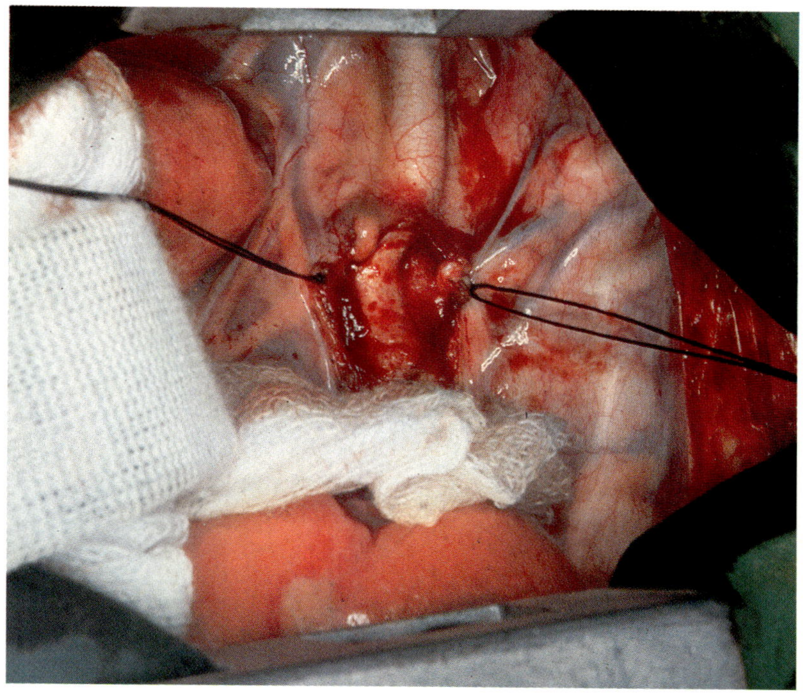

4 and 5 The left superior intercostal vein is divided between ligatures.

6

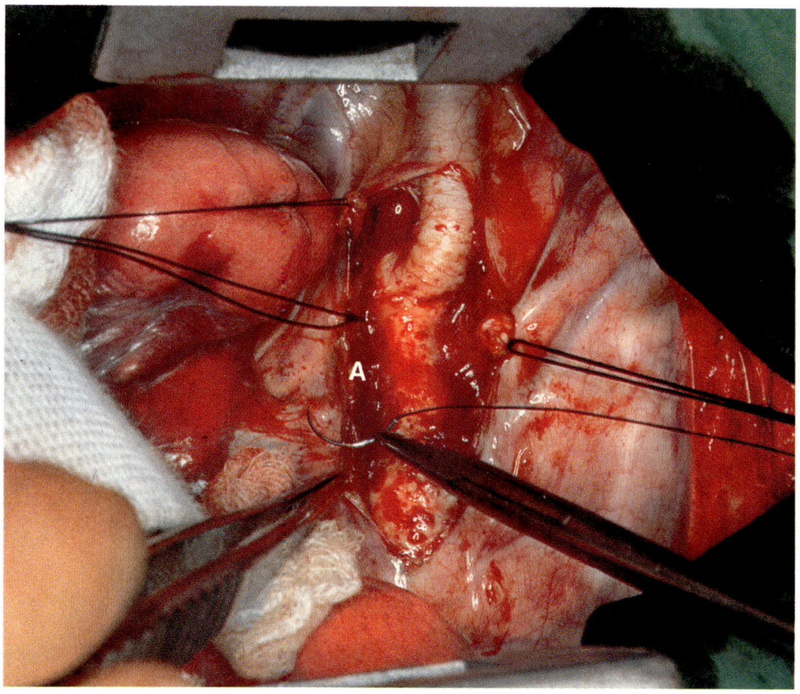

6 Three stay-sutures are placed in the pleura anteriorly to provide retraction. Care must be taken not to place them too deeply to avoid damage to the vagus nerve (**A**).

7

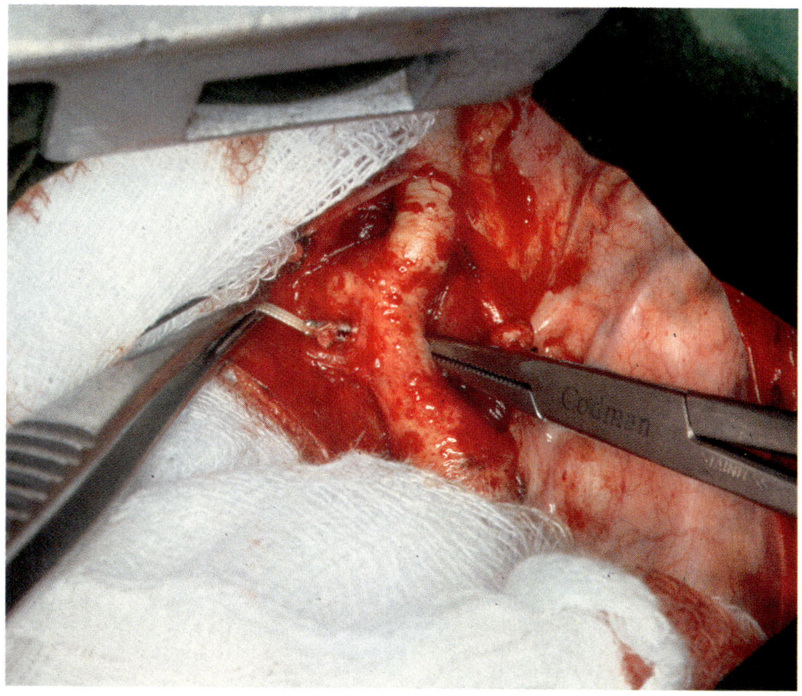

7 The narrowed area of the aorta containing the coarctation has been dissected free and a tape is placed around the aorta just above the ligamentum arteriosum.

8
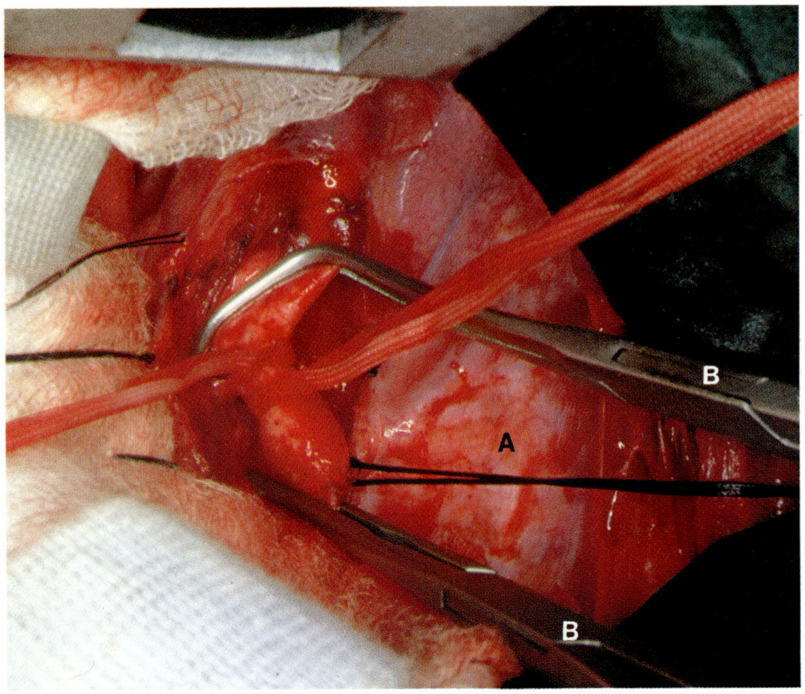

9
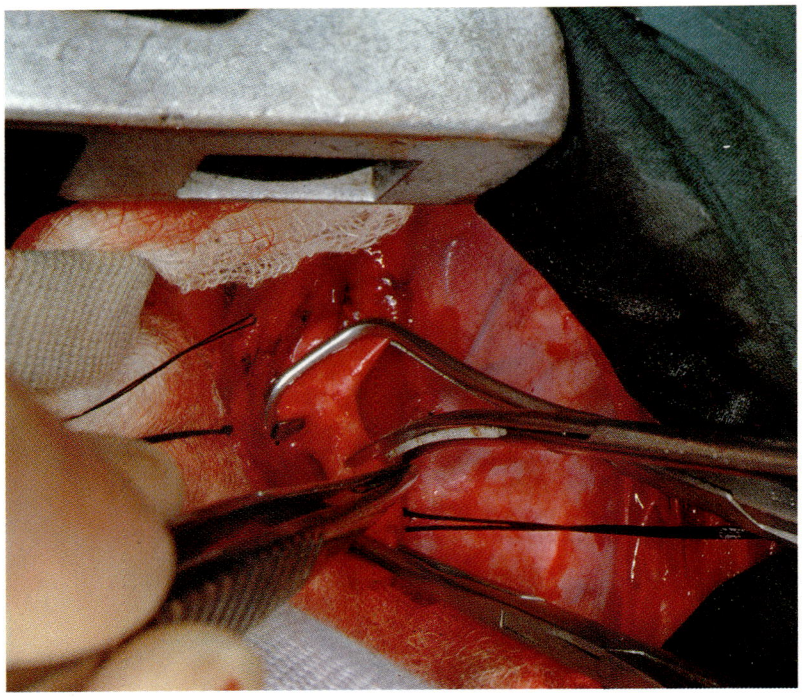

8 Another tape has been placed around the aorta to help dissection and a temporary ligature placed around an intercostal artery (**A**). Clamps (**B**) have been applied across the aorta above and below the coarctation.

9 The aorta is then transected, with a pair of scissors, below the coarctation.

10
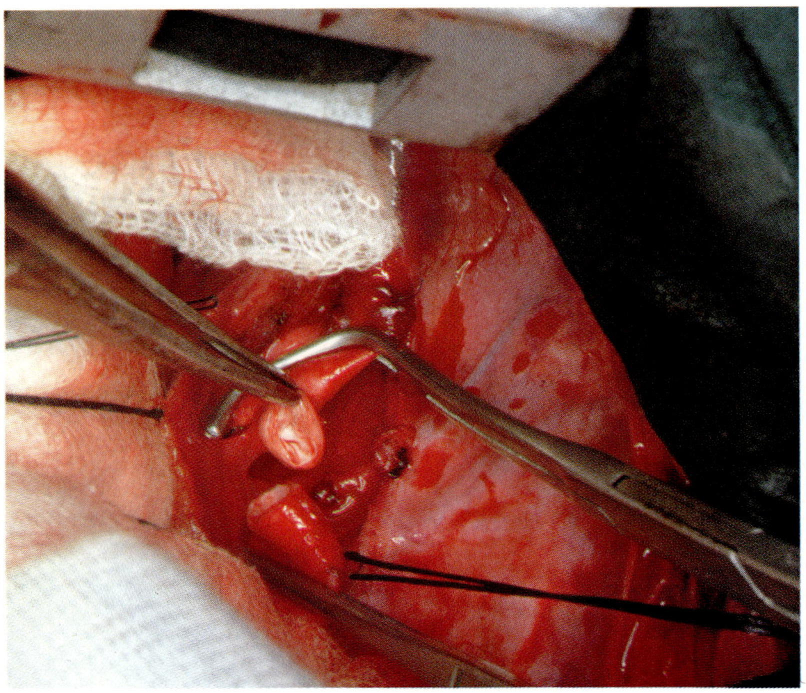

11
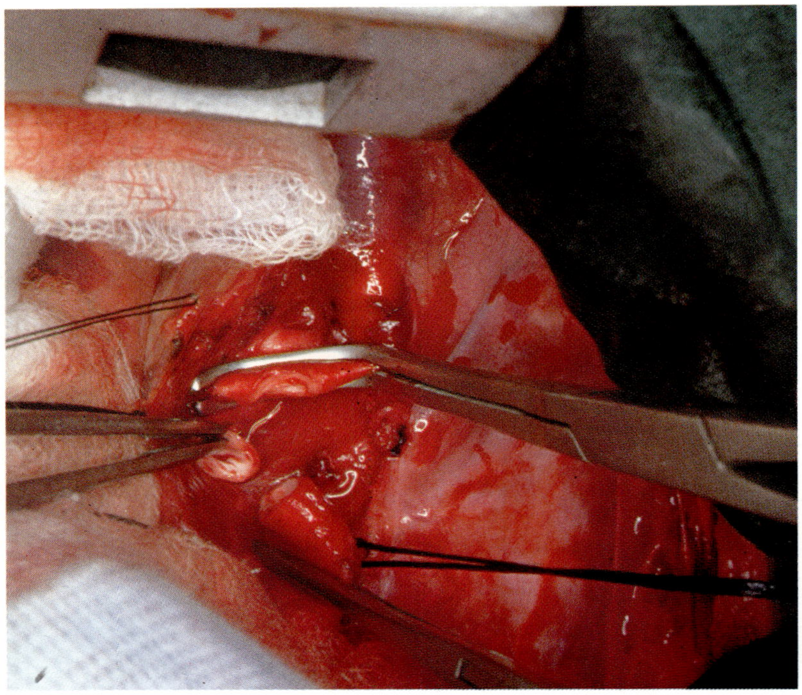

10 and 11 The very severe narrowing of the aorta can be seen and the coarcted segment, now detached from the aorta above and below, can be removed after cutting the aortic end of the ligamentum arteriosum.

12

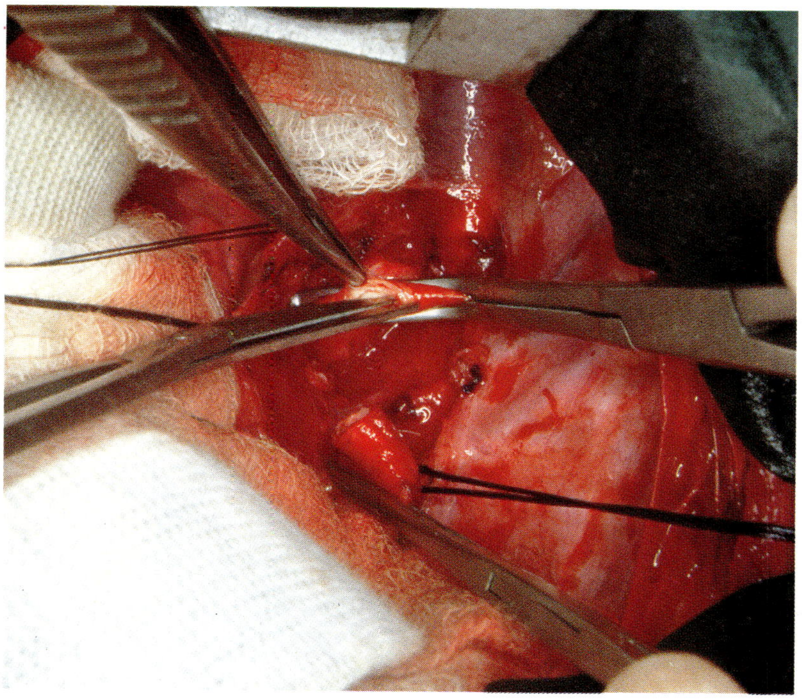

13

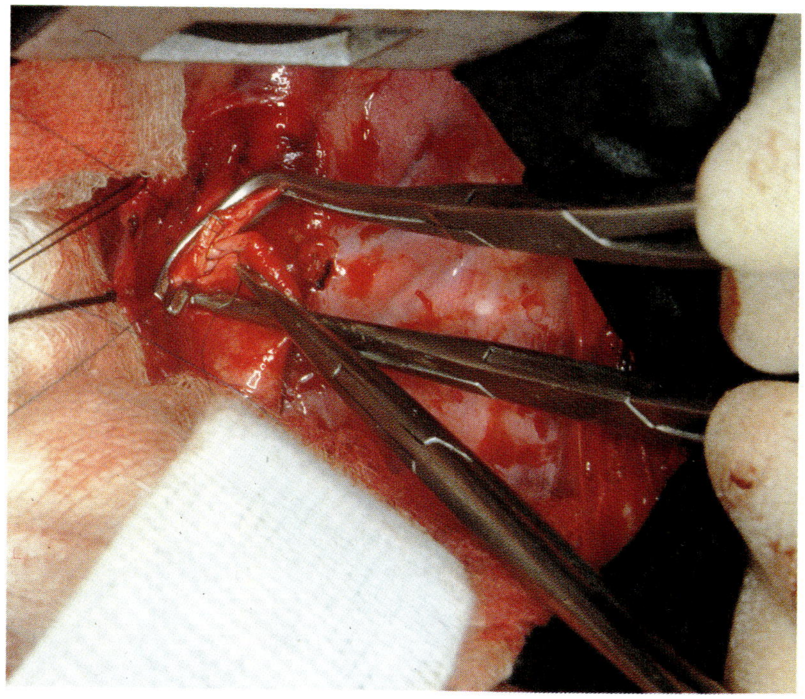

12 The upper clamp has been applied also across the base of the left subclavian artery and it is therefore possible to extend the upper arteriotomy with a pair of scissors so that the anastomosis can be as wide as possible.

13 The posterior part of the anastomosis is performed with continuous Prolene.

14

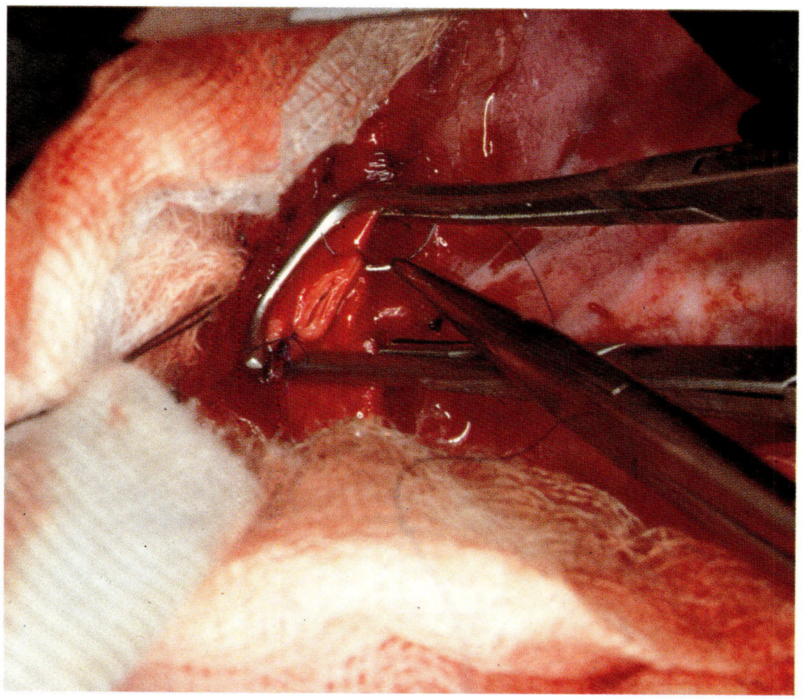

15

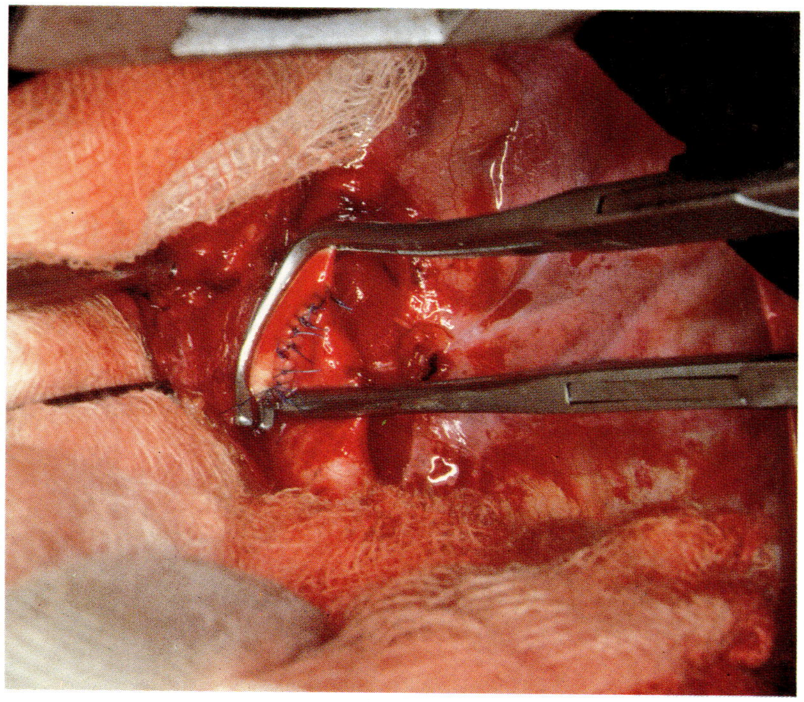

14 and 15 The anterior suture line is completed with interrupted sutures to allow for growth.

16

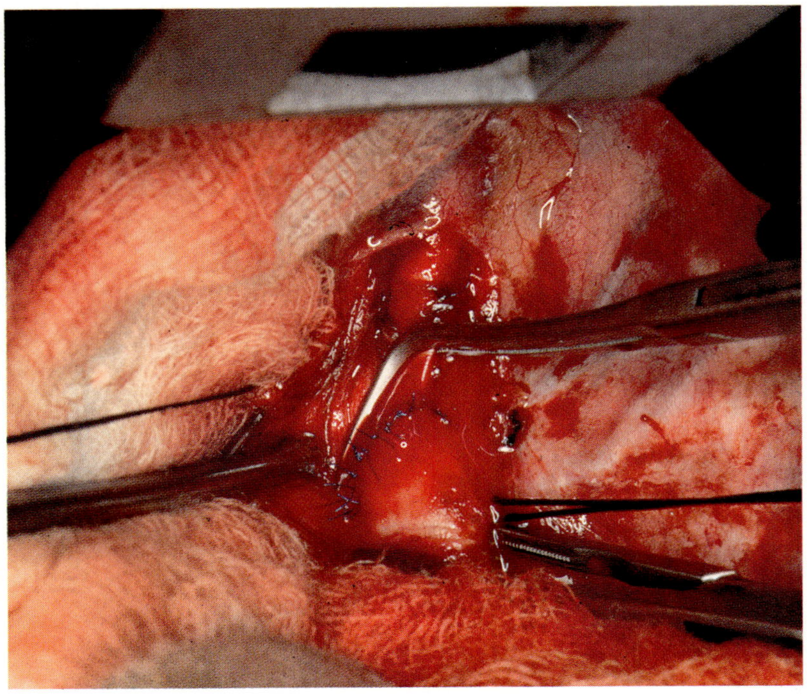

16 When the anastomosis is complete, the lower clamp is released first and any air escapes from the suture holes followed by some inevitable bleeding.

17

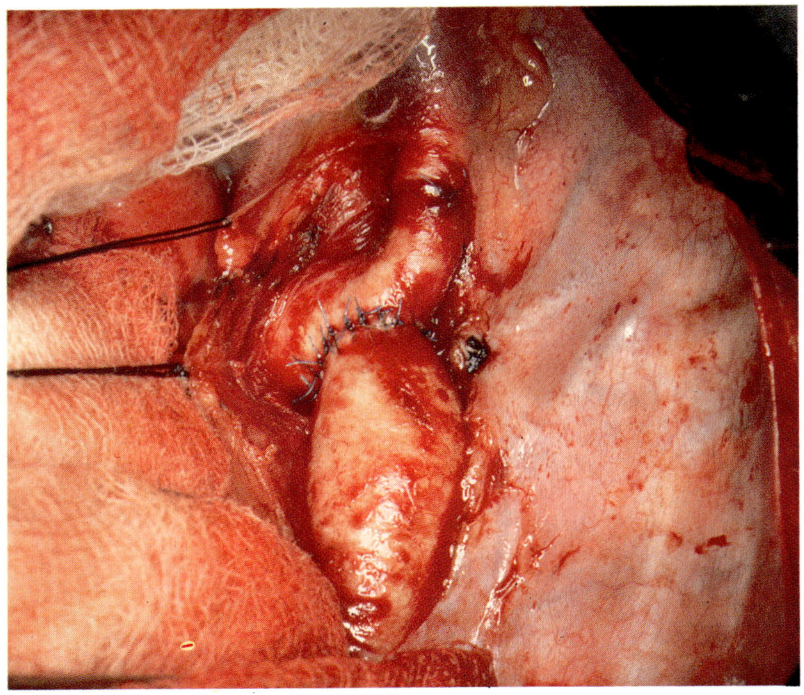

17 When the upper clamp is released, blood can flow through the now wide lumen of the aorta and, with pressure from a swab, the bleeding soon stops.

18

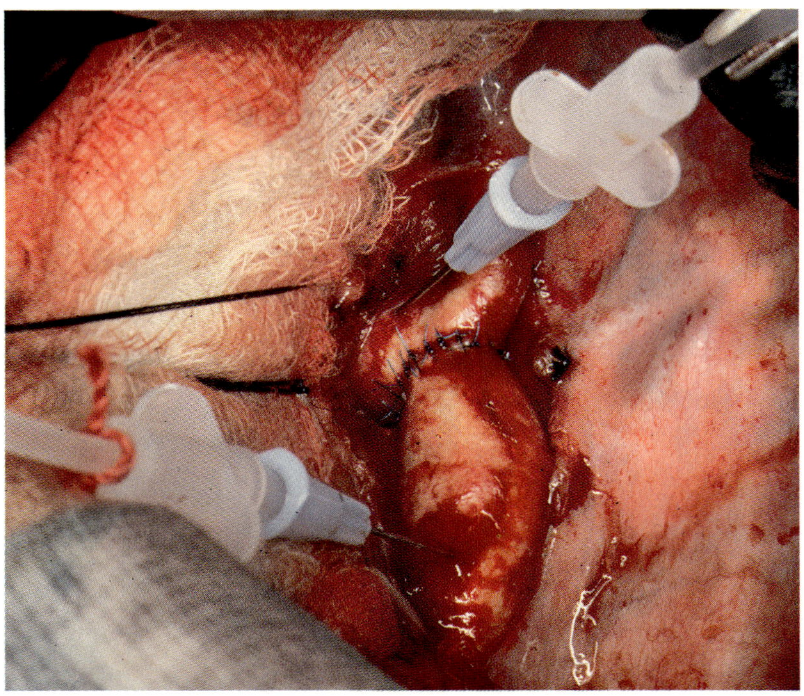

18 Simultaneous pressure measurements are made above and below the anastomosis to confirm complete relief of the stenosis.

19

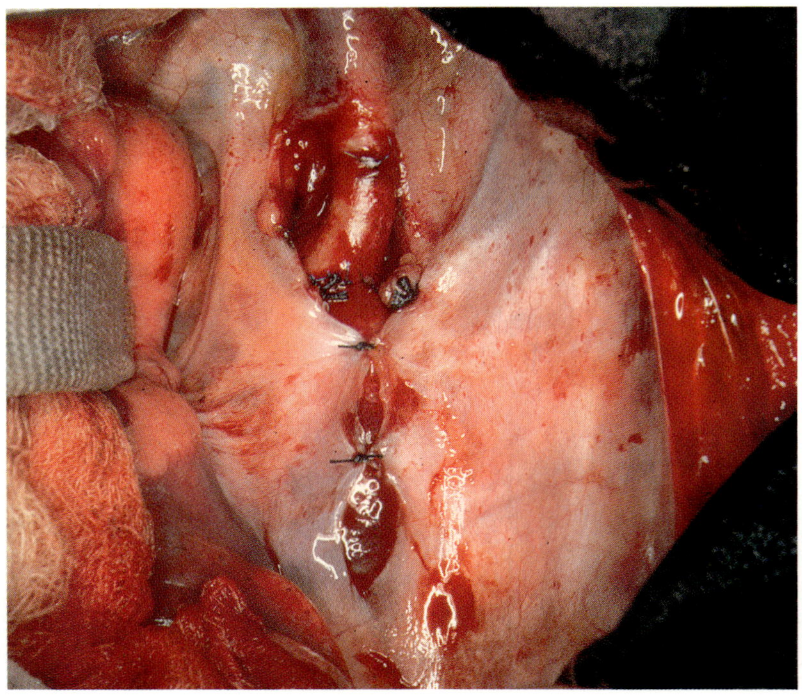

19 The pleura can be loosely closed over the aorta, but care must be taken not to constrict the anastomosis.

Patch insertion

20

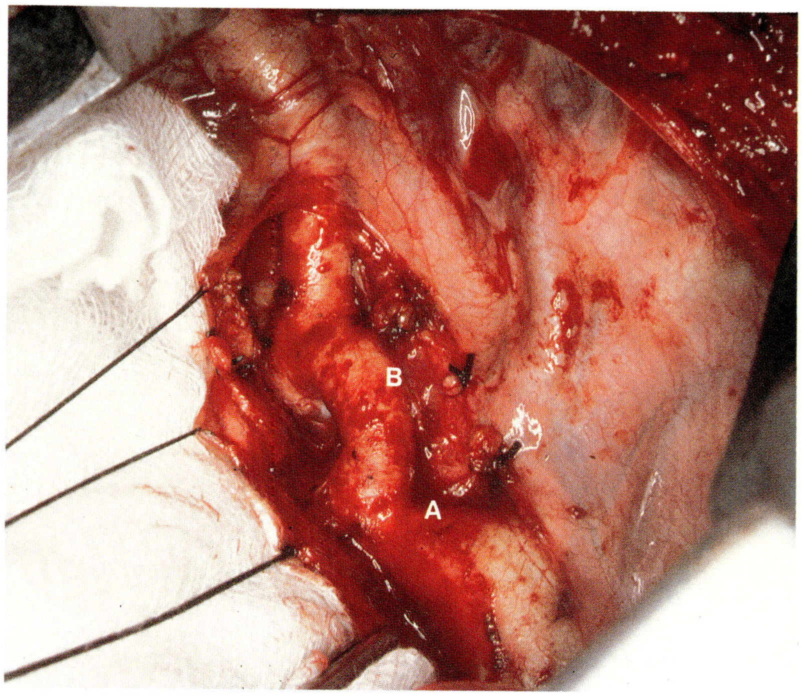

20 In this patient the coarctation (**A**) is distal to a narrow aortic isthmus (**B**) and end-to-end anastomosis would be difficult.

21

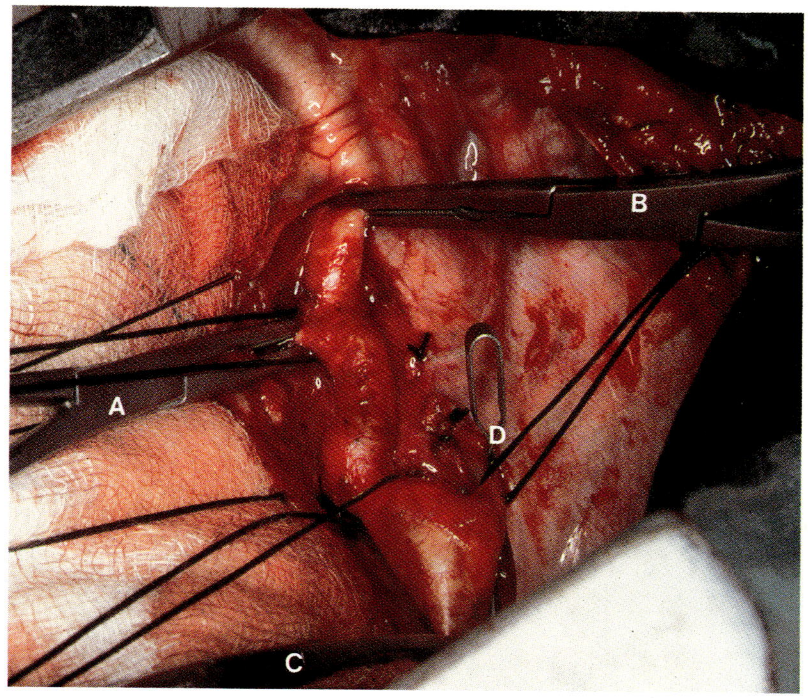

21 Clamps have been applied to the aortic arch (**A**), left subclavian artery (**B**) and descending aorta distal to the coarctation (**C**). In addition, a large intercostal artery has been temporarily occluded with a bulldog-clamp (**D**).

22

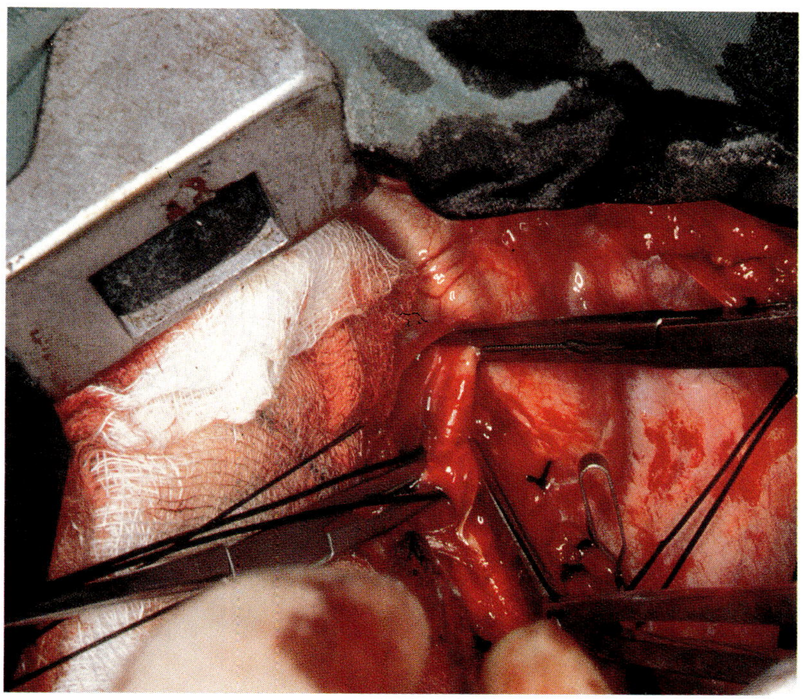

23

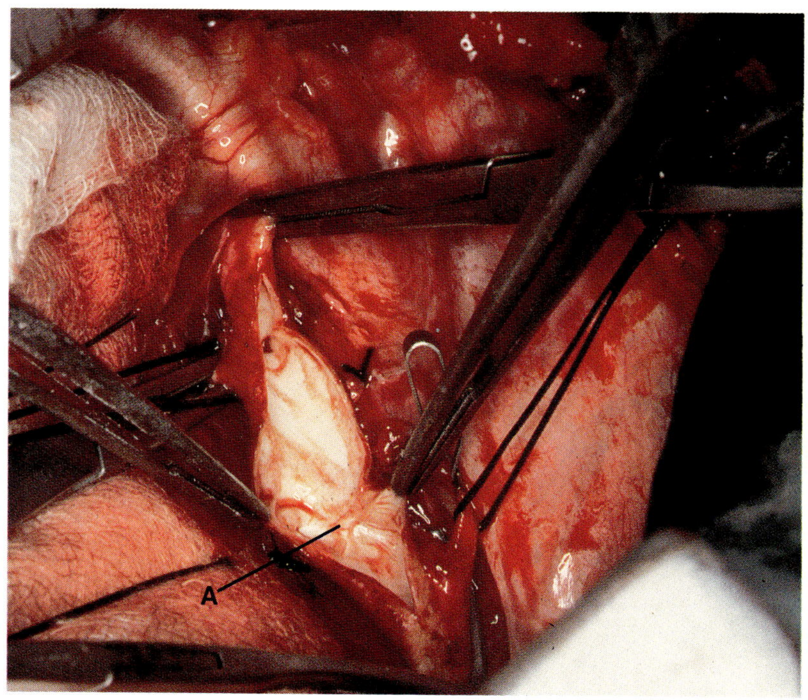

22 and 23 The aorta is incised longitudinally and the site of the coarctation is seen clearly (**A**).

24

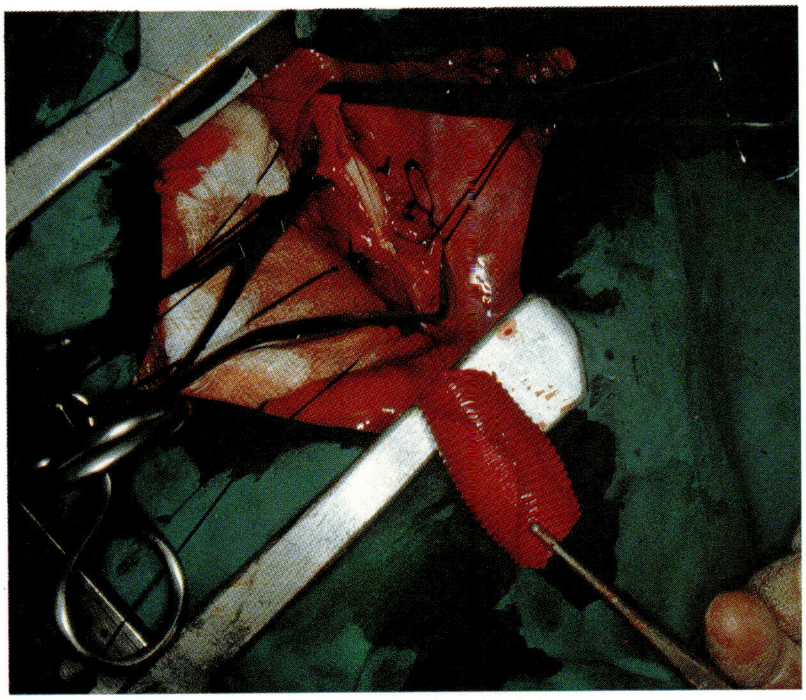

25

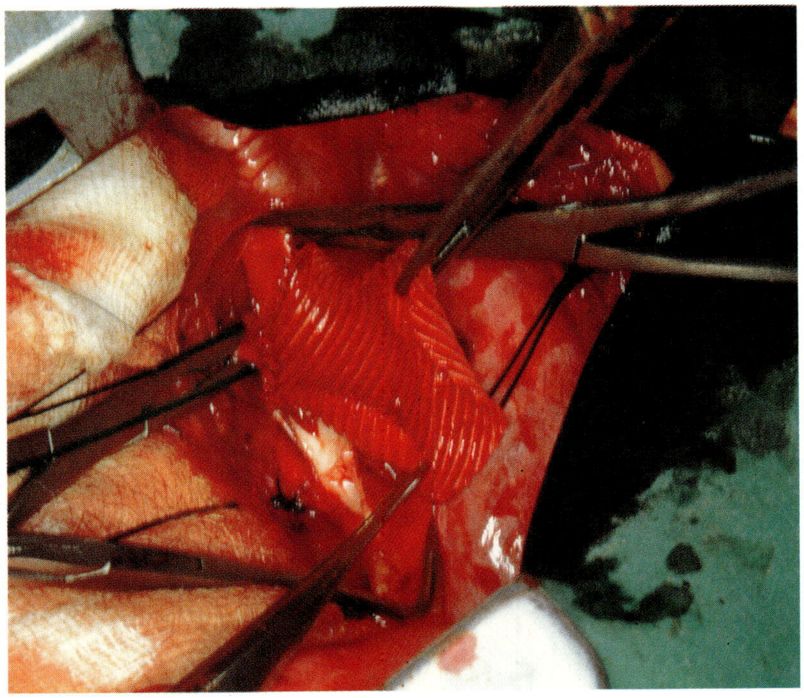

24 to 27 A diamond-shaped piece of preclotted woven dacron cut from a tube graft is then sutured in with continuous Prolene. It is helpful to place the graft inside out so that the edges are easier to pick up for placing the sutures.

26

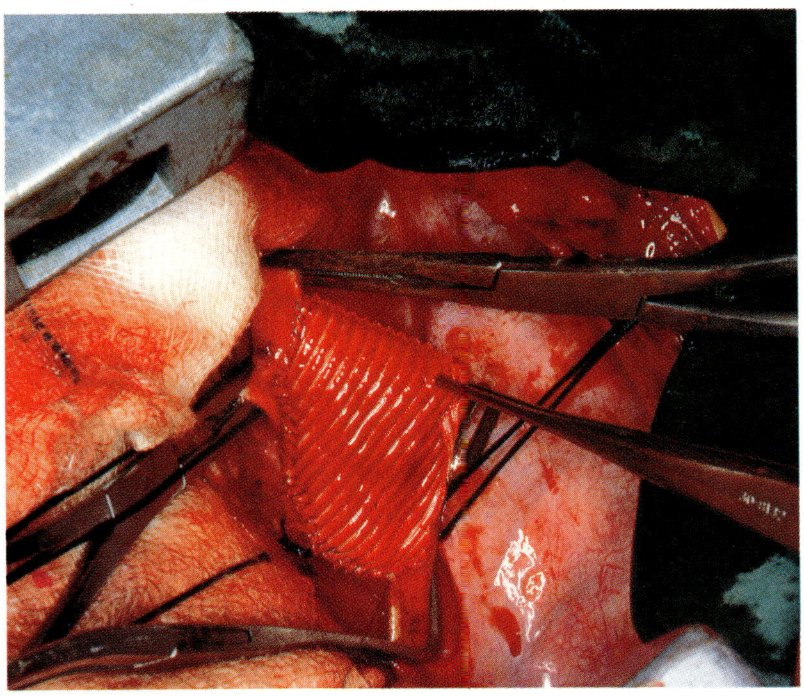

27

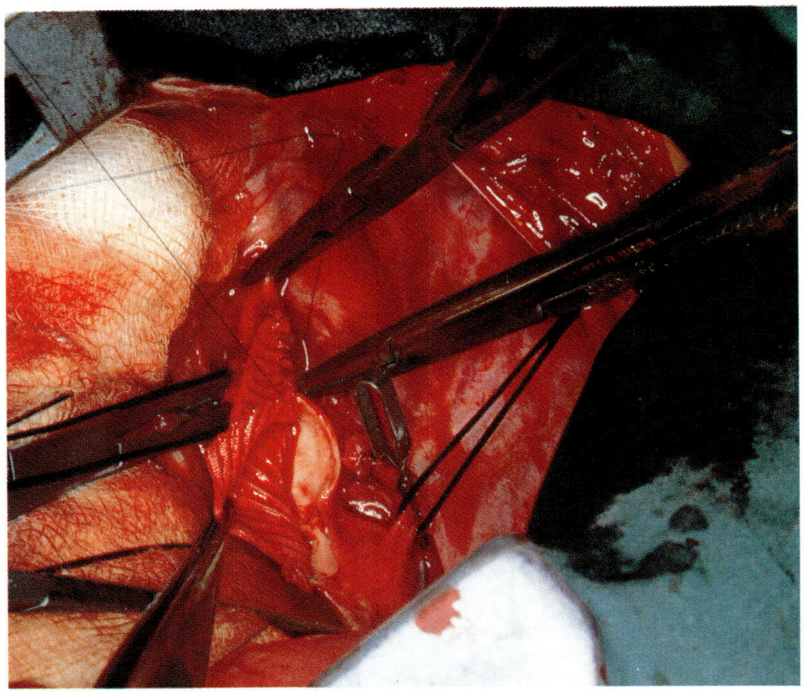

28

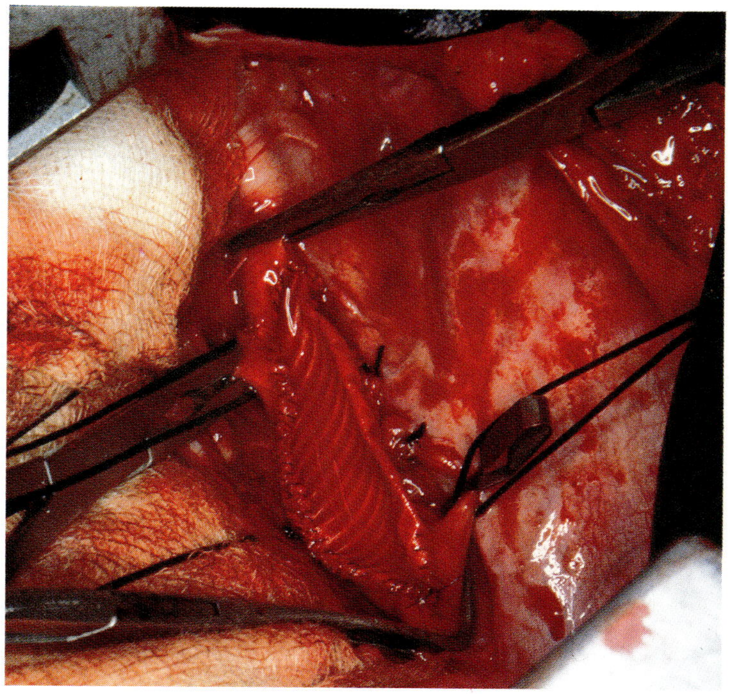

28 The suturing is complete and the clamps can be removed.

29

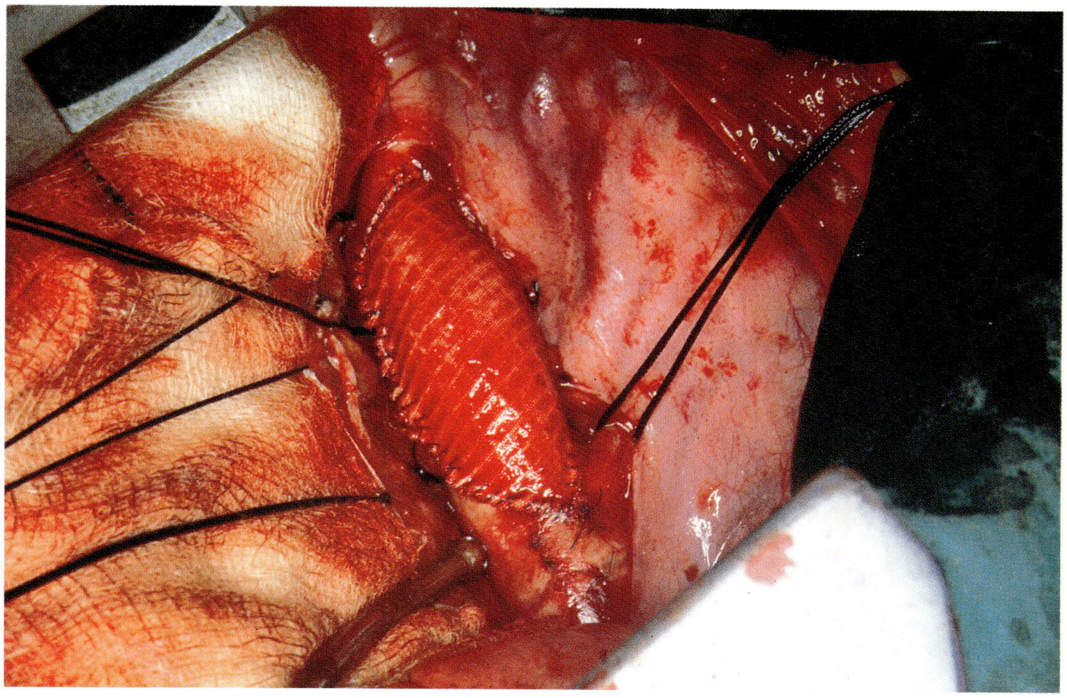

29 When the clamps are removed and the graft filled out by the aortic pressure, it can be seen that the stenosis caused by the coarctation has been satisfactorily relieved.

Insertion of dacron tube graft in parallel

30

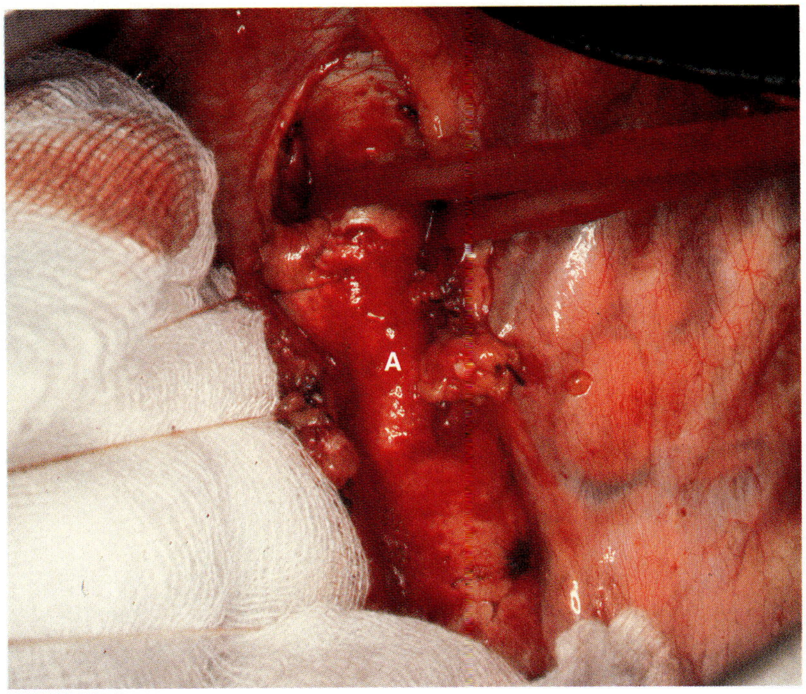

30 This patient with coarctation was thought to have a poor collateral supply to the descending thoracic aorta and therefore, rather than use cardiopulmonary bypass, the simpler insertion of a graft in parallel was used. The long, narrow segment of aorta can be seen (**A**).

31

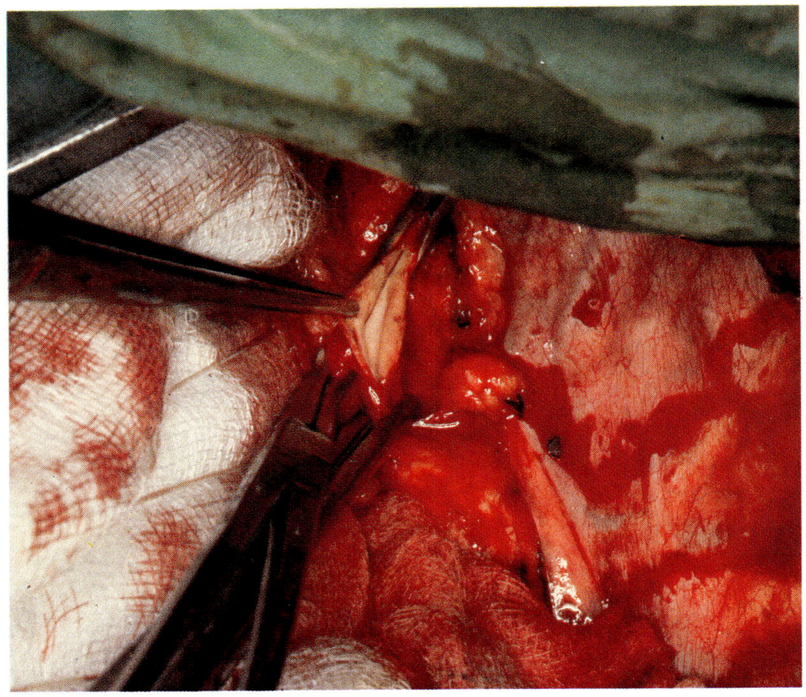

31 A side-clamp is placed on the left subclavian artery and an arteriotomy made.

32

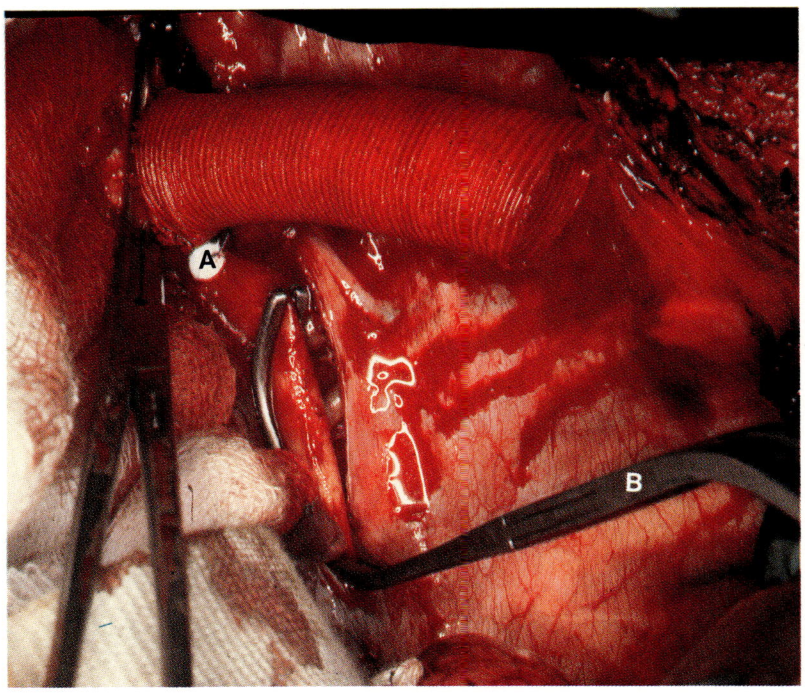

32 The upper anastomosis is performed with continuous Prolene which has been tied over a teflon felt pledget (**A**). A side-clamp (**B**) has been applied to the aorta below the coarctation but blood can still pass through the coarctation and past the side-clamp.

33

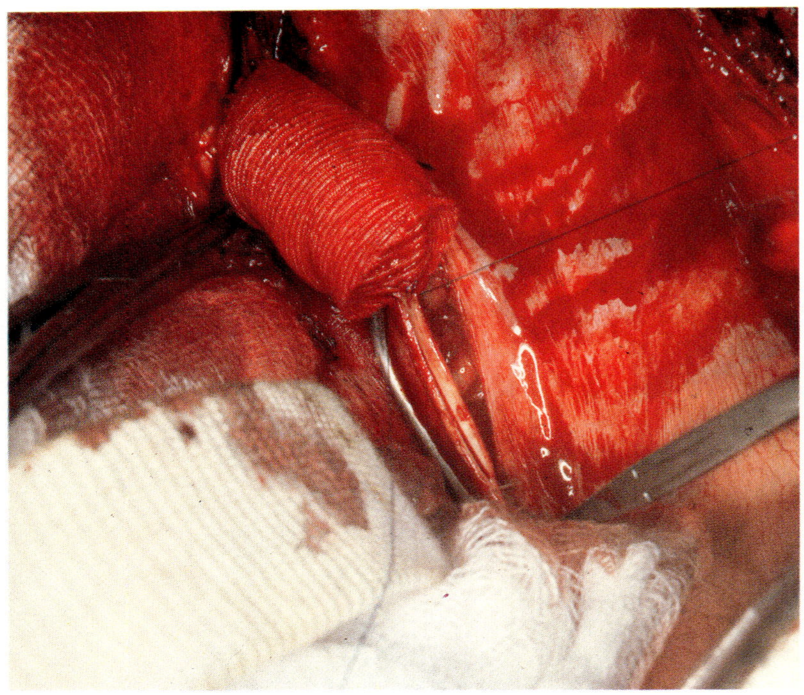

33 The lower end of the dacron tube is now sutured to the arteriotomy in the descending thoracic aorta.

34

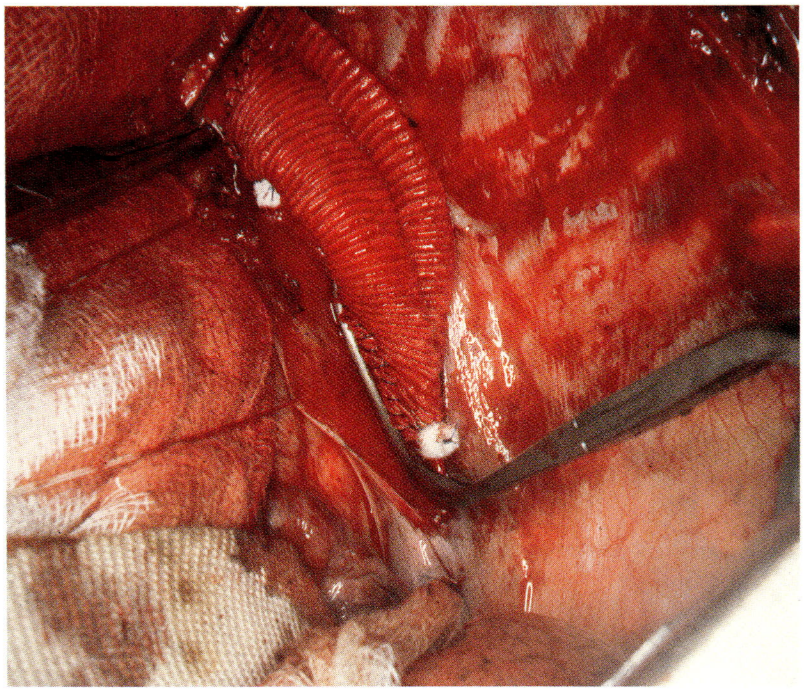

34 The lower anastomosis is complete and ready for removal of the clamps.

35

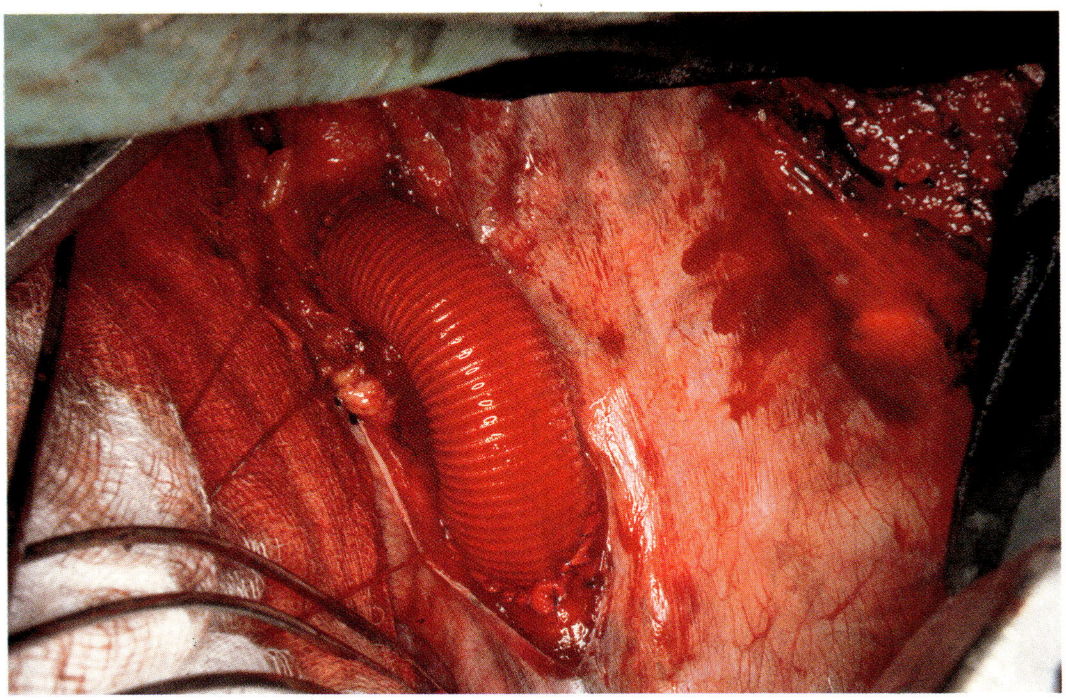

35 With the clamps removed, the tube fills out and it can now be seen that there is a very adequate way for blood to reach the descending aorta.

Subclavian flap

36

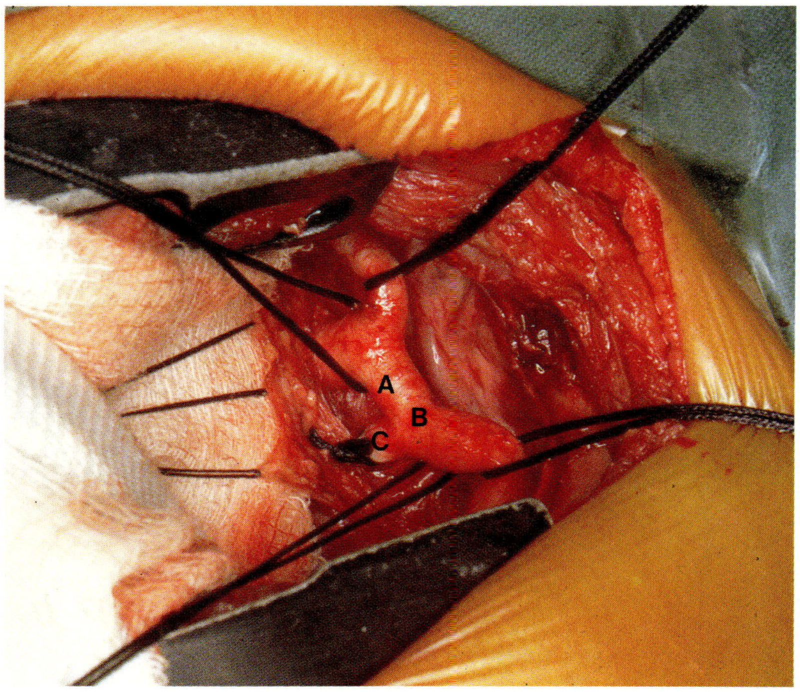

37

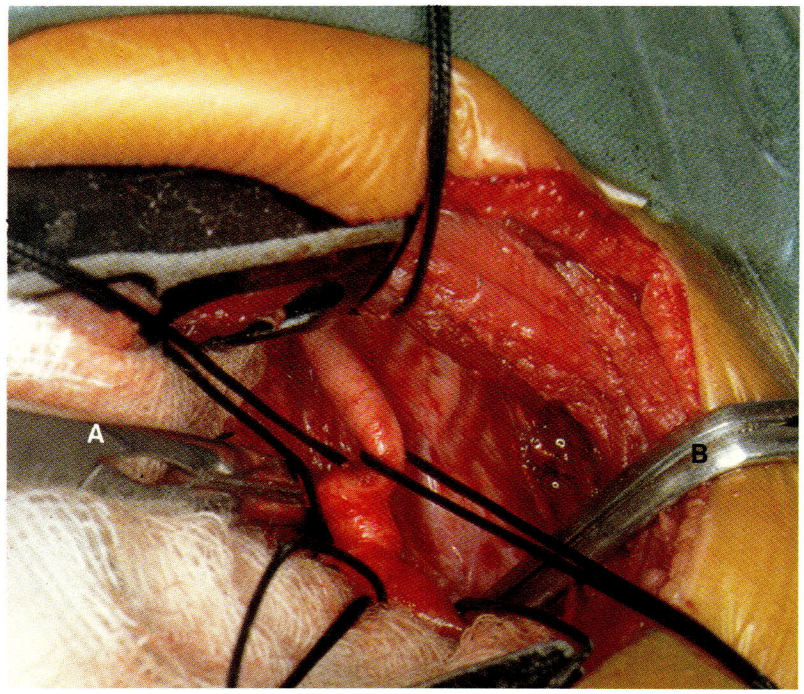

36 In this small infant there is a long, narrow aortic isthmus (**A**) and the main coarctation (**B**) is opposite the ductus arteriosus (**C**) which has been ligated.

37 Clamps have been placed across the aortic arch proximal to the subclavian artery (**A**) and across the descending aorta, well below the coarctation (**B**). The subclavian artery is being pulled down before dividing it.

38

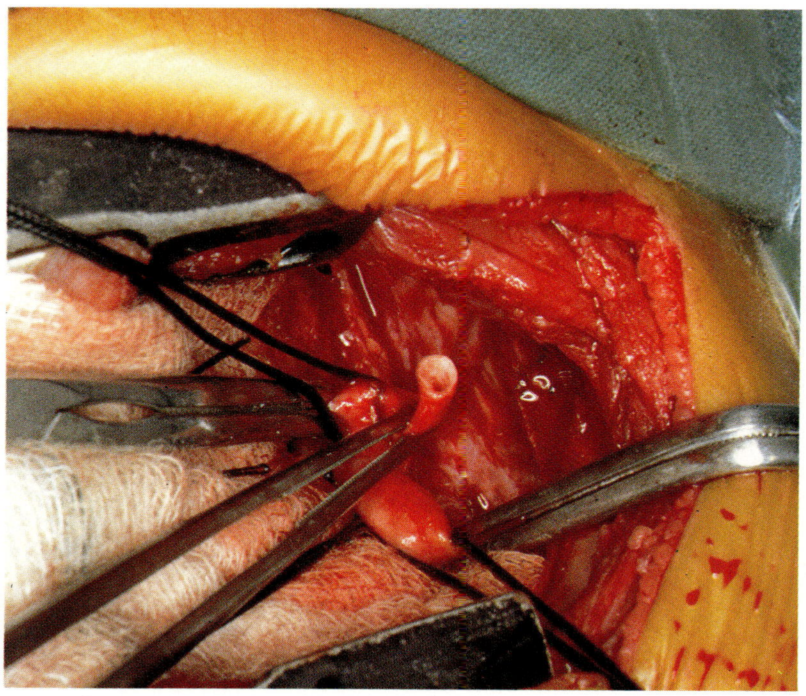

39

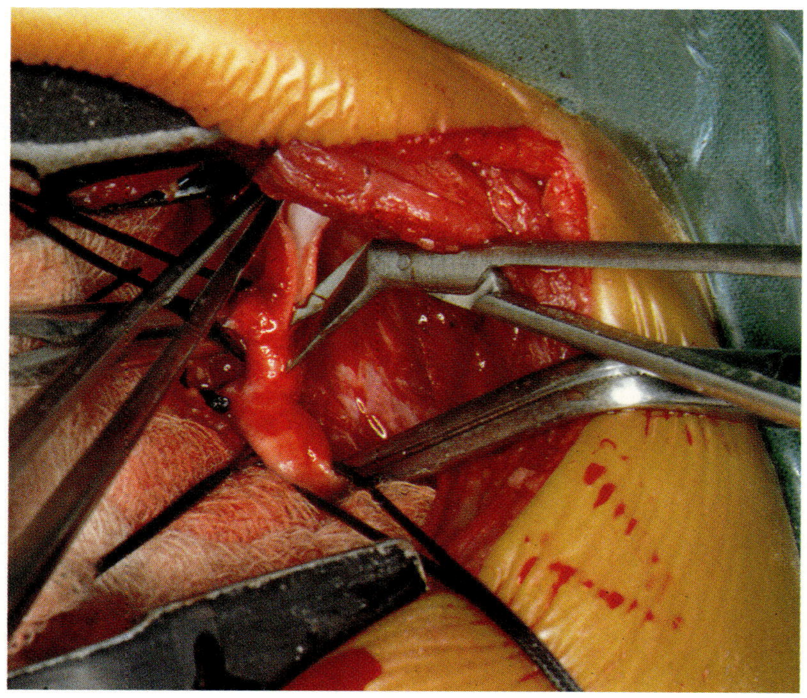

38 and 39 The subclavian artery has been divided and is incised downwards.

40

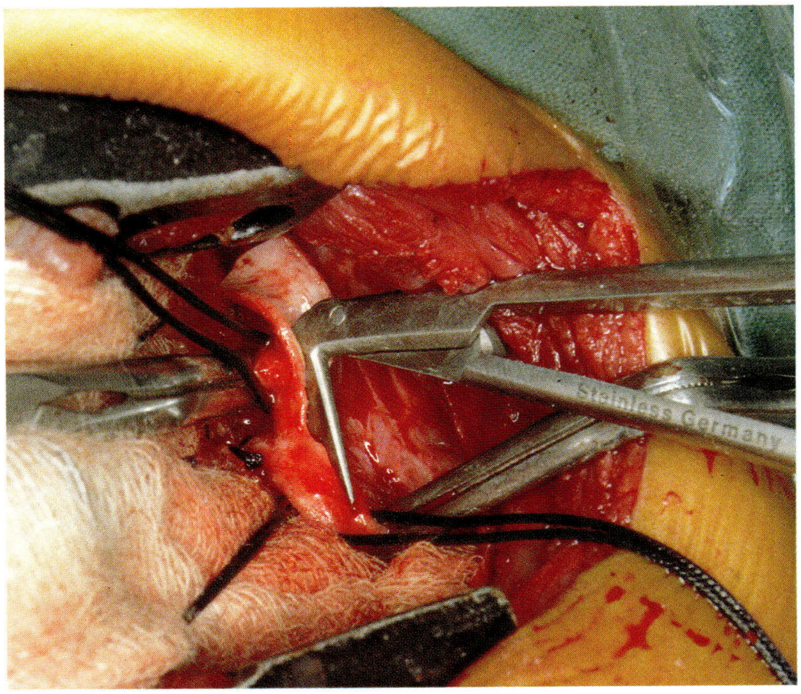

41

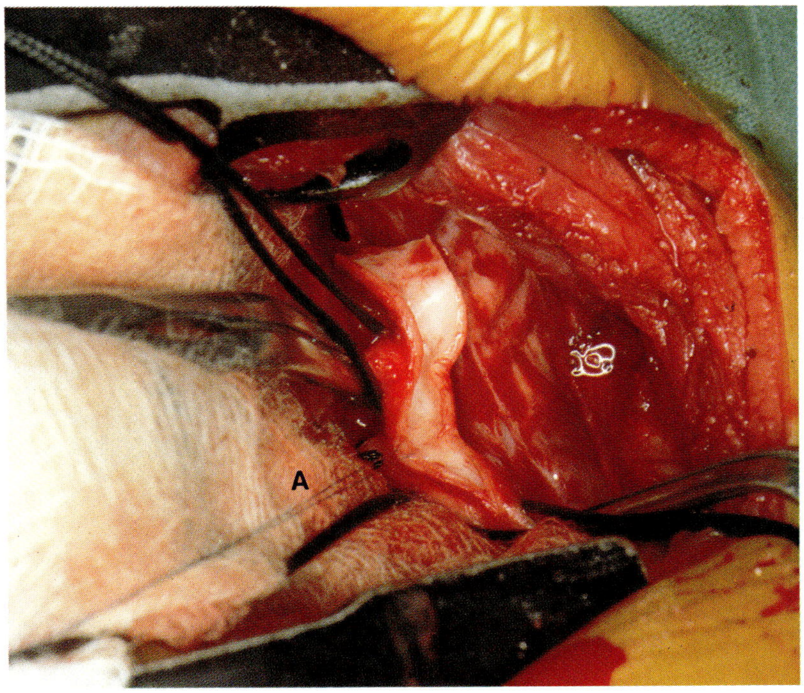

40 and 41 The incision is continued down into the aorta and past the site of the coarctation, which is being retracted with a fine suture (**A**). Any ridge of coarctation that remains posteriorly can be excised.

42

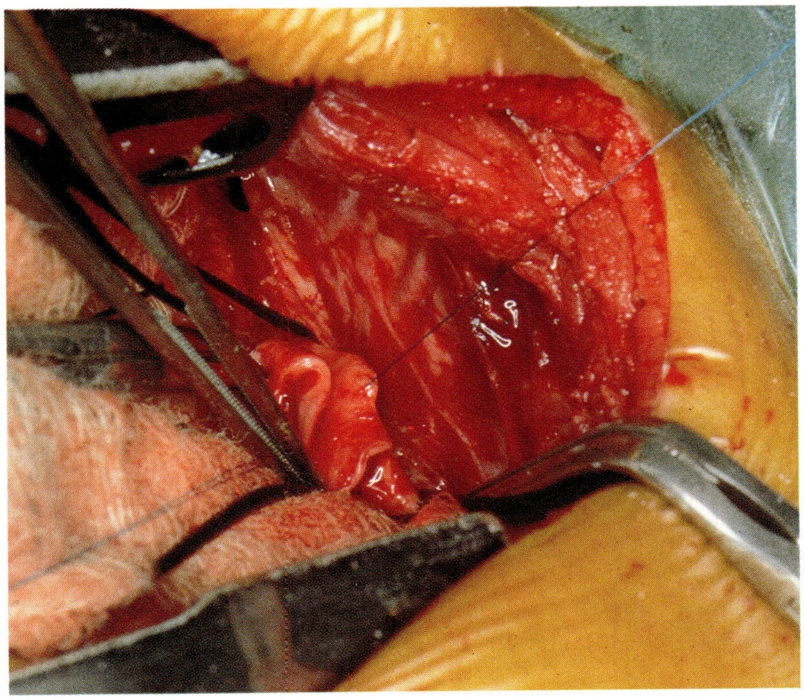

43

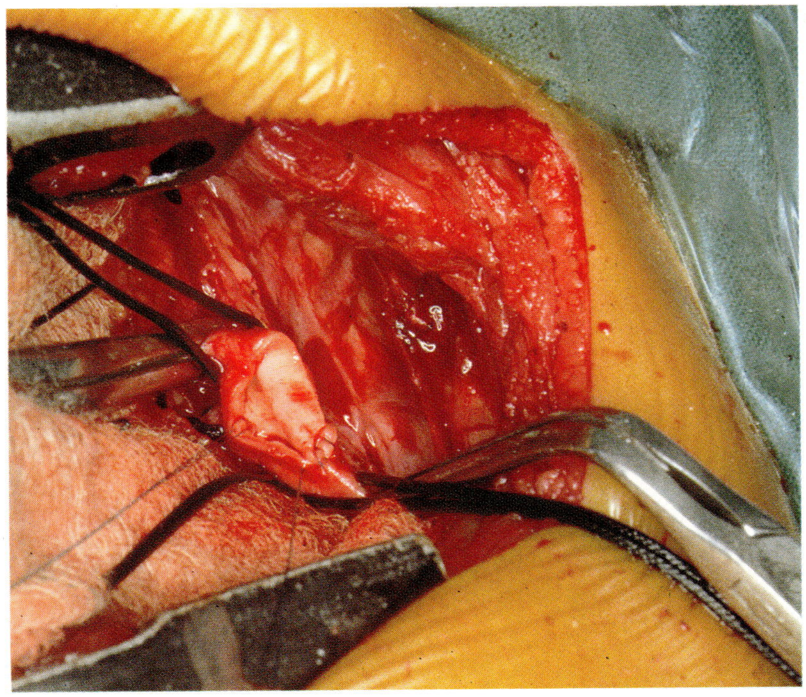

42 and 43 A continuous, fine Prolene suture is started superiorly and taken down the lateral side of the flap.

44

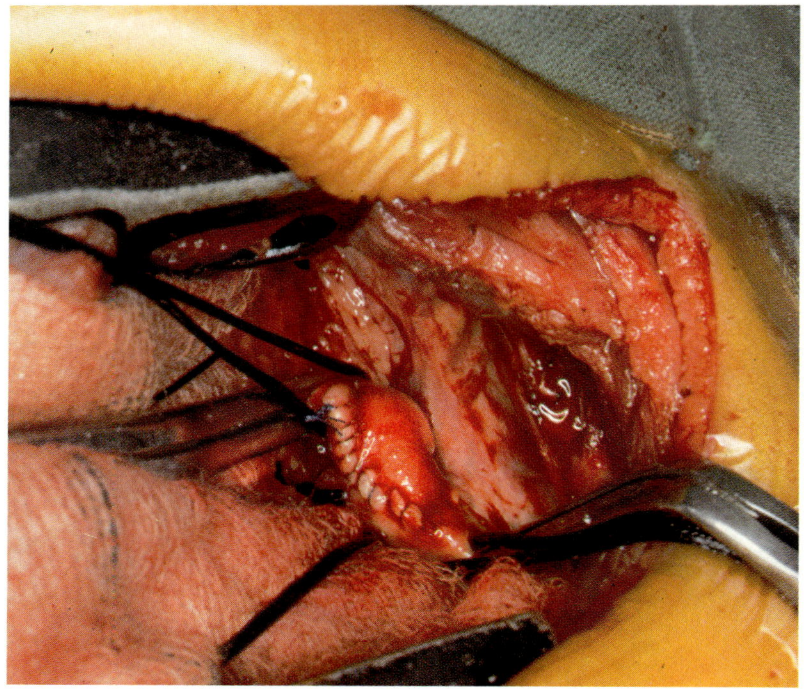

44 The suture is continued up the medial side, taking care not to pull too tight and narrow the anastomosis.

45

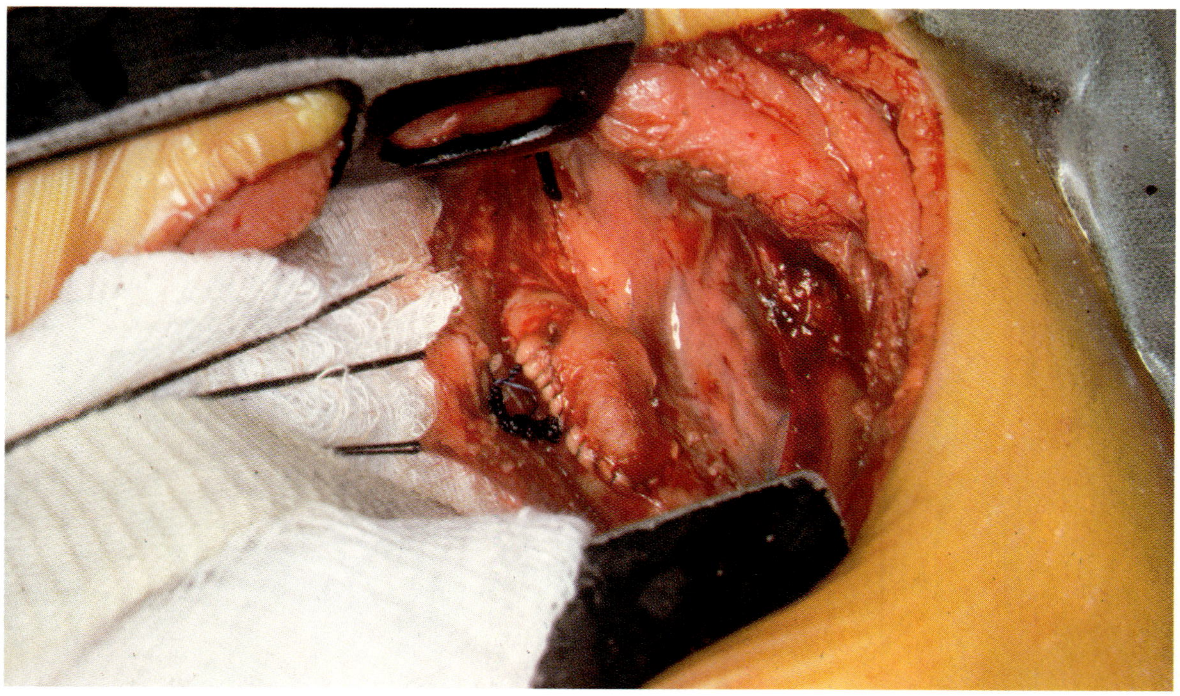

45 The clamps are removed and a wide lumen is produced and, furthermore, the flap can grow as well as the back wall of the aorta, thus reducing the chance of restenosis.

6: The Blalock-Taussig shunt

In 1945 Blalock and Taussig[1] reported the first successful shunt procedure for cyanotic heart disease. The subclavian artery was divided and turned down to be anastomosed to the right pulmonary artery (see diagram **A**). The same operation is used today for palliation of certain conditions that are unsuitable for correction. The size of the subclavian artery limits the flow of blood to the lungs so that they do not become flooded, and, as the subclavian artery grows with the patient, the amount of blood going to the lungs increases.

To avoid sacrificing the subclavian artery, a 'modified' Blalock-Taussig shunt may be performed with a synthetic tube graft such as Goretex (see diagram **B**). Again, as the graft is anastomosed to the subclavian artery, the size of the shunt is limited.

The approach is through a thoracotomy on the appropriate side (see Chapter 3). When the definitive procedure is performed, the Blalock-Taussig shunt must be closed, and better still divided as this will not tend to kink up the pulmonary artery as the child grows.

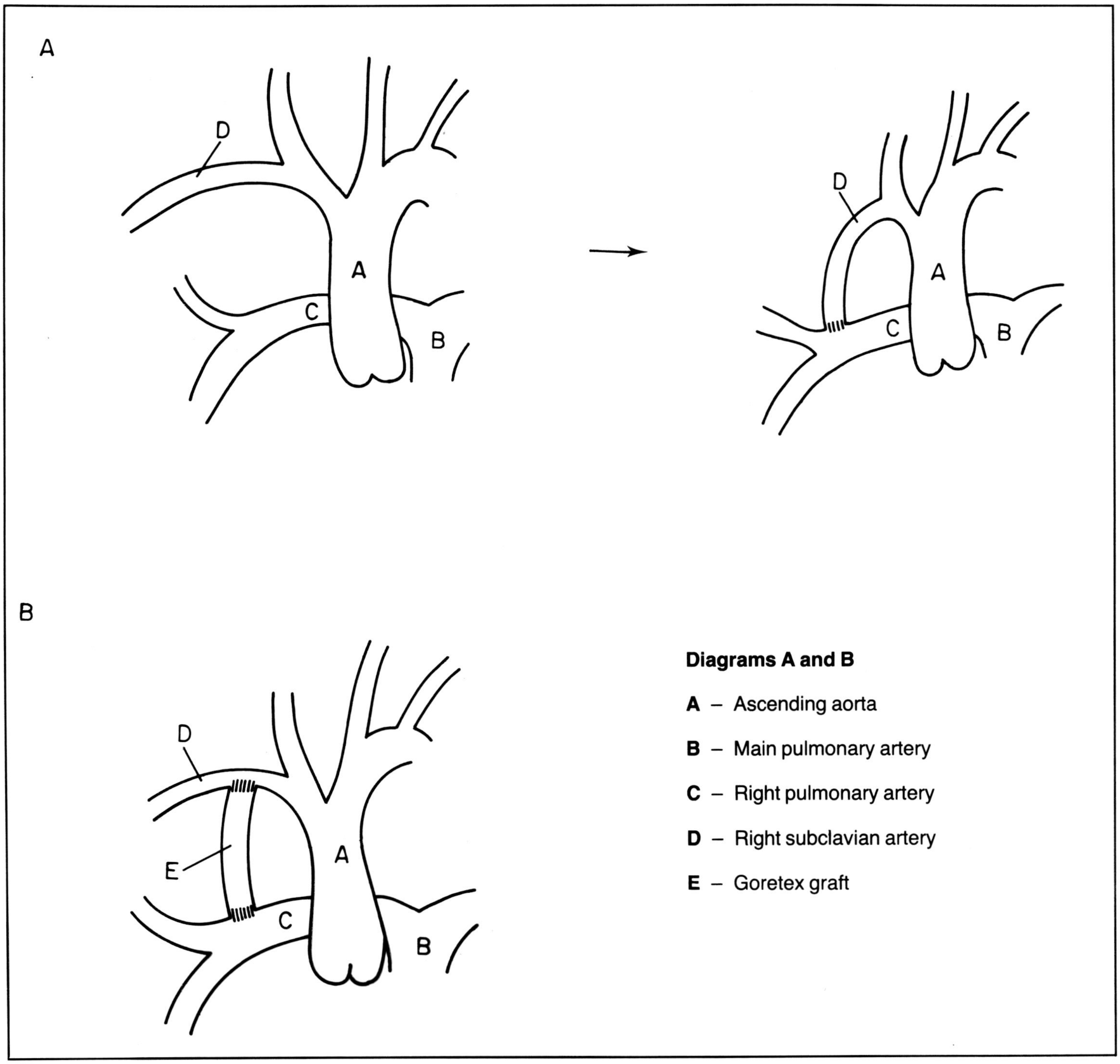

Diagrams A and B

A – Ascending aorta

B – Main pulmonary artery

C – Right pulmonary artery

D – Right subclavian artery

E – Goretex graft

1
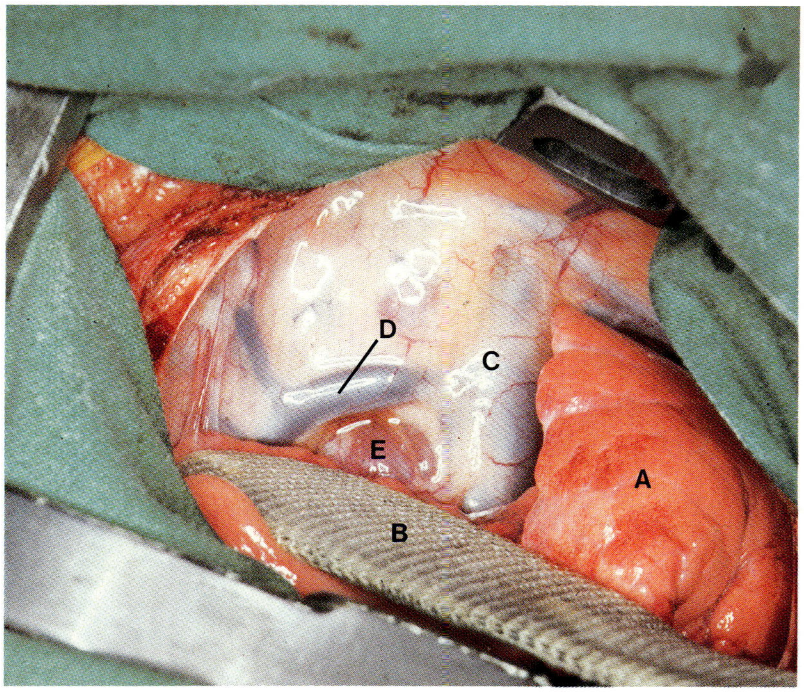

1 A right thoracotomy has been performed and the lung (**A**) retracted downwards with a malleable retractor (**B**). The superior vena cava (**C**), azygos vein (**D**) and right pulmonary artery (**E**) can be seen.

2
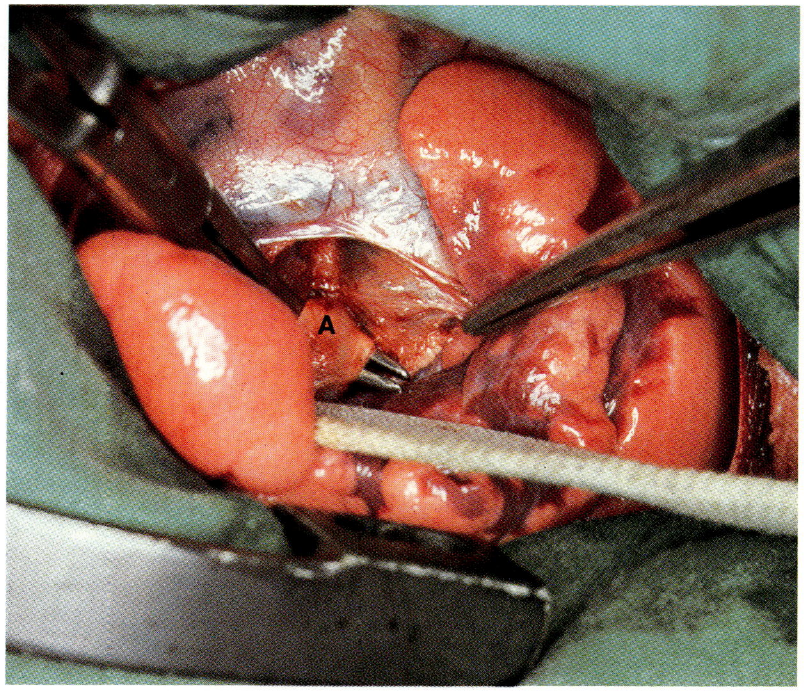

2 The right pulmonary artery (**A**) has been dissected out and an instrument is passed behind it in order to pass a heavy silk thread around it.

3
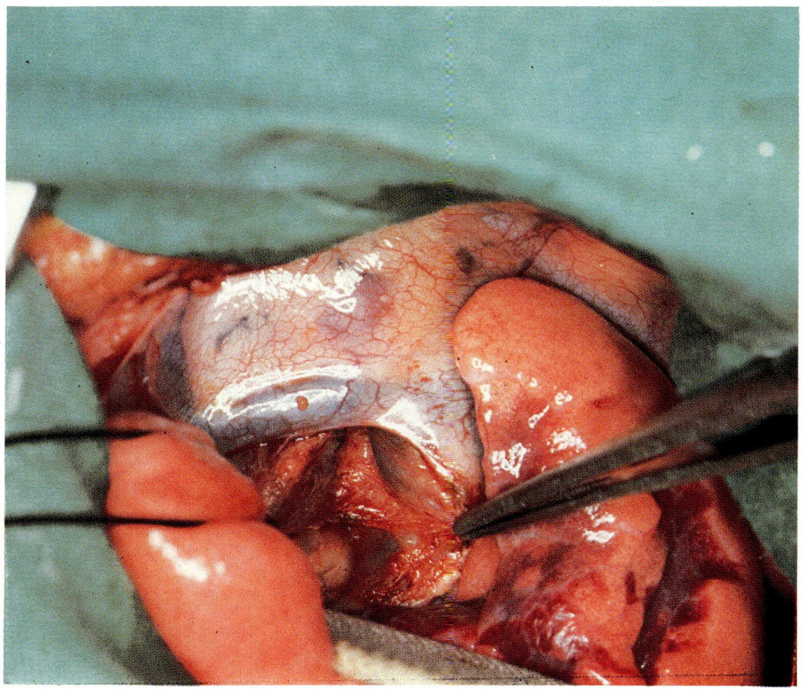

3 The silk thread passes around the right pulmonary artery which is now ready for the anastomosis.

4
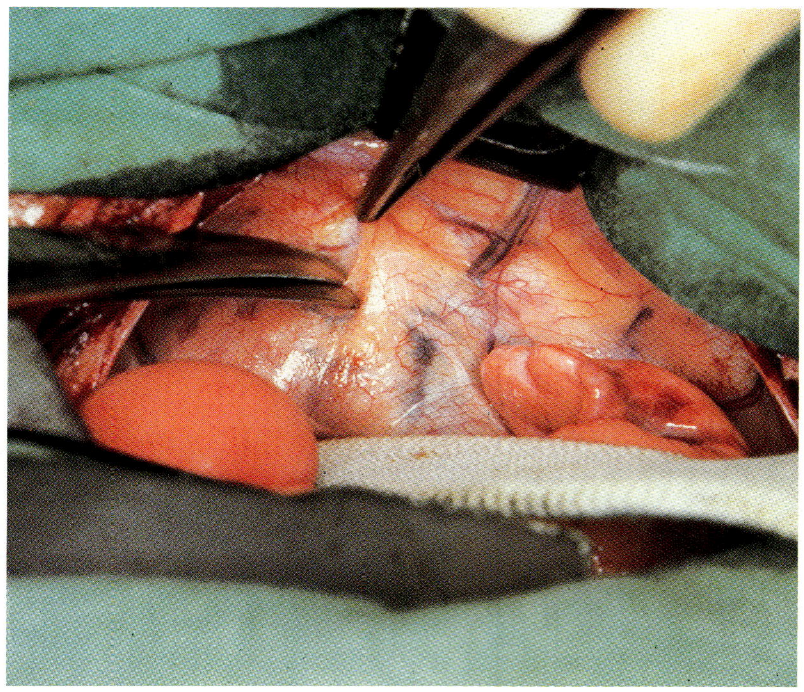

4 The pleura is incised over the right subclavian artery.

5

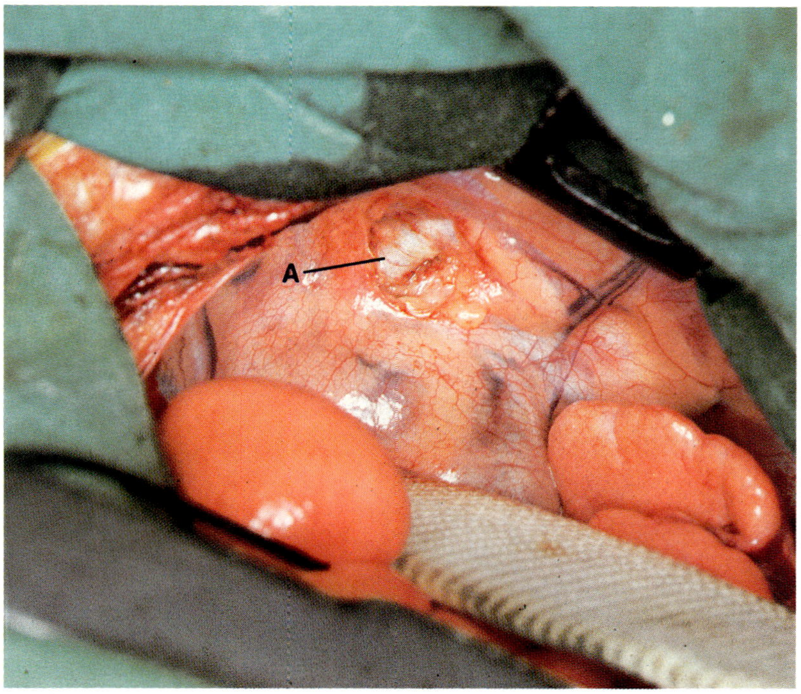

6

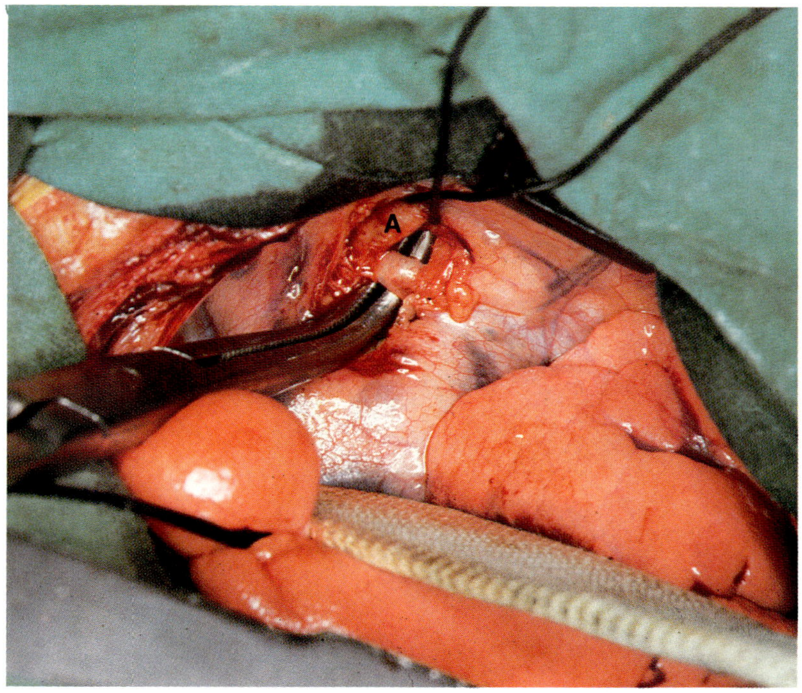

5 The pleura has been incised to reveal the subclavian artery (**A**).

6 A silk thread has been passed around the subclavian artery (**A**) to help dissection. The branches of the subclavian artery are dissected out and divided. Here an instrument passes behind the internal mammary artery before its division.

7

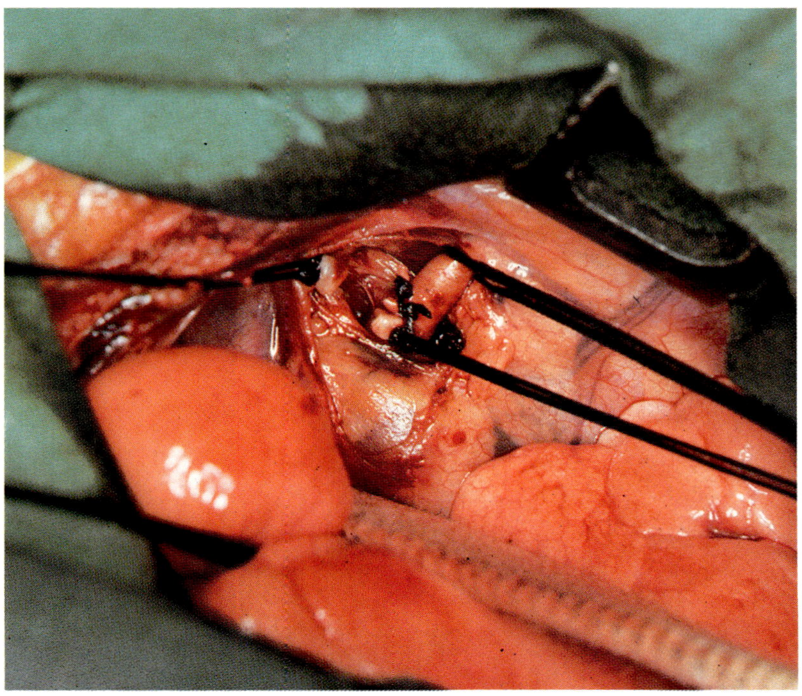

8

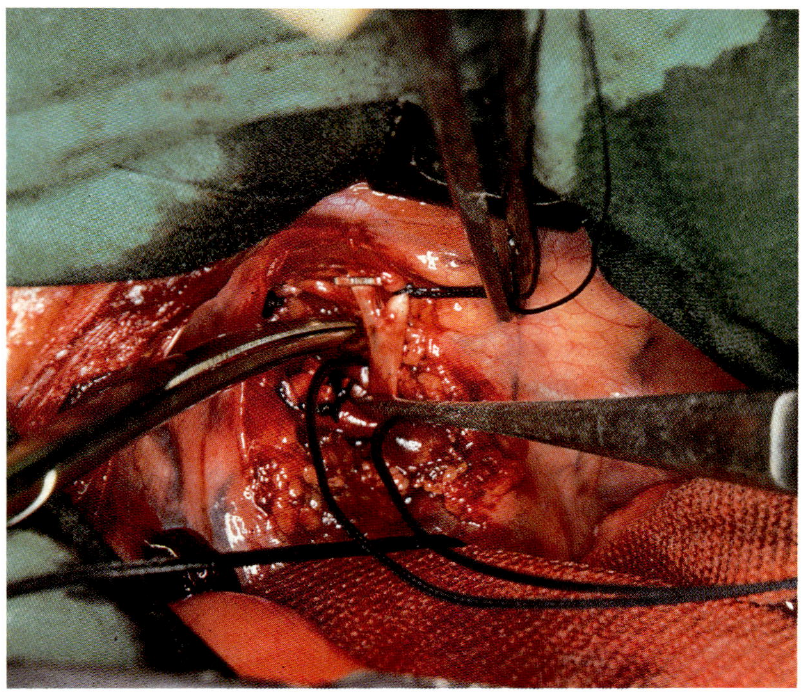

7 The branches have now been divided.

8 The subclavian artery and a further branch are tied and clipped before dividing the subclavian artery as far out as possible.

9
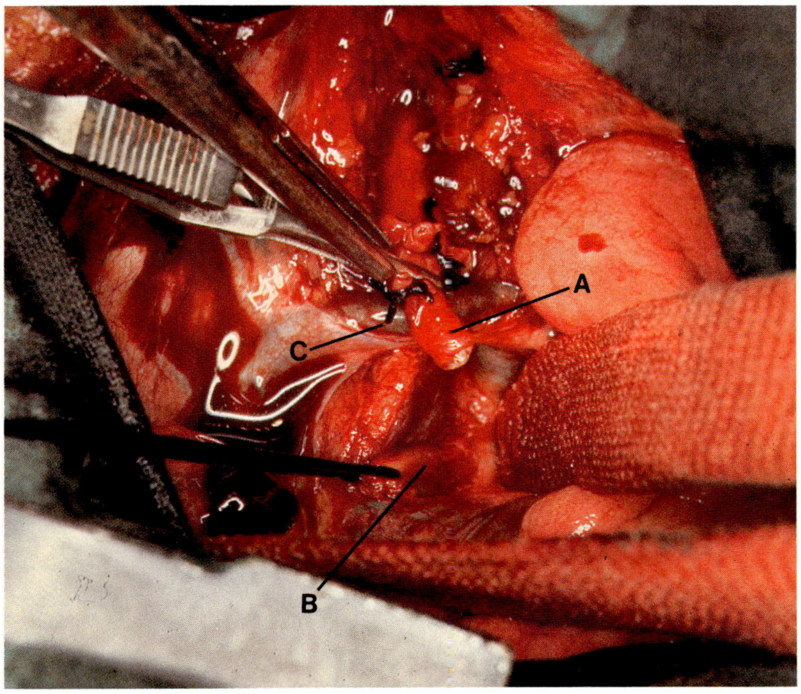

9 The divided subclavian artery (**A**) is turned down toward the pulmonary artery (**B**). As is often the case the azygos vein (**C**) is rather in the way and should be divided.

10
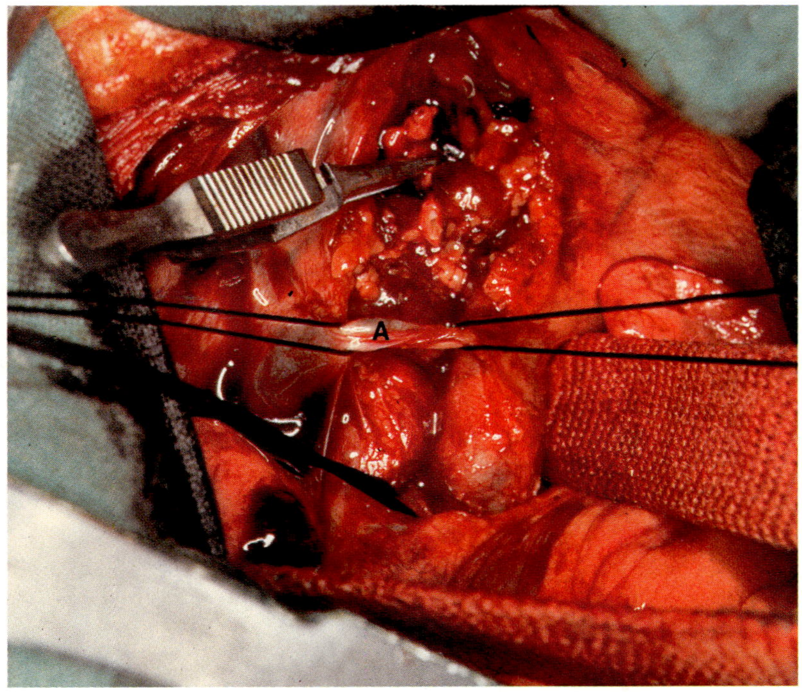

10 The azygos vein (**A**) has had two ligatures passed around it.

11
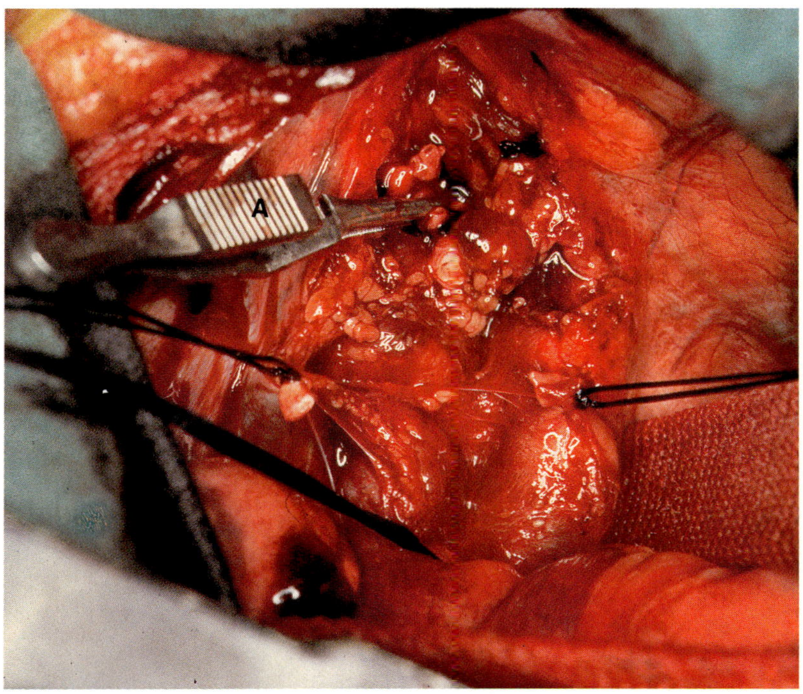

11 The azygos vein has been divided. The subclavian artery has meanwhile been occluded with a bulldog-clamp (**A**). It is advisable to partially heparinise the patient to avoid clot-formation in the subclavian artery.

12
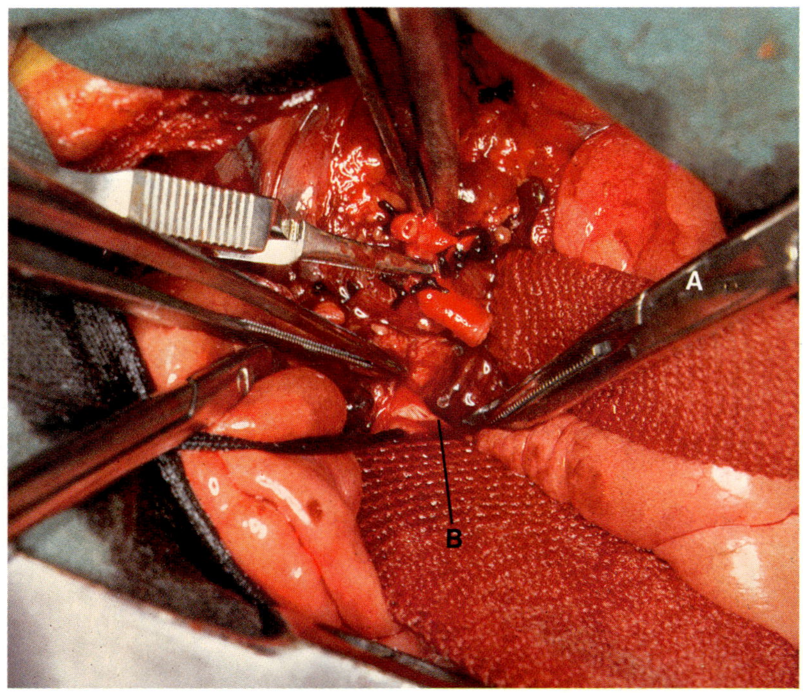

12 A side-clamp (**A**) has been applied to the pulmonary artery which has been incised longitudinally (**B**).

13

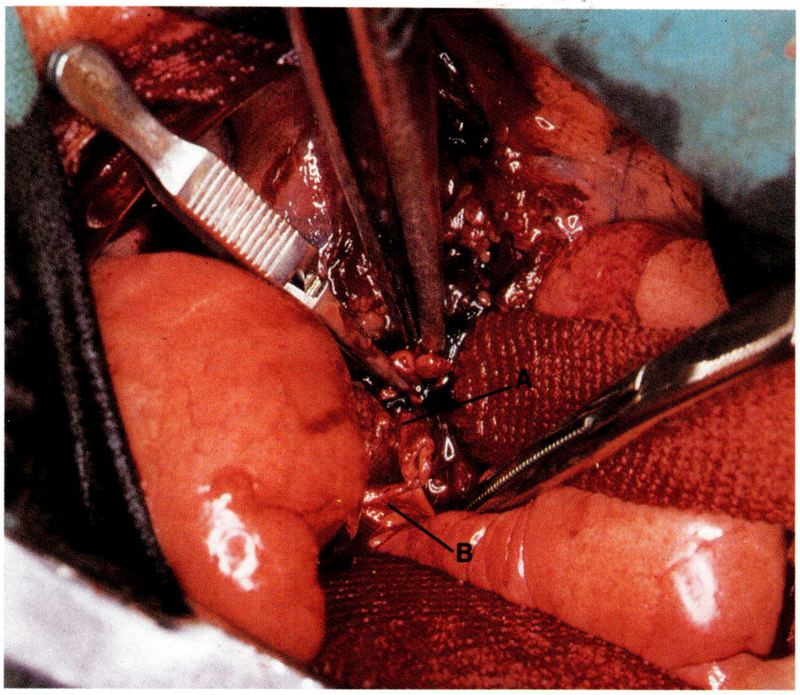

14

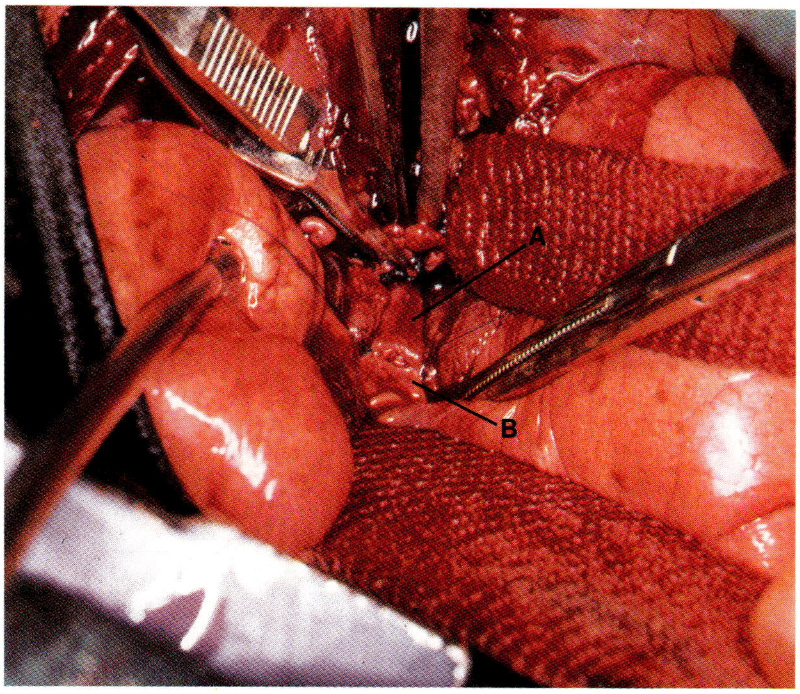

13 and 14 The distal end of the subclavian artery (**A**) is anastomosed to the pulmonary artery (**B**) using continuous Prolene posteriorly and interrupted sutures anteriorly to allow for some growth.

15

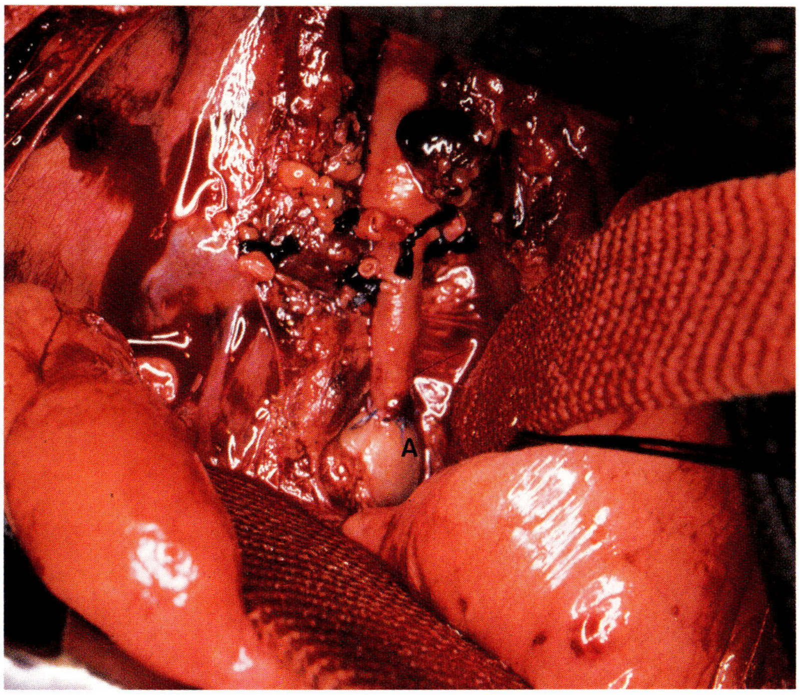

15 The anastomosis has been completed and the clamps released. The subclavian artery is seen to be well-filled (**A**).

Modified Blalock-Taussig shunt with Goretex graft

16

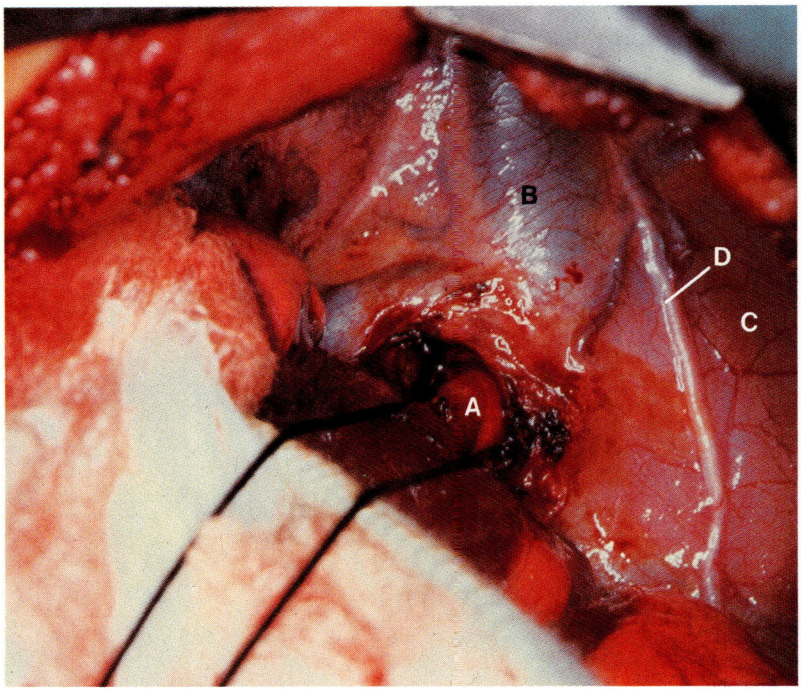

16 Through a right thoracotomy, the lung has been retracted and the right pulmonary artery (**A**) dissected out and silk thread passed around it. The superior vena cava (**B**), pericardium (**C**) and phrenic nerve (**D**) are seen clearly.

17

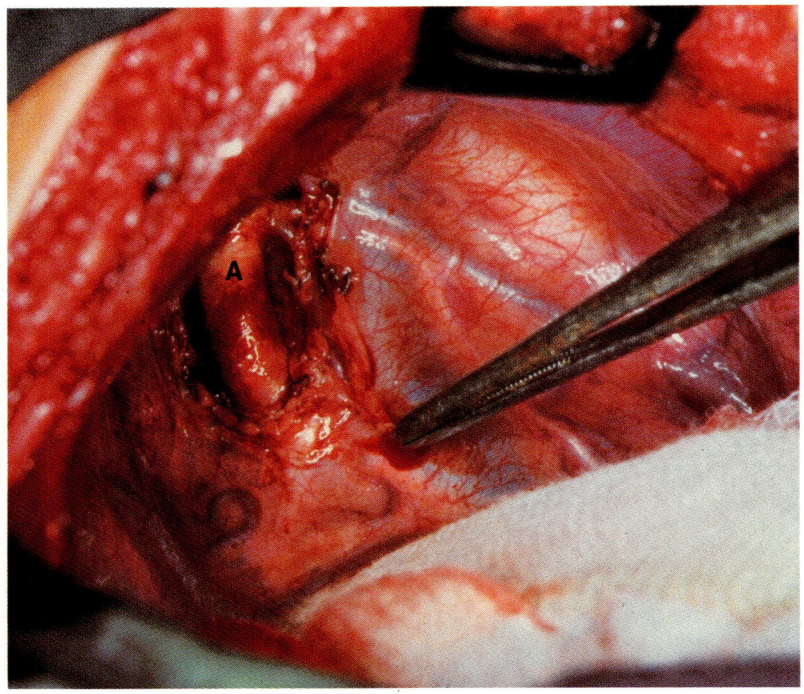

17 The pleura has been incised and the subclavian artery (**A**) dissected free.

18

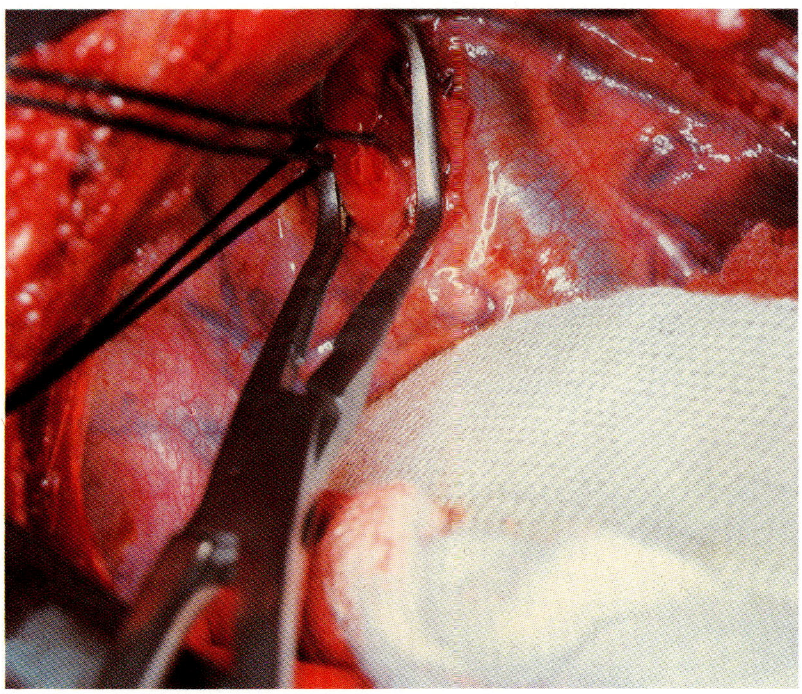

19

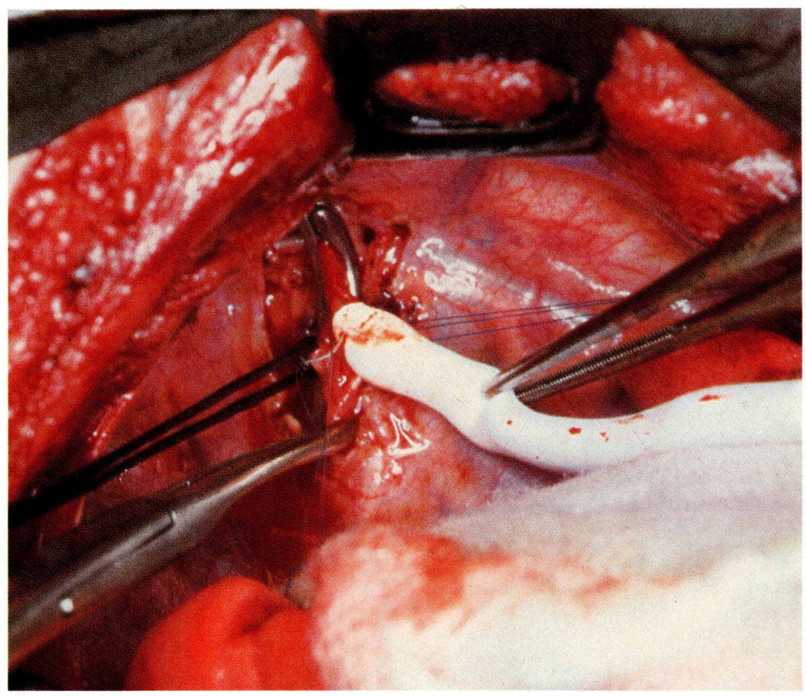

18 and 19 A side-clamp is placed on the subclavian artery and an end-to-side anastomosis performed using 6 mm diameter Goretex tube graft. Fine, continuous Prolene sutures are used.

20

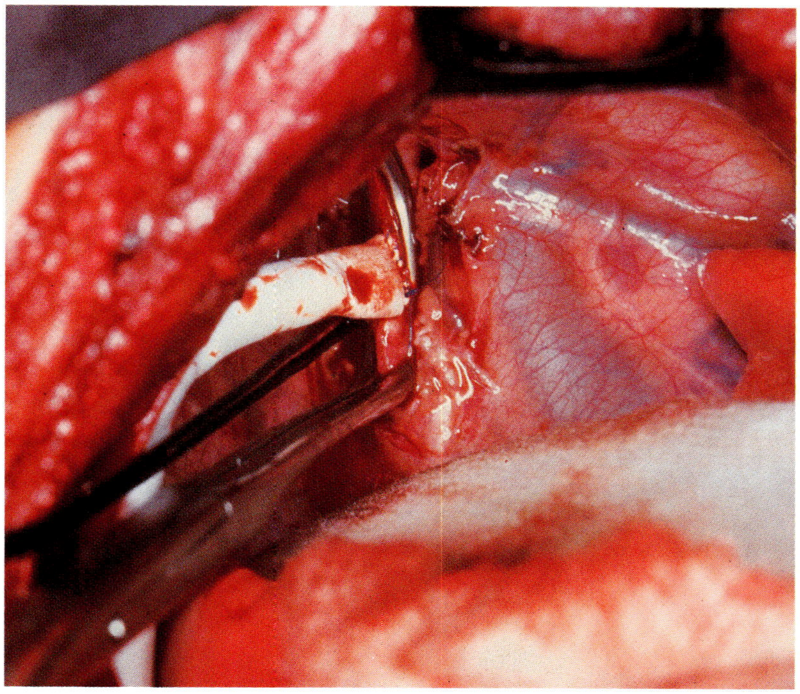

20 The upper anastomosis is now complete.

21

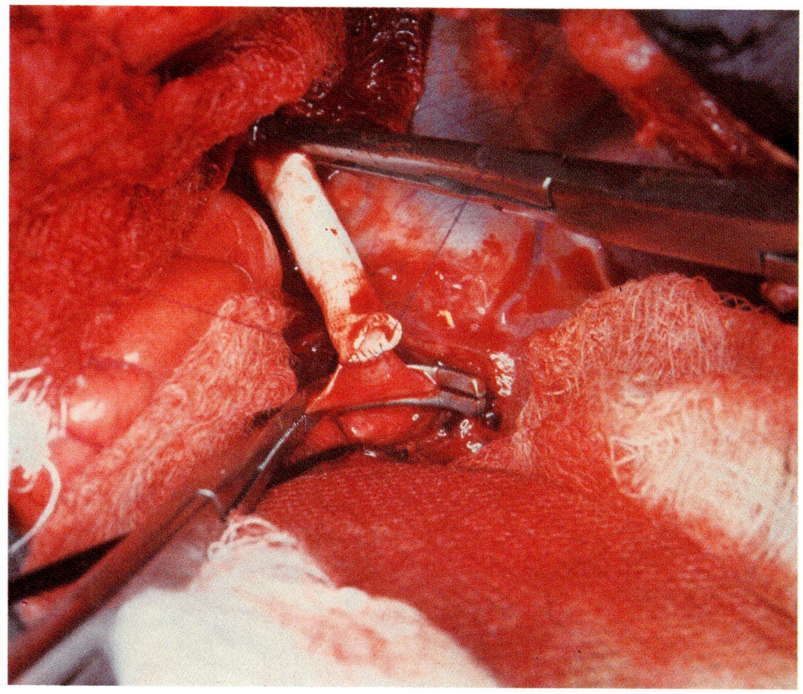

21 A side-clamp has been placed on the right pulmonary artery and a longitudinal incision made in it. The lower end of the Goretex graft is anastomosed, again using fine, continuous Prolene sutures.

22

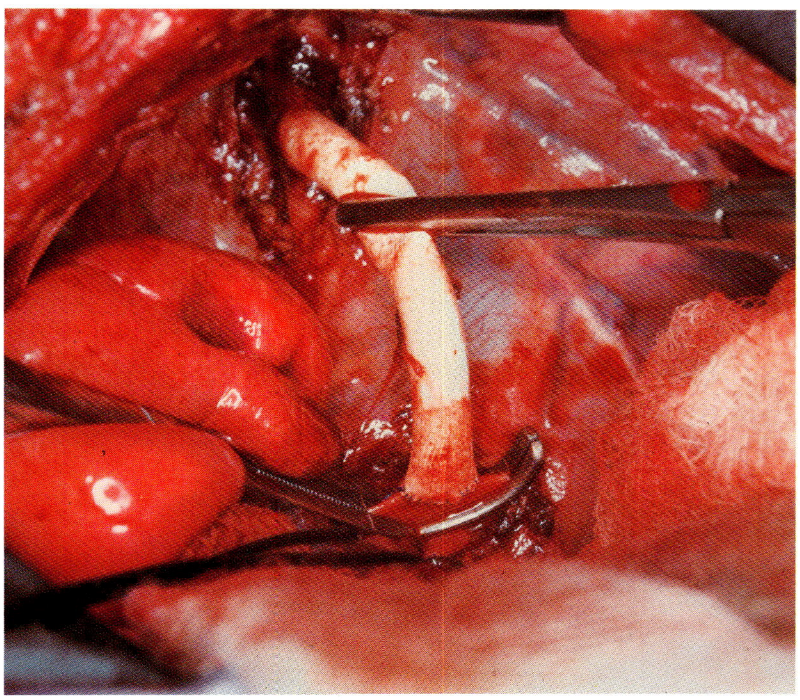

23

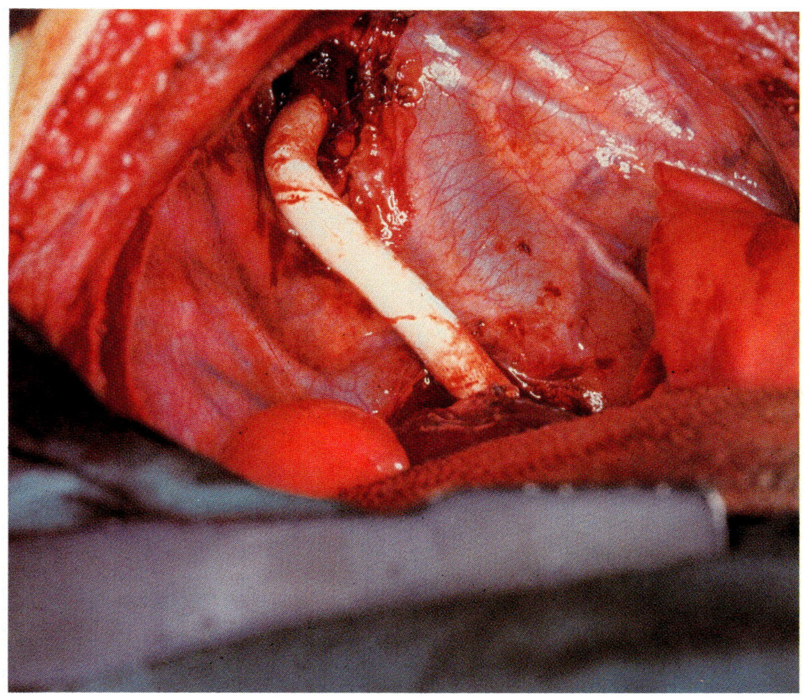

22 and 23 When the anastomosis is complete, the clamps are released and blood allowed to flow through the graft. A marked thrill can be felt with the finger placed on the pulmonary artery. In fact, it is probably better to leave a side-clamp on the subclavian artery, rather than clamp the graft itself, as this may predispose to thrombosis in the graft.

7: The Waterston shunt

This operation was first performed by Waterston in 1962[1] and subsequently popularised by Cooley[2]. It is designed to increase the flow of blood to the lungs in cyanosed babies who are otherwise unsuitable for correction of their heart condition. The shunt is produced by anastomosing the right pulmonary artery to the back of the ascending aorta (diagram **A**) and cardiopulmonary bypass is not used. Unlike the Blalock-Taussig procedure where the amount of blood flowing through the lungs is limited by the size of the subclavian artery, with the Waterston procedure the size of the communication is critical and it is easy to make the anastomosis too large. Furthermore, it may grow too large subsequently and the development of pulmonary vascular disease can be a worry. It is also quite common for the pulmonary artery to become kinked, particularly on the left side, so that unequal flow to the lungs may be produced.

For these reasons it is usually preferable to perform a Blalock-Taussig shunt where feasible, but in very small infants the Waterston may be technically easier. It is usual to perform the Waterston anastomosis through a right anterolateral thoracotomy using the fourth intercostal space.

When the definitive procedure is performed, it is necessary to close the Waterston anastomosis. This can be achieved either by closing the defect from inside the aorta, providing there is no kinking or narrowing of the right pulmonary artery, or by detaching the right pulmonary artery from the back of the aorta and closing both holes. A patch can be inserted into the pulmonary artery to widen it if necessary; both methods are shown in this chapter.

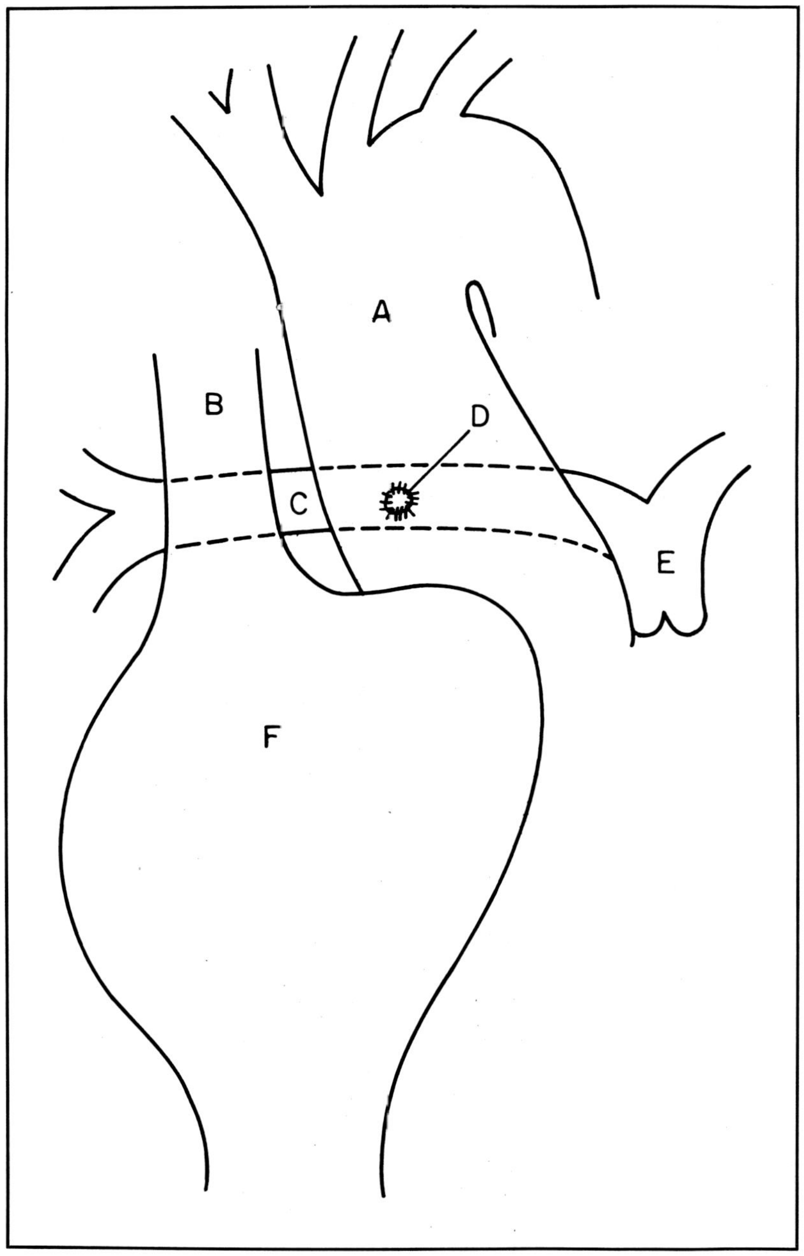

Diagram A

A – Ascending aorta

B – Superior vena cava

C – Right pulmonary artery

D – Waterston anastomosis

E – Main pulmonary artery

F – Right atrium

1
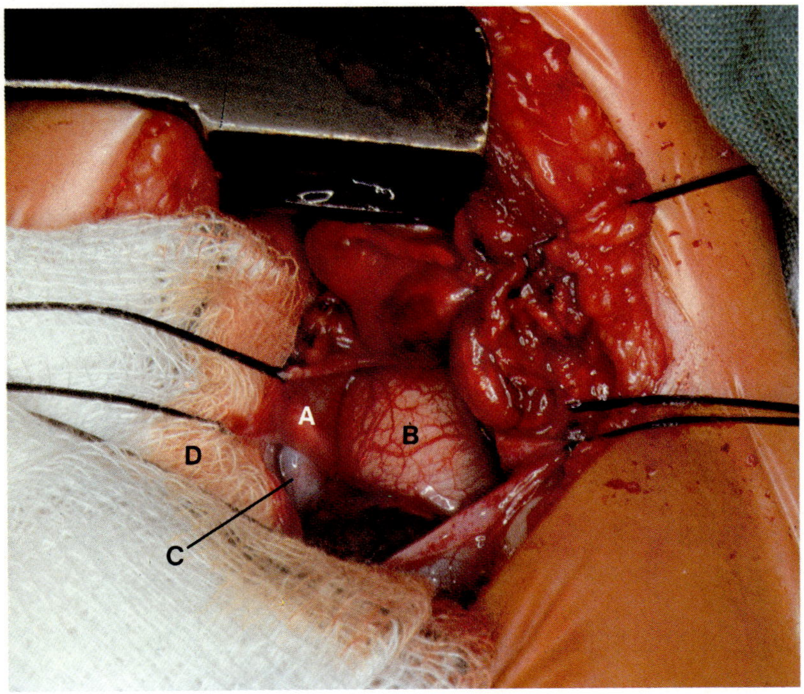

1 The chest has been opened through a right thoracotomy and the pericardium (**A**) incised and retracted with stay-sutures. The ascending aorta (**B**) and superior vena cava (**C**) are seen. The right pulmonary artery runs across behind both and must be dissected out. The lung has been held out of the way with a swab (**D**).

2
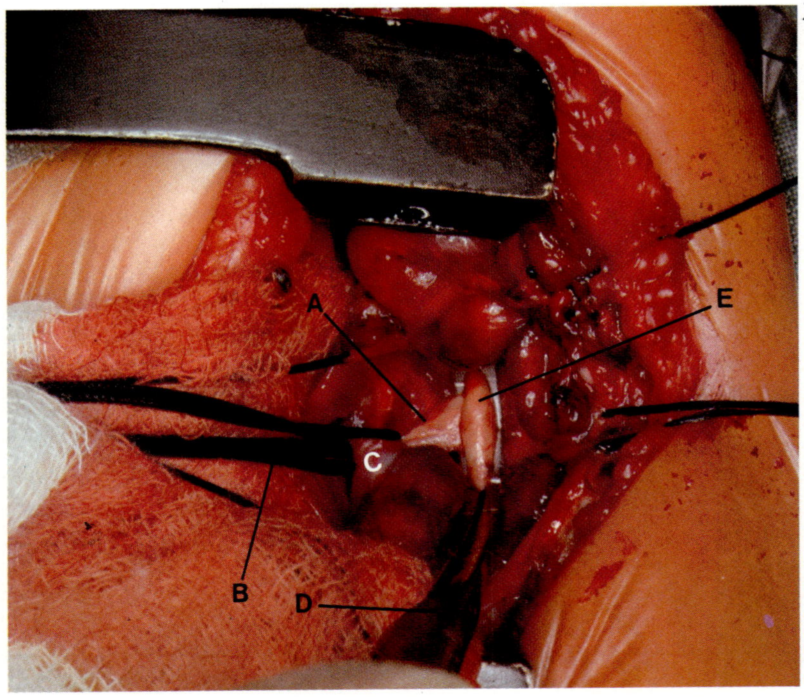

2 The pulmonary artery (**A**) has been dissected out and a temporary ligature (**B**) placed around it lateral to the superior vena cava (**C**). A side-clamp (**D**) has been placed so as to occlude the right pulmonary artery proximally and, in the same bite, a portion of the ascending aorta (**E**).

3
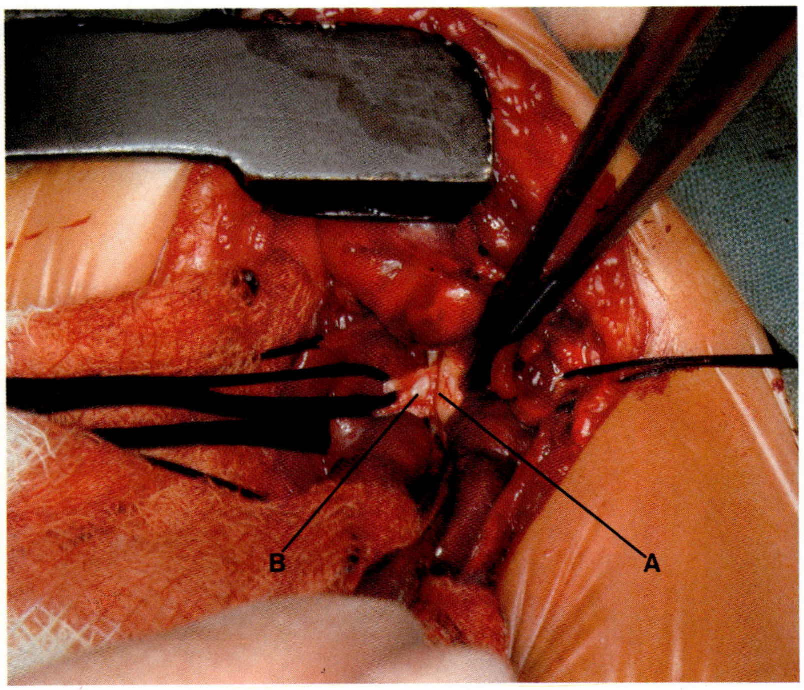

3 Matching incisions are made longitudinally in the aorta (**A**) and transversely in the pulmonary artery (**B**). Care must be taken not to make the incisions too big, particularly in the pulmonary artery where the tissue tends to stretch.

4
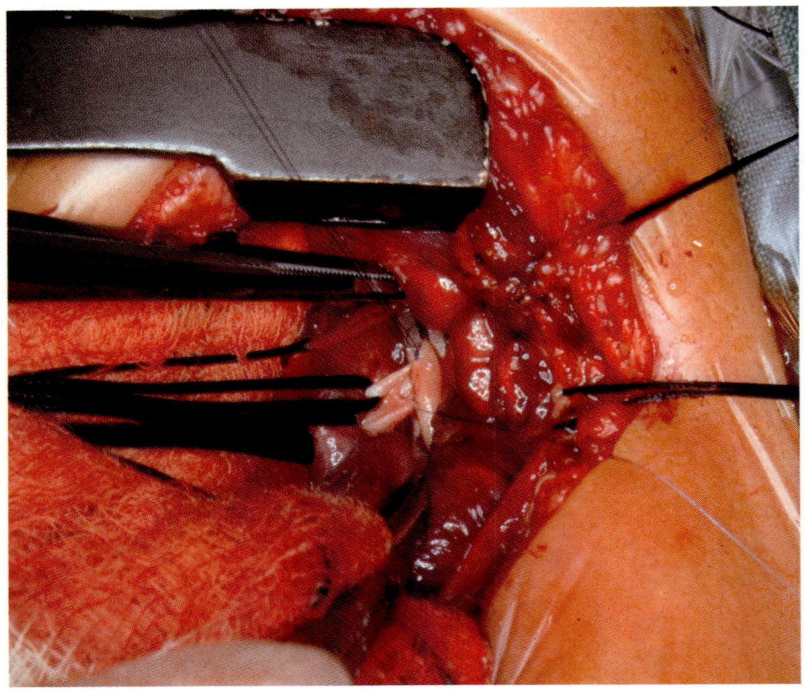

4 The posterior layer of the anastomosis is then performed with continuous Prolene.

5
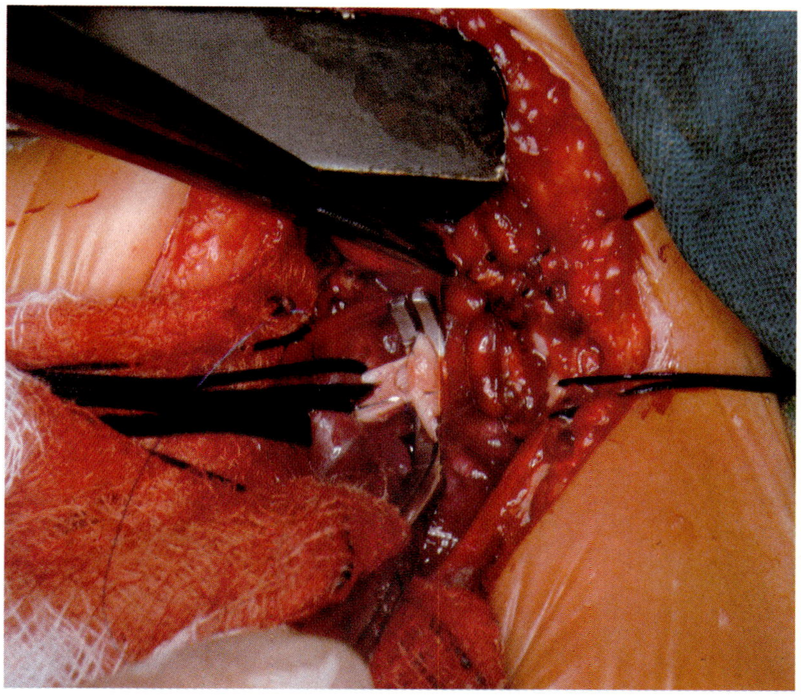

5 The anterior suture line can be performed with interrupted sutures to allow for growth, and in this picture the needle can be seen passing through the edge of both pulmonary artery and aorta.

6
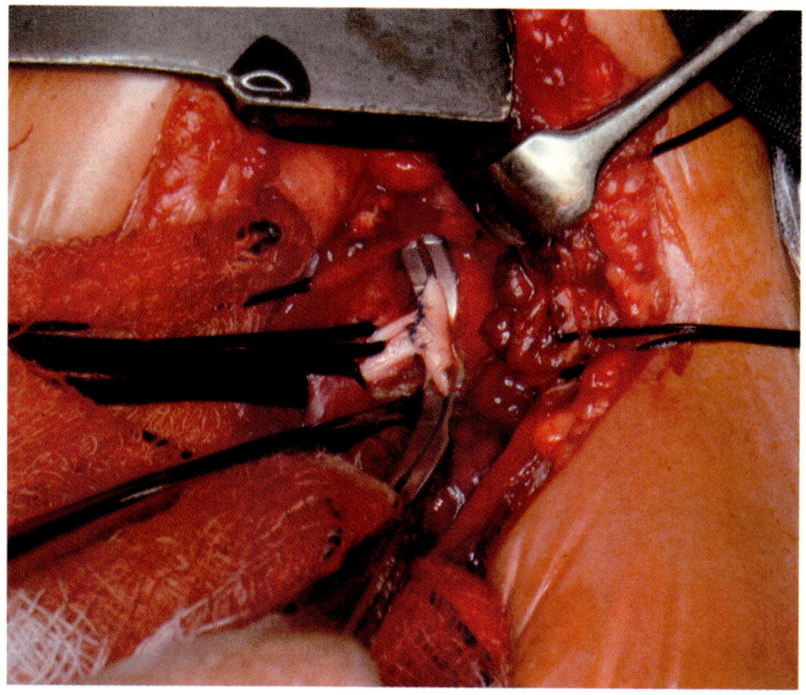

6 The completed anastomosis is seen with no blood as yet in the pulmonary artery.

7
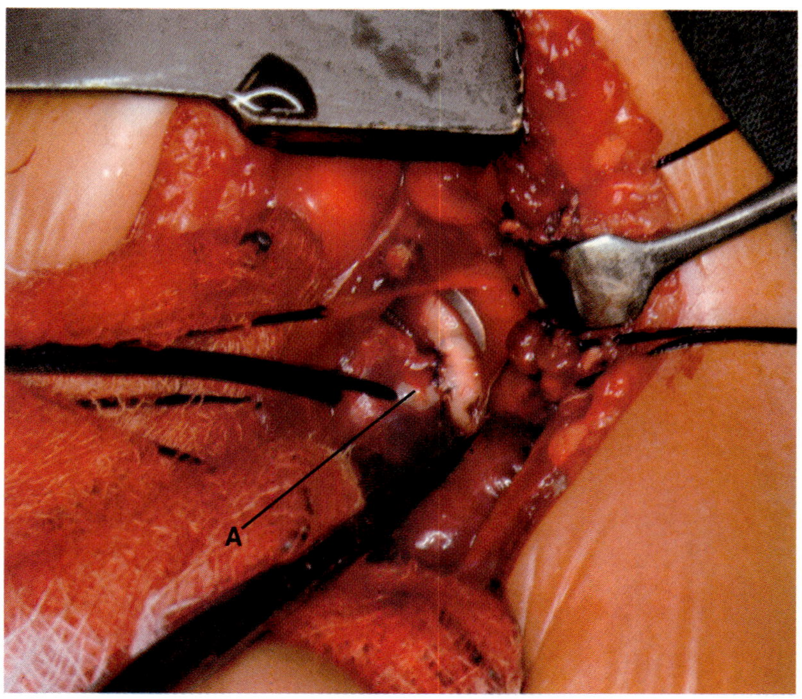

7 The temporary ligature around the distal right pulmonary artery has been removed so that the pulmonary artery (**A**) is filled with blood at low pressure to check the anastomosis.

8
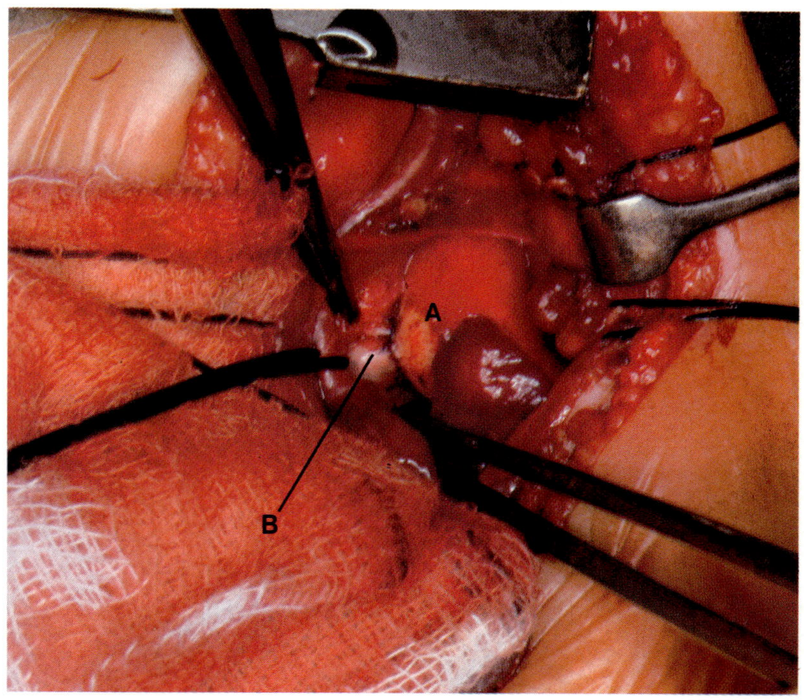

8 The side-clamp has been removed and blood can now flow from the aorta (**A**) into the right pulmonary artery (**B**).

Closure through the ascending aorta

9

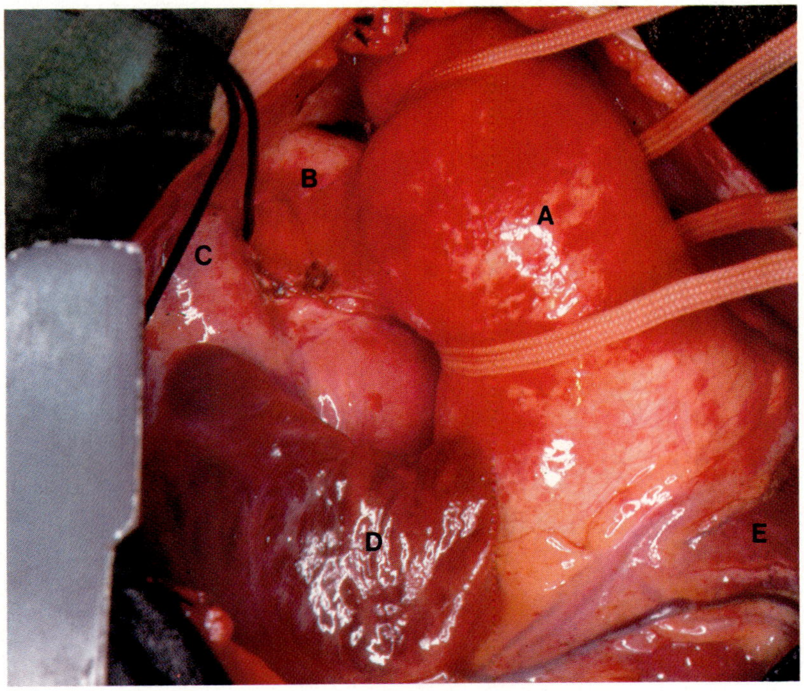

9 This patient coming to correction has had a previous Waterston shunt. The ascending aorta (**A**) has been dissected and tapes placed around it, above and below the level of the anastomosis to the right pulmonary artery (**B**). The superior vena cava (**C**), right atrial appendage (**D**) and right ventricle (**E**) are also seen.

10

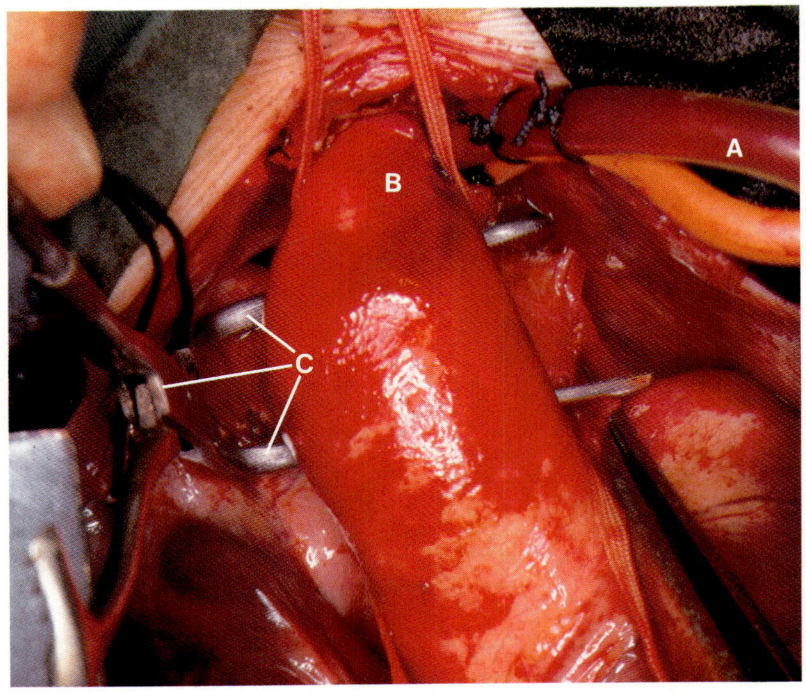

10 A cannula (**A**) has been inserted into the ascending aorta (**B**) and, just as cardiopulmonary bypass is commenced, the Waterston anastomosis is occluded with a clamp (**C**).

11

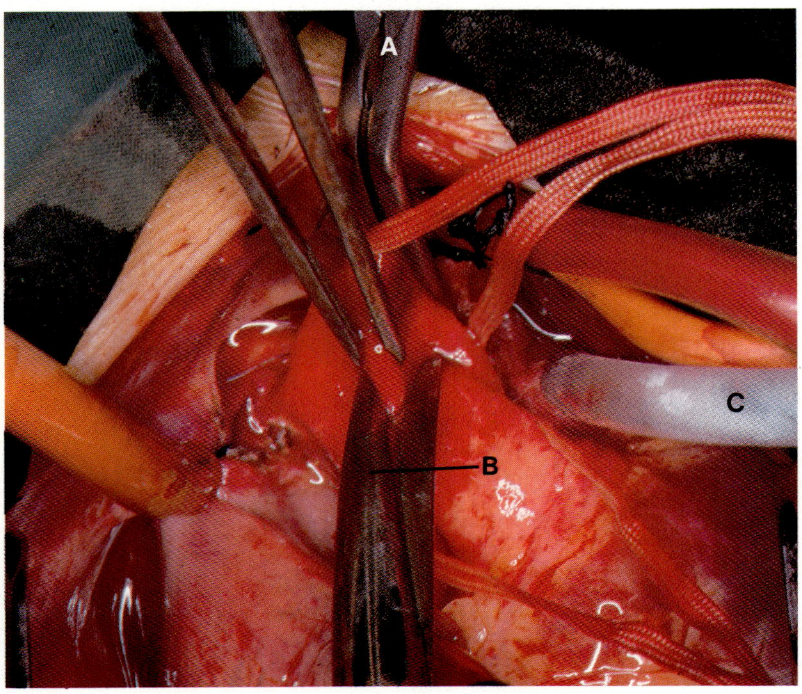

11 A clamp (**A**) has been placed on the ascending aorta and cardioplegic fluid infused into the ascending aorta while the clamp is still occluding the anastomosis. The aorta is incised transversely with scissors (**B**). The heart is being cooled externally with fluid passing through the tube (**C**).

12

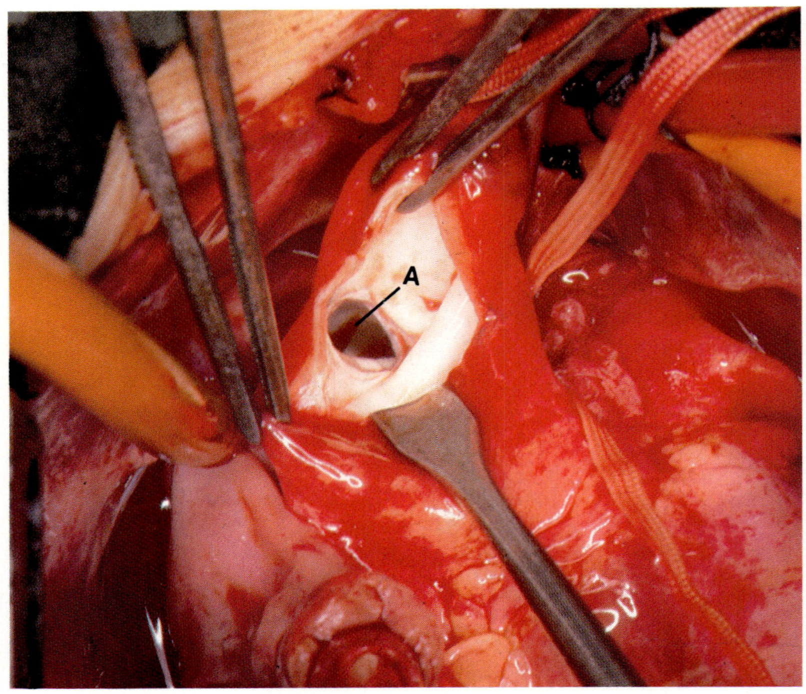

12 The aorta has been opened to reveal the large anastomosis (**A**) with the right pulmonary artery in its back wall.

13

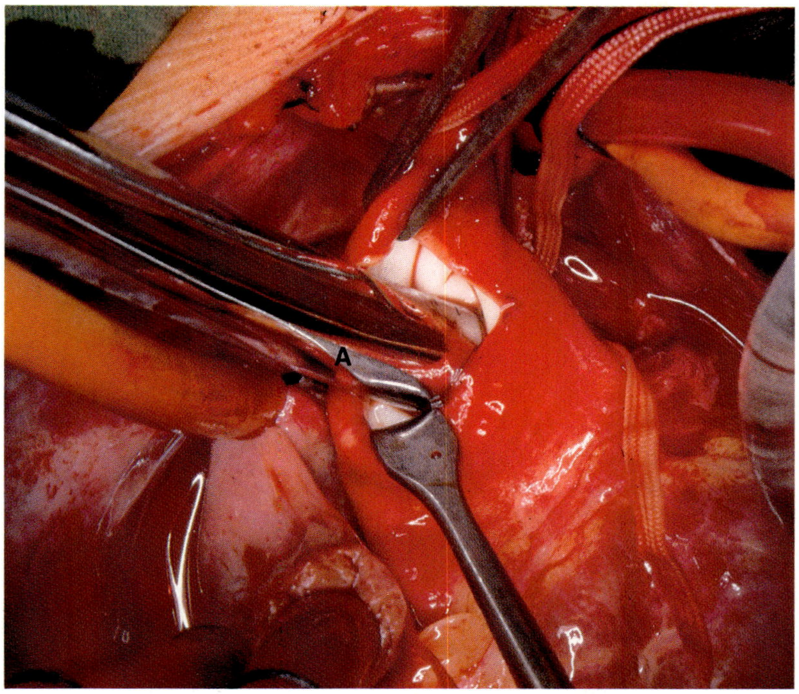

14

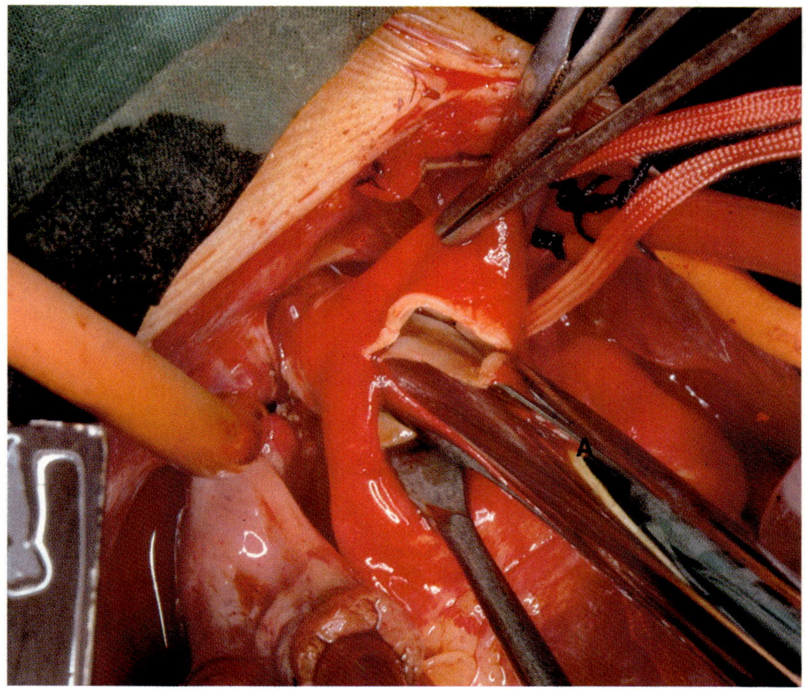

13 and 14 The easy passage of a large Hegar dilator (**A**) into both the proximal and distal right pulmonary artery confirms that there is no stenosis and that it is safe to close the anastomosis from inside the aorta.

15

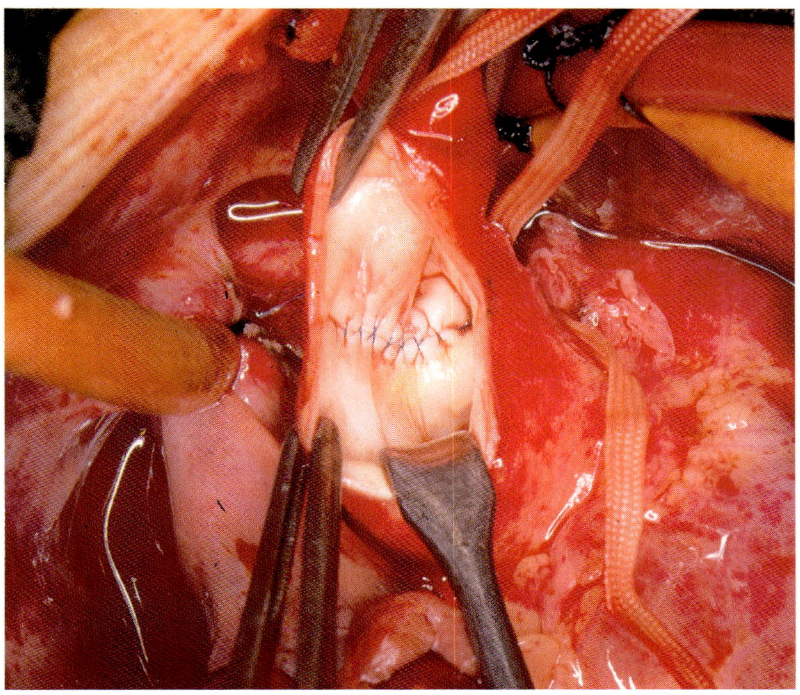

16

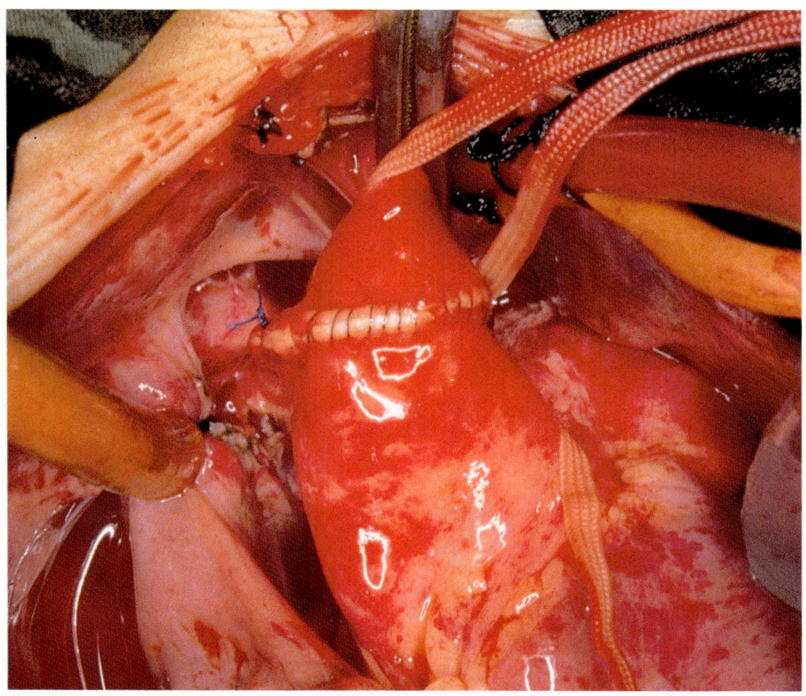

15 The Waterston anastomosis has been closed with a double layer of continuous Prolene.

16 The transverse aortotomy has been closed with continuous Prolene and it is now safe to proceed with correction of the main defect.

Closure by detaching the right pulmonary artery

17
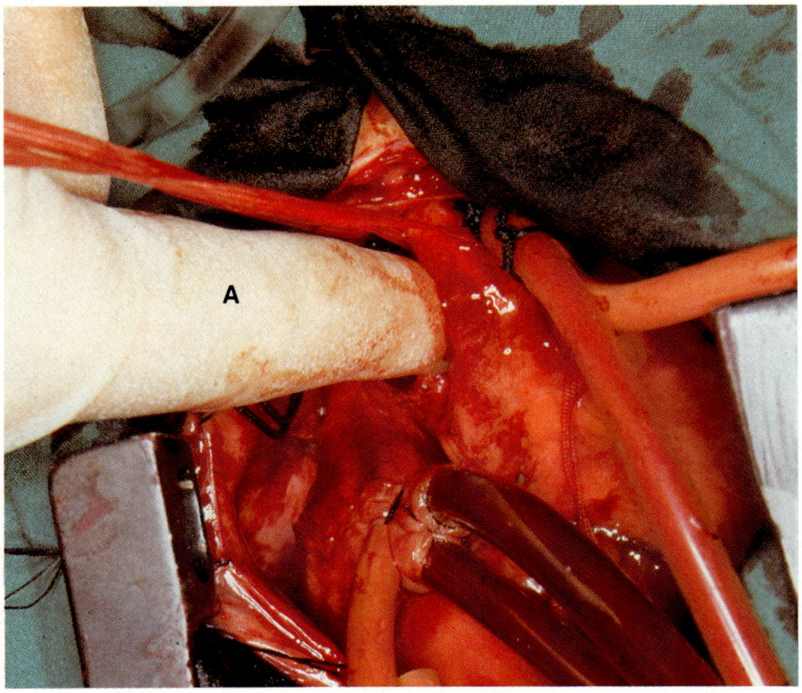

18
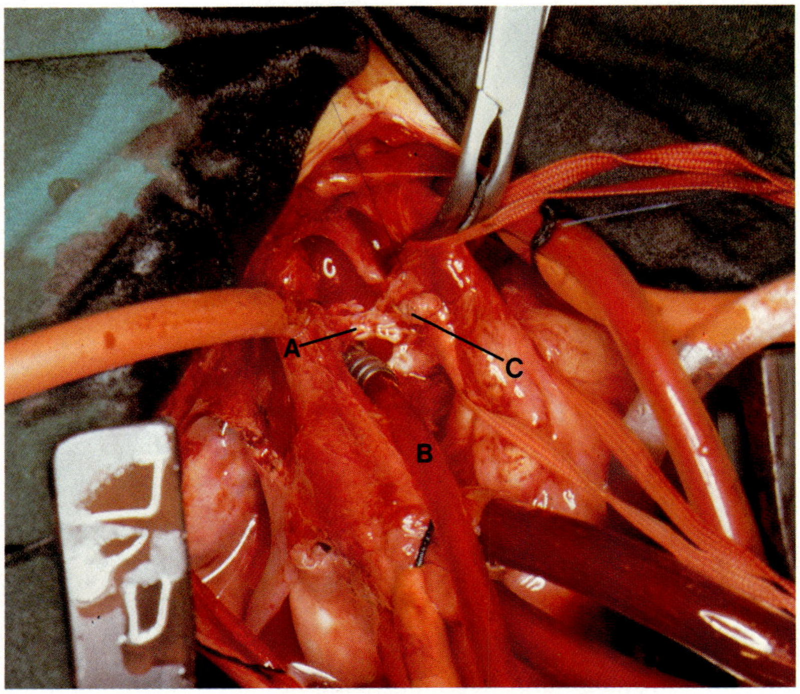

17 In this patient, who had had a previous Waterston anastomosis, it was thought safer to detach the right pulmonary artery from the back of the aorta, as to suture it direct might narrow the pulmonary artery. Here, the anastomosis is closed when cardiopulmonary bypass is commenced by pressing on the back of the ascending aorta with a finger (**A**).

18 The right pulmonary artery (**A**) has been detached from the back of the aorta and a sucker (**B**) placed in it through the site of the previous anastomosis returns blood to the bypass machine. The hole in the back of the aorta is closed directly with Prolene sutures (**C**).

19
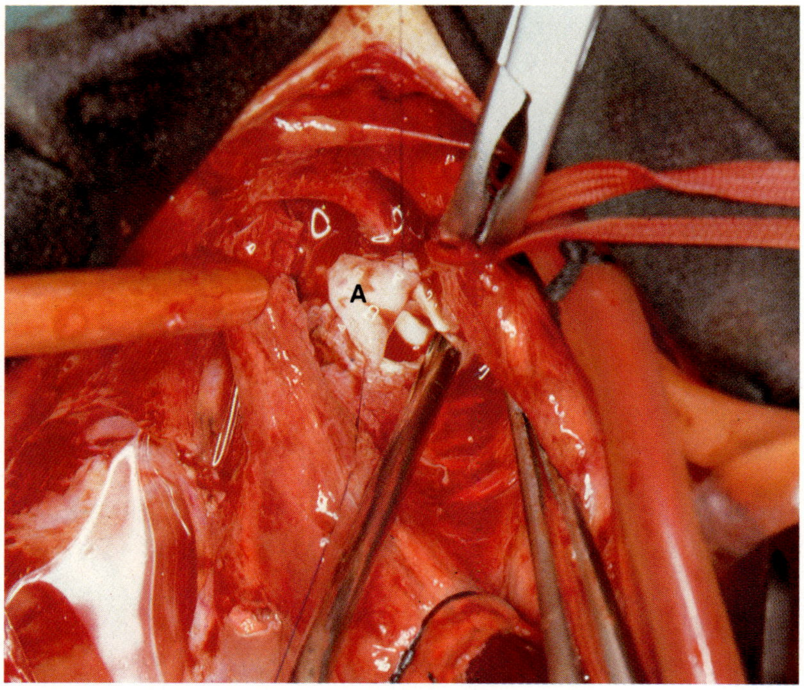

20
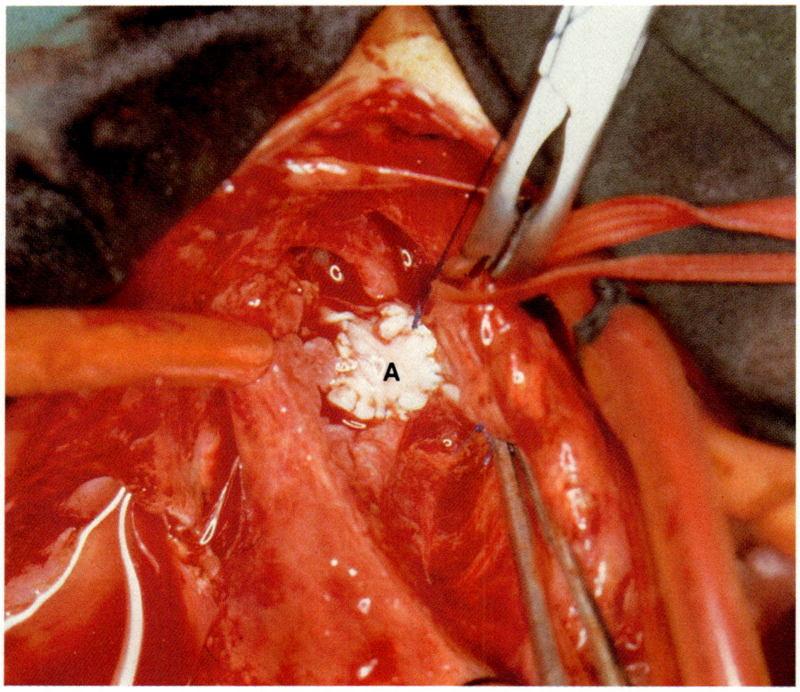

19 and 20 The defect left in the anterior surface of the right pulmonary artery has been closed with a small pericardial patch (**A**) as direct suturing might have narrowed the pulmonary artery.

8: Pulmonary artery banding

Banding of the pulmonary artery was first described by Muller and Damman in 1952[1] for treating certain congenital malformations with excessive pulmonary blood flows. It involves tying a tape around the main pulmonary artery (see diagram **A**) so as to partially occlude it. Before open-heart surgery was available, this was therefore the only surgical treatment that could be offered for conditions with a large left-to-right shunt, such as ventricular septal defect. Indeed, in small infants with a large ventricular septal defect, banding was still being practised instead of closure of the defect until quite recently. However, there are certain conditions with large left ro right shunts resulting in a high pulmonary blood flow, such as univentricular heart without pulmonary stenosis, where correction is not advisable early in life and, therefore, there is still a place for pulmonary artery banding.

The approach depends on whether the pulmonary artery is to the left or right of the aorta. Obviously the left is much the commonest and the usual incision is therefore through the left fourth intercostal space (see Chapter 3). However, occasionally the pulmonary artery is to the right of the aorta, as in the case illustrated in this chapter, and therefore the right chest should be opened. Pulmonary artery banding can be performed at the same time as repair of coarctation of the aorta, and when coarctation coexists with some condition causing a large left to right shunt, this may be considered the appropriate treatment.

The degree of narrowing of the pulmonary artery needed can be difficult to judge, as one is trying to diminish the blood flow to the lungs to near-normal levels. Usually if the pressure in the pulmonary artery distal to the band is half or just less than half systemic, this proves about right.

It is, of course, necessary to remove the band at the definitive operation and this can be facilitated by using teflon tape which slips out easily. However, there is often a narrowing and it may be necessary to widen the site of the band with a patch. This is particularly so if the band has slipped distally on the pulmonary artery and the left or right pulmonary artery has been compromised.

Diagram A

A – Main pulmonary artery

B – Band

C – Left pulmonary artery

D – Right pulmonary artery

E – Ascending aorta

F – Right atrium

G – Right ventricle

H – Left ventricle

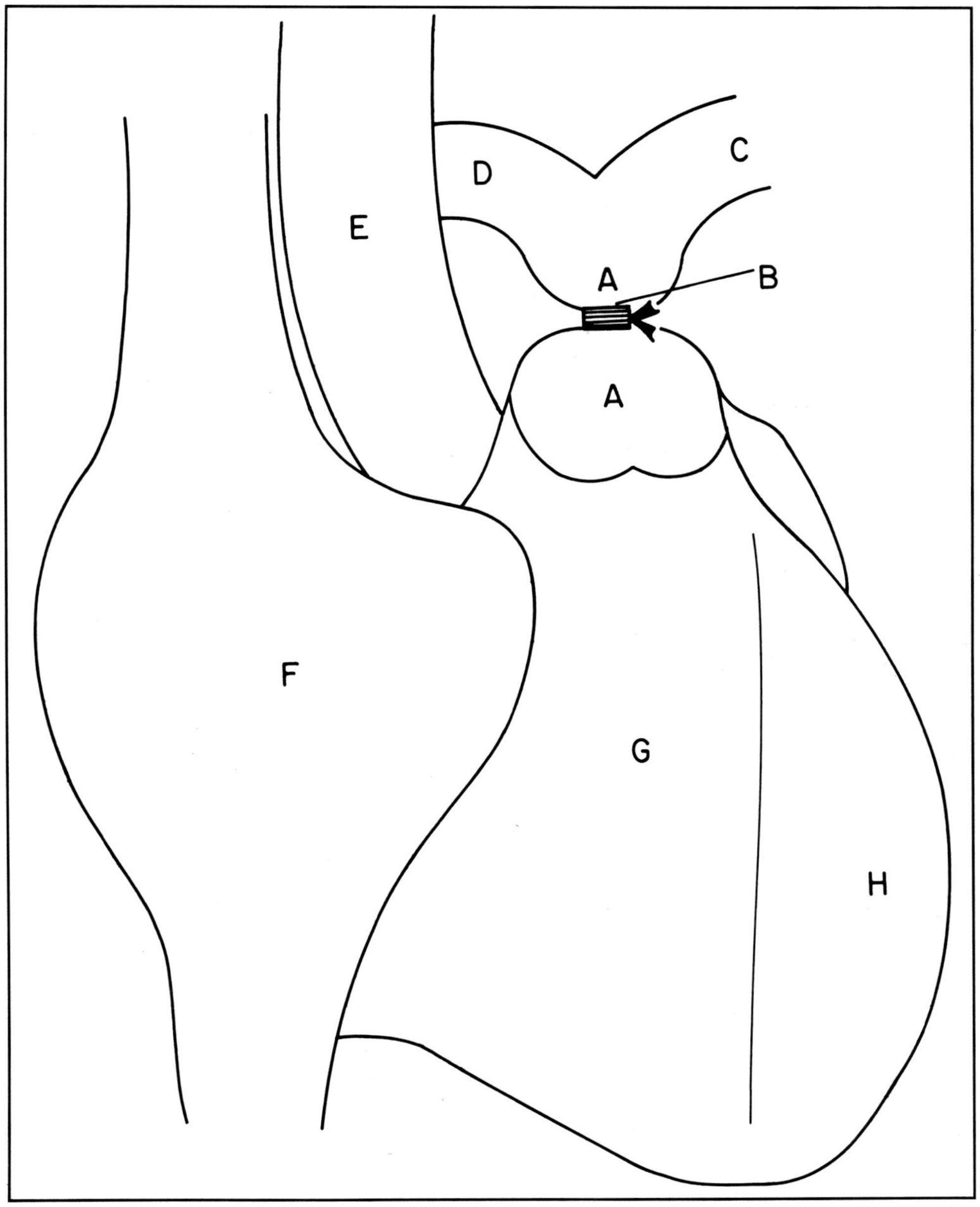

1

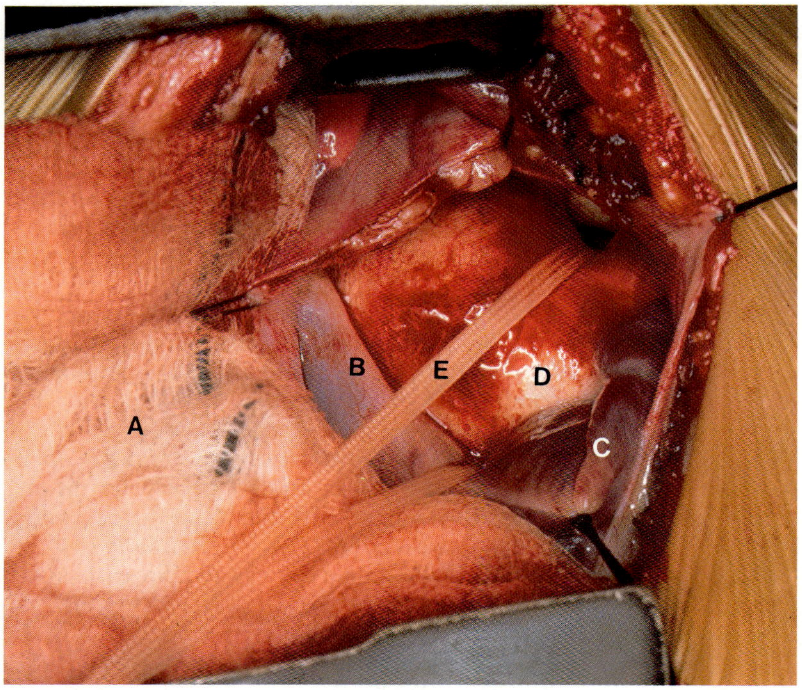

1 The chest has been opened through the right side, the pericardium opened and retracted with stay-sutures to hold the lung beneath the swab (**A**). The superior vena cava (**B**), right atrial appendage (**C**) and main pulmonary artery (**D**) can be seen. A tape (**E**) has been passed around the pulmonary artery.

2

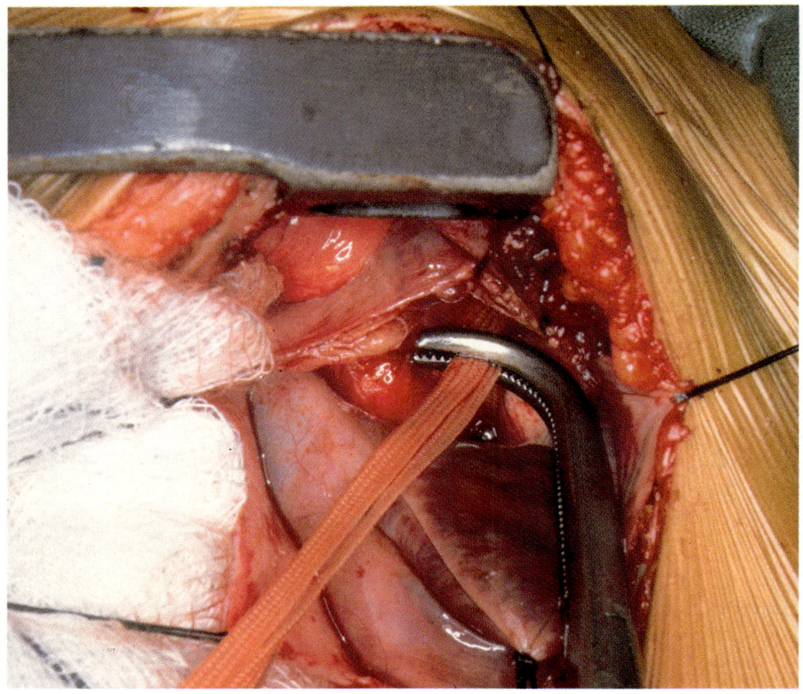

2 The tape is initially being tightened around the pulmonary artery being held with forceps at what seems the right degree of tightness.

3

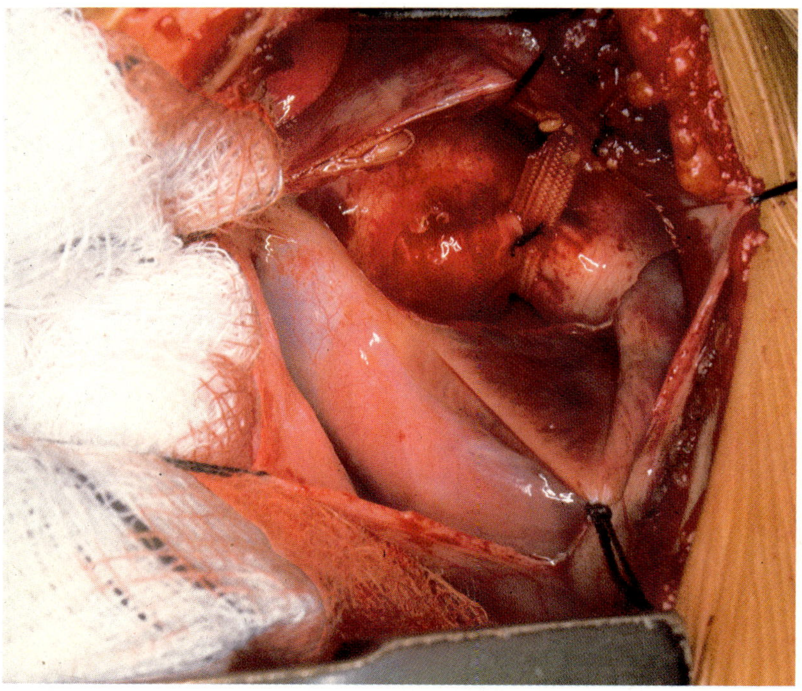

3 A suture has been placed through the tape to hold it at the appropriate degree of tightness and extra sutures can be added progressively to tighten it further if necessary.

4

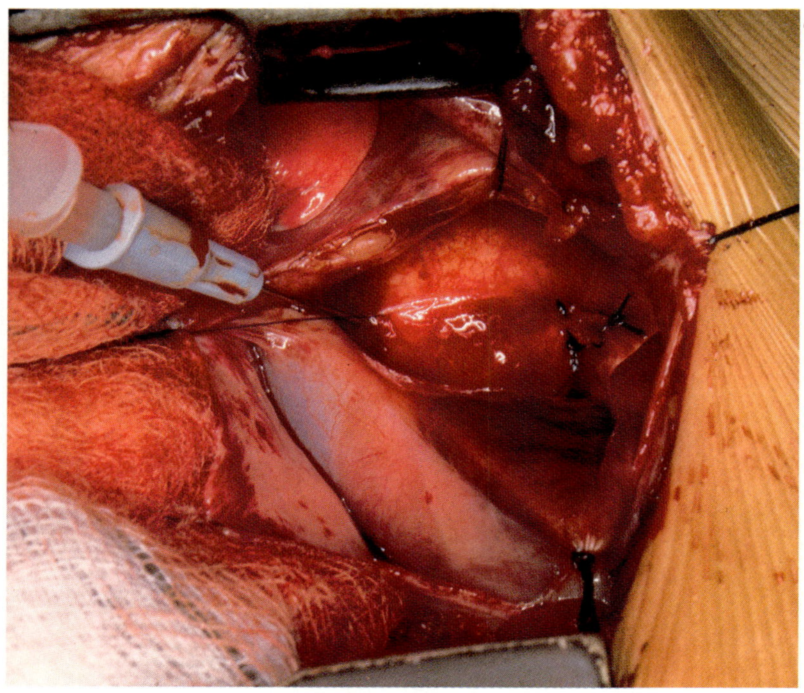

4 The pressure in the pulmonary artery distal to the band is being measured by a needle connected by tubing to a pressure transducer. This pressure is compared with the systemic pressure, in this case being measured in the radial artery. The band can be tightened further by placing more sutures to achieve a distal pressure just less than half systemic.

Removal of the band

5
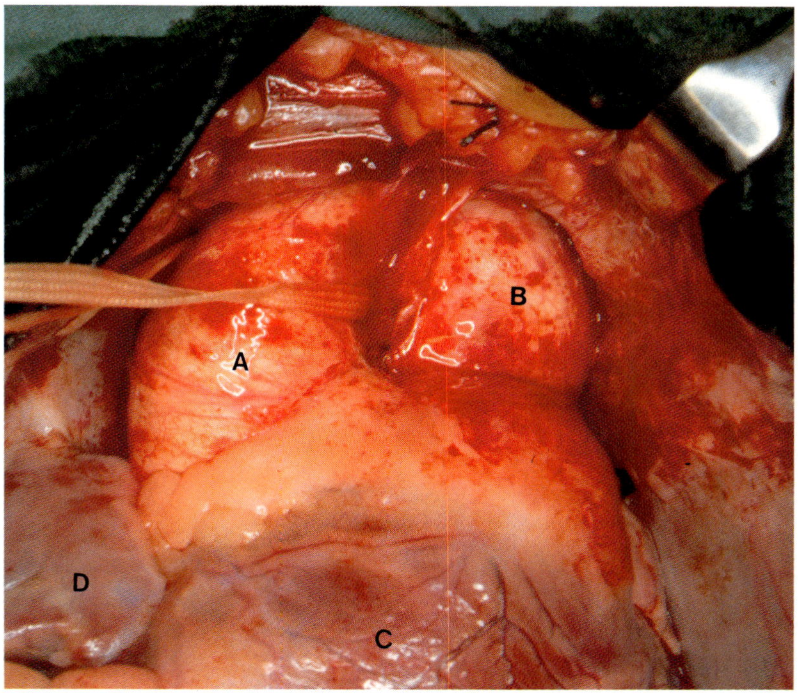

6
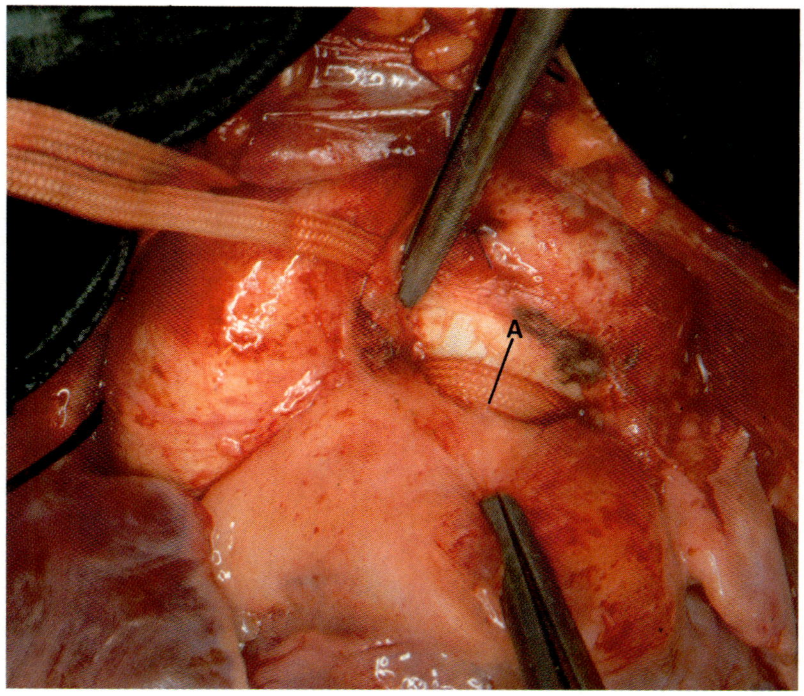

5 This picture, taken from the front, shows the aorta **(A)**, pulmonary artery **(B)**, right ventricle **(C)** and right atrium **(D)** in a patient being operated on for total correction, who had previously had banding of the pulmonary artery.

6 The band **(A)** has been exposed by dissection.

7
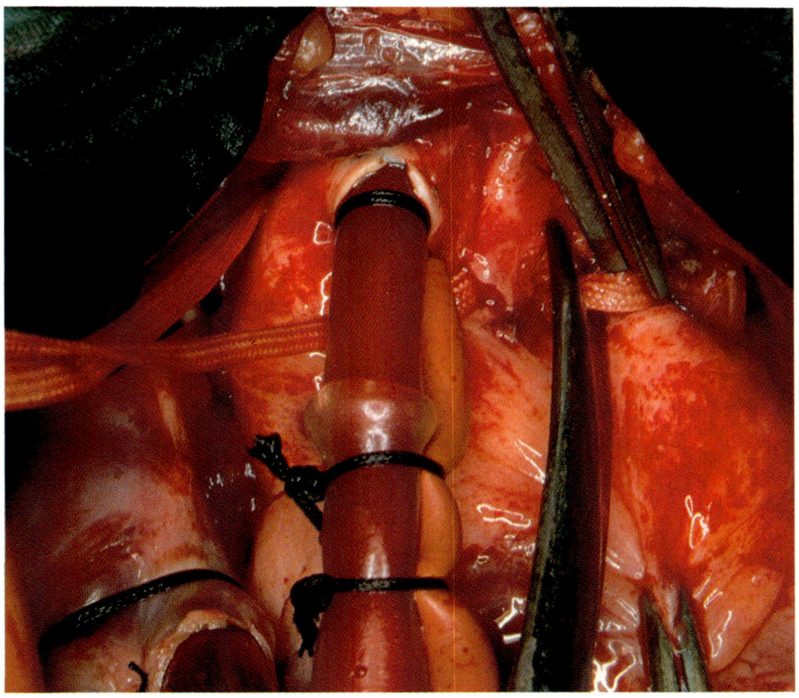

8
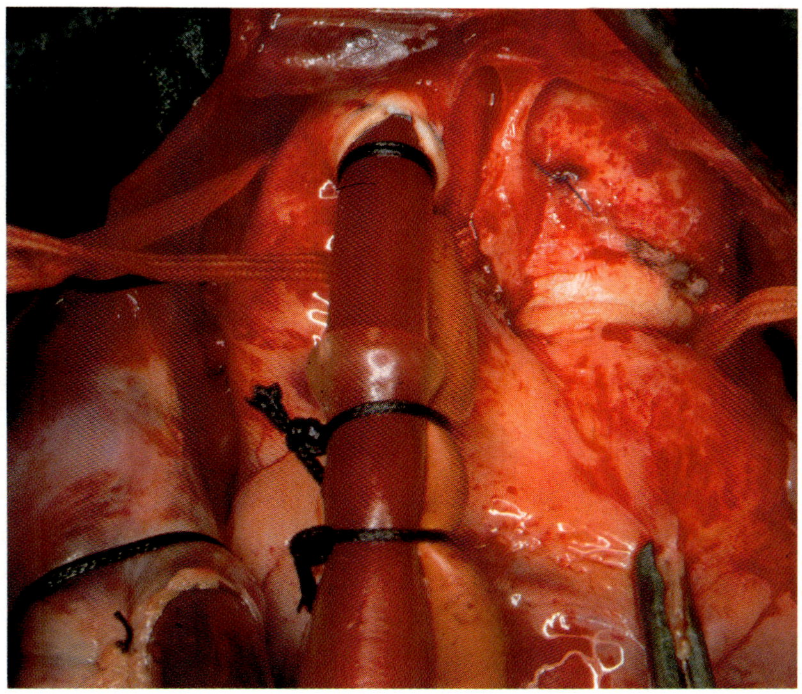

7 and 8 The band is cut and pulled out, allowing the pumonary artery to expand and relieve the obstruction.

9: Closure of atrial septal defect

Secundum atrial septal defects are the commonest and these, together with sinus venosus atrial septal defects, are described in this chapter. Ostium primum defects or partial atrioventricular defects are described in Chapter 10. In the developing heart, failure of the descending septum secundum to meet the septum primum leaves a centrally placed defect, the secundum defect (see diagram **A**). If, during development, the septum secundum breaks away superiorly, the so-called sinus venosus defect is produced (see diagram **A**). This defect is close to the entrance of the superior vena cava and frequently, the right upper pulmonary vein drains into the lower end of the superior vena cava.

Closure of an atrial septal defect is one of the most straightforward intracardiac procedures and was first successfully performed by Lewis in 1952[1], using in-flow occlusion and moderate hypothermia. The following year, Gibbon first successfully closed an atrial septal defect using cardiopulmonary bypass[2] and this method is now always used with two vena caval cannulae.

Most secundum defects in children can be closed directly with a continuous suture, but in adults and large defects it is better to use a patch as there might otherwise be undue tension, which could cause the defect to reopen. Pericardium or dacron can be used. When repairing a sinus venosus defect, a patch should always be used because it is necessary to redirect the pulmonary venous return without compromising the superior vena cava.

The only real risk with this operation is of air embolus, as air can be trapped in the left side of the heart. Care must therefore be taken to fill the left atrium with blood as the closing suture is pulled tight, and also the apex of the heart should be aspirated and a needle placed in the ascending aorta to allow escape of any trapped air.

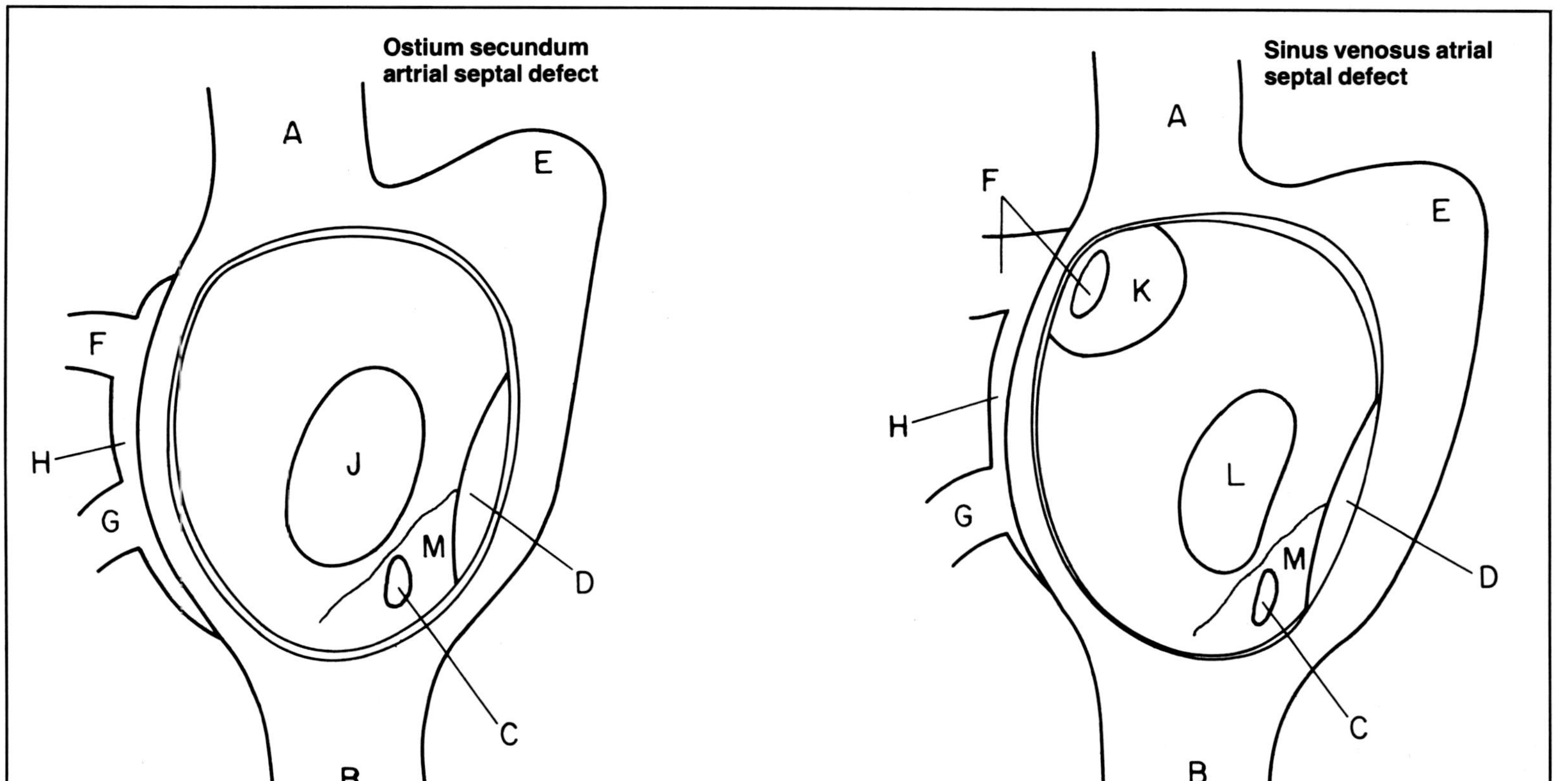

Diagram A

A –	Superior vena cava	**G** –	Right inferior pulmonary vein
B –	Inferior vena cava	**H** –	Left atrium
C –	Coronary sinus	**J** –	Ostium secundum atrial septal defect
D –	Tricuspid valve	**K** –	Sinus venosus atrial septal defect
E –	Right atrial appendage	**L** –	Fossa ovalis
F –	Right superior pulmonary vein	**M** –	Position of atrioventricular node

Closure of ostium secundum atrial septal defect by direct suture

1

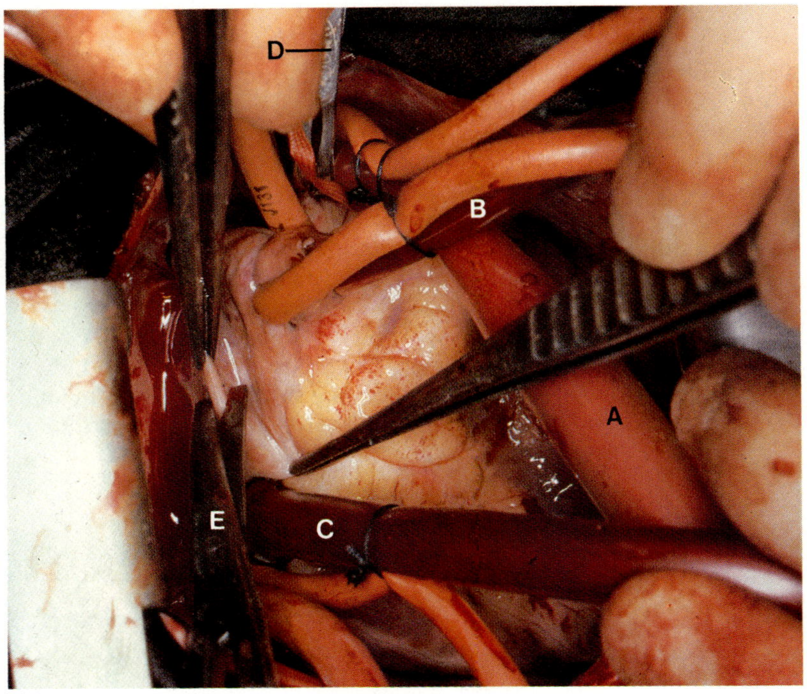

1 A cannula (**A**) has been placed in the ascending aorta. Two venous cannulae have been inserted, one (**B**) into the superior vena cava via the atrial appendage, and the other (**C**) directly through the right atrial wall into the inferior vena cava. An aortic cross-clamp (**D**) has been applied and the right atrium is being opened with a pair of scissors (**E**).

2

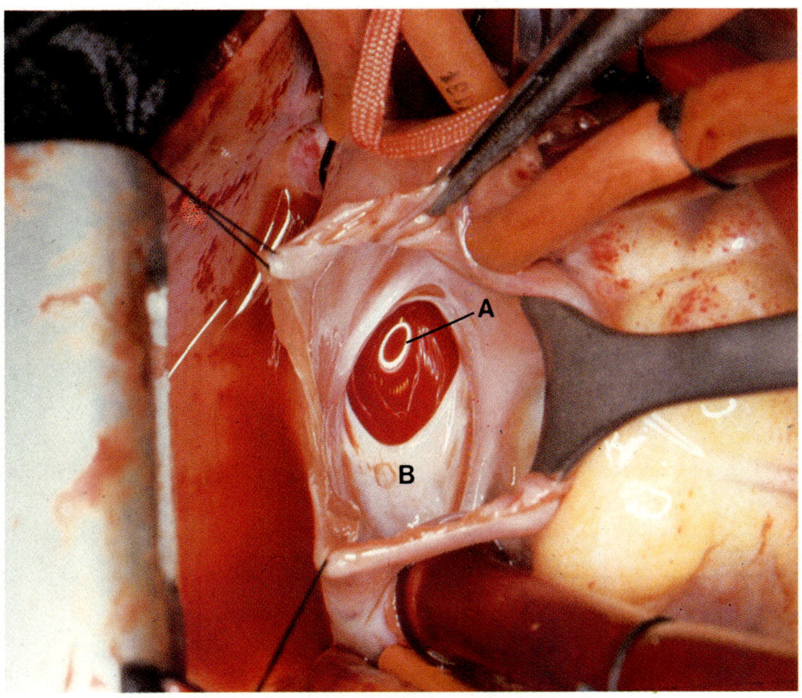

3

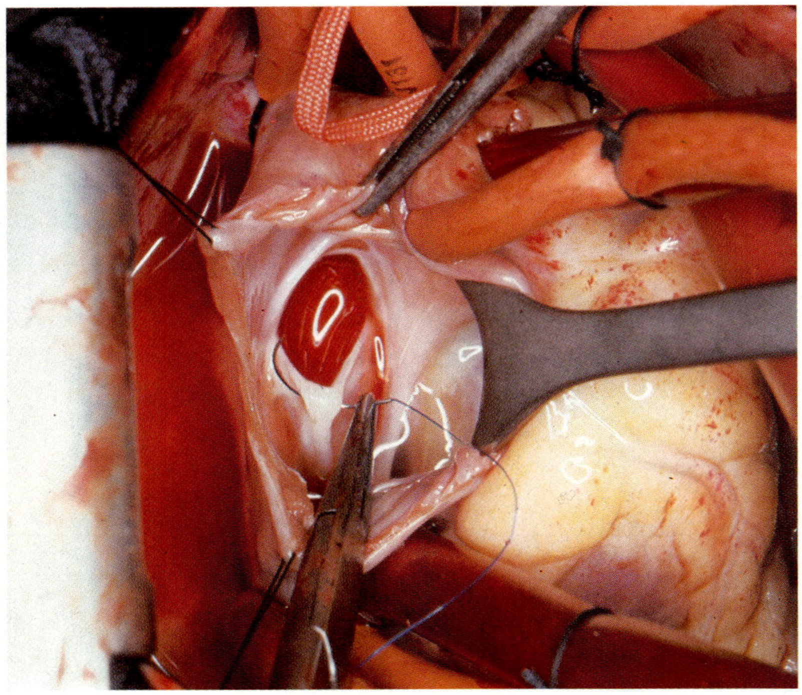

2 and 3 When the right atrium has been adequately opened and retracted, the secundum atrial septal defect is clearly seen with blood in the left atrium beyond (**A**). Most of the atrial septum (**B**) lies below the defect and the continuous Prolene suture is started at the lowest point of the defect.

4

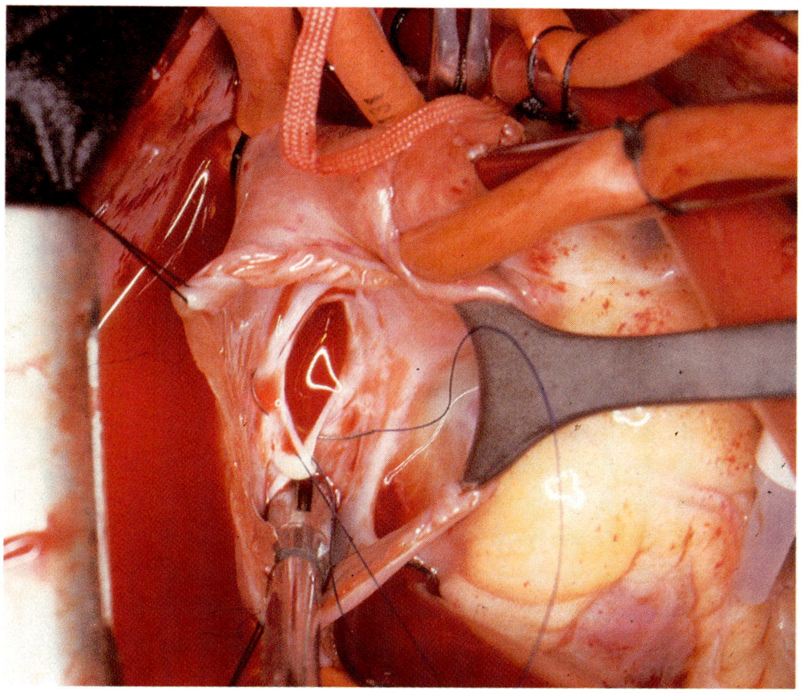

5

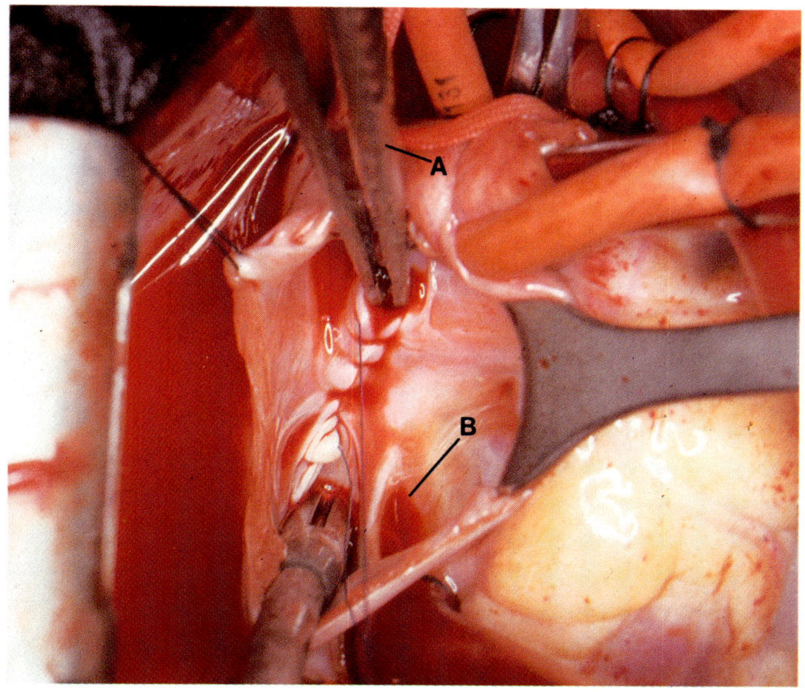

4 and 5 The suture is continued upwards and, as the defect is nearly closed, any air in the left atrium can be squeezed out gently by the anaesthetist gently inflating the lungs while the last part of the defect is held open with forceps (**A**). The coronary sinus is also well seen in this picture (**B**).

6

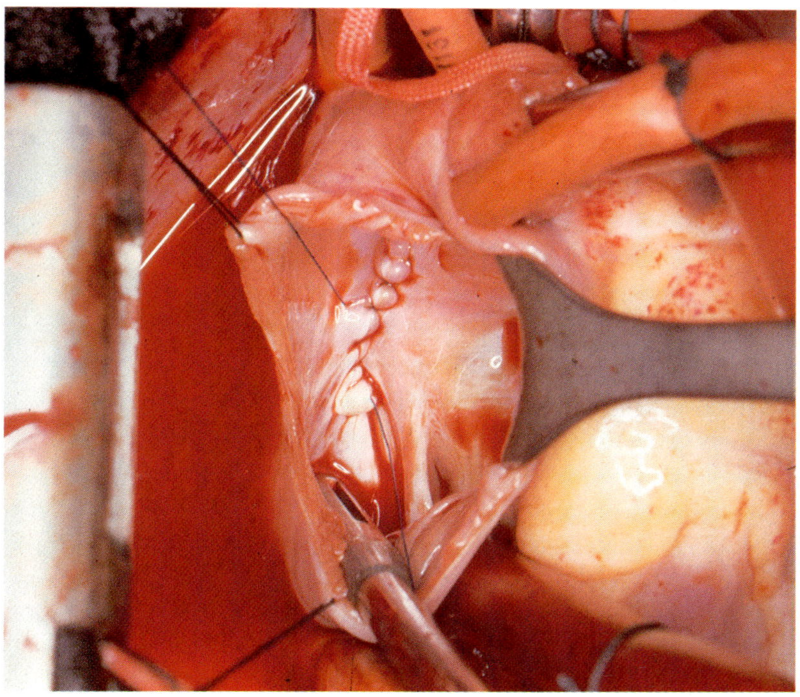

7

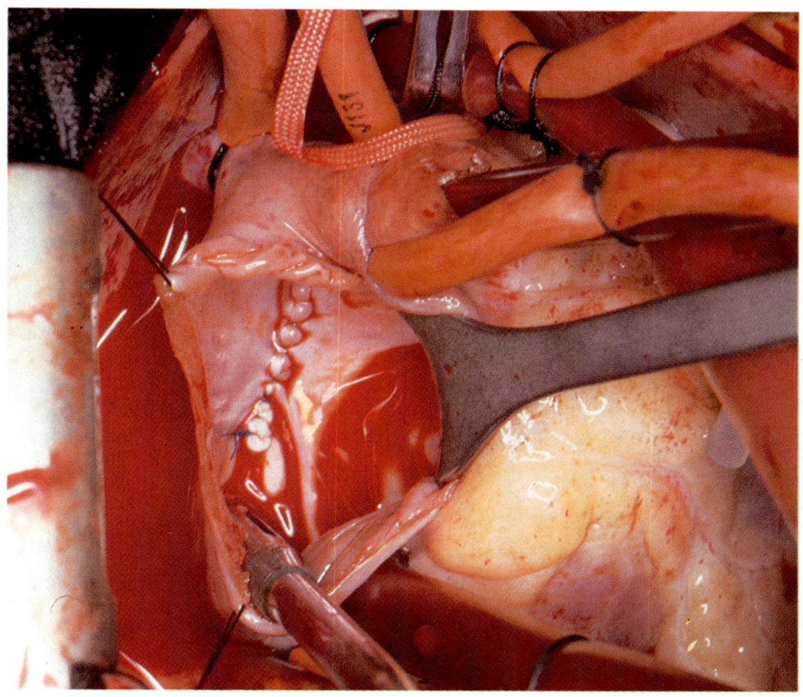

6 and 7 The same suture is then run down to reinforce the suture line and tied at the lower end.

8

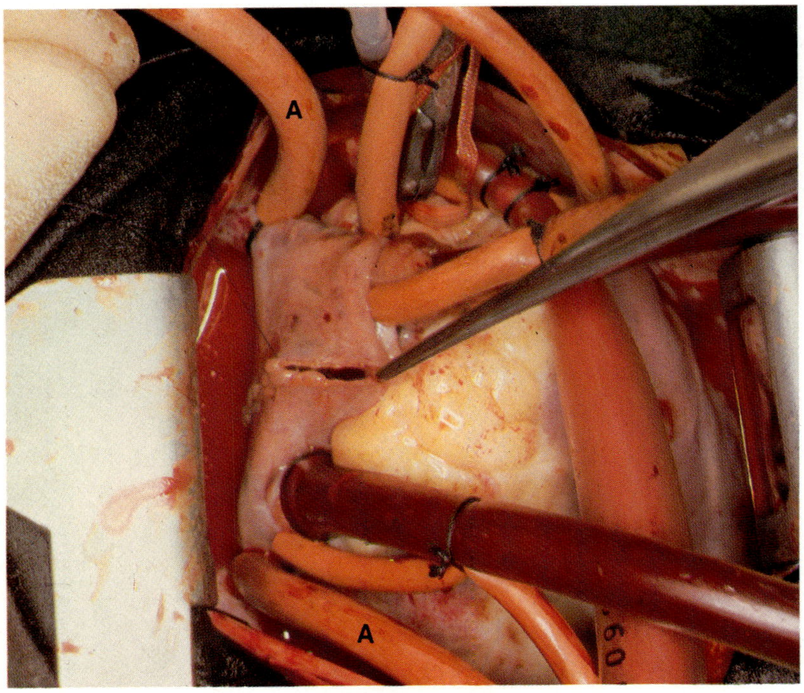

9

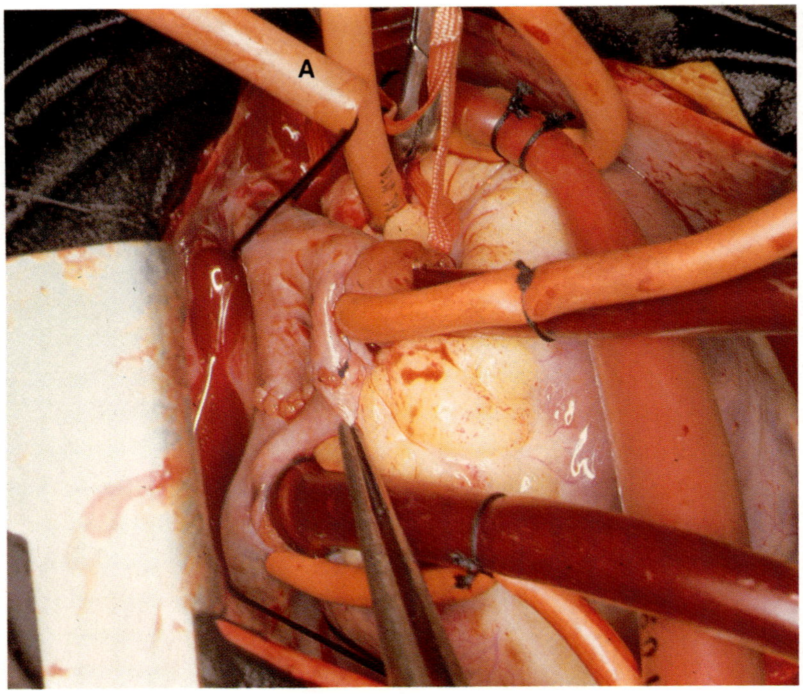

8 and 9 The atrial suture line is then closed with continuous Prolene and the caval snares (**A**) released to allow the right atrium to fill before finally closing the atrium. Any residual air is then removed by aspirating the left atrium and the left ventricular apex before the aortic clamp is released. The aortic clamp can be released once the defect is closed and the atriotomy closed while the heart is recovering, with an open sucker in the atrium to return blood from the coronary sinus to the cardiopulmonary bypass machine.

Closure of ostium secundum atrial septal defect with dacron patch

10

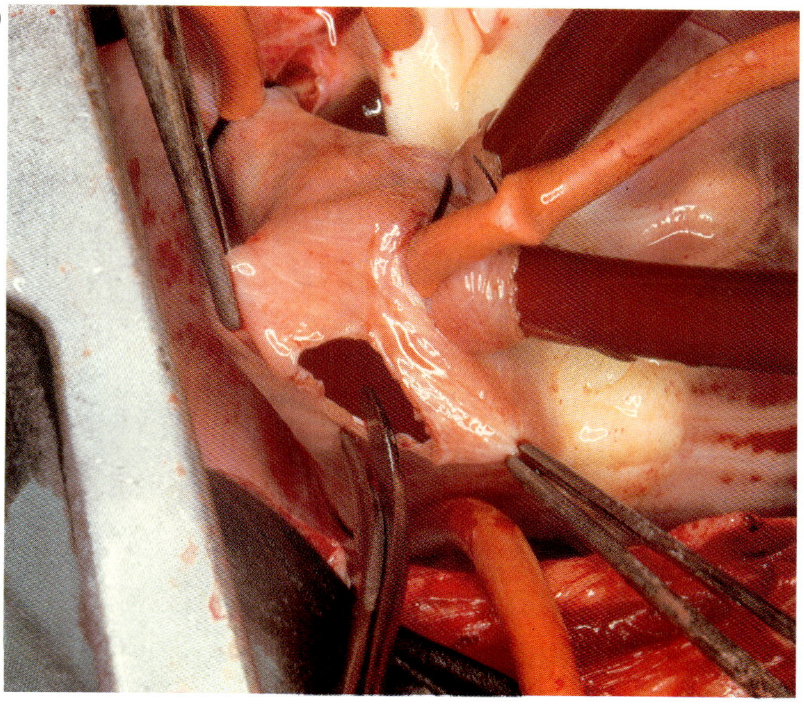

11

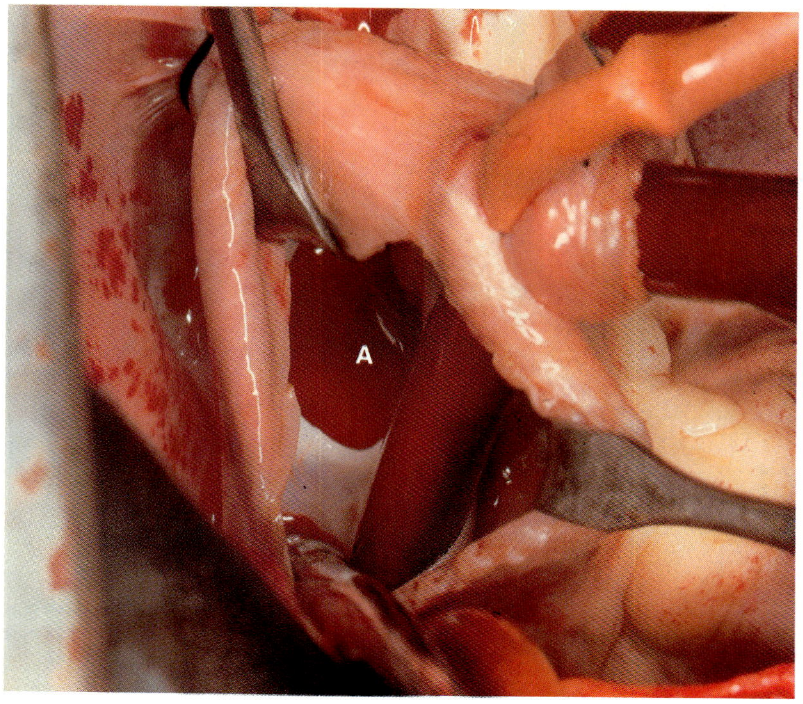

10 and 11 The right atrium is opened in this adult patient to reveal a large secundum atrial spetal defect (**A**).

12

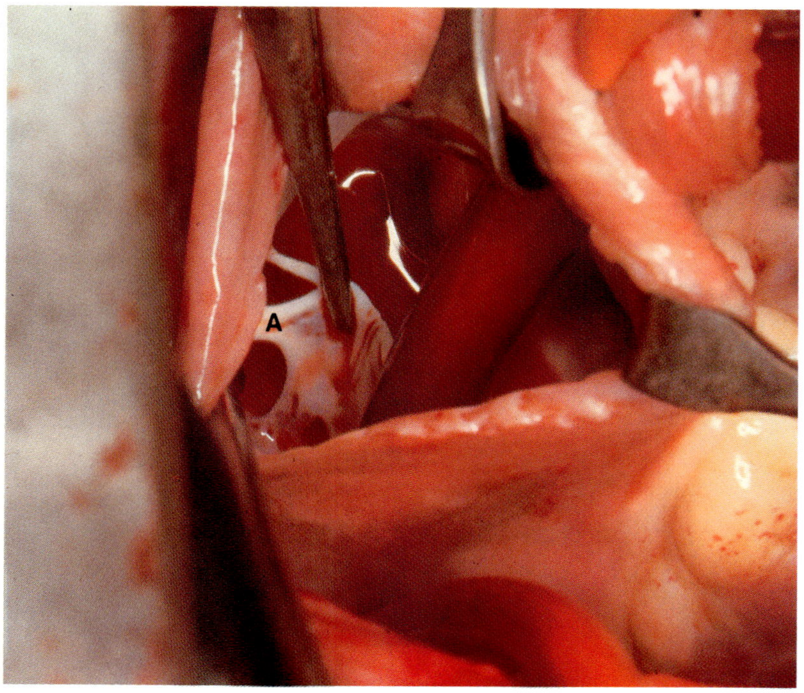

13

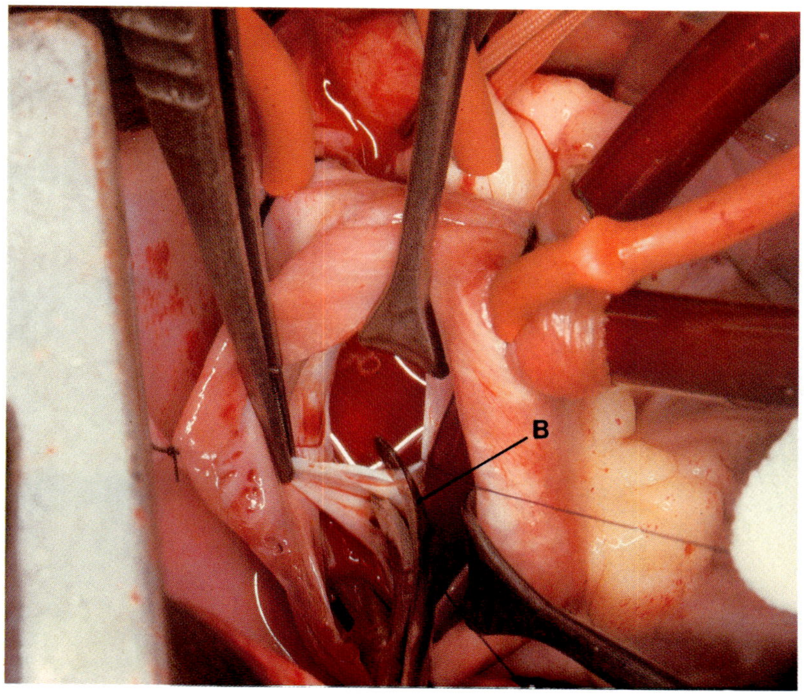

12 and 13 The lower part of the atrial septum is thin and fenestrated (**A**) and is therefore removed with scissors (**B**).

14

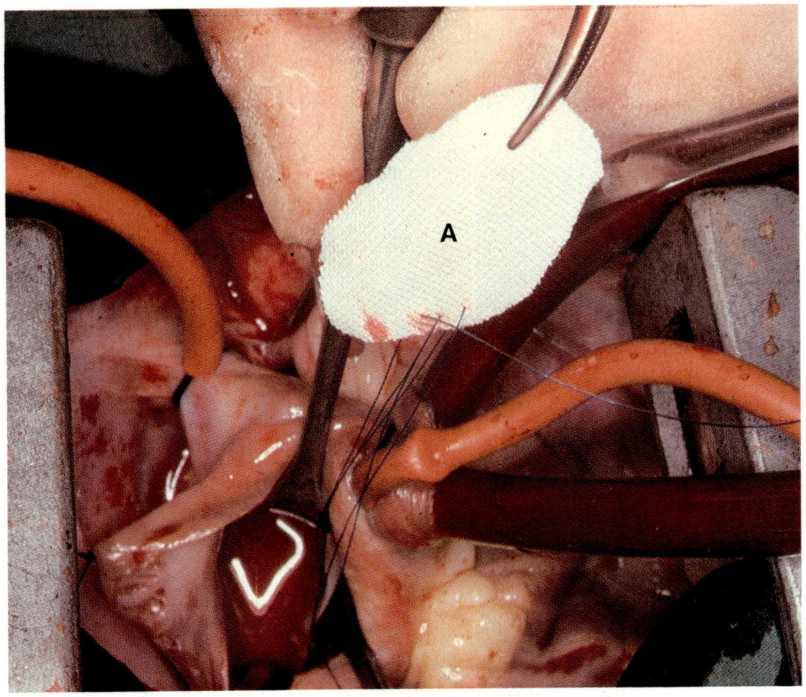

15

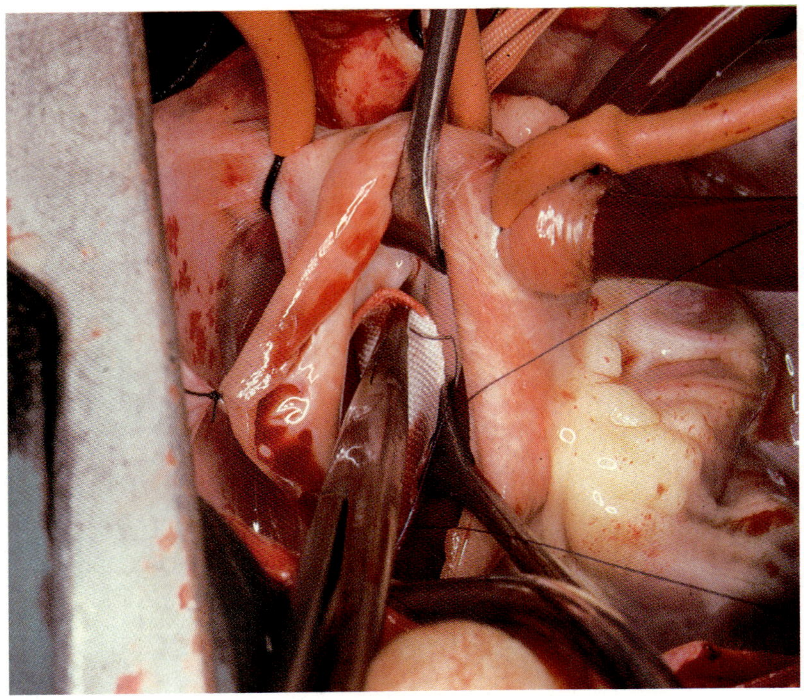

14 The defect is much too large to close directly without undue tension and therefore a dacron cloth patch (**A**) is used, although pericardium would also be very satisfactory. The patch is inserted with a continuous Prolene suture and three stitches have been placed into the lower margin of the defect before sliding the patch down.

15 The dacron patch has been lowered into position but before running the two ends of Prolene up from below, a separate suture is placed to secure the patch at the upper end of the defect.

16

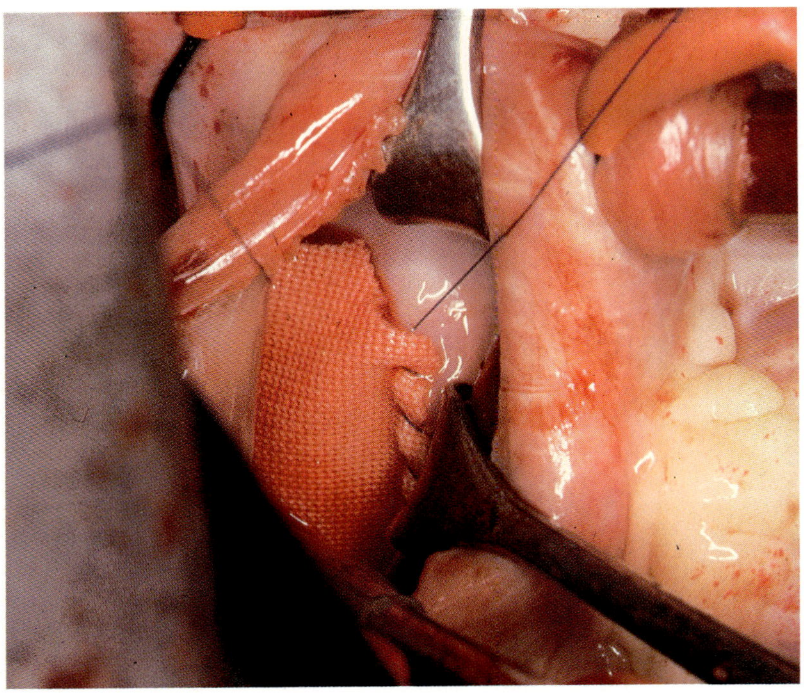

17

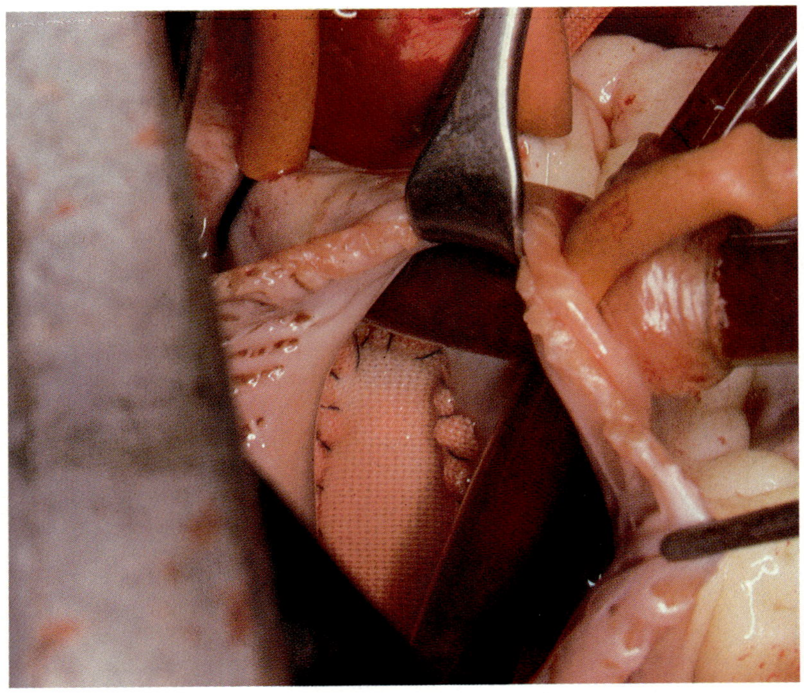

16 and 17 The remaining continuous sutures are then inserted and the patch can be seen securely closing the defect.

Closure of sinus venosus atrial septal defect with pericardial patch

18

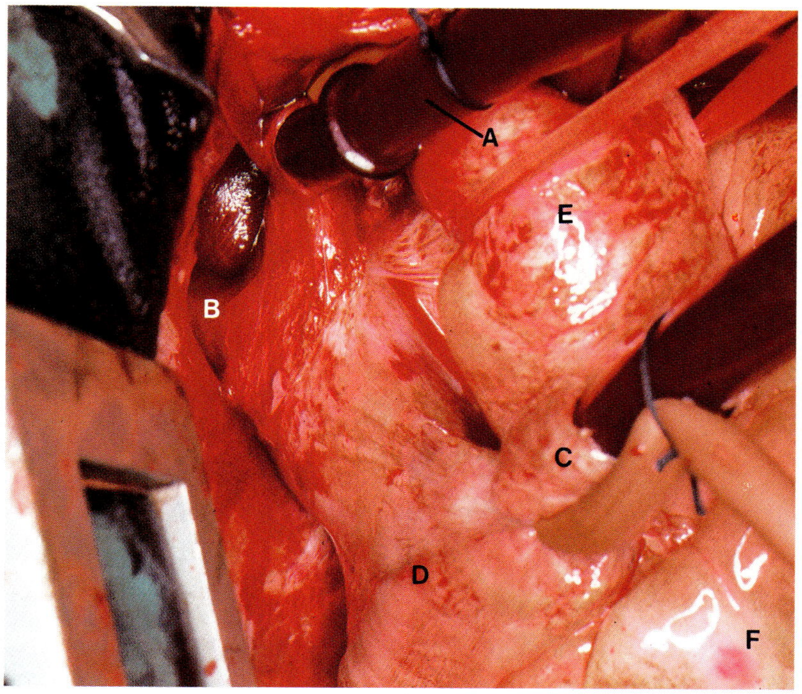

18 The superior vena caval cannula (**A**) has been placed directly into the superior vena cava, well above the entry of the right upper pulmonary vein (**B**). The inferior vena caval cannula is inserted through the atrial appendage (**C**). The right atrium (**D**), aorta (**E**) and right ventricle (**F**) can be seen.

19

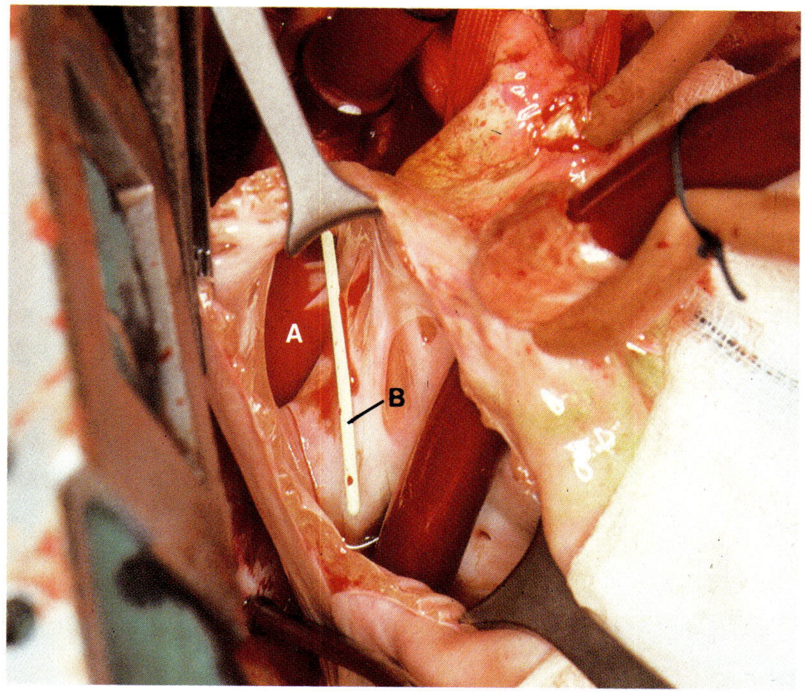

19 The right atrium has been opened and the defect (**A**) seen in the upper right part of the atrial septum. The central venous cannula (**B**), inserted percutaneously through the internal jugular vein by the anaesthetist, is seen lying in the middle of the right atrium.

20

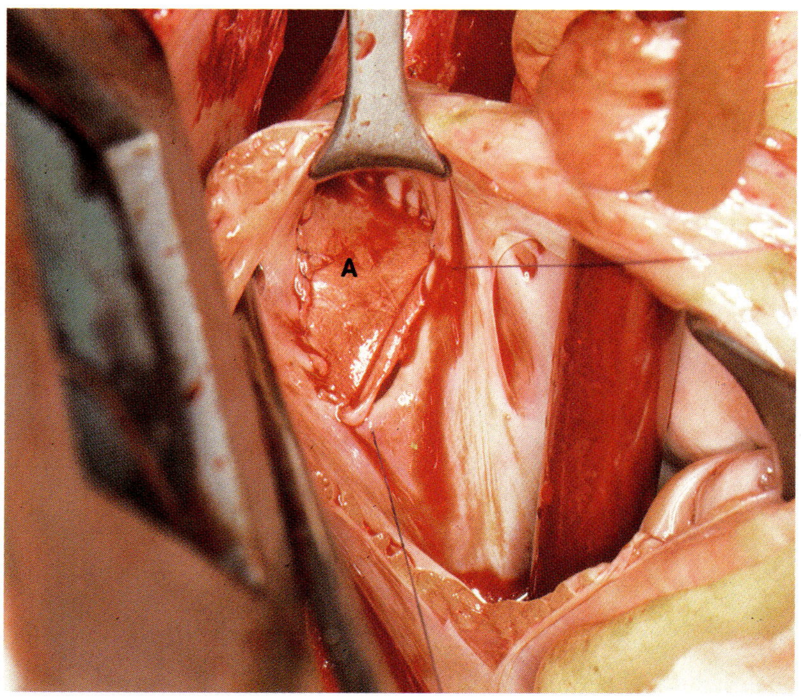

21

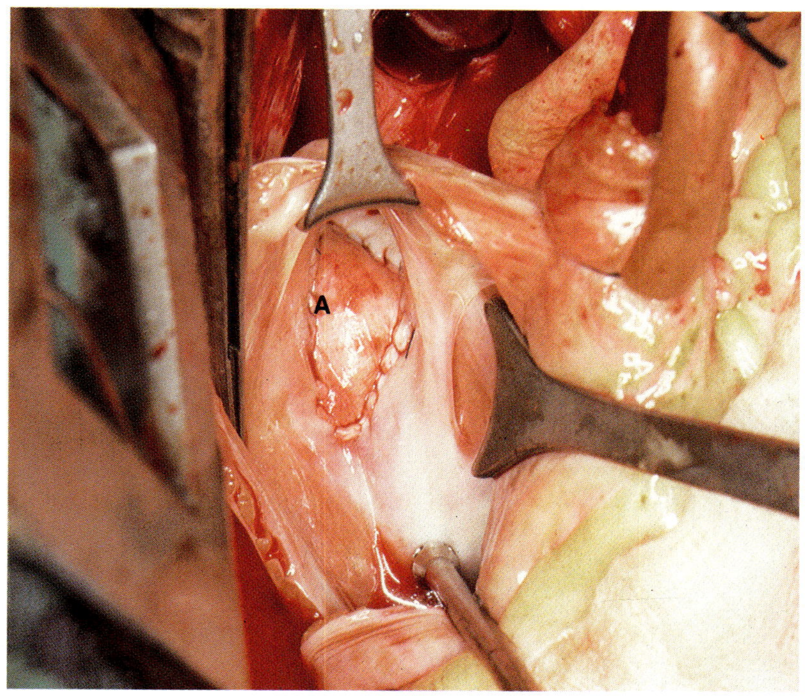

20 and 21 The high defect is closed with a pericardial patch (**A**) using continuous Prolene. Care must be taken at the upper end of the defect not to compromise the superior vena cava or upper pulmonary vein. It is for this reason that a patch is needed and it is much easier with the superior vena caval cannula well above this region.

10: Repair of atrioventricular canal defects

This chapter is divided into two parts, first the repair of the partial atrioventricular defect, or ostium primum defect, and secondly the complete atrioventricular defect. These are difficult lesions to deal with and have been the subject of continuing discussion and advance. In both types of defect, the atrioventricular valves fail to develop normally as well as the atrial and ventricular septa. The partial defect (diagram **A**) results from a failure of the septum primum to descend adequately and meet the endocardial cushions. This results in a low defect just above the atrioventricular valves. There is a cleft in the 'anterior' leaflet of the mitral valve always associated with the atrial septal defect.

In the complete defect (diagram **B**) page 92, the ventricular septum also fails to meet the endocardial cushions when developing, and this results in a ventricular septal defect as well as an atrial septal defect and marked valve abnormality. Components of both the mitral and tricuspid valves join to form anterior and posterior bridging leaflets. Rastelli[1] described three main types, depending on whether the anterior bridging leaflet was divided and on its attachments to the ventricular septum.

Repair of the mitral valve is most crucial to the success of the operation and Carpentier[2] has contributed greatly to the understanding of the unusual anatomy of the mitral valve in this condition and its repair as a tri-leaflet rather than bi-leaflet structure. This applies to both forms of atrioventricular defect, but late mitral regurgitation remains a formidable problem.

In repairing a partial defect, the right atrium is opened and the mitral valve assessed and repaired through the atrial septal defect. The atrial septal defect must always be closed with a patch, and pericardium is the most convenient material to use. However, the conduction mechanism of the heart must be guarded and the author's preference is to take the patch along the base of the tricuspid leaflet and well around the atrioventricular node. However, it is possible to place the sutures into the base of the mitral leaflet tissue.

When repairing a complete defect, again the right atrium is opened and the anatomy assessed. The anterior bridging leaflet may or may not be cleft and its attachment to the septum is variable. It is usual to first approximate the centre of the anterior and posterior bridging leaflets to assess the mitral valve. Traditionally, if the anterior bridging leaflet was intact, it would be divided so as to allow closure of the ventricular component of the defect with a dacron patch and re-attachment of the valve tissue at an appropriate level to the patch. The atrial component of the defect would then be closed with the same patch, as described in this chapter. However, as many of the patients requiring correction of this difficult defect are in the first year of life, tissues are friable and avoidance of division of the anterior bridging leaflet is an advantage. It is therefore probably better to close the ventricular component with a dacron patch and, again, great care must be taken to avoid the conduction tissue. The atrial component is then closed with pericardium as for a partial defect and, by attaching this tissue along the centre of the repair, it reinforces the sutures used to fix the dacron to the valve leaflets.

The mitral valve can be tested for competence before the atrial defect is closed and extra sutures placed as necessary. However, the difficulty in achieving lasting mitral competence, particularly in the presence of deficient valve tissue, the complexity of the remaining repair with what is often poor tissue and the avoidance of damage to the conduction mechanism, make this one of the most challenging lesions to correct.

Cardiopulmonary bypass is used with two venous cannulae.

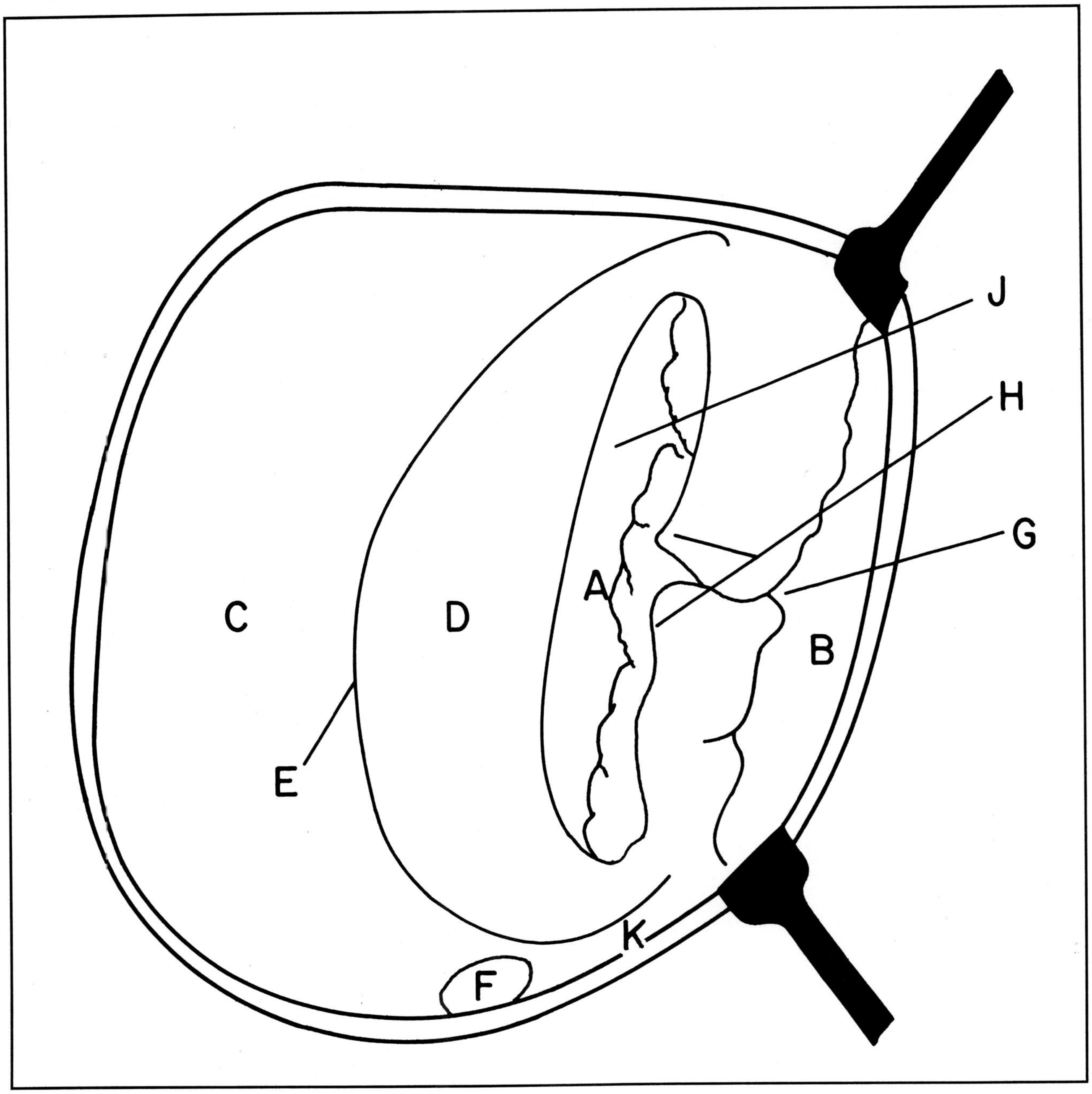

Diagram A – Partial atrioventricular canal defect

A – Mitral valve orifice

B – Tricuspid valve orifice

C – Atrial septum

D – Posterior wall of left atrium

E – Margin of ostium primum defect

F – Coronary sinus

G – Interventricular septum

H – Cleft 'anterior' leaflet of mitral valve

J – Posterior leaflet of mitral valve

K – Position of atrioventricular node

Partial atrioventricular defect

1

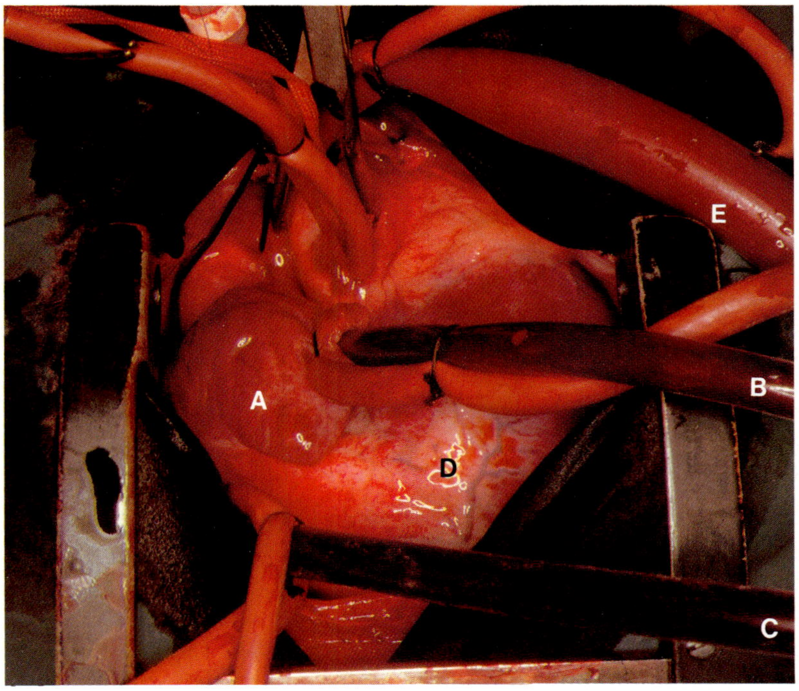

1 This overall view of the heart shows the right atrial appendage (**A**) with the superior vena caval cannula (**B**) inserted into it. The inferior vena caval cannula (**C**), right ventricle (**D**) and aortic cannula (**E**) are shown.

2

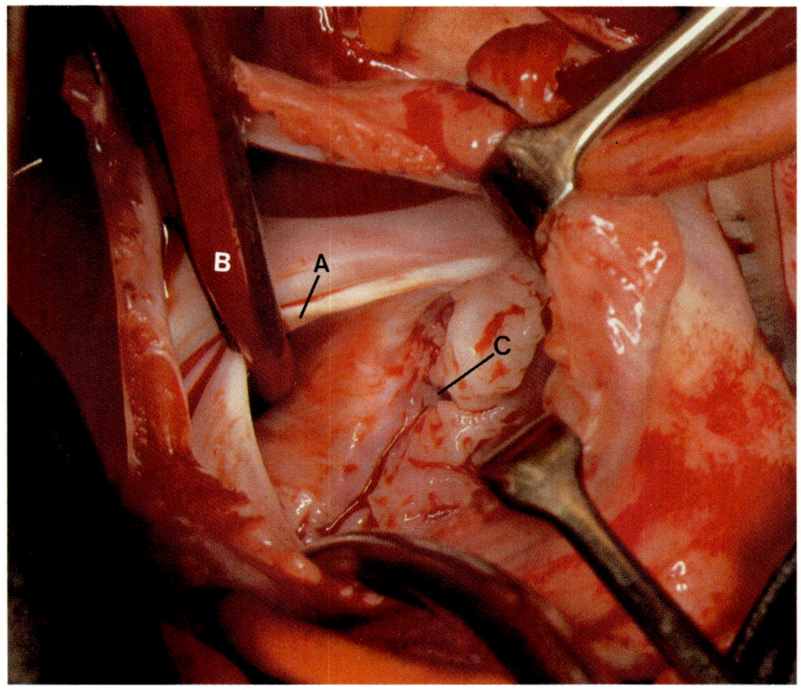

2 The right atrium has been widely opened and retracted. The crescentic upper margin of the defect (**A**) is being partially retracted by a suction tube (**B**) placed into the left atrium. The cleft (**C**) in the 'anterior' leaflet of the mitral valve and other features are seen as illustrated in diagram **A.**

3

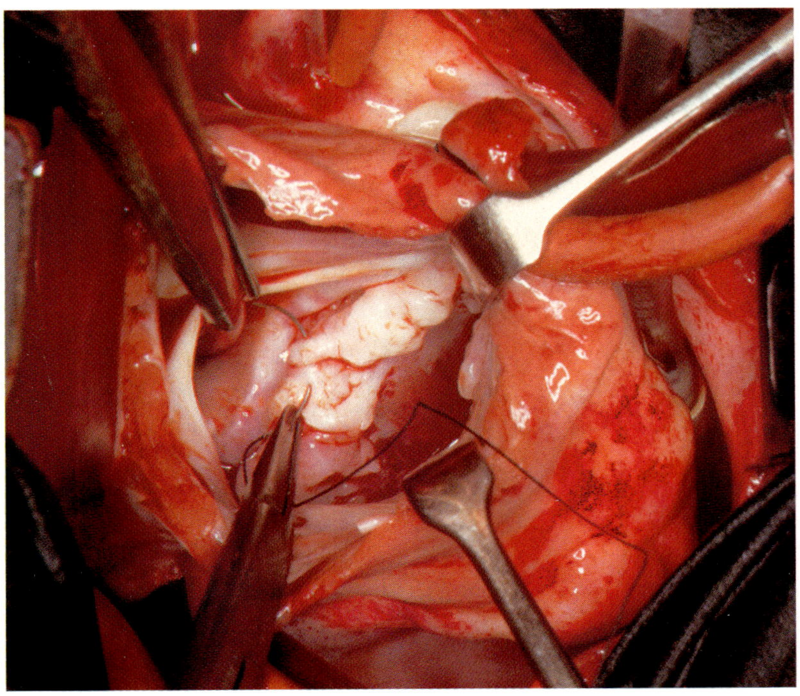

4

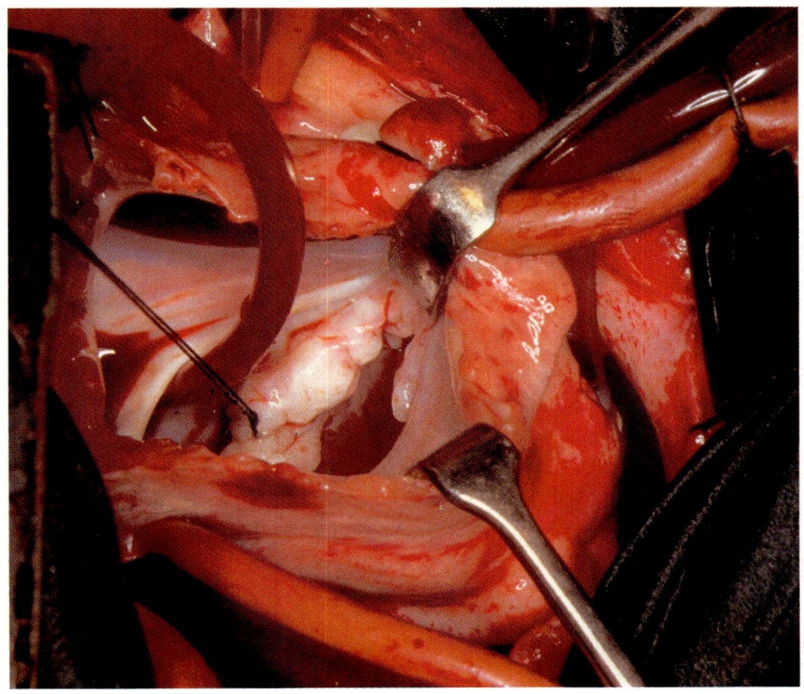

3 and 4 A suture has been placed so as to bring together the opposing surfaces of the anterior mitral valve leaflet either side of the cleft.

5

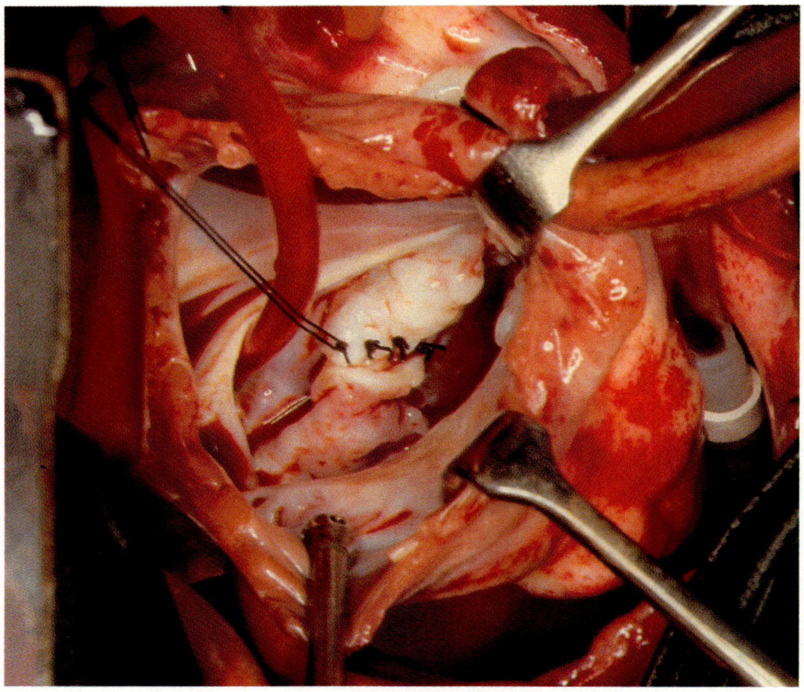

6

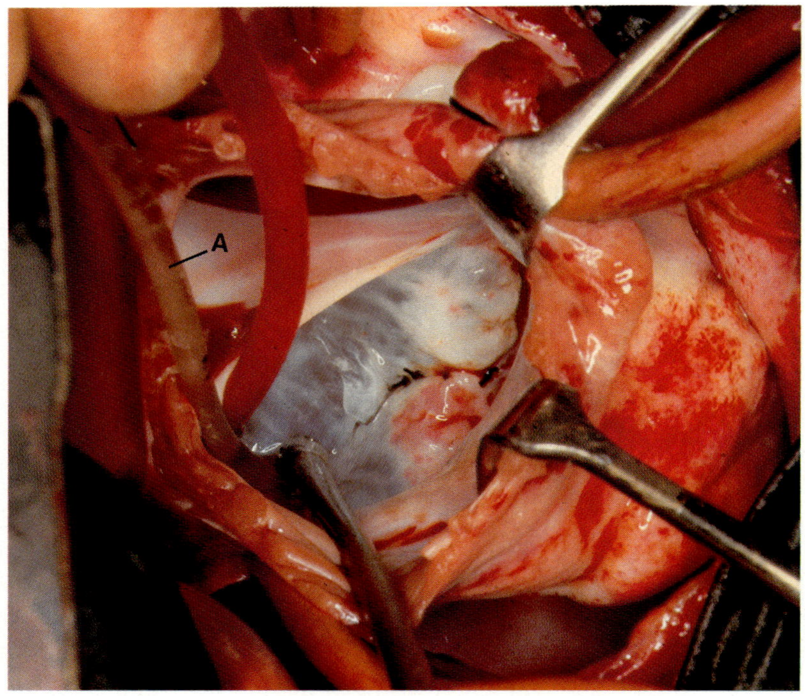

5 The cleft in the anterior leaflet of the mitral valve has been closed with interrupted silk sutures. However, it is often better to only approximate the two parts of the anterior leaflet of the mitral valve at the proximal end of the cleft.

6 Clear fluid is being injected through a tube (**A**) into the left ventricle to distend the mitral valve and test it for competence.

7

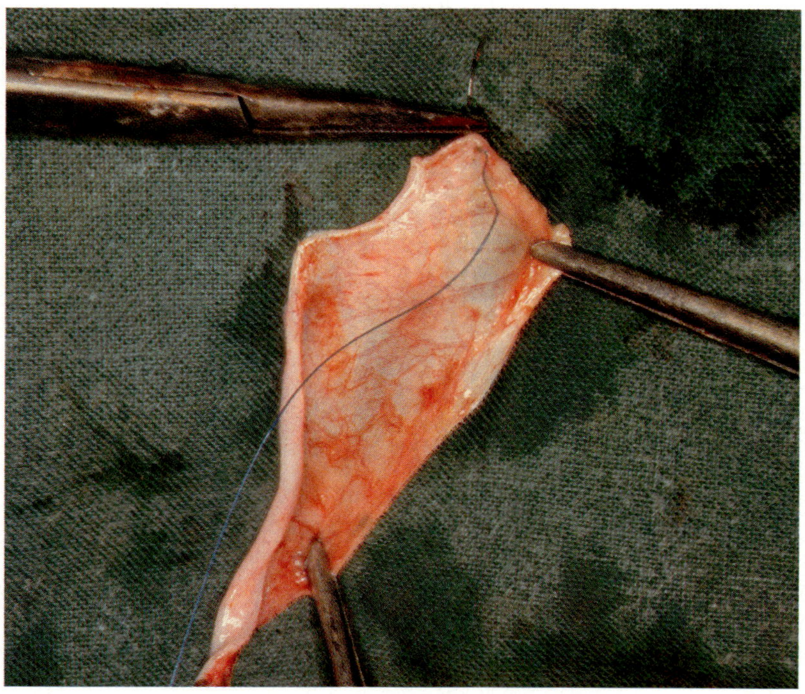

8

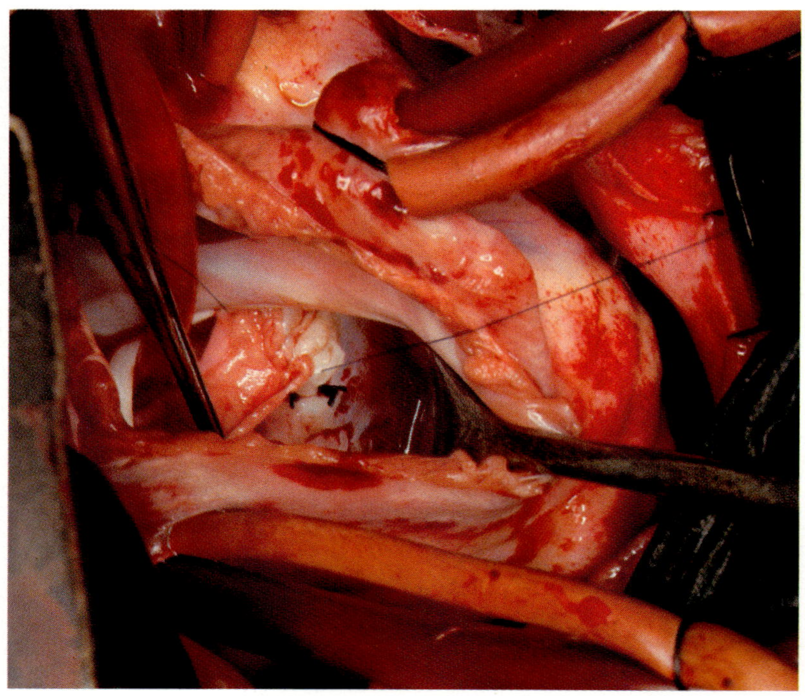

7 and 8 The atrial septal defect is now closed with a pericardial patch. The first suture is placed in the edge of the patch which is then lowered down into the atrium and the continuous suture started at the upper border of the defect where it joins the tricuspid valve and working in a clockwise direction.

9

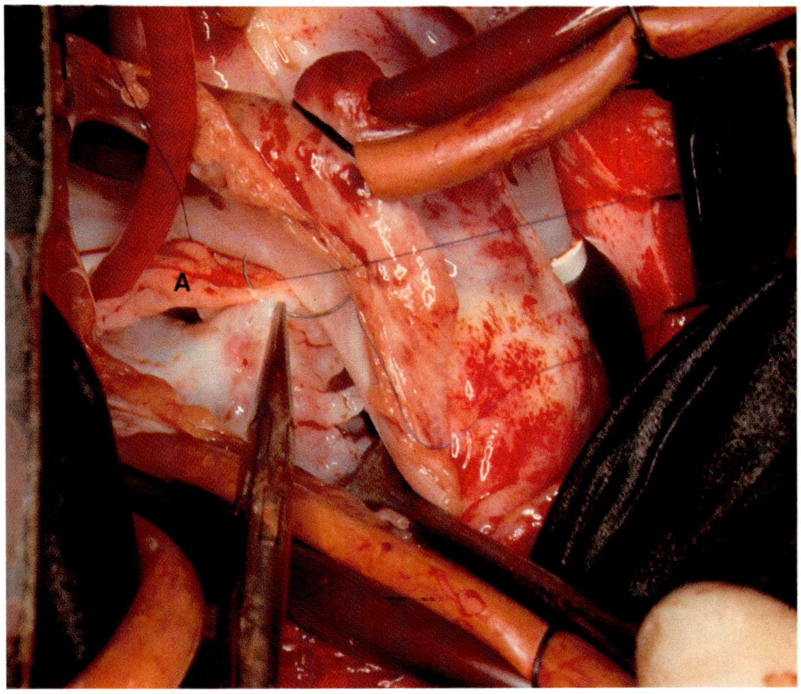

10

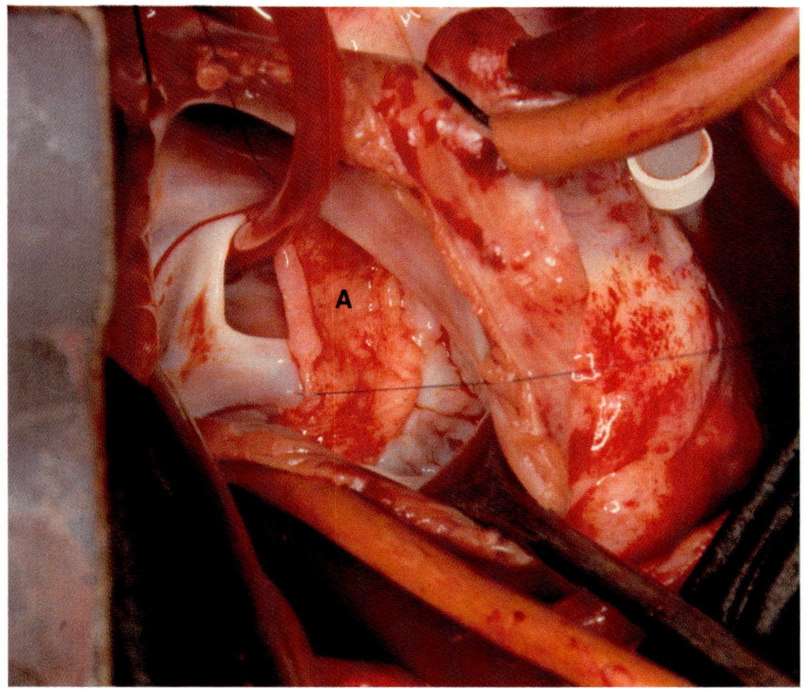

9 and 10 The pericardial patch (**A**) is sutured to the base of the tricuspid valve leaflets and the line of attachment continued well around the atrioventricular node and into the tip of the coronary sinus. It is also possible to suture the patch around the coronary sinus leaving it draining into the left atrium.

11

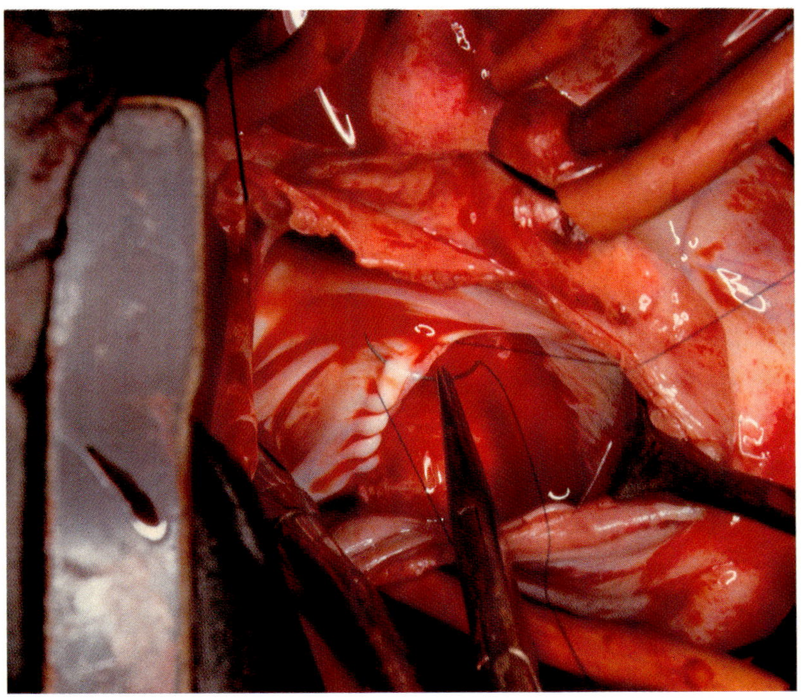

12

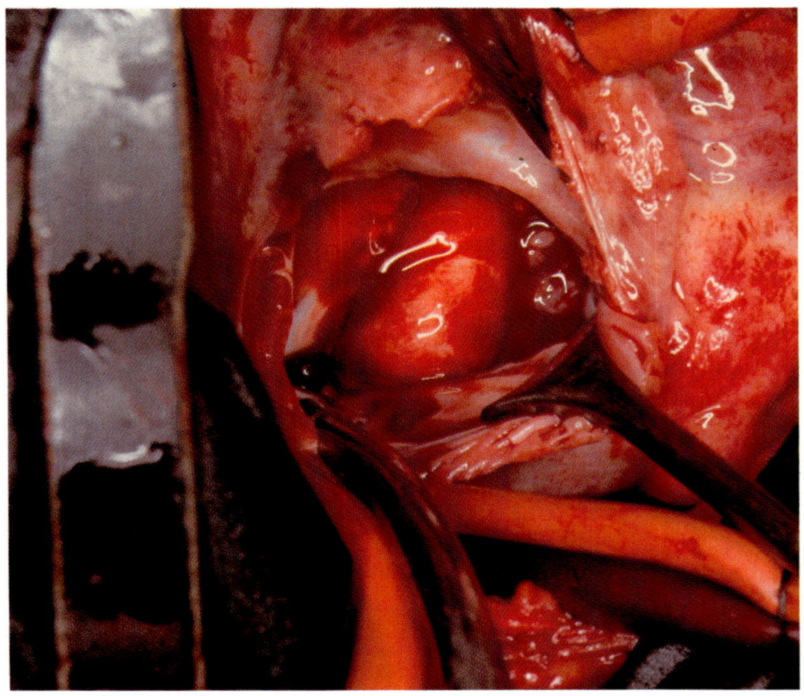

11 and 12 The final sutures are placed and the defect completely closed by a pericardial patch.

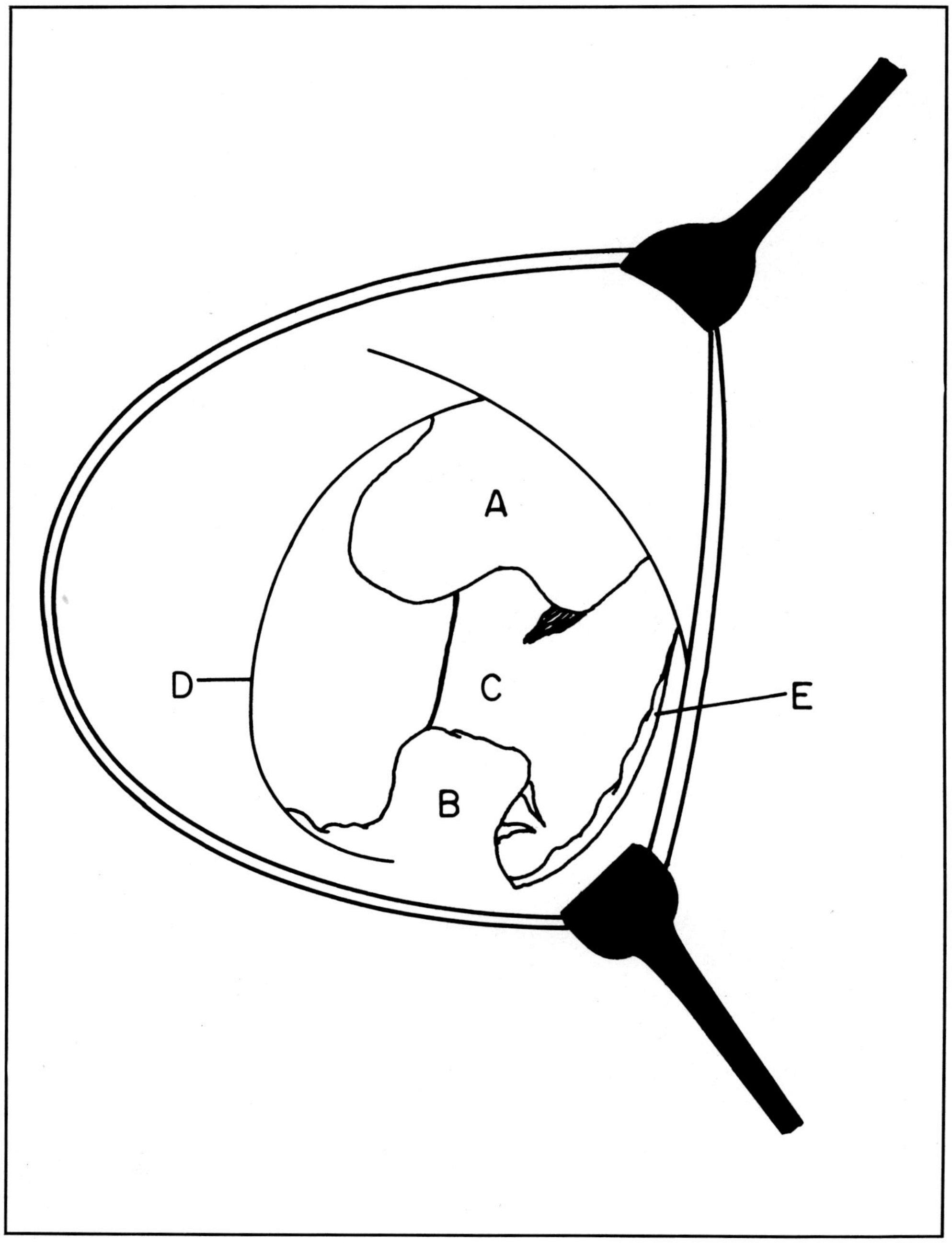

Diagram B – Complete atrioventricular canal defect

A – Anterior bridging leaflet

B – Posterior bridging leaflet

C – Ventricular septum

D – Lower margin of atrial septum

E – Anterior part of tricuspid valve ring

Complete atrioventricular defect

13

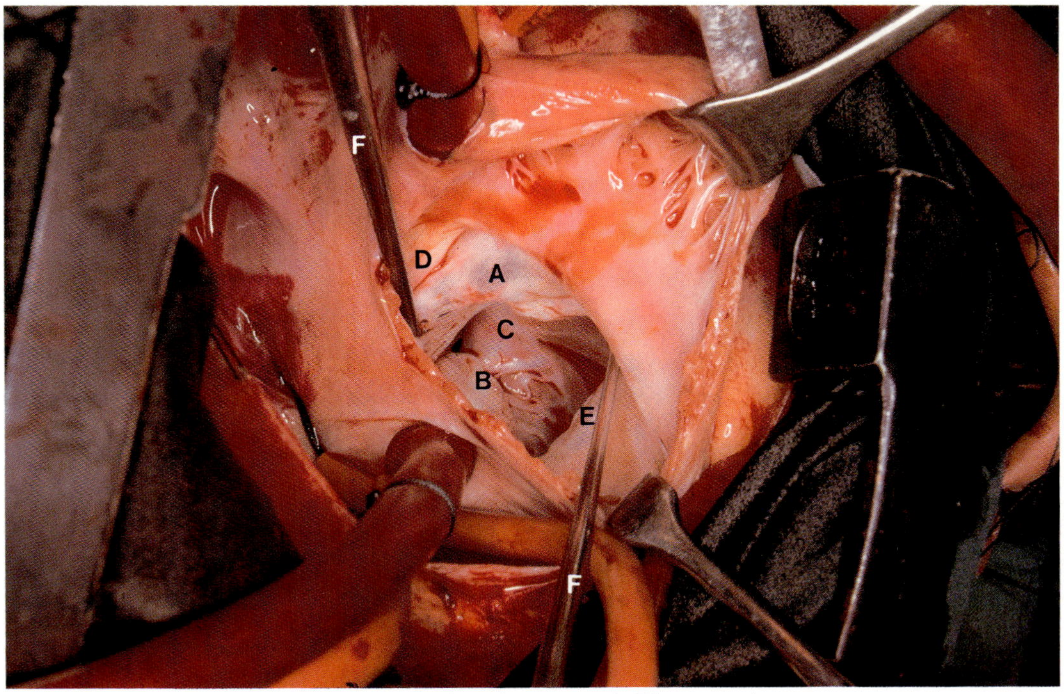

13 The right atrium has been opened and retracted. The anterior bridging leaflet (**A**) and posterior bridging leaflet (**B**) are widely separated showing the thick muscular ventricular septum (**C**) beneath. The crescentic lower edge of the atrial septum (**D**) and anterior part of the tricuspid valve ring (**E**) are shown as in diagram **B**. The anterior bridging leaflet has been spread out by fine hooks (**F**).

14

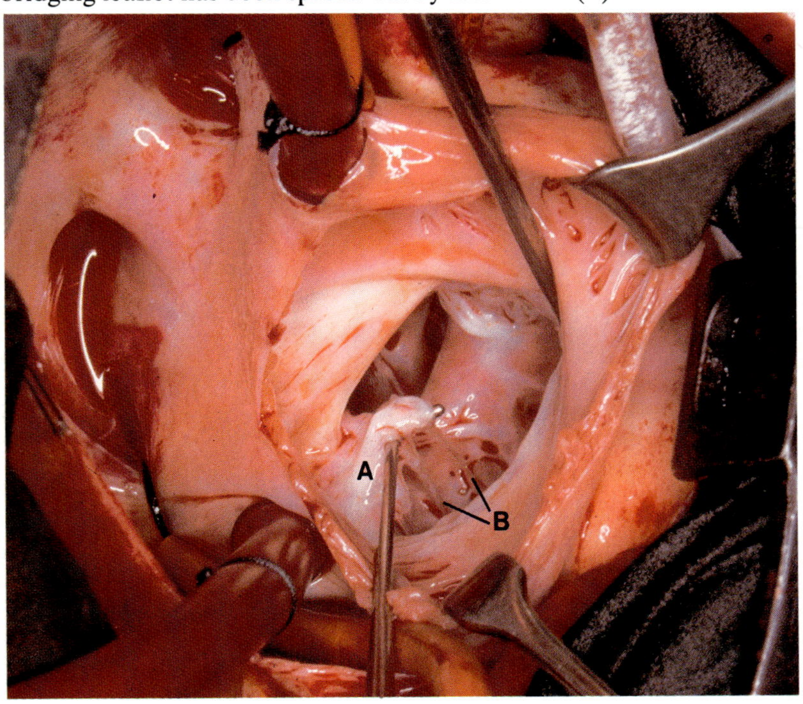

14 The anterior bridging leaflet has been released and the posterior bridging leaflet (**A**) has been hooked forward, showing the chordae (**B**).

15

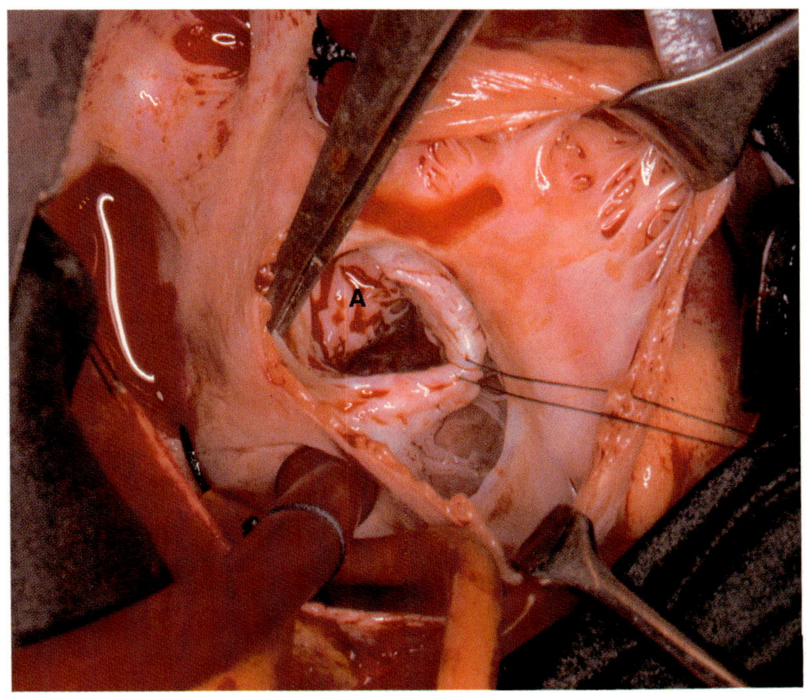

15 The anterior and posterior bridging leaflets have been approximated with a suture. The posterior leaflet (**A**) of the mitral valve can also be seen.

16

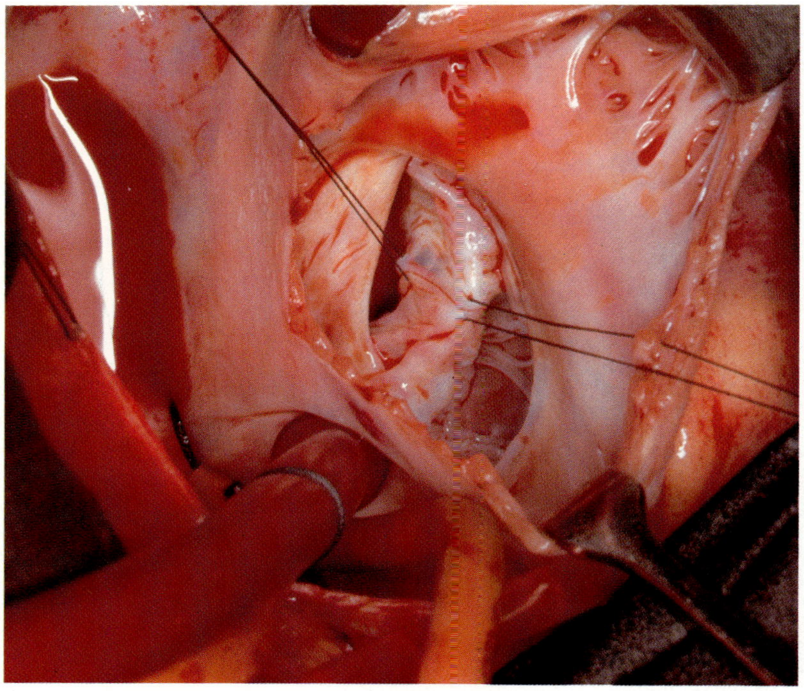

17

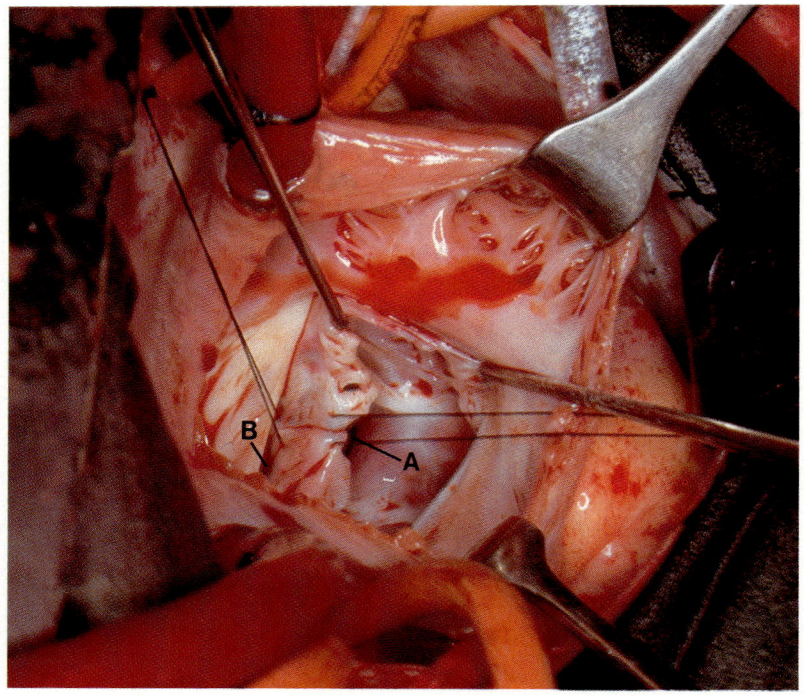

16 and 17 A second suture has been placed to demonstrate adequate mitral leaflet tissue. When the approximated leaflets are pulled up, it can be seen that the ventricular component of the defect **(A)**is large, but the atrial component relatively small **(B)**.

18

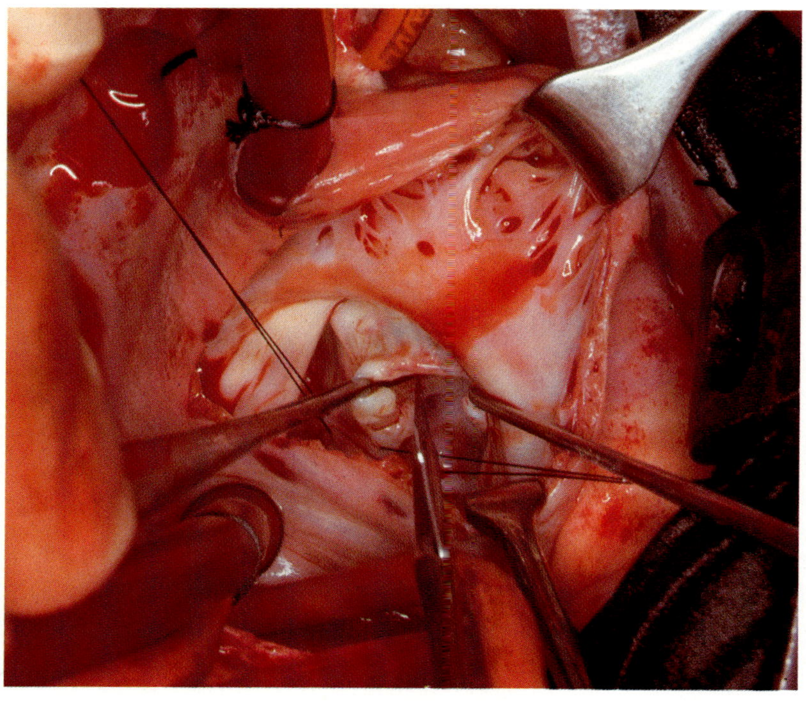

19

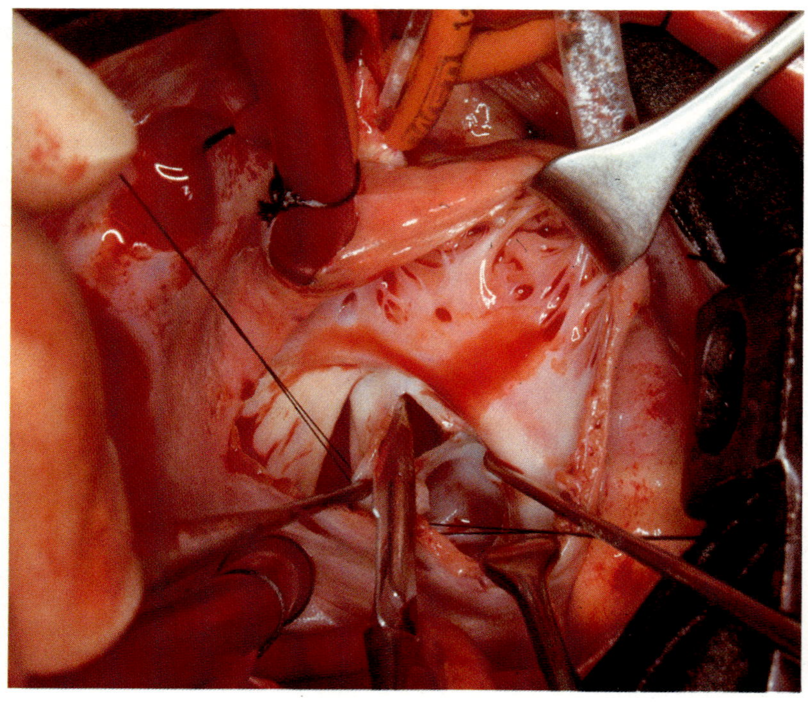

18 and 19 The anterior bridging leaflet is incised to divide it into its mitral and tricuspid components. This must be done in the traditional repair when a single patch is used, but particularly in infants, where the tissue is rather thin, the anterior bridging leaflet may be left intact and a separate patch used to close the ventricular and atrial components of the defect.

20

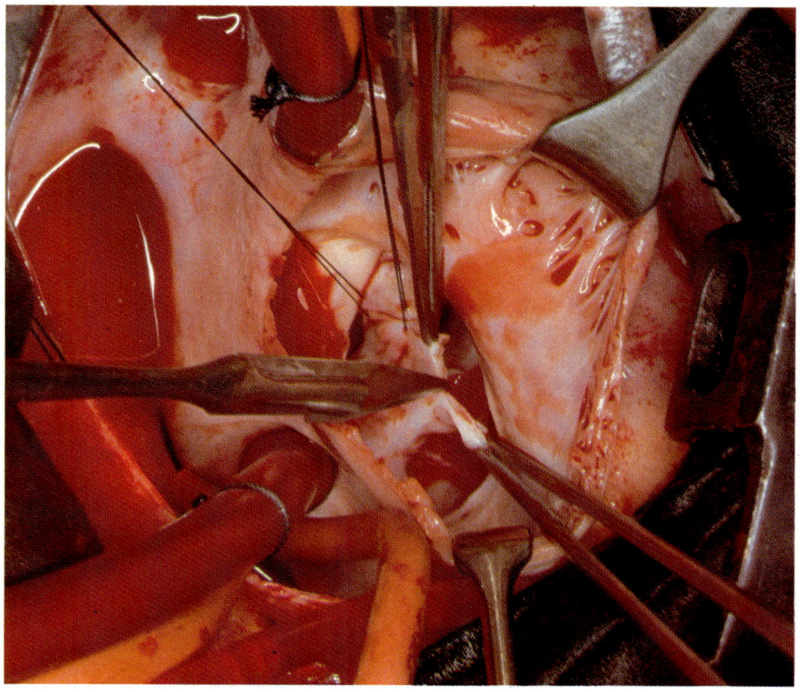

21

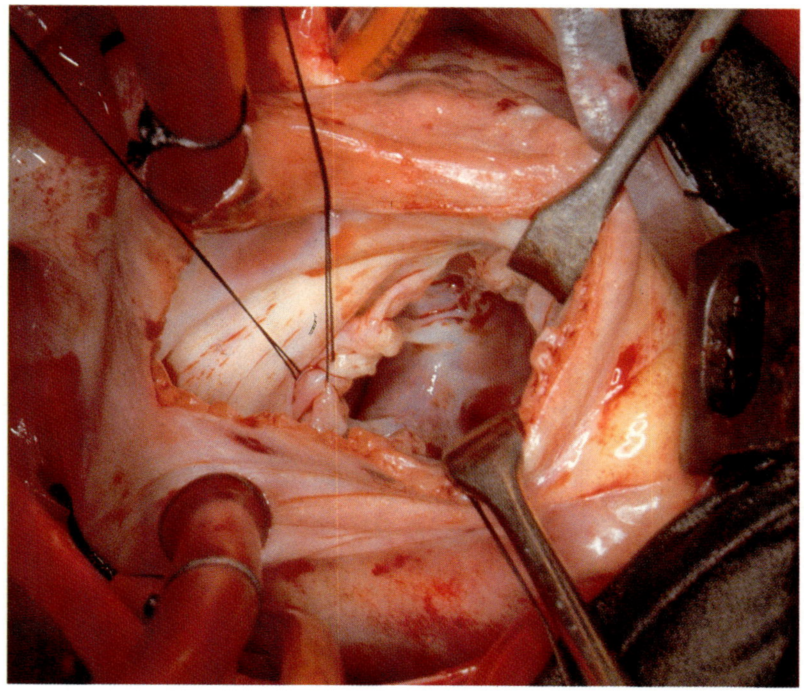

20 The posterior bridging leaflet is also incised.

21 With both the anterior and posterior bridging leaflets divided, an extensive view of the crest of the ventricular septum is achieved in preparation for patch insertion.

22

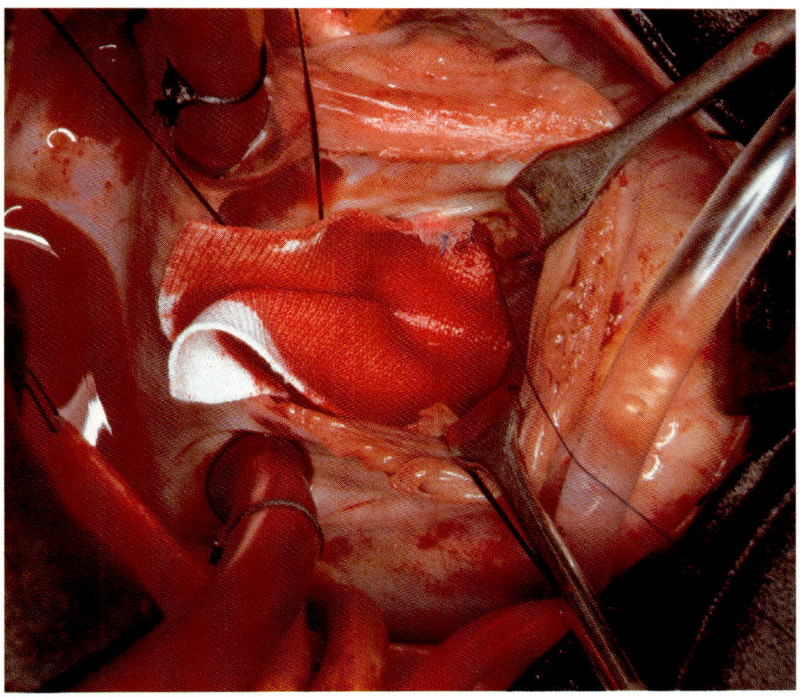

23

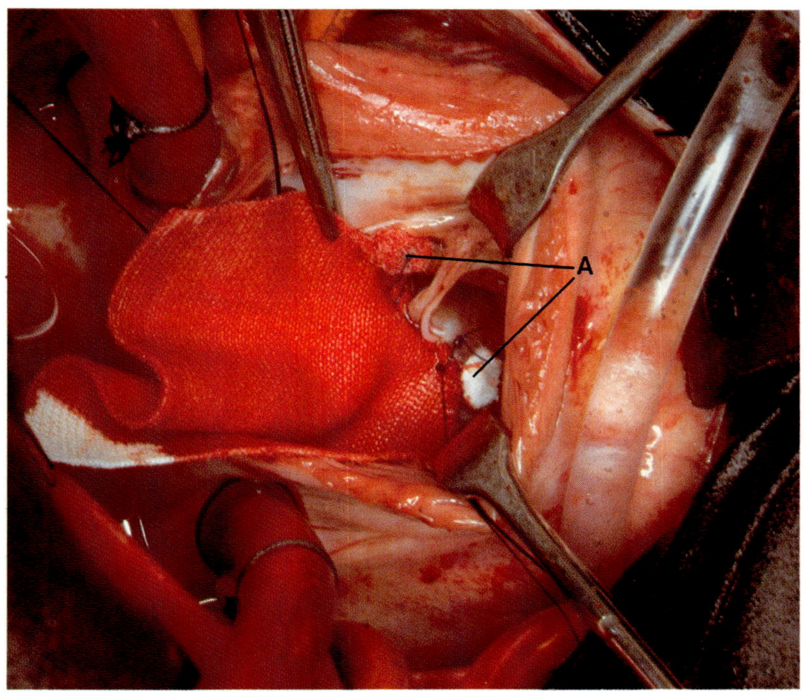

22 and 23 The dacron cloth patch is sutured to the crest of the ventricular septum starting anteriorly using continuous Prolene sutures. Two extra sutures on pledgets of teflon felt (**A**) have been inserted for extra strength.

24

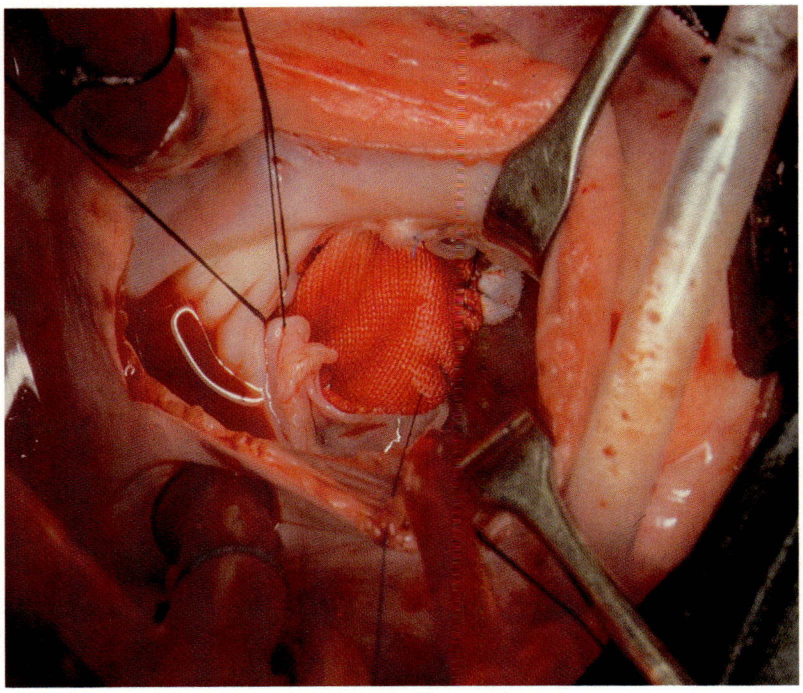

25

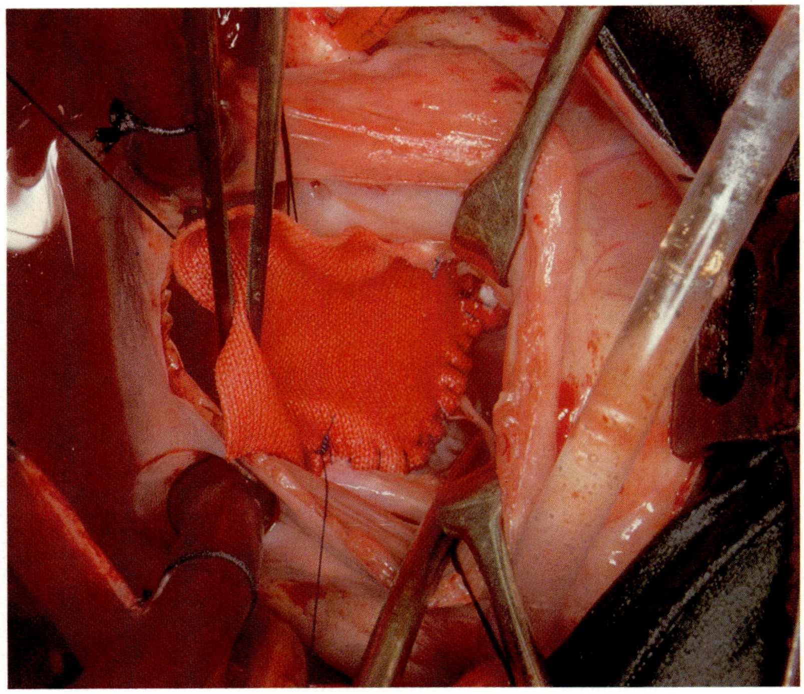

24 and 25 From the mid-point of the crest of the ventricular septum back, care is taken to insert the sutures on the right side of the septum, as if sutures are placed through the crest of the septum or left side, the conduction mechanism might be damaged.

26

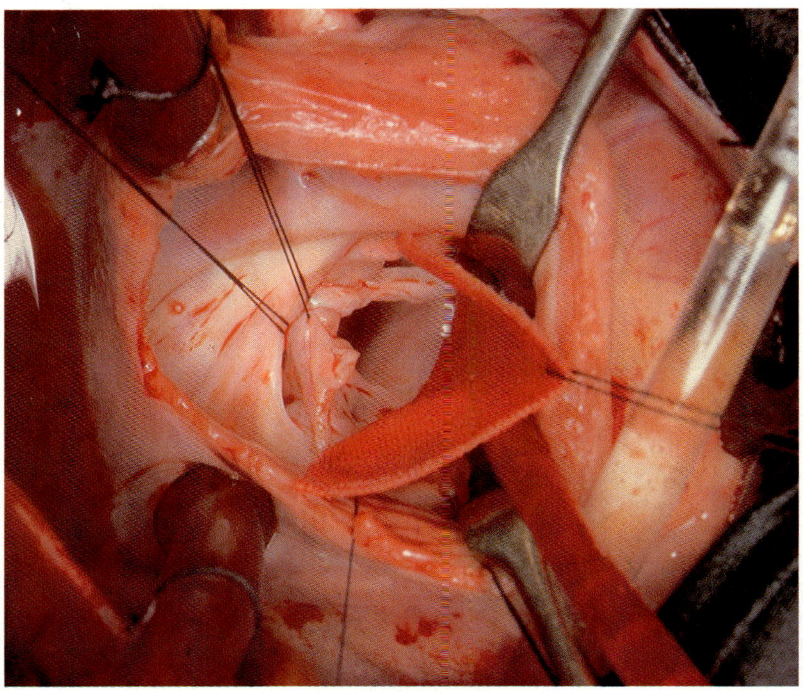

27

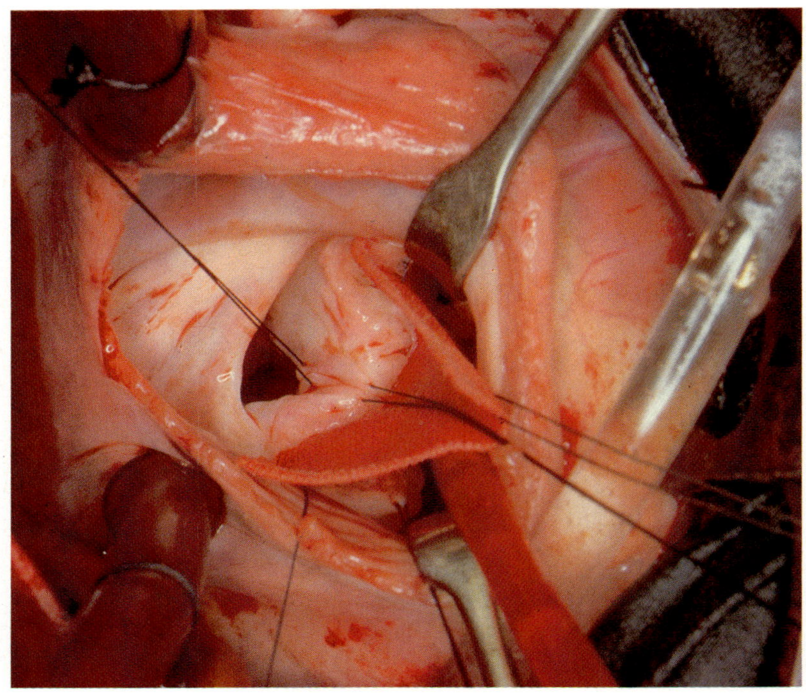

26 and 27 The view from the left side shows the dacron patch fixed to the ventricular septum and the mitral valve leaflets can be pulled up appropriately to judge where they should be resuspended and fixed to the dacron patch.

28

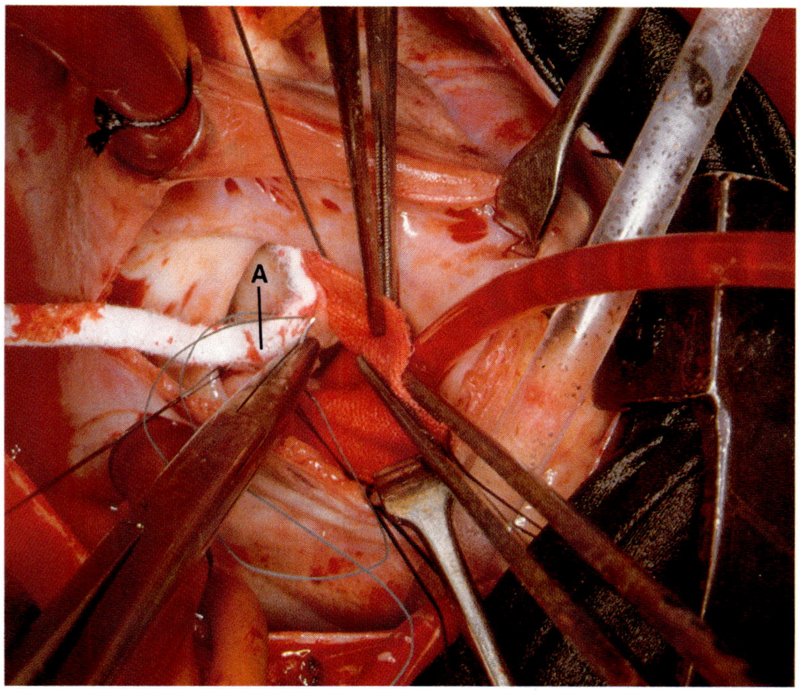

29

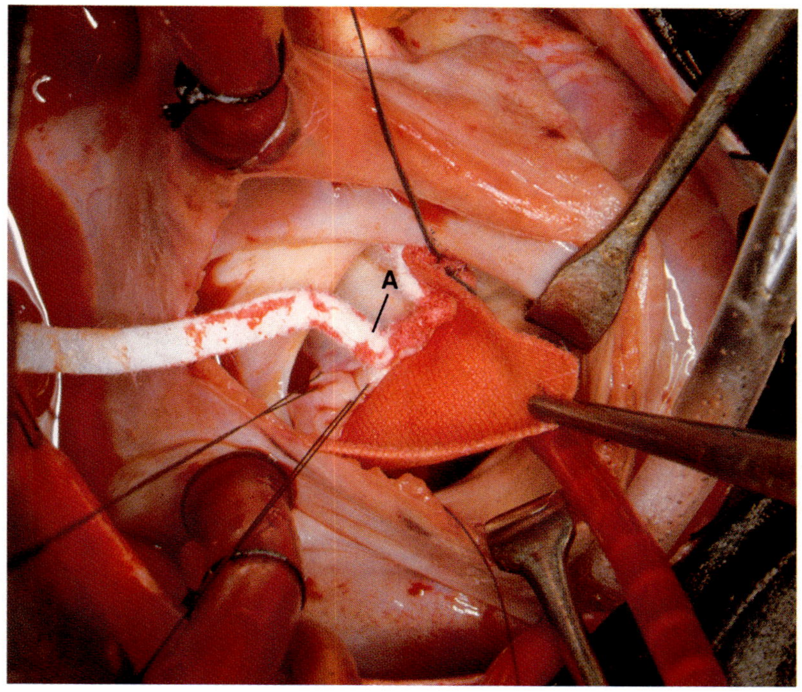

28 and 29 The mitral and tricuspid valve leaflets are sutured to the dacron patch at what is judged to be the correct level. In this case a strip of teflon felt (**A**) is being incorporated on the left side to reinforce the valve tissue.

30

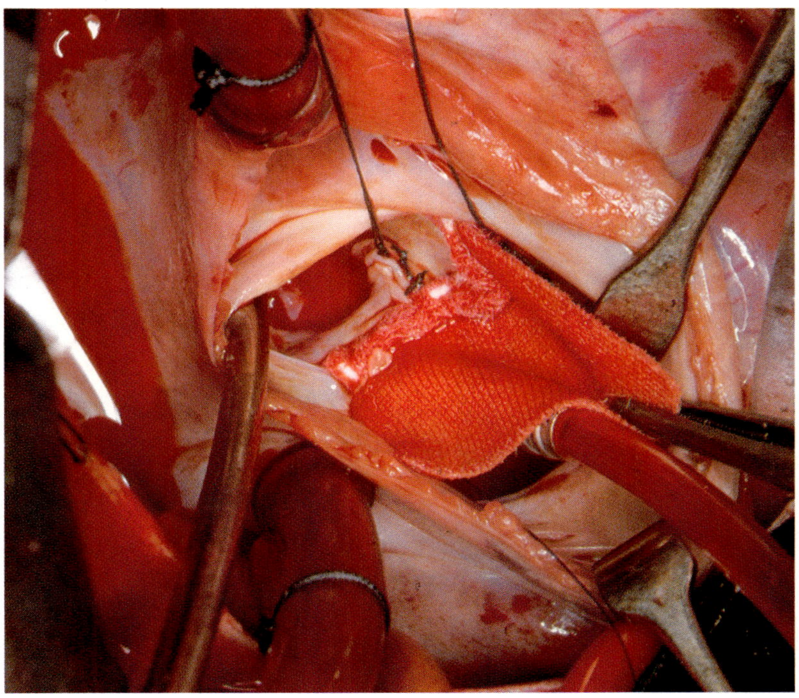

31

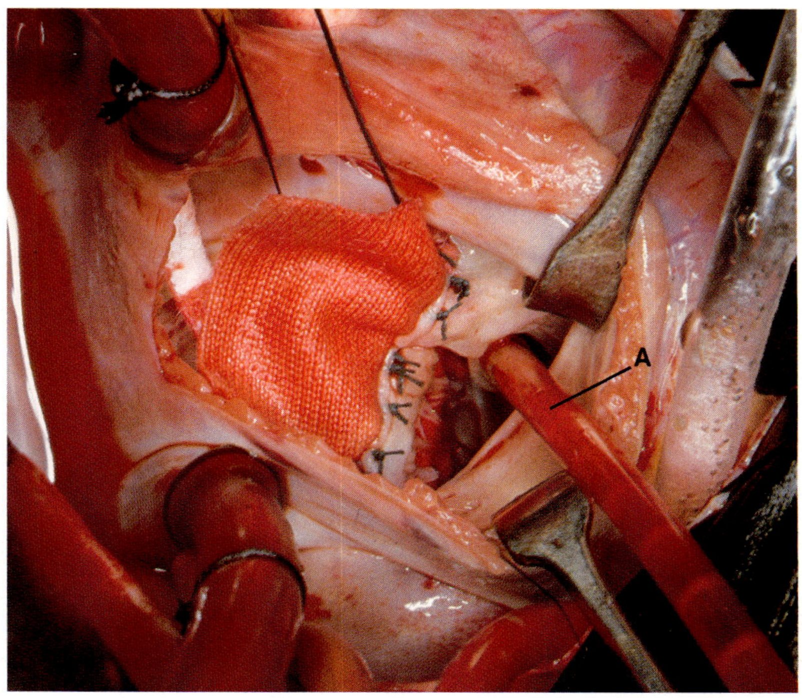

30 The final view from the left side shows the mitral valve 'anterior' leaflet reconstituted and attached to the new septum made of the dacron patch. The 'cleft' has also been closed with interrupted sutures. This is often not necessary and testing the valve helps the surgeon to decide.

31 The view from the right side shows the tricuspid valve attached to the dacron by interrupted sutures which have already been used to attach the mitral valve. A sucker (**A**) has been placed through the tricuspid valve orifice into the right ventricle.

32

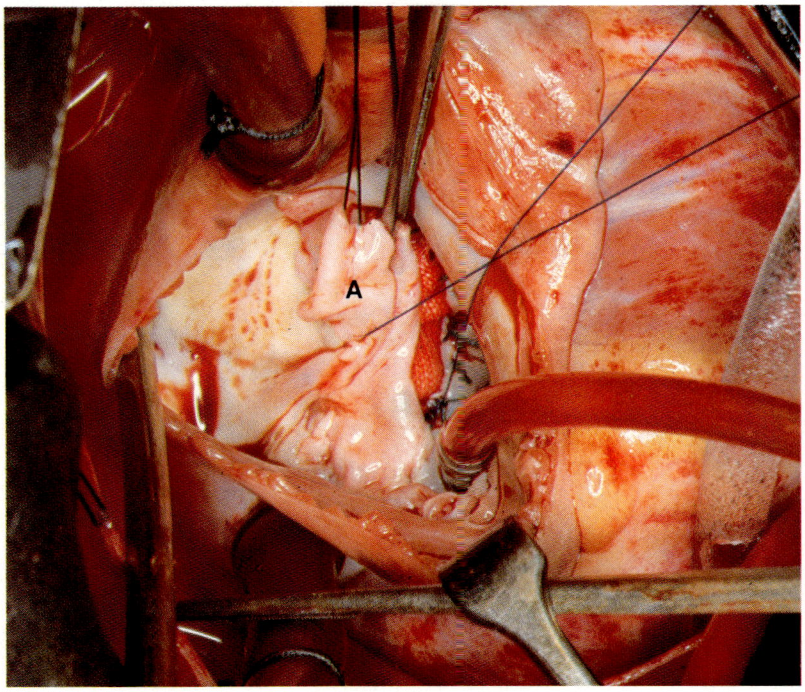

33

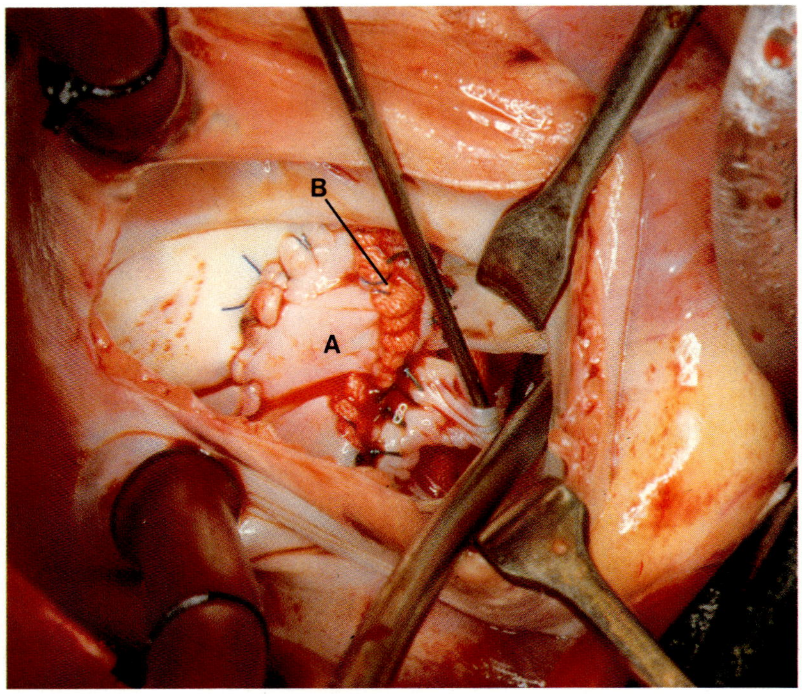

32 It would have been possible to close the atrial component of the defect with the remainder of the dacron patch. However, it was thought better in this case to use a separate piece of pericardium which is easier to suture around the region of the atrioventricular node, as for closure of a partial atrioventricular defect. The dacron has been cut just above the level of the valves and the pericardium (**A**) sutured to it.

33 The atrial component of the defect has now been completely closed by the pericardial patch (**A**). The rim of the dacron (**B**) remaining above the level of the valves can be seen and the new 'septal' leaflet of the tricuspid valve is being held forward by a hook.

34

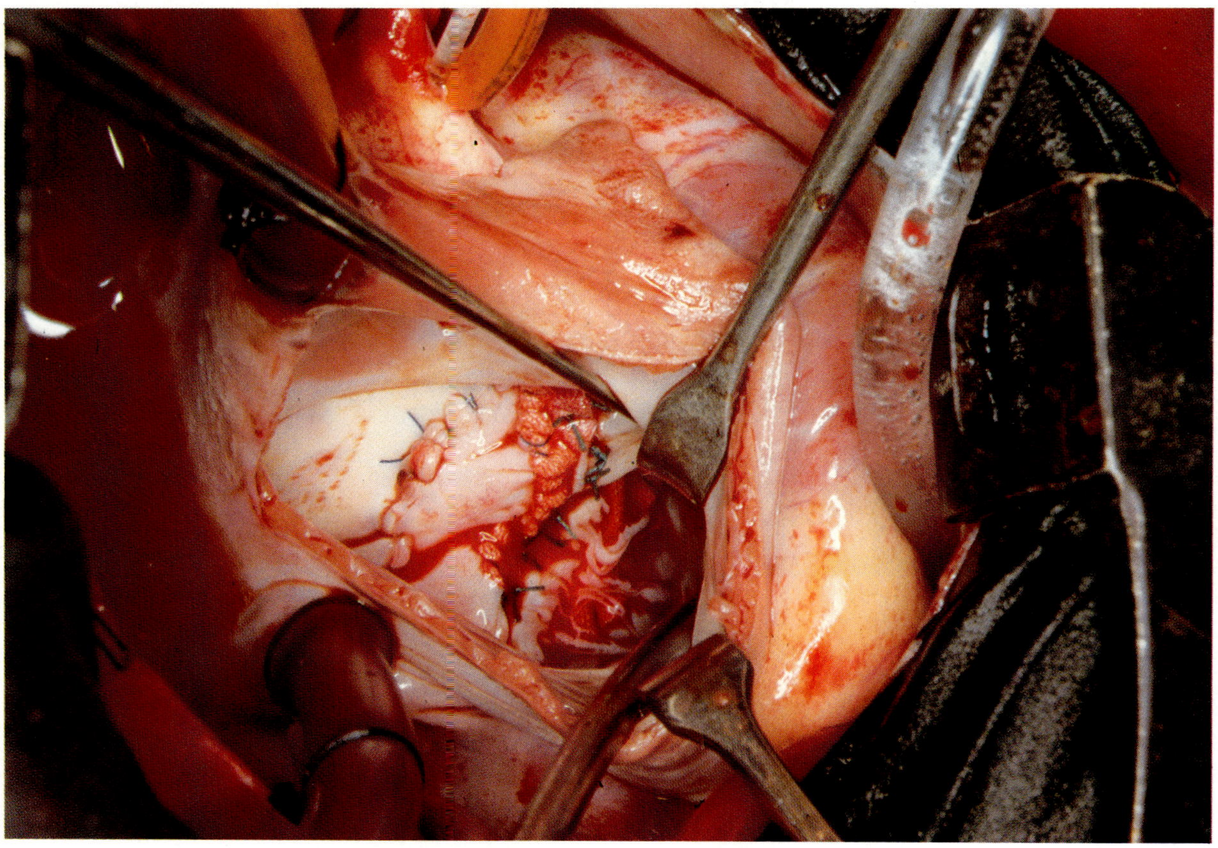

34 The final view of the repair is seen before closure of the right atrium.

11: Closure of ventricular septal defect

Ventricular septal defects can be single or multiple and situated in different positions in the ventricular septum as shown in diagram **A**. The approach for closure is most commonly through the right atrium and tricuspid valve which is particularly suitable for most perimembranous defects, and those in the inlet septum. Alternatively, the now less frequently used ventricular approach through the right ventricle gives good exposure for perimembranous defects and high subpulmonary defects. It is also possible to close sub-arterial defects through the pulmonary valve and apical defects are closed most effectively through an incision in the apex of the left ventricle.

Small defects can be closed by direct suture but most defects should be closed with a patch of some suitable material such as dacron cloth. Some surgeons use interrupted sutures for all or part of the closure, but the author's preference is for a continuous Prolene suture; this method is illustrated. However, the bundle of His runs very close to the inferior margin of perimembranous defects and sutures are placed into the base of the septal leaflet of the tricuspid valve so as to avoid this area and possible heart block.

Cardiopulmonary bypass is used with venous cannulae inserted into the superior and inferior vena cavae which are snugged.

Diagram A

- **A** – Sub-arterial ventricular septal defect
- **B** – Perimembranous ventricular septal defect
- **C** – Muscular ventricular septal defect
- **D** – Tricuspid valve ring
- **E** – Right atrium
- **F** – Aorta
- **G** – Pulmonary artery
- **H** – Inlet septum
- **J** – Outlet septum
- **K** – Trabecular septum

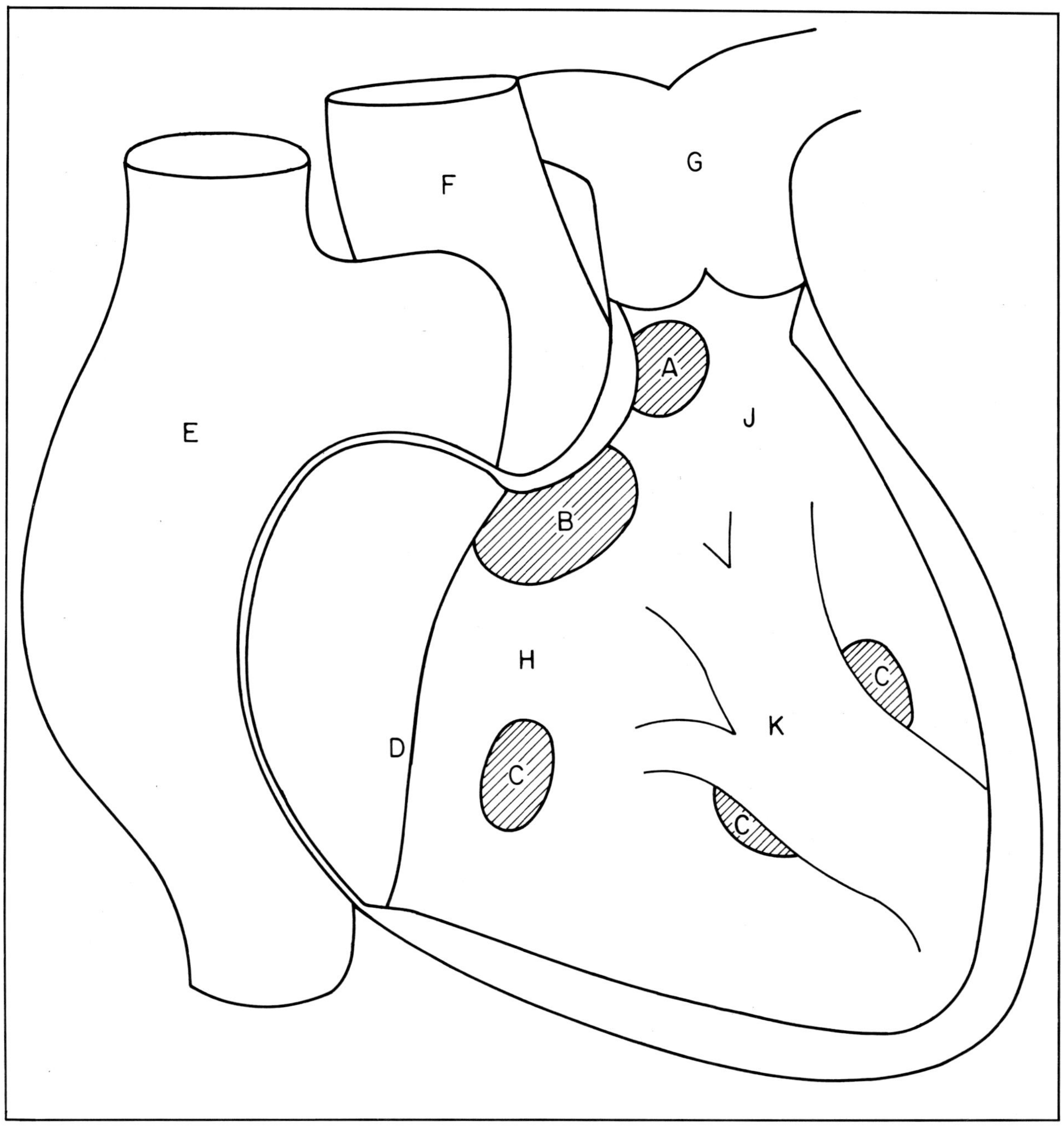

Transatrial approach – perimembranous defect

1

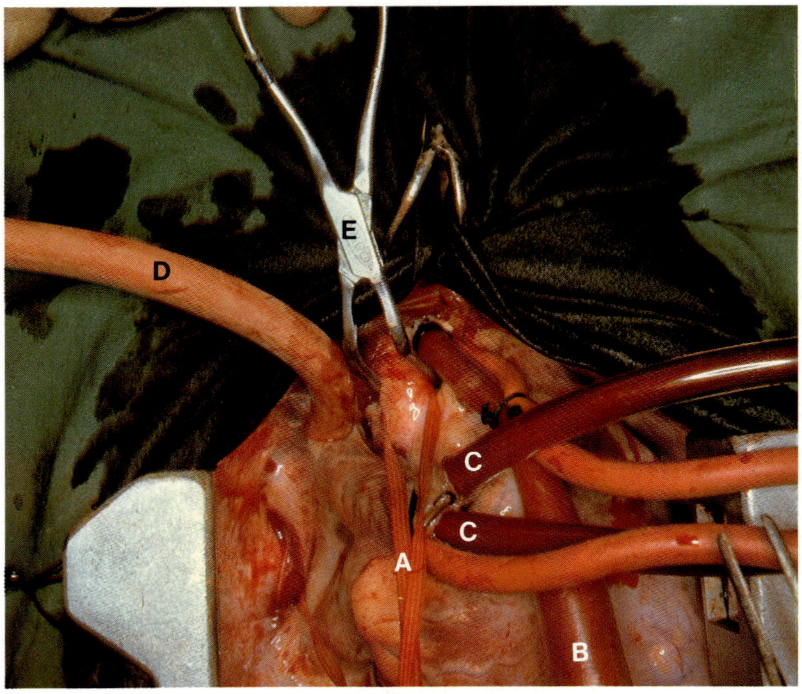

2

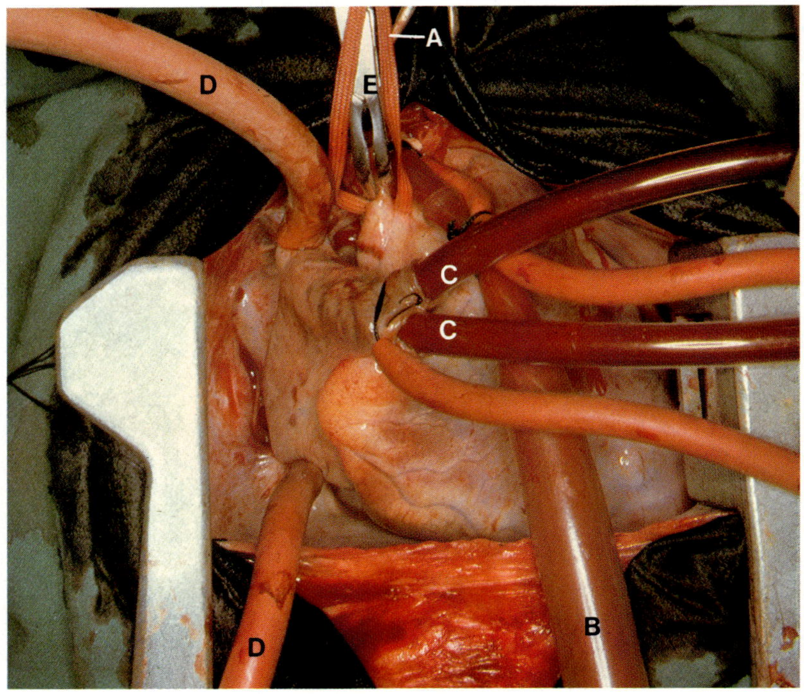

1 and 2 A tape **(A)** has been placed around the aorta and the aortic cannula **(B)** inserted. Two venous cannulae **(C)** have been inserted into the right atrial appendage and cardiopulmonary bypass commenced. The caval snuggers **(D)** have been tightened to occlude the cavae around the cannulae and the aortic cross-clamp is applied. **(E)**.

3

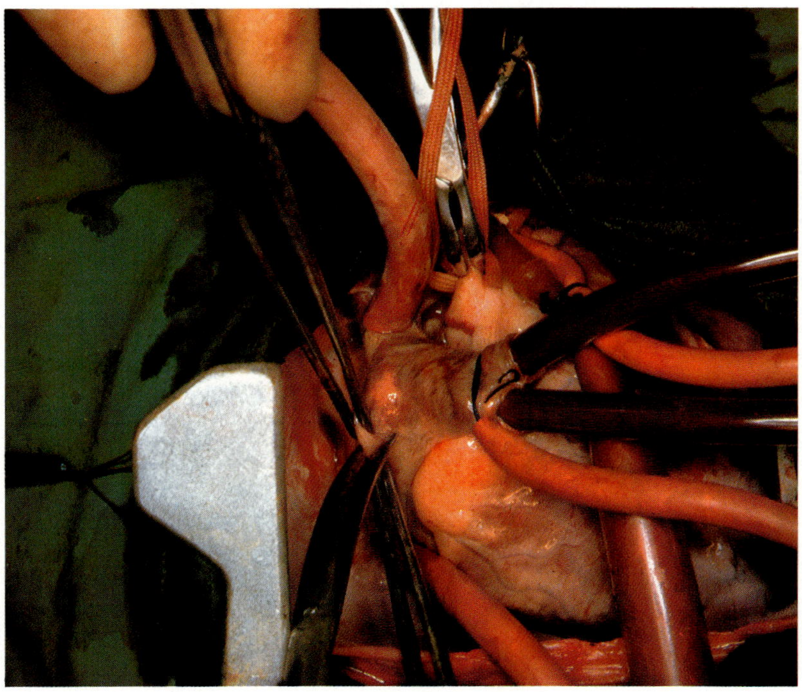

4

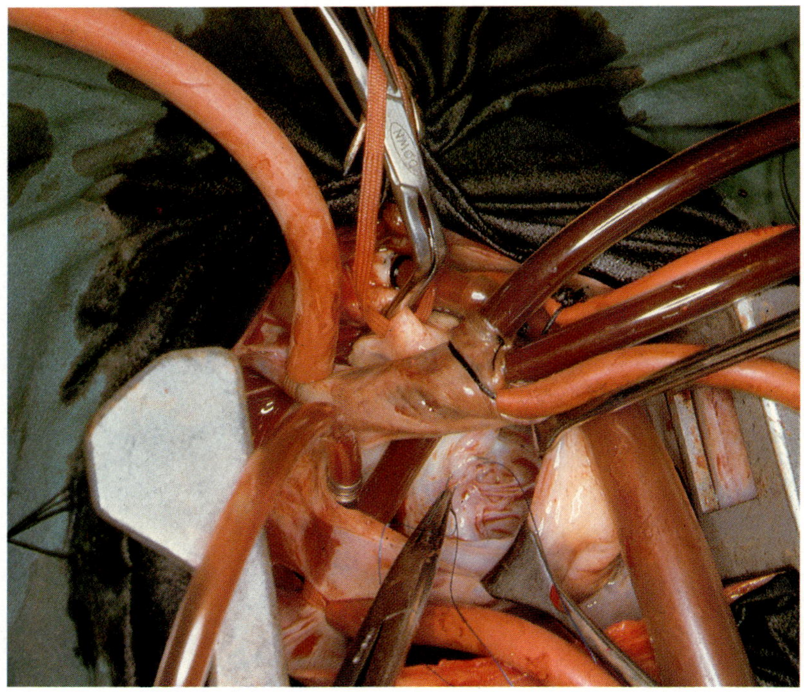

3 The right atrium is opened with scissors.

4 The right atrium has been widely opened and retracted. Cardioplegic fluid has been infused into the ascending aorta (see Chapter 1) and sucked from the coronary sinus. A stay-suture is being inserted into the septal leaflet of the tricuspid valve to help expose the ventricular septal defect.

5

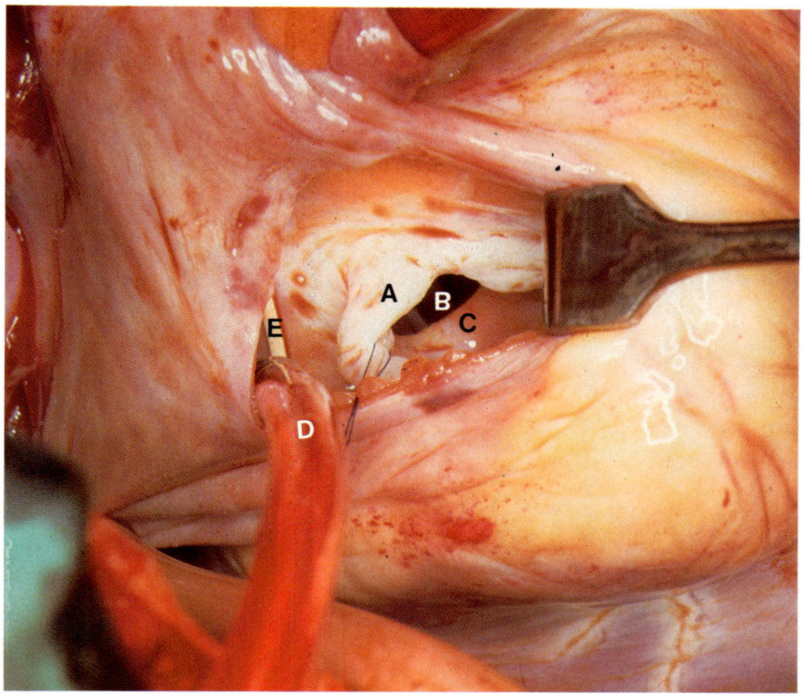

6

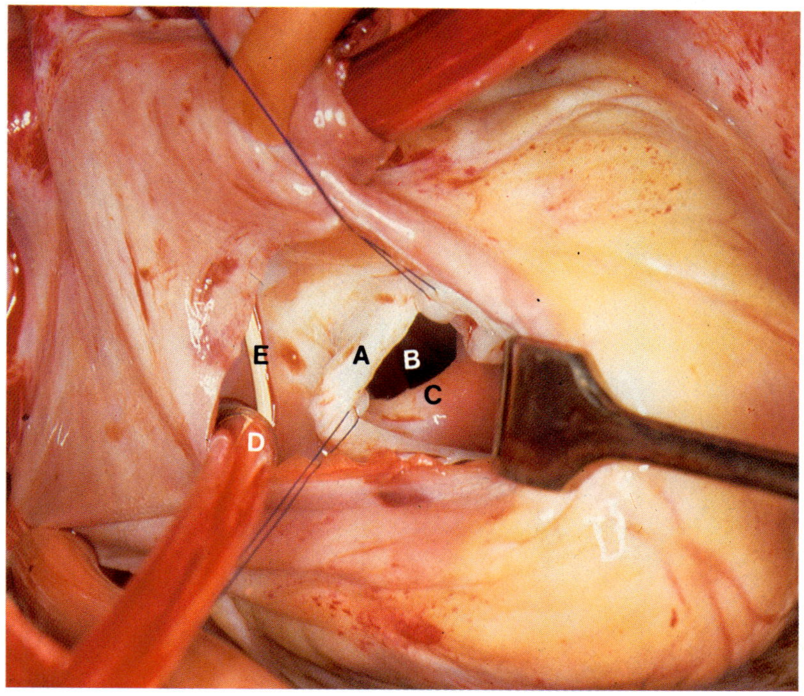

5 and 6 A second mattress suture has been inserted into the septal leaflet of the tricuspid valve **(A)** and, with retraction, most of the ventricular septal defect **(B)** is seen behind it. The lower margin of the defect **(C)**, an open sucker **(D)** and the anaesthetist's central venous line **(E)** are also seen.

7

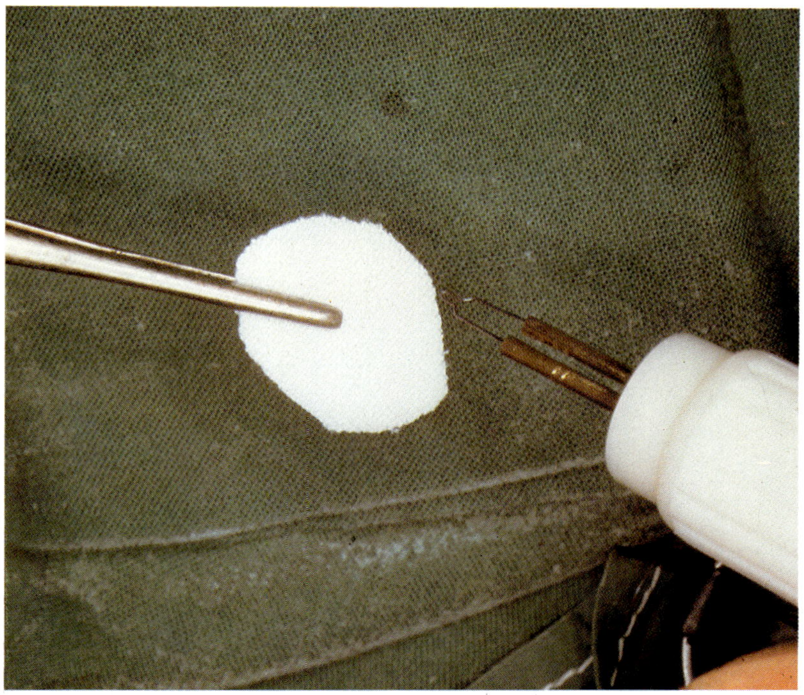

7 A suitably sized piece of dacron cloth is cut out and it is helpful to seal the edges with a disposable cautery to stop fraying.

8

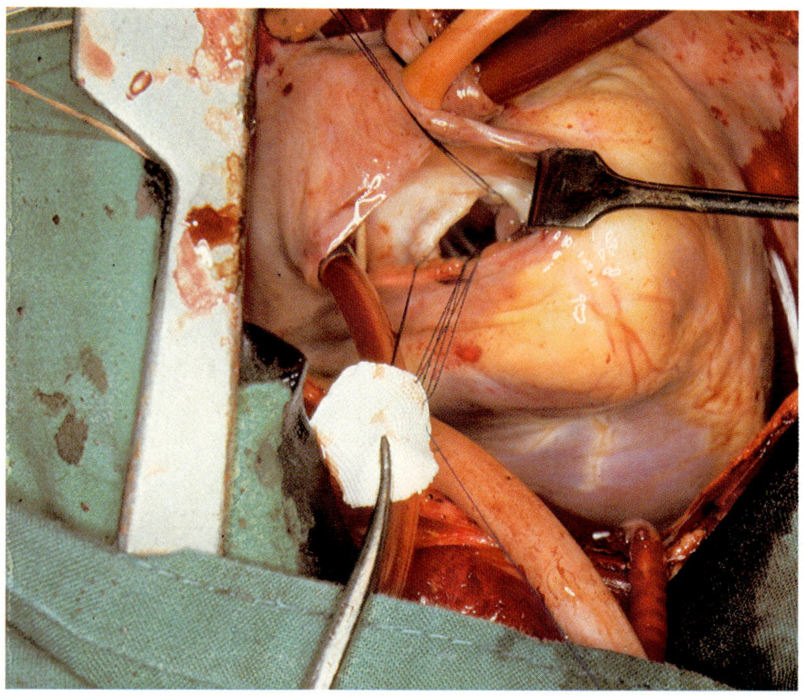

8 The patch is then sutured into position using a continuous Prolene suture. The first stitch has been inserted into the rim of the defect furthest away and then several further sutures placed in an anticlockwise direction before sliding down the patch. Gentle traction on the sutures pulls the upper rim of the defect down into view.

9

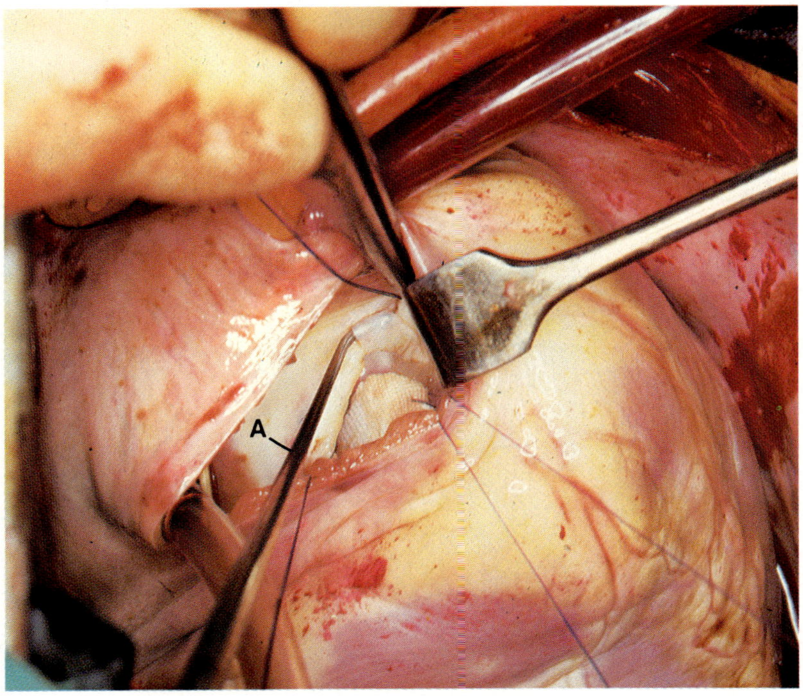

10

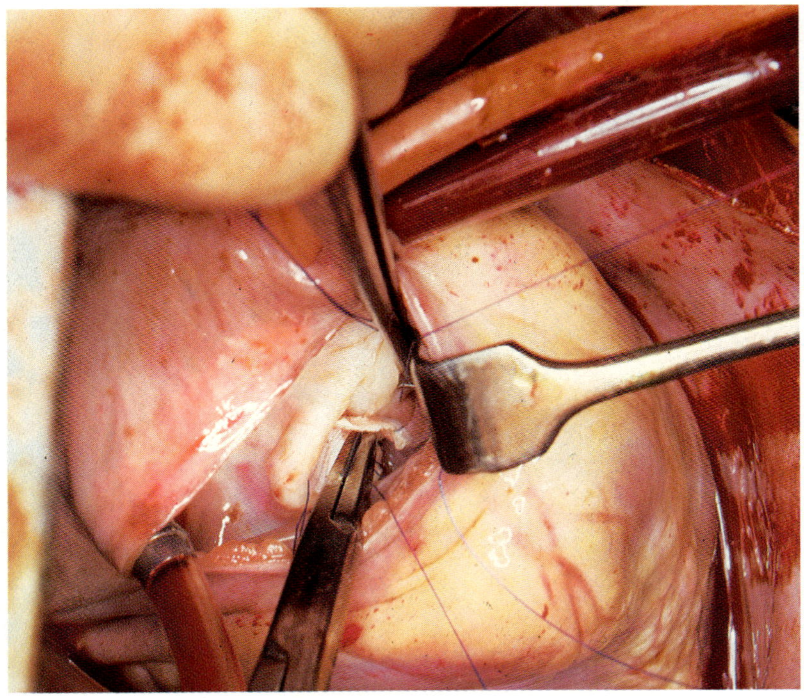

9 Great care must be taken to avoid damage to the aortic valve cusps which can be rather in the way. One cusp is here seen being held up carefully by the Blalock hook (**A**).

10 The suture is continued along the upper rim of the defect.

11

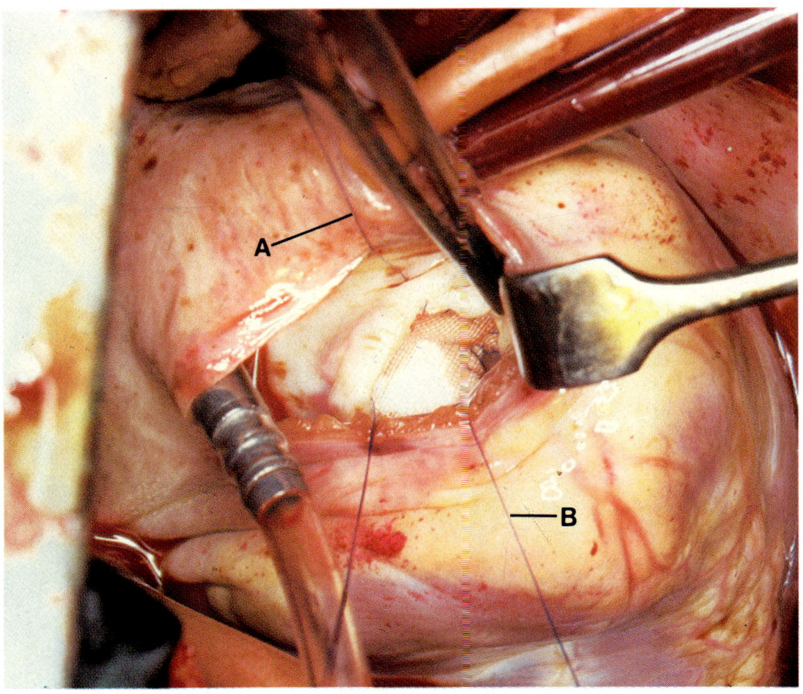

12

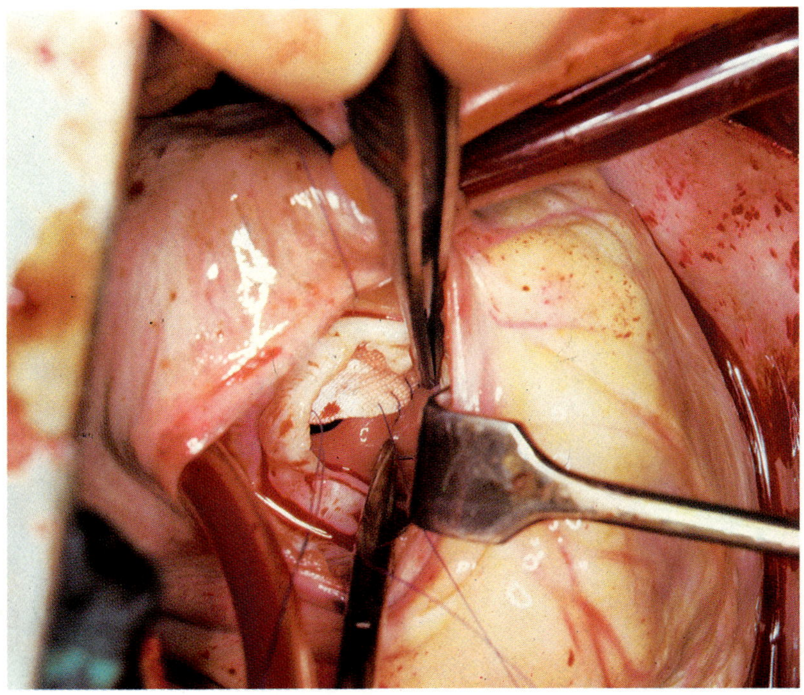

11 When the septal leaflet is reached, the suture (**A**) is taken through the septal leaflet and held. The other end of the same suture (**B**) has been held since the patch was slid down into position.

12 The other end of the suture is continued in a clockwise direction towards the tricuspid valve. At first, good bites of muscle can be taken.

13

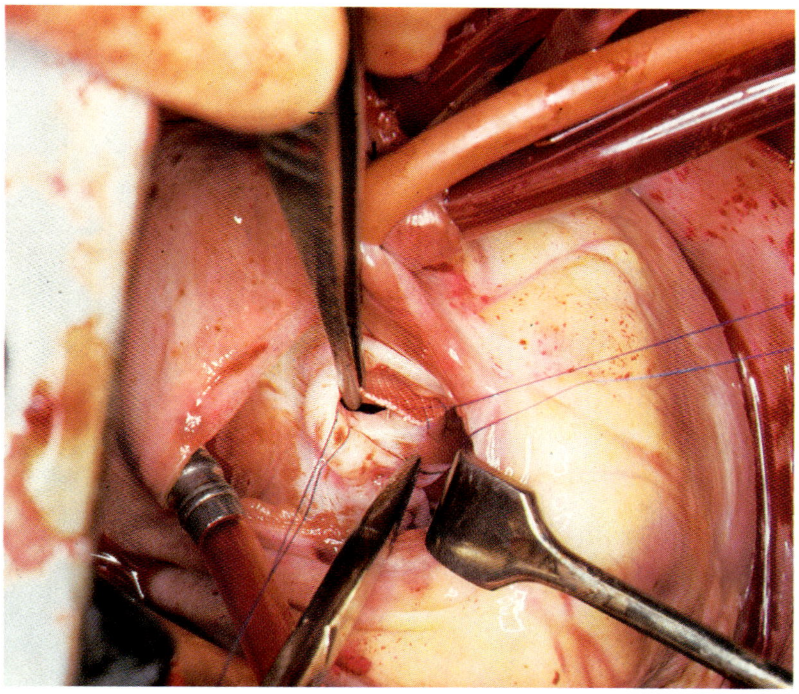

13 As the suture nears the tricuspid valve, the lower margin becomes a danger area because of the proximity of the bundle of His, and damage to this structure, which is, in fact, indistinguishable to the naked eye from other tissue, will cause heart-block. The needle is therefore inserted beneath the lower rim of the defect on the right side of the septum, avoiding the rim.

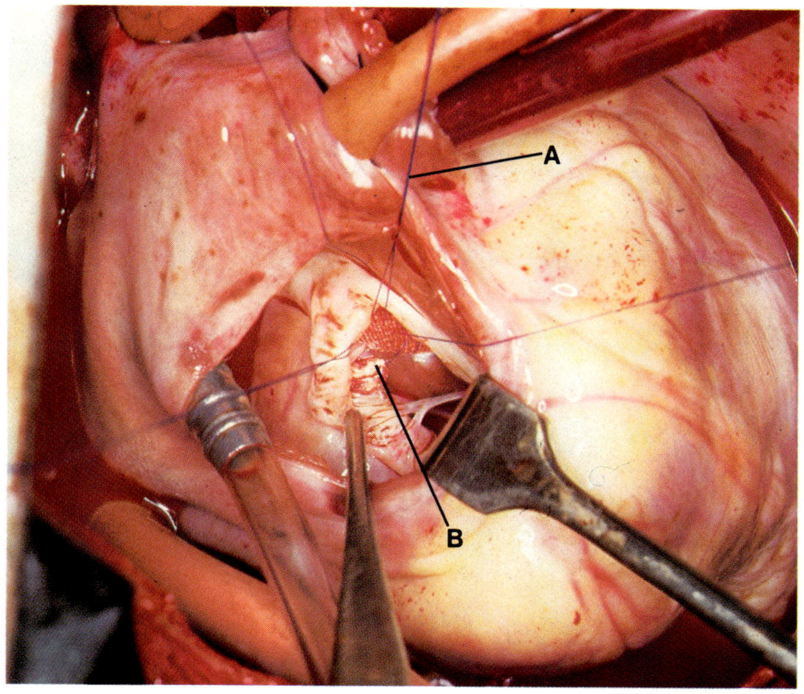

14

14 In this patient an extra mattress suture (**A**) on a pledget of teflon felt (**B**) has been inserted near the corner of the defect close to the tricuspid valve. This gives extra support at what might otherwise have been a weak point in the continuous suture and reduces the risk of a residual defect, but is not necessary in most cases.

15

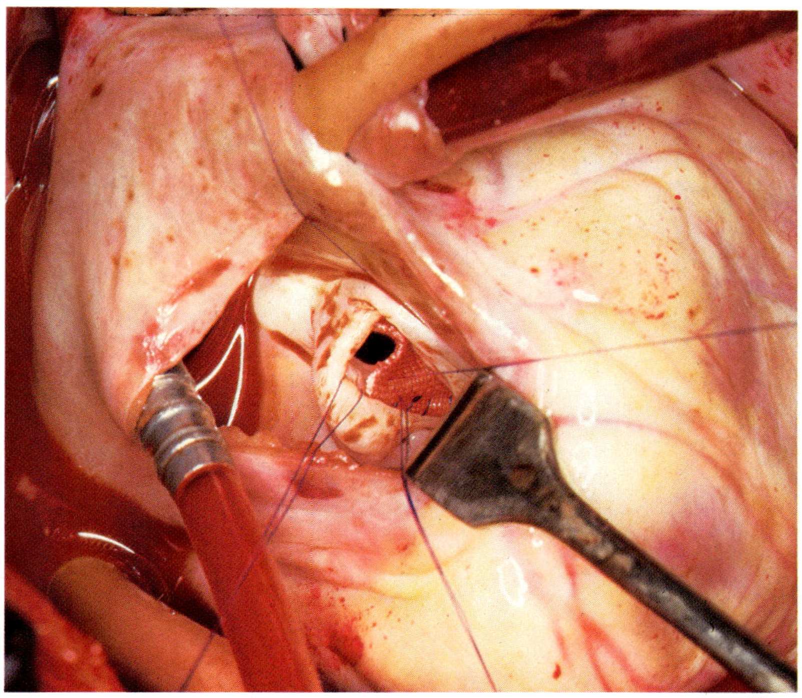

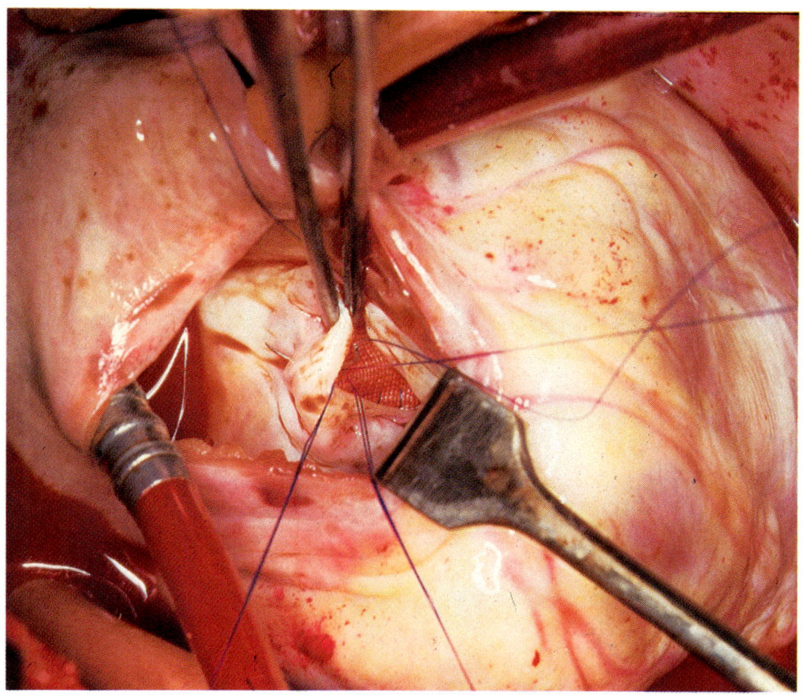

16

15 and 16 The patch is now sutured by continuous mattress sutures to the septal leaflet of the tricuspid valve which contains no conduction mechanism.

17

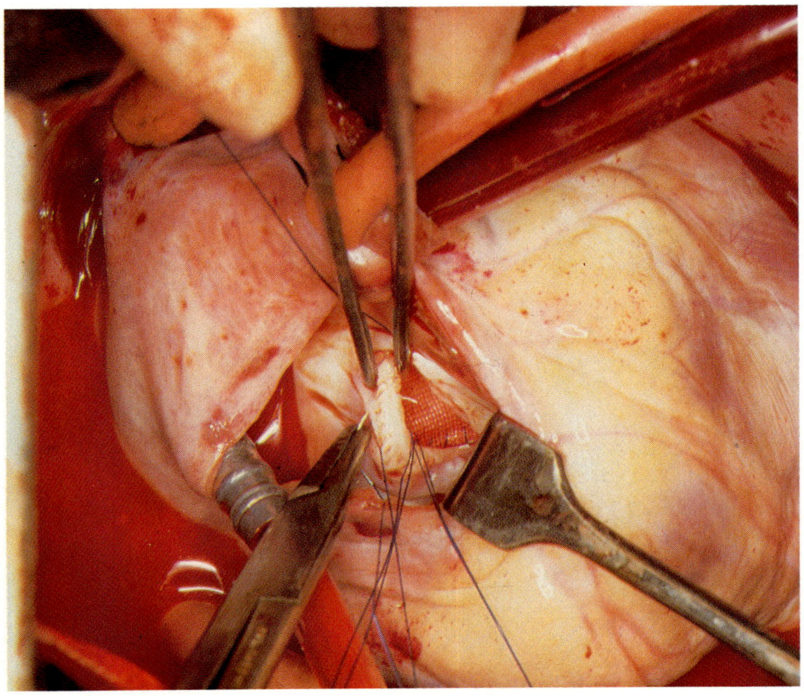

18

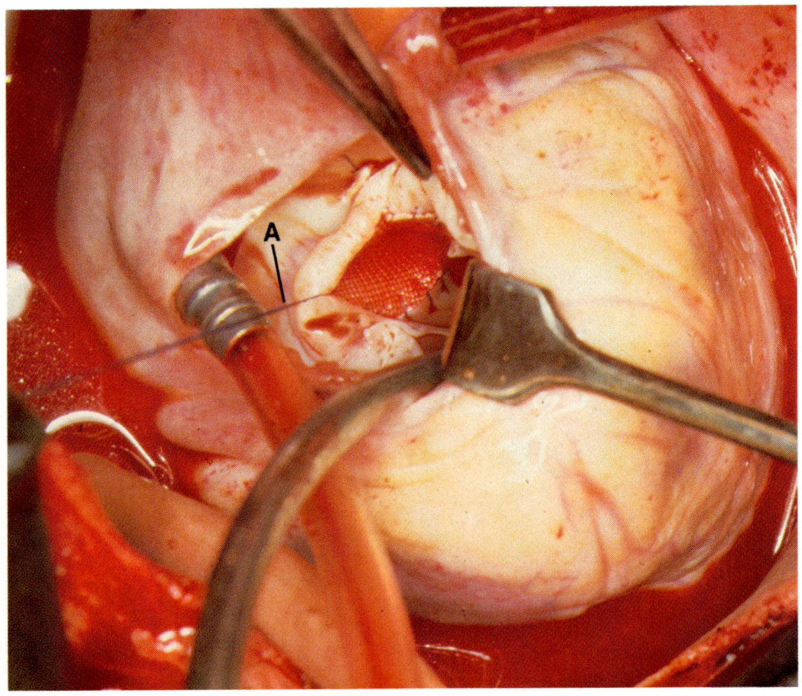

17 and 18 The suture is continued back and forth through the septal leaflet of the tricuspid valve until the other end of the suture is reached, when the suture is tied and the defect closed completely. The stay-suture (**A**) which has been so helpful in displaying the defect is removed.

19

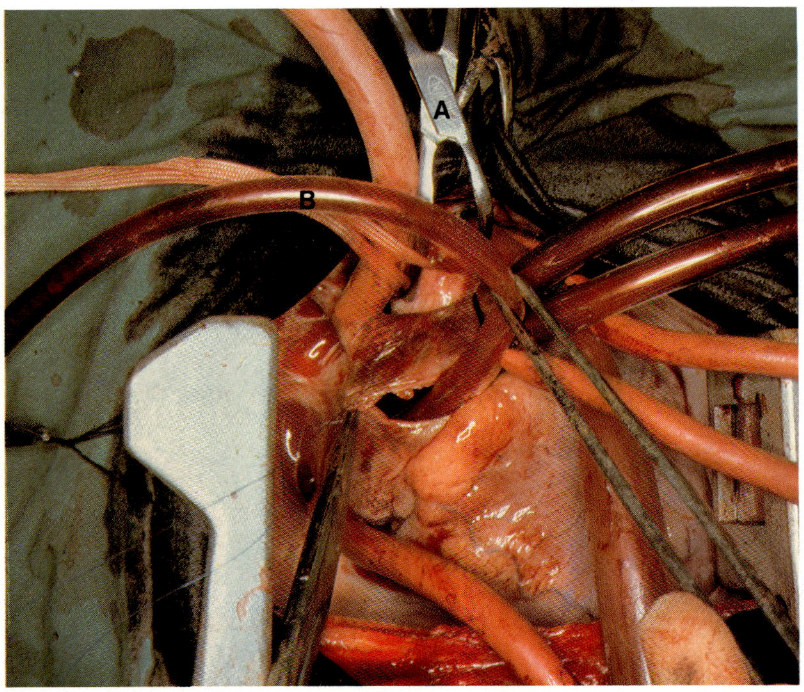

20

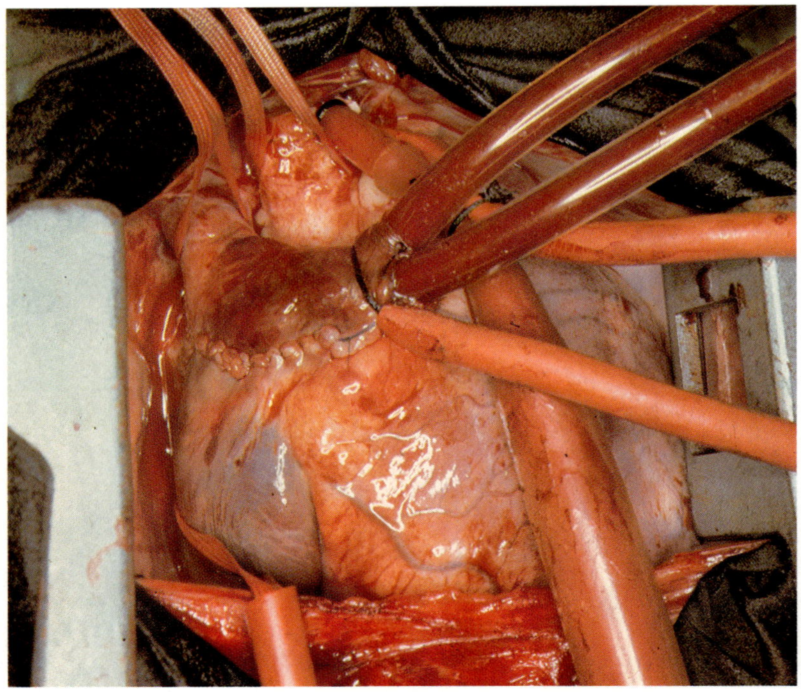

19 and 20 Air is removed from the left ventricle by upending the heart and venting the apex and then the aortic clamp (**A**) is released. Blood returning to the right atrium is returned to the cardiopulmonary bypass machine through the tube (**B**) and the right atrium is closed.

Transatrial approach – inlet defect

21

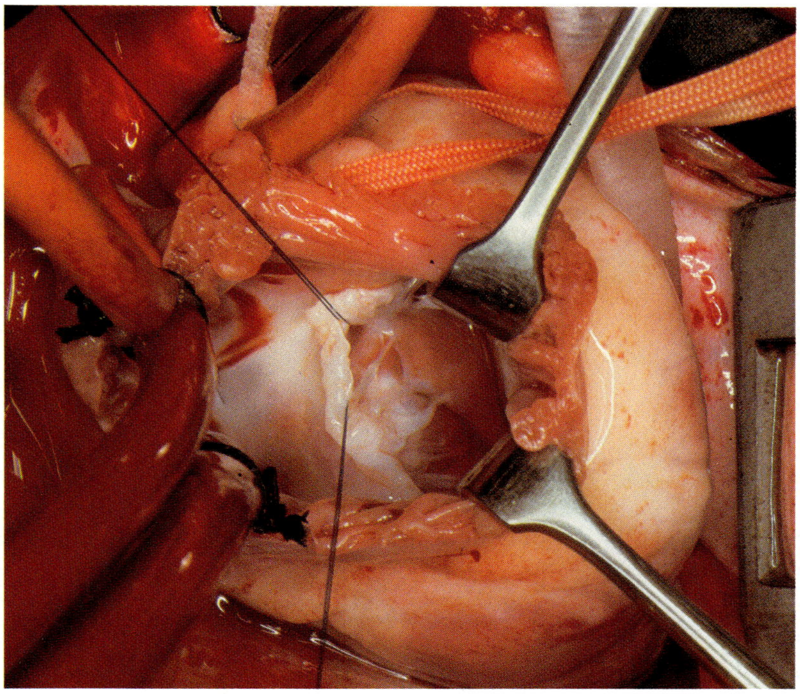

22

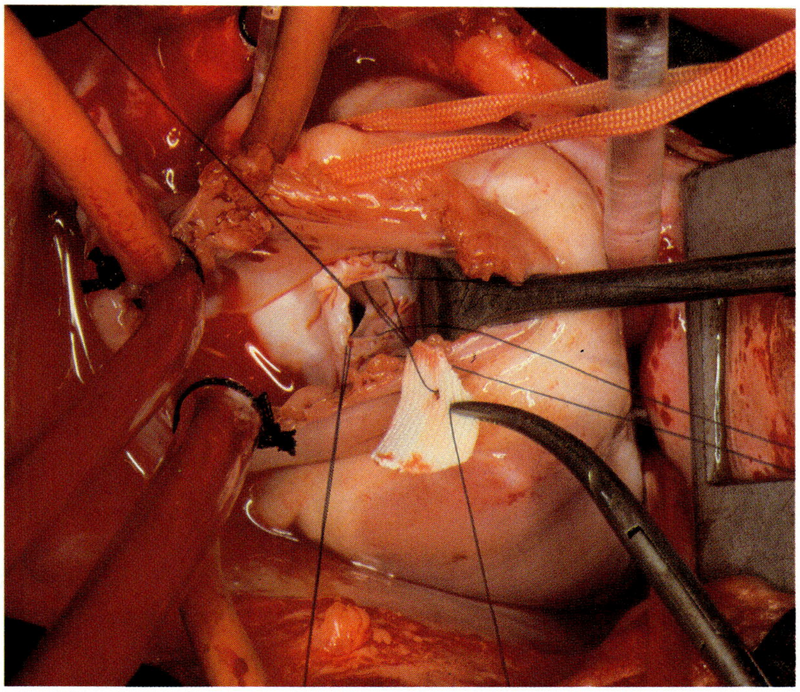

21 The transatrial approach is also suitable for inlet defects, which, as in this case, are positioned rather inconveniently behind the septal leaflet of the tricuspid valve. Again, two stay-sutures in the septal leaflet of the tricuspid valve help to expose the defect.

22 The defect is lower than the perimembranous defect illustrated previously and, although the technique of insertion is the same, it can be difficult weaving in and out of the chordae tendinae of the tricuspid valve. Here some sutures have been inserted before sliding the dacron patch into position. In low inlet defects, the conduction mechanism may run above rather than below the defect.

23

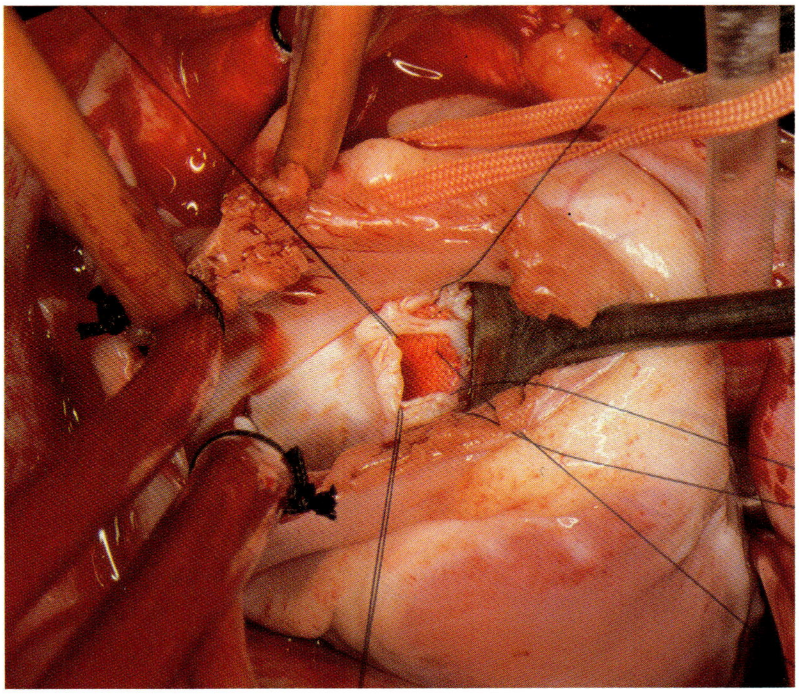

24

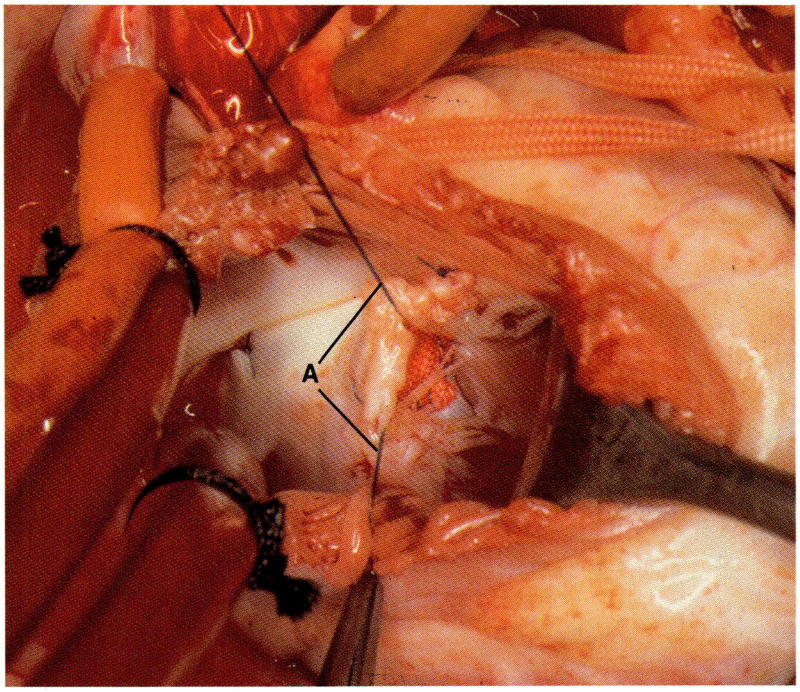

23 and 24 The remainder of the patch is sutured in with a continuous Prolene suture and the knot tied. The stay-sutures (**A**) are removed before closing the atrium.

Transatrial approach — muscular defect

25 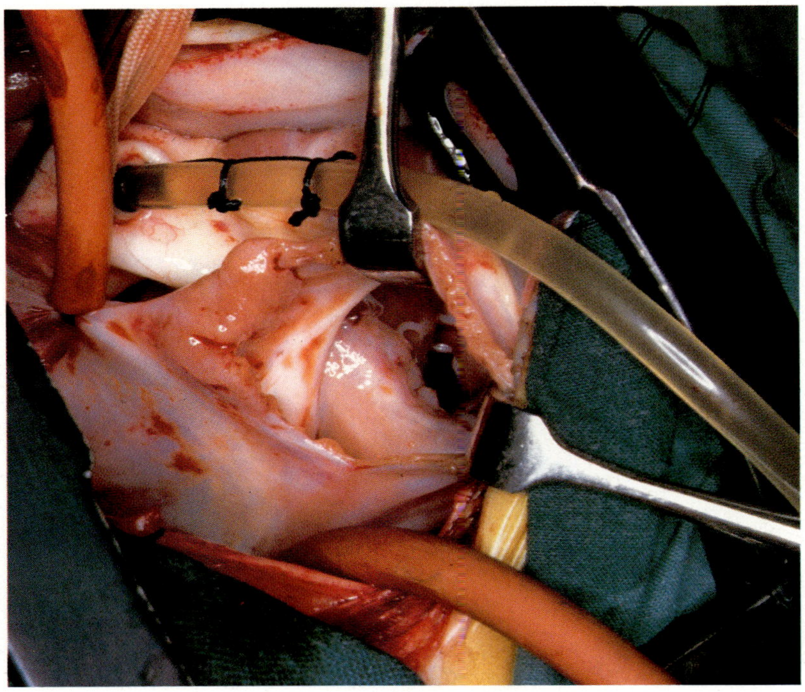

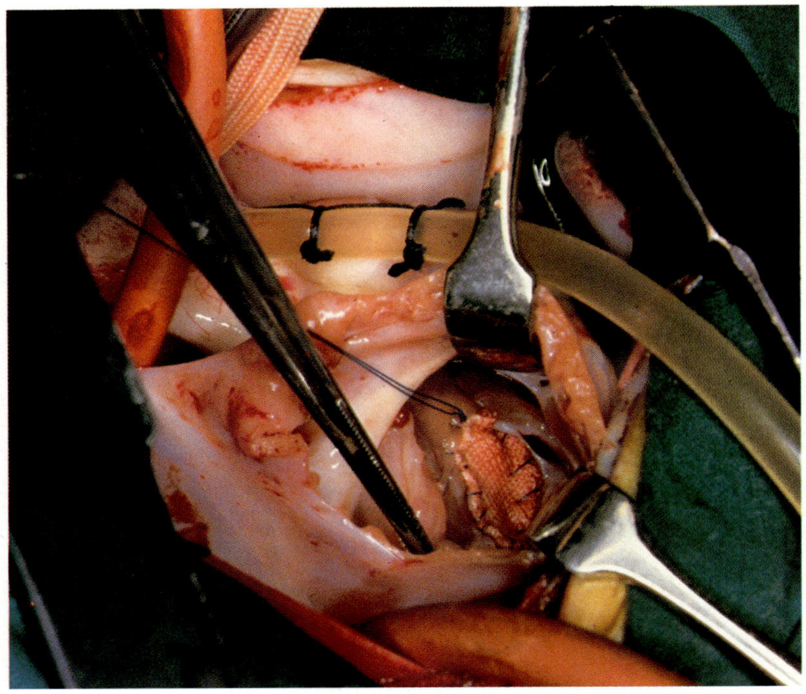 26

25 and 26 The muscular defect is situated well away from the tricuspid valve ring and has been closed with a dacron patch and continuous Prolene suture.

Transventricular approach

27

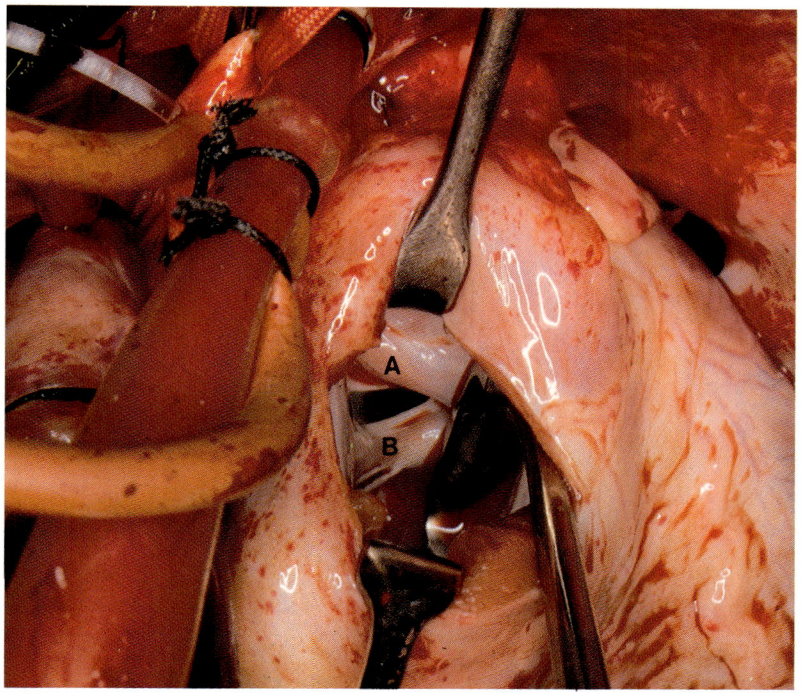

28

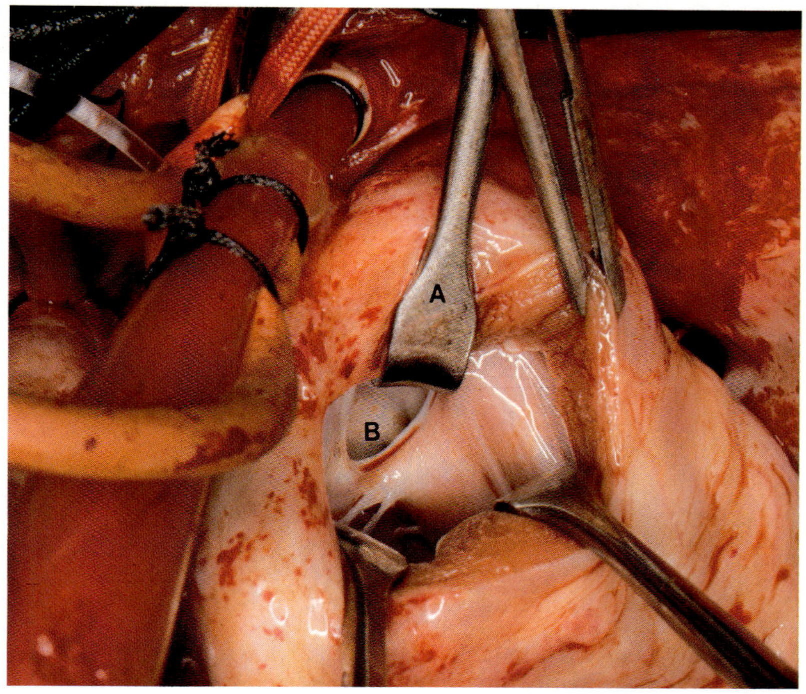

27 The ventricular septal defect is exposed through a transverse right ventriculotomy. The conus septum (**A**) (crista supraventricularis) forms the upper margin of the defect. The papillary muscle of the conus (**B**), which is rather small in this patient, is seen just below the lower margin of the defect.

28 A retractor (**A**) has been placed carefully in the upper part of the defect which gives good exposure of the defect, through which the anterior leaflet of the mitral valve (**B**) can be seen in the left ventricle.

29

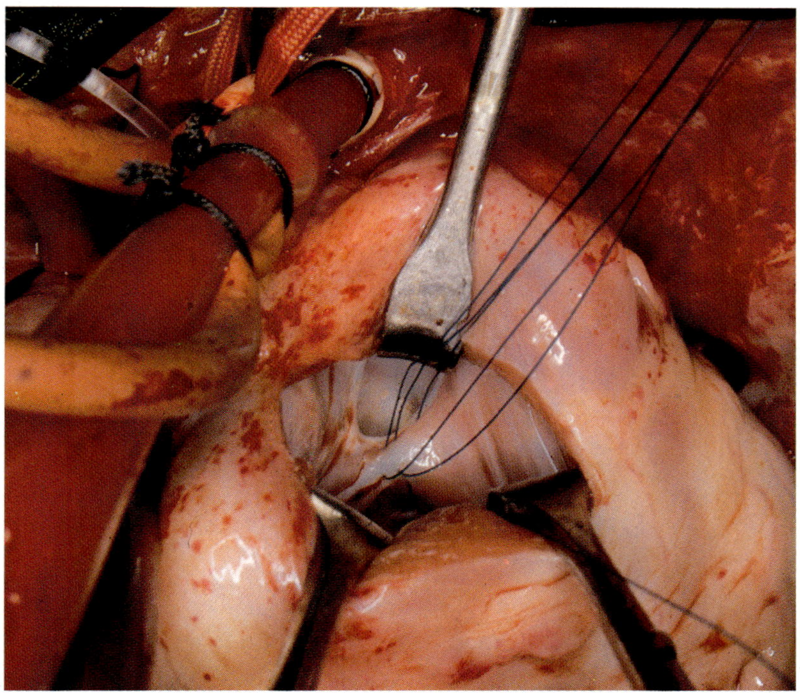

30

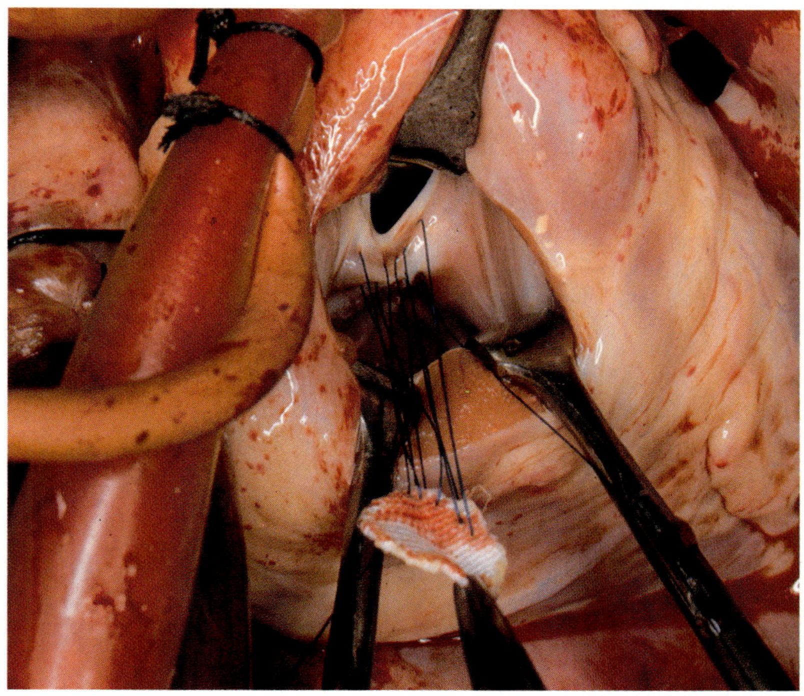

29 and 30 A continuous Prolene suture is started at the lower left corner of the defect and several sutures are inserted before the dacron patch is slid down into position. Care is taken in placing the sutures to stay on the right side of the septum, thus avoiding the bundle of His and left bundle branch.

31

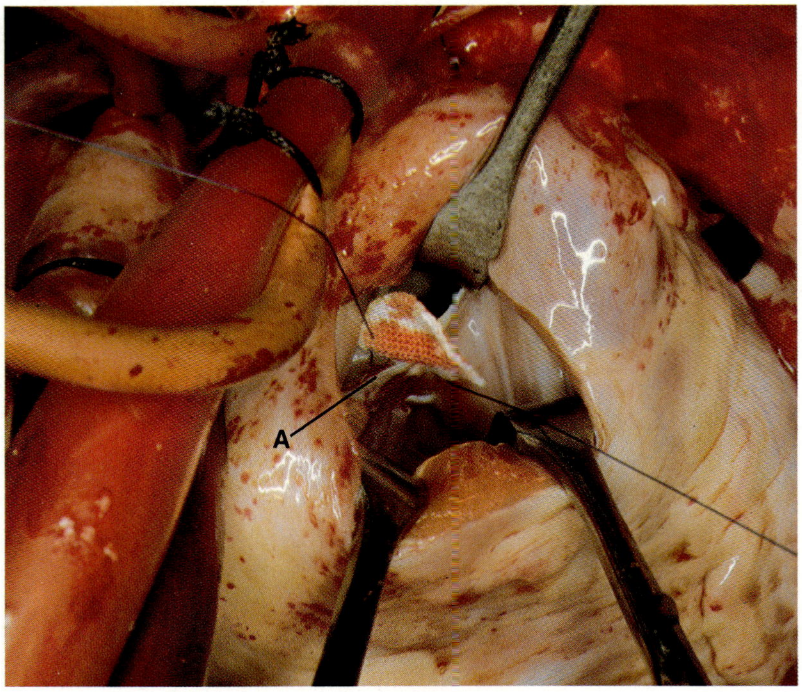

32

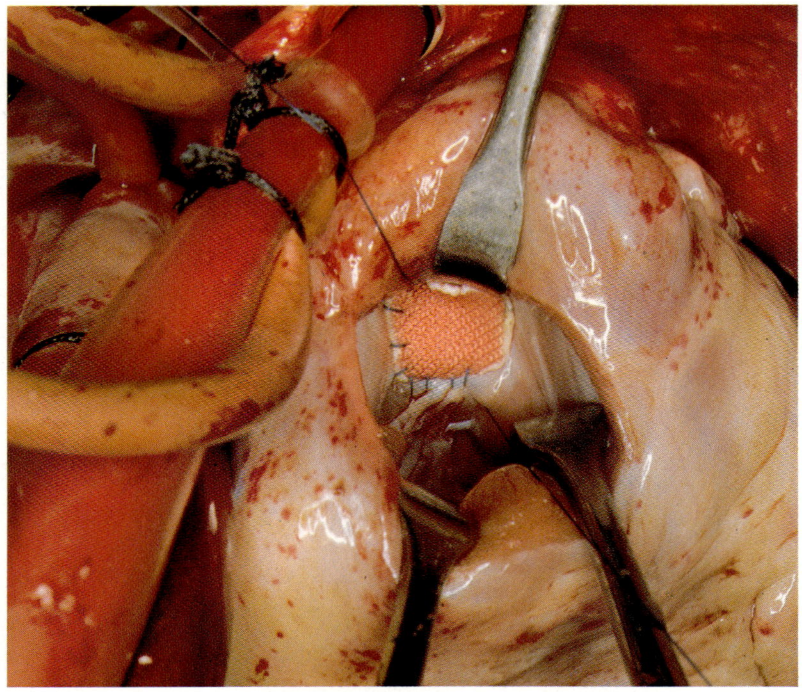

31 and 32 The dacron patch is carefully slid down into position and the Prolene suture tightened. The right-hand end of the suture is then continued in a clockwise direction until the superior part of the defect is reached. Great care must be taken not to damage the aortic valve cusps when placing these superior sutures. This defect is high and therefore the tricuspid valve (**A**) is below the defect and the bundle is well away from its inferior margin.

33

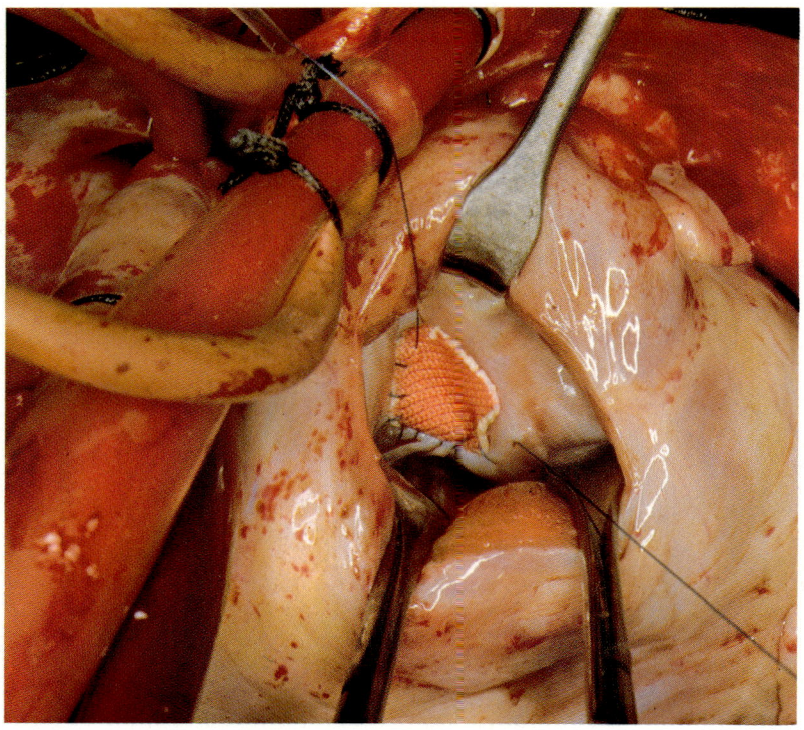

34

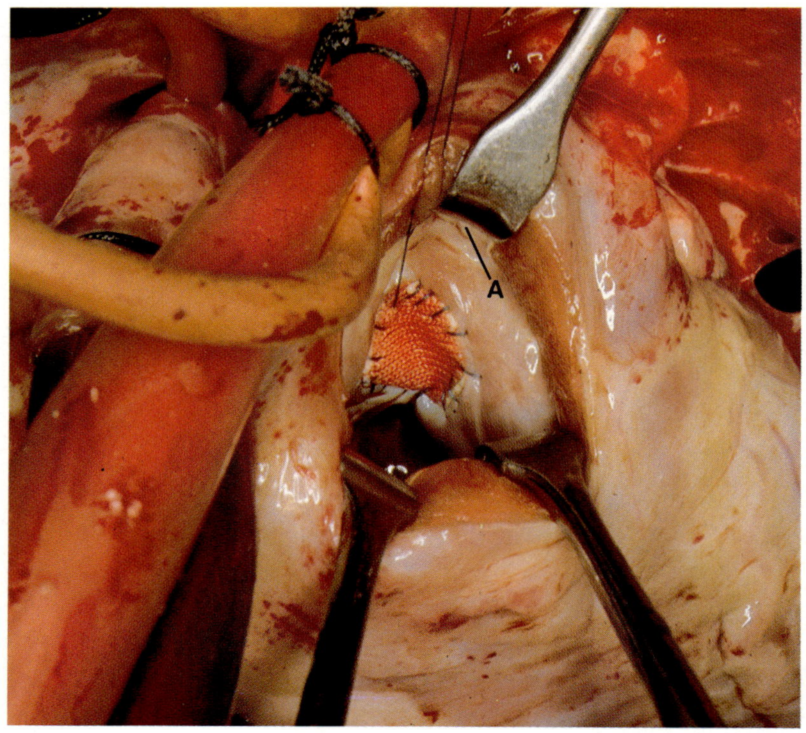

33 and 34 The other end of the Prolene suture is now continued in an anti-clockwise direction and the two suture ends tied to complete closure of the defect. The pulmonary valve (**A**) can just be seen.

12: Correction of Fallot's tetralogy

The combination of pulmonary outflow tract obstruction, ventricular septal defect, overriding of the aorta and right ventricular hypertrophy comprise the condition described by Fallot in 1888[1]. The first successful correction of this condition was reported by Lillehei in 1955[2]. Some patients with this condition may not be suitable for correction and therefore a palliative procedure, such as a Blalock-Taussig or a Waterston shunt, may have to be performed initially, and correction delayed until later in childhood. However, correction in infancy can be performed successfully, although this may well result in a high incidence of outflow patching.

The operation is to close the ventricular septal defect and relieve the pulmonary outflow tract obstruction (see diagram **A**). It is important to achieve an adequate relief of outflow tract obstruction, even at the expense of the better tolerated pulmonary regurgitation. Resection of the obstructing infundibular muscle and relief of any valve stenosis are a routine part of the operation. However, if the pulmonary valve ring is too narrow, this will cause an obstruction which the right ventricle may not be able to tolerate post-operatively. The decision whether to widen the outflow tract with a transannular patch can be difficult and is based on the pre-operative angiography[3], the operative findings[4] and the measurement of pressures after correction. If the right ventricular pressure is at or near left ventricular pressure at the end of the operation, then it is probably better to go back and insert a transannular patch. Ideally, the right ventricular pressure should be less than half systemic, but, to preserve pulmonary valve competence, a higher right-to-left ventricular pressure ratio may be accepted.

To perform the correction, an incision is made in the right ventricle and its direction depends on whether a transannular patch is likely to be needed. If it is unlikely to be needed, a transverse ventriculotomy can be made[5]. However, if a transannular patch is likely to be needed, the ventriculotomy should be vertical so that the incision can be extended across the pulmonary valve ring and up into the main pulmonary artery. In planning the incision, the presence of coronary arteries over the right ventricle must be considered.

Patching may be performed with pericardium, dacron, homologous dura mater and other materials, but they will all leave a regurgitant valve. To get over this problem, particularly in infants, patching can be performed with a single cusp from an antibiotic sterilised homograft as illustrated in this chapter (see diagram **B**). As the patient grows, the valve will become regurgitant but this is well-tolerated after the initial post-operative phase.

To perform correction, cardiopulmonary bypass is necessary with two venous cannulae, except in small infants where use of the deep hypothermia technique only requires one. It is also advisable to close any patent foramen ovale or atrial septal defect at the same operation.

Diagram A – Before correction

- **A** – Right atrium
- **B** – Right ventricle
- **C** – Ventricular septal defect
- **D** – Left ventricle
- **E** – Ascending aorta
- **F** – Pulmonary artery
- **G** – Infundibular muscular obstruction
- **H** – Stenosed pulmonary valve

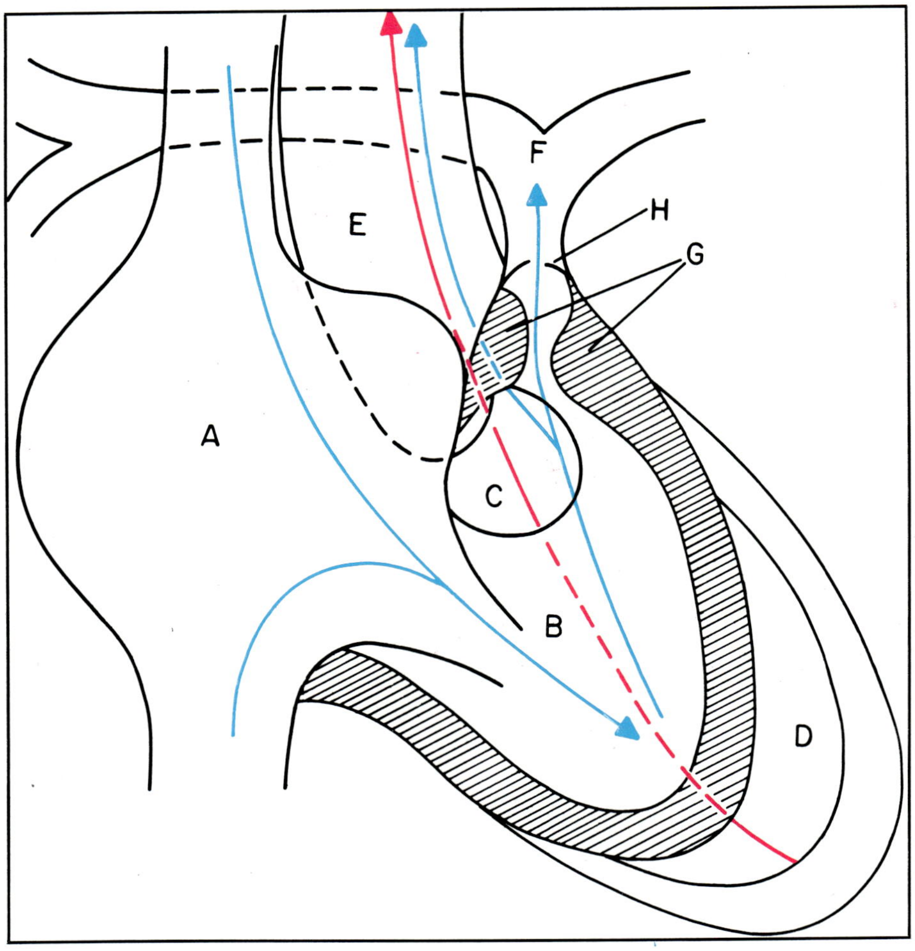

The desaturated blood returning through the right atrium (**A**) to the right ventricle (**B**) is ejected partly into the pulmonary artery (**F**), but because the outflow tract is obstructed by muscle (**G**), some blue blood passes from right to left through the ventricular septal defect (**C**). This desaturated blood joins the red saturated blood coming from the left ventricle (**D**) resulting in cyanosis. The pulmonary valve (**H**) is usually stenosed as well.

Diagram B – After correction

- **A** – Right atrium
- **B** – Right ventricle
- **C** – Dacron patch closing ventricular septal defect
- **D** – Left ventricle
- **E** – Ascending aorta
- **F** – Pulmonary artery
- **G** – Unicusp homograft outflow patch

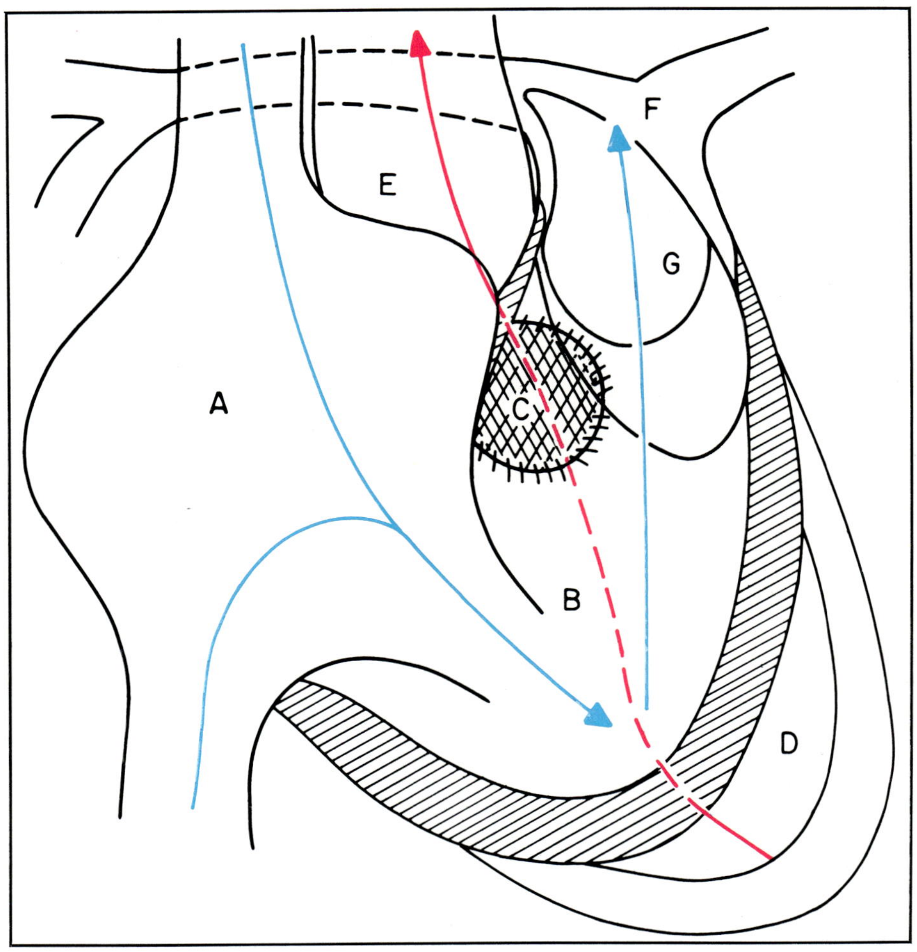

The ventricular septal defect has been closed with a dacron patch (**C**), so all the desaturated blood flows to the pulmonary artery (**F**). The outflow tract has been widened by resection of infundibular muscle and the insertion of a transannular patch, which in this illustration is a unicusp homograft (**G**). No blue desaturated blood enters the systemic circulation and the patient is no longer cyanosed.

With pericardial patch to outflow tract

1

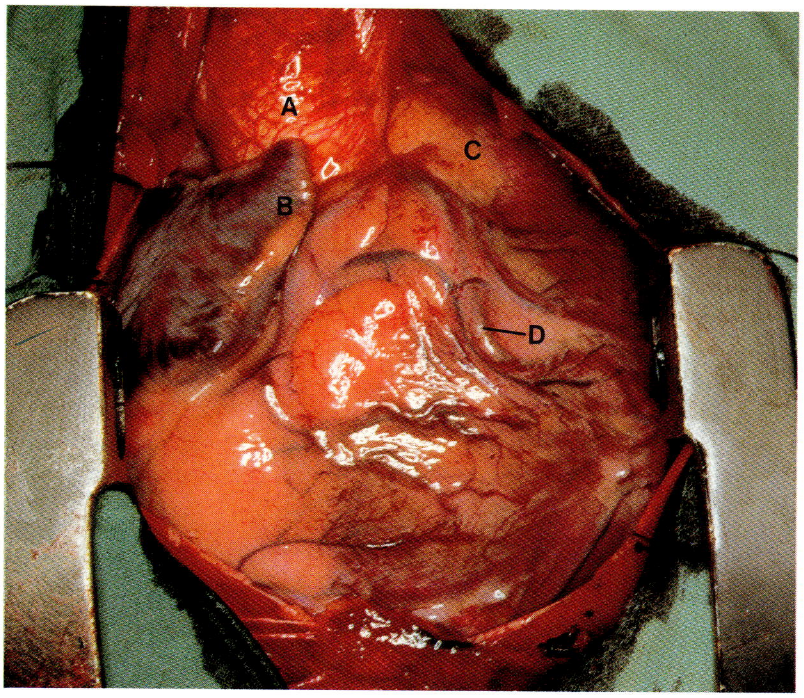

1 The overall view of the heart shows the large aorta (**A**), the right atrial appendage (**B**) and the pulmonary outflow tract (**C**) with a large ventricular branch of the right coronary artery (**D**).

2

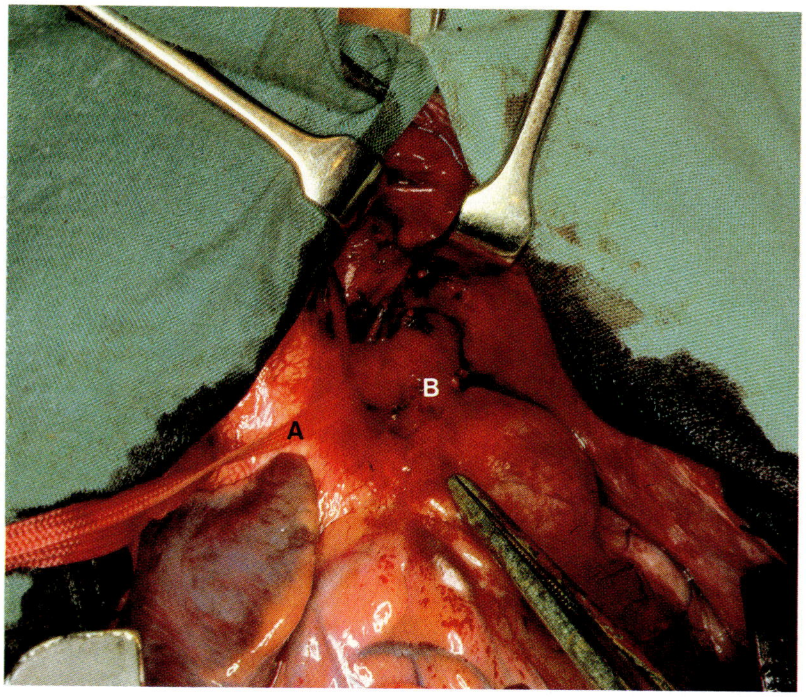

2 The aorta has been retracted by a tape around it (**A**) to demonstrate the narrowed main pulmonary artery (**B**).

3

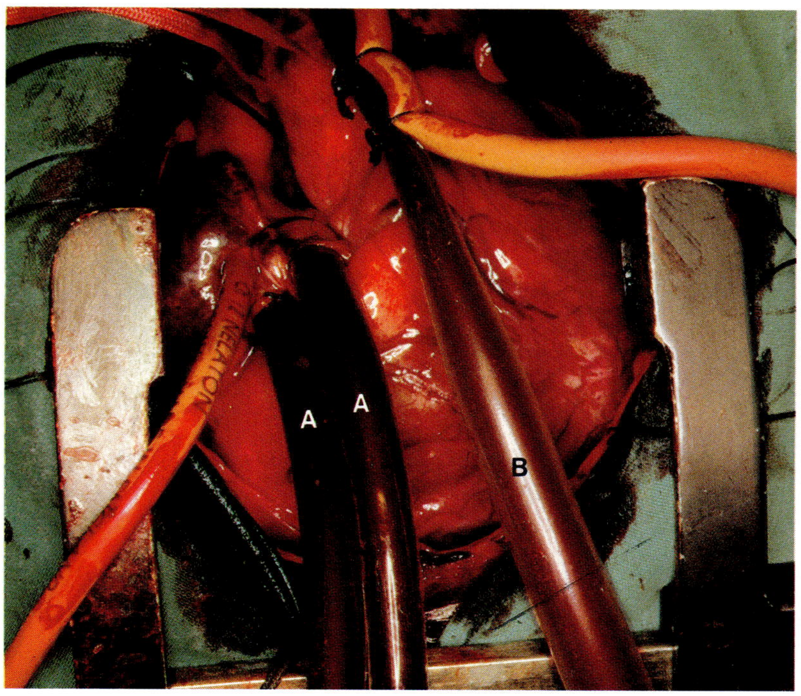

3 Two venous cannulae (**A**) have been inserted into the right atrium and placed into the vena cavae. An aortic cannula (**B**) has been inserted and markedly desaturated blood has come back up into the cannula.

4

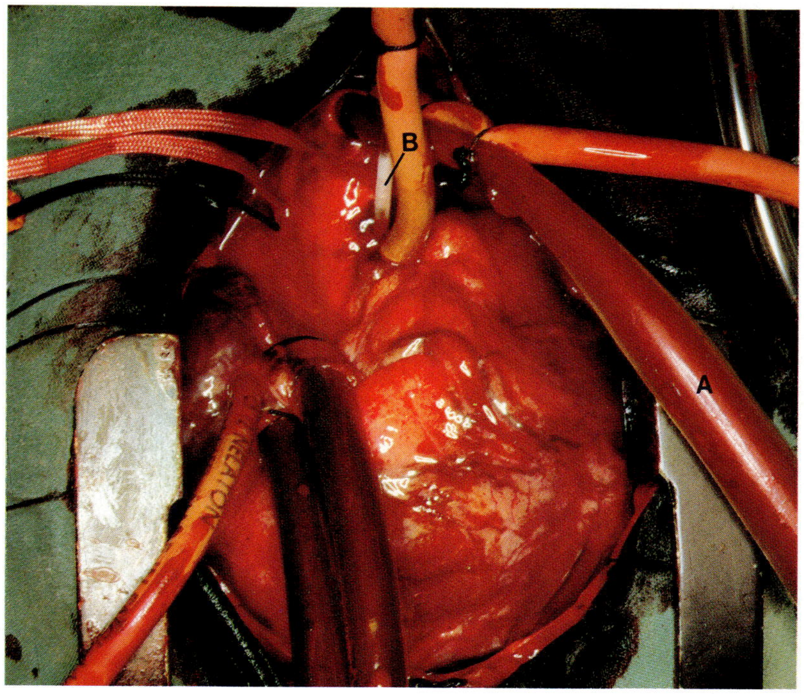

4 Bypass has now been commenced and saturated blood from the cardiopulmonary bypass machine can be seen in the aortic cannula (**A**). A separate small cannula (**B**) has been inserted more proximally into the aorta, for infusion of cardioplegic fluid.

5

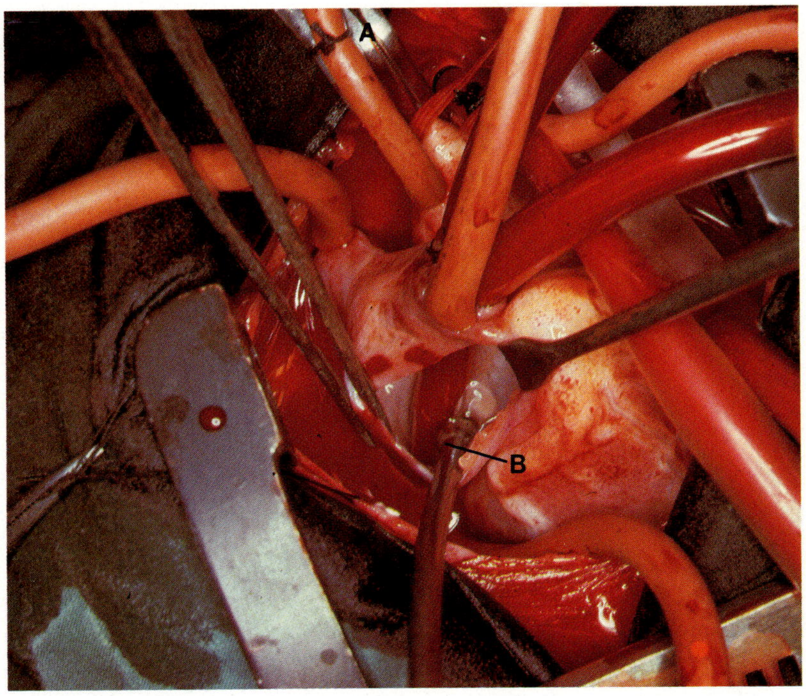

6

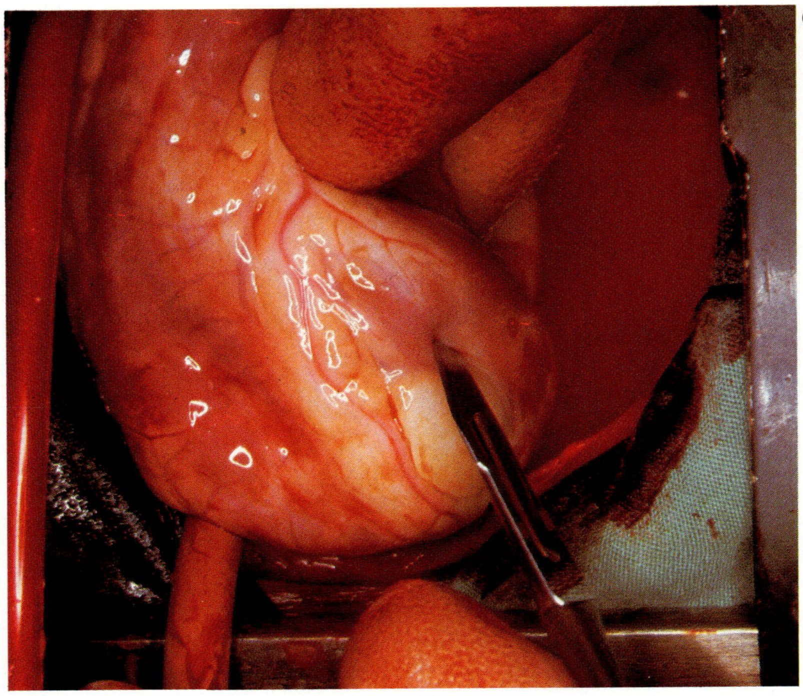

5 A clamp (**A**) has been placed on the aorta proximal to the aortic cannula, the right atrium has been opened and a sucker (**B**) removes the cardioplegic fluid which is being infused through the ascending aorta. A search is made for a patent foramen ovale which is closed if found, and the right atrium is then closed.

6 and 7 After clamping the aorta, a small incision is made in the apex of the left ventricle and a sucking vent inserted to remove any blood returning to the heart which would otherwise interfere with closure of the ventricular septal defect.

7

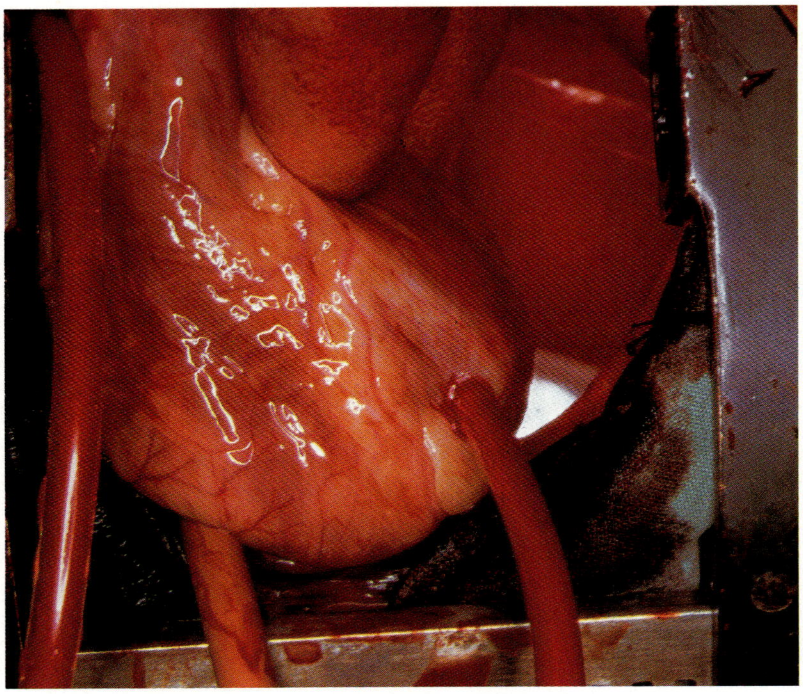

8

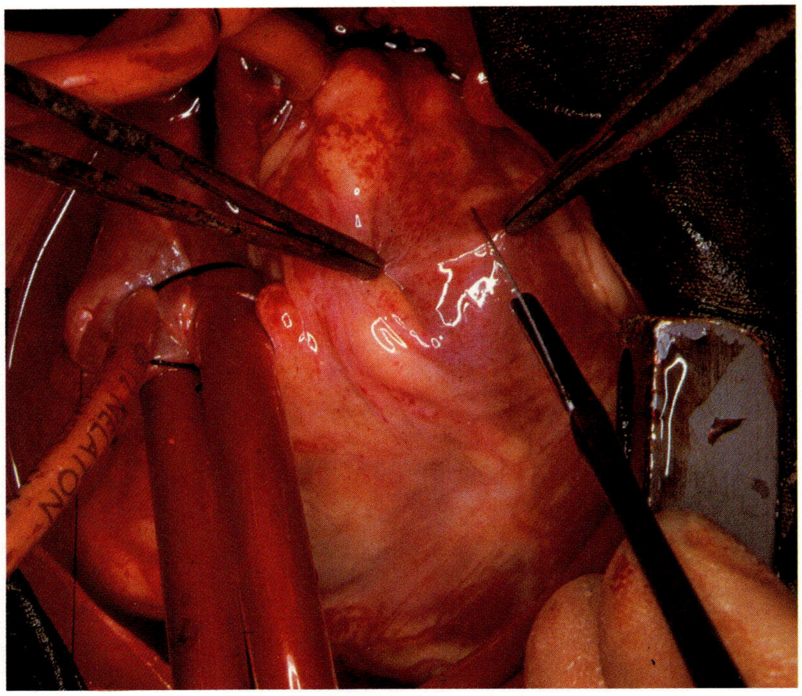

8 In this patient it has been decided that the pulmonary valve ring is likely to be too small and, as a transannular patch will be needed, a vertical incision is made in the right ventricle.

9

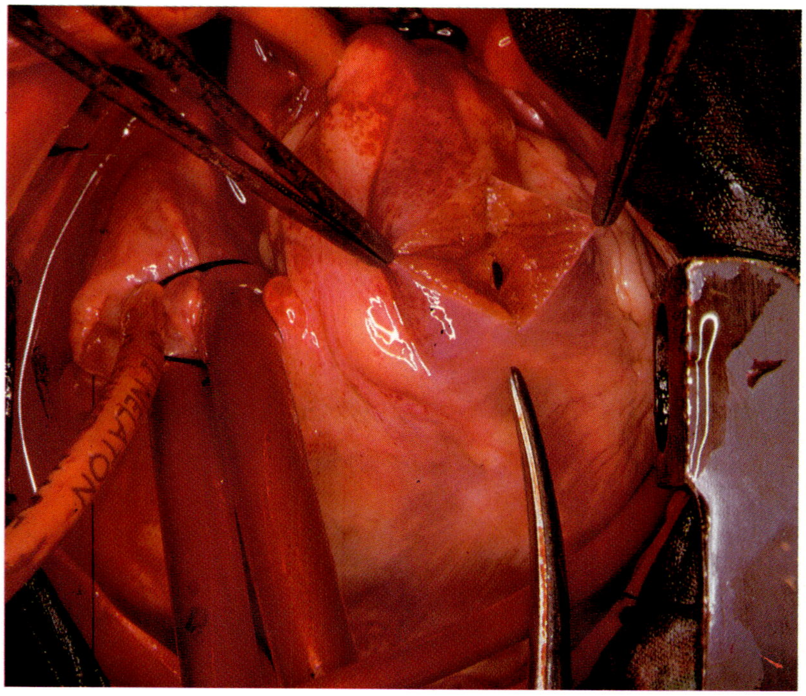

10

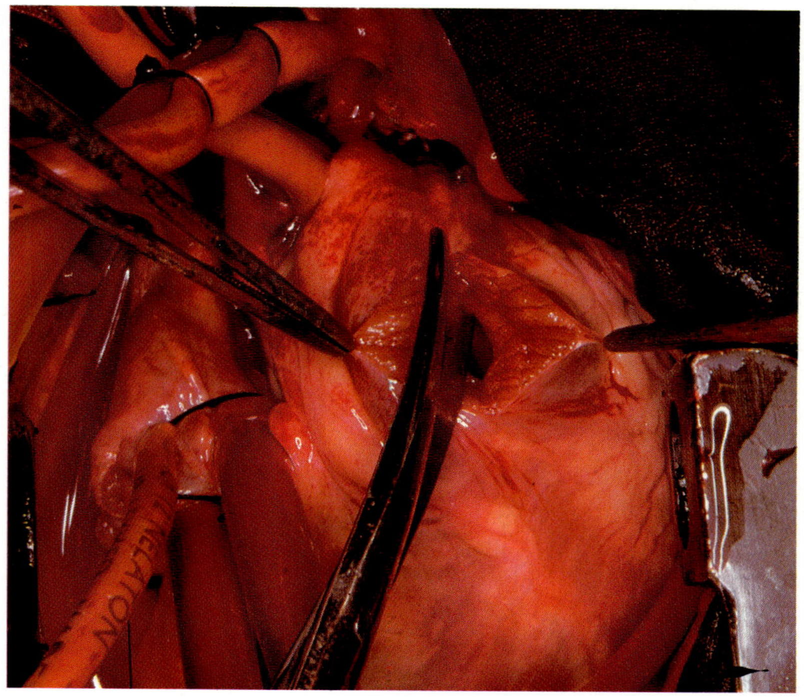

9 and 10 The small incision made with the knife is then enlarged with scissors.

11

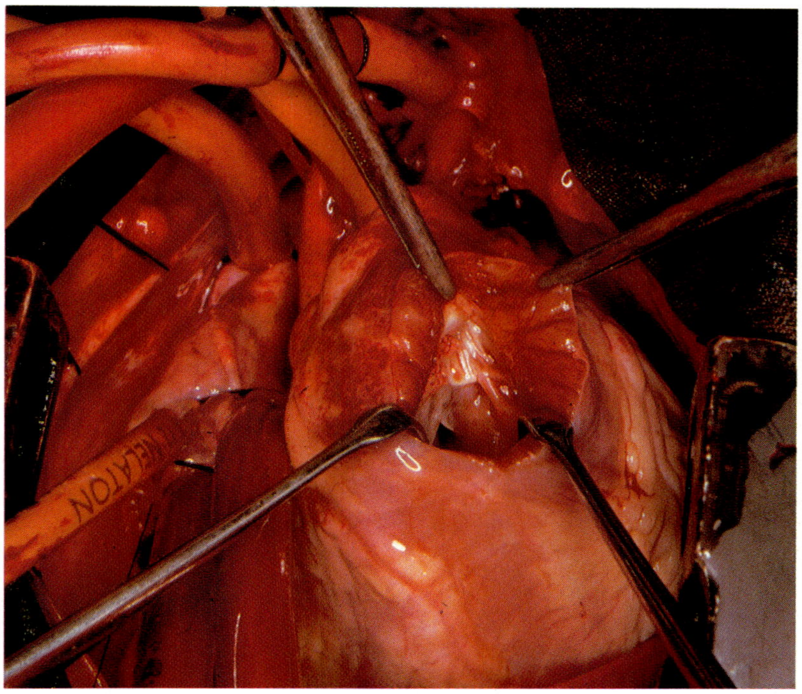

12

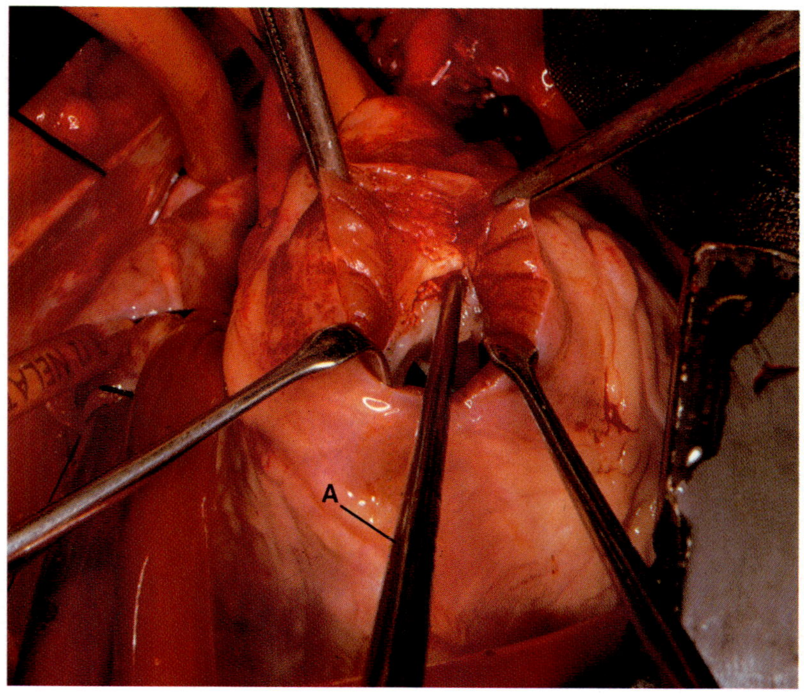

11 and 12 Having opened up the outflow tract further, a tight, fibrous infundibular narrowing is seen and the valve is explored with a probe (**A**).

13

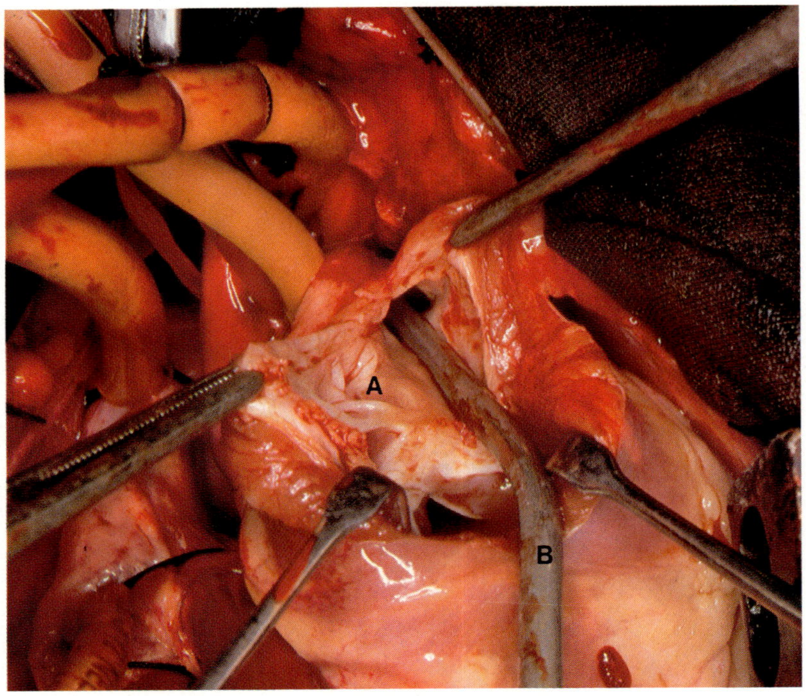

14

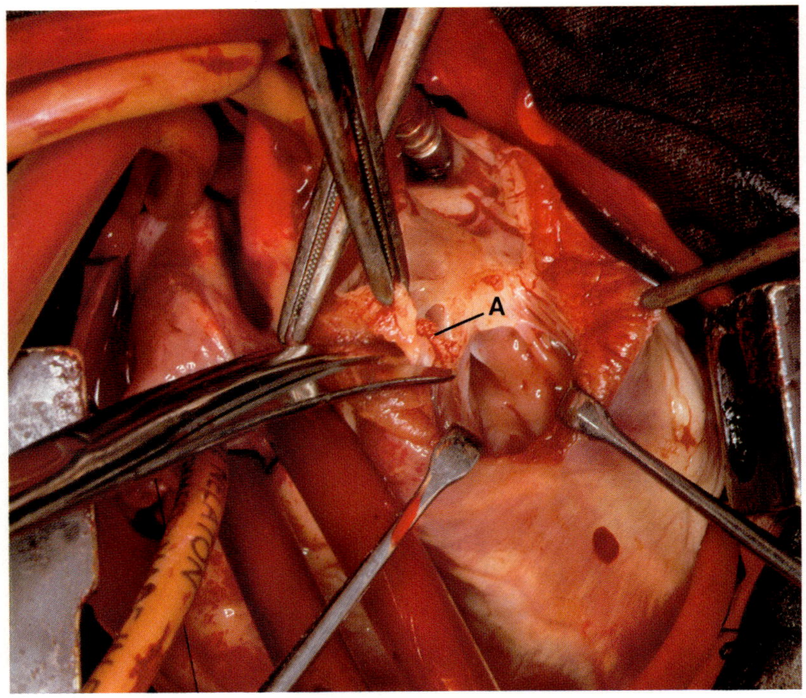

13 The very narrowed outflow tract was too small and therefore a longitudinal incision has been made through the pulmonary valve (**A**) and into the pulmonary artery. A sucker (**B**) lies in the pulmonary artery returning blood to the bypass machine.

14 Some of the obstructing fibrous tissue is removed with scissors, together with some fresh, but adherent, fibrin (**A**) that has formed on the fibrous tissue.

15

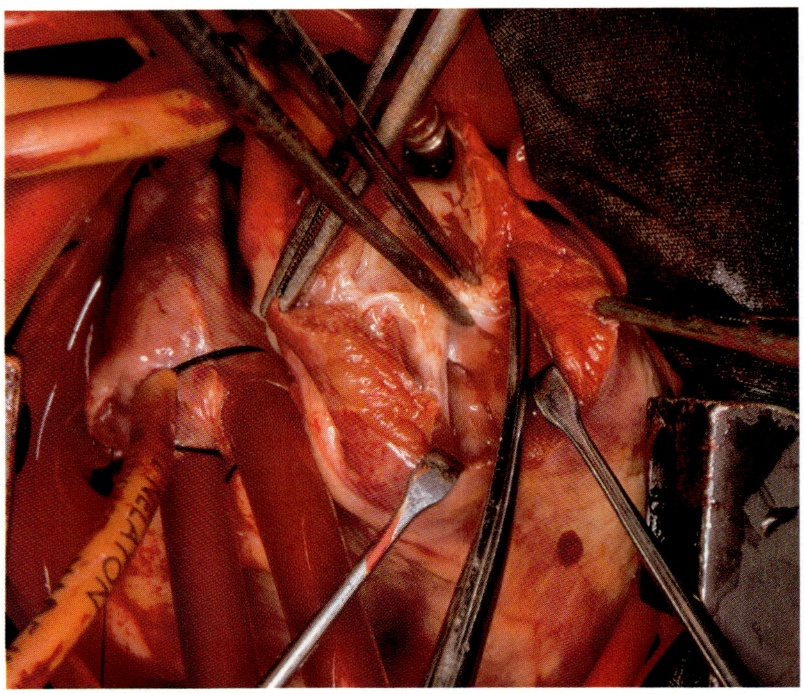

16

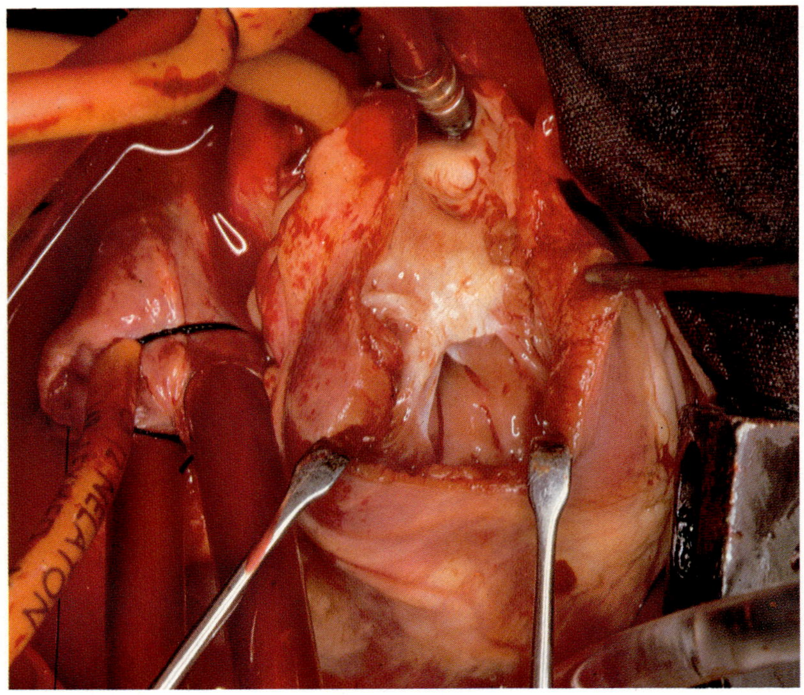

15 and 16 More fibrous tissue and muscle is excised from the left side of the outflow tract, thus opening it up widely.

17
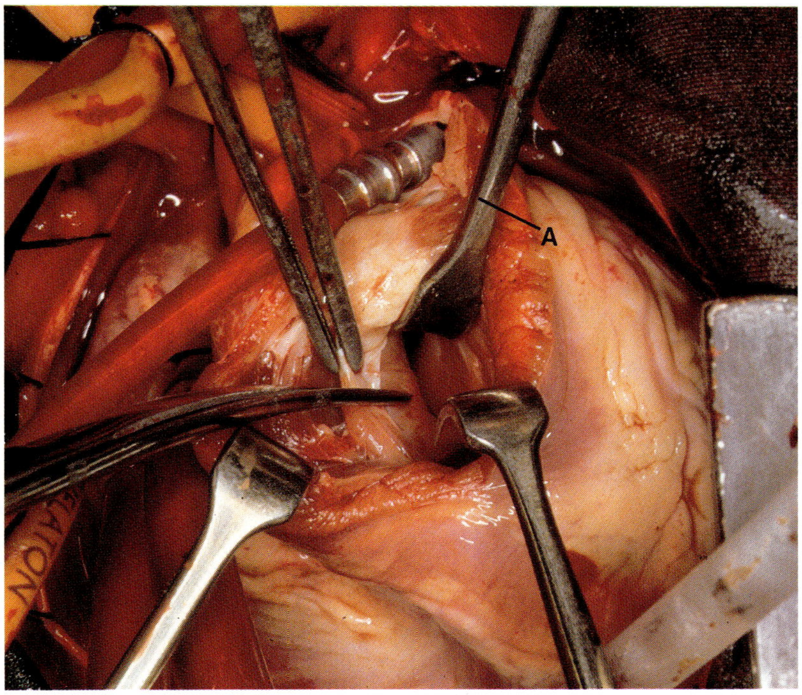

18
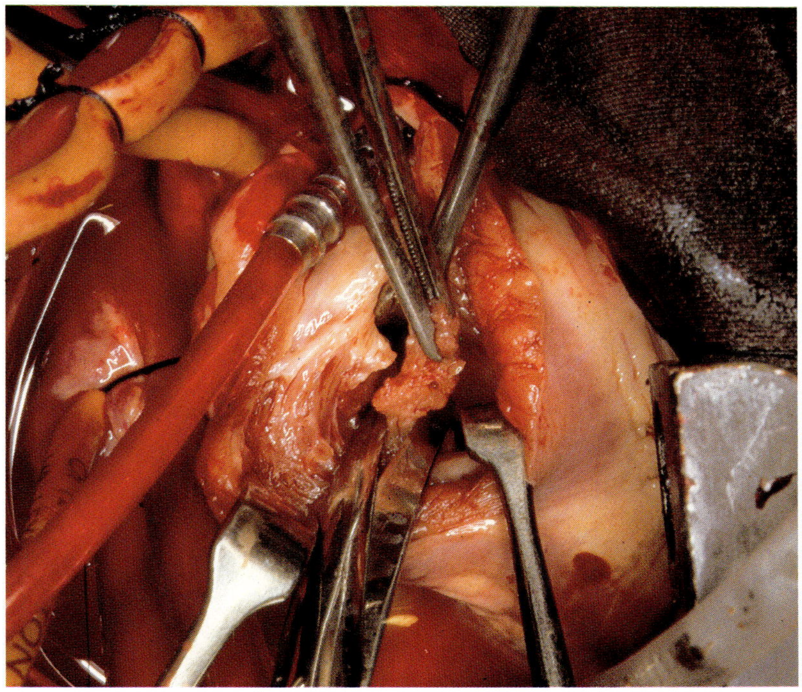

17 and 18 A retractor (**A**) retracts the upper margin of the ventricular septal defect which is formed by the conus septum (crista). Obstructing muscle forming the parietal insertion of the conus septum is incised and removed. If the septal insertion of the conus septum is also obstructing, then this too should be removed. However, when a longitudinal patch is being inserted, this will greatly relieve the obstruction and therefore it may be possible to remove less muscle.

19
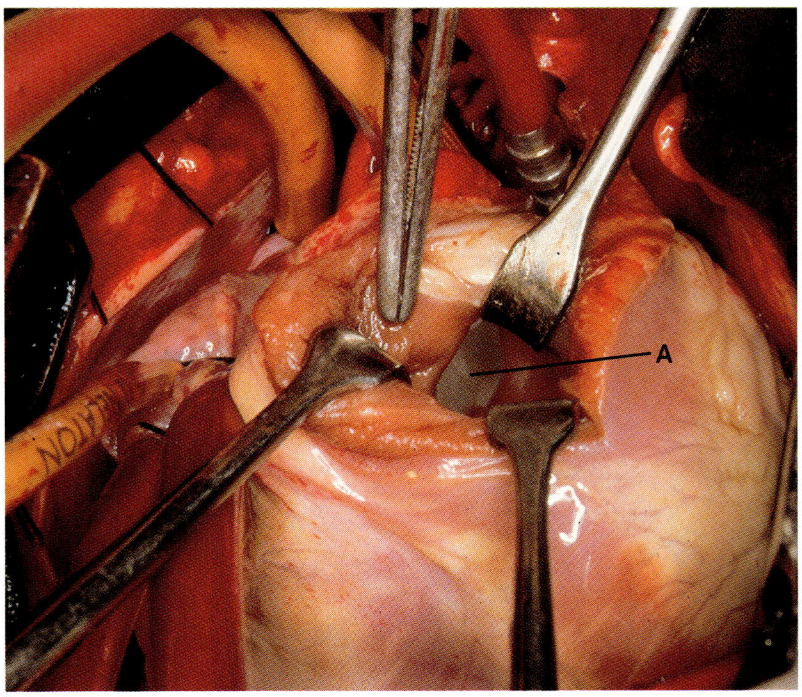

19 With retraction, a good view of the ventricular septal defect (**A**) is obtained, with the lighter coloured left ventricle beyond.

20
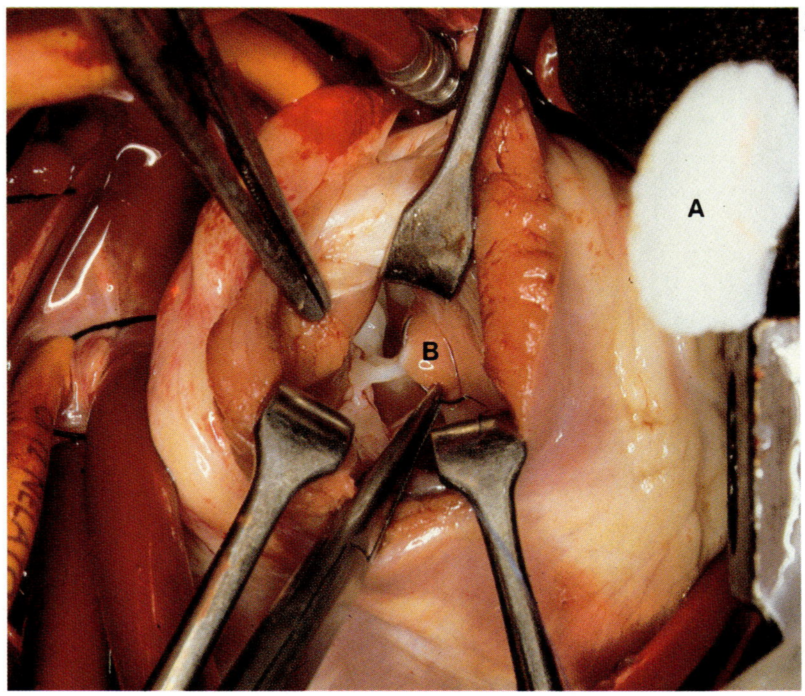

20 The defect is closed with a patch of dacron cloth (**A**) using a continuous Prolene suture. The first stitch is placed at the base of the papillary muscle of the conus (**B**).

21

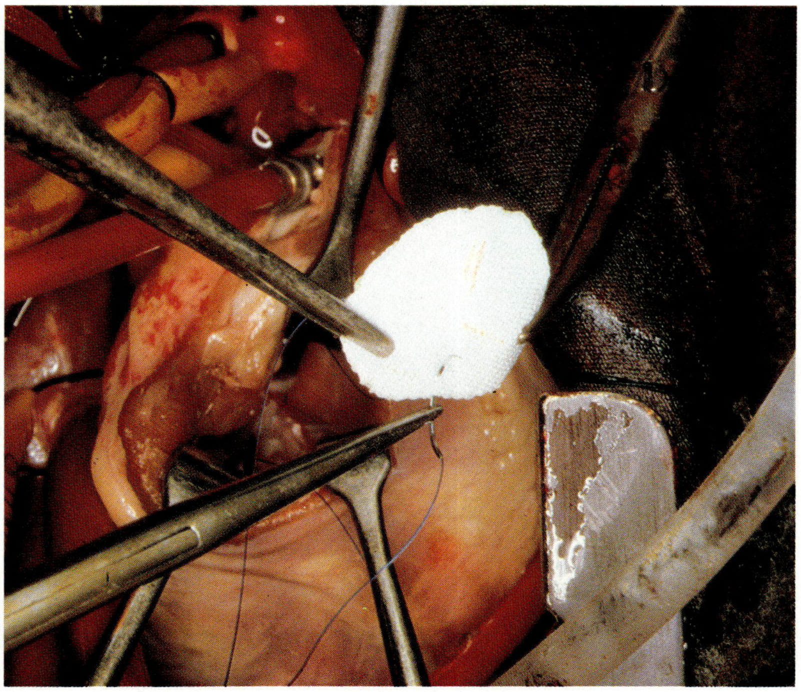

21 The suture is then placed through the patch and, to help with the careful placement of the stitches along the lower margin of the defect, several stitches are placed through both the patch and defect margin before sliding the patch down into position.

22

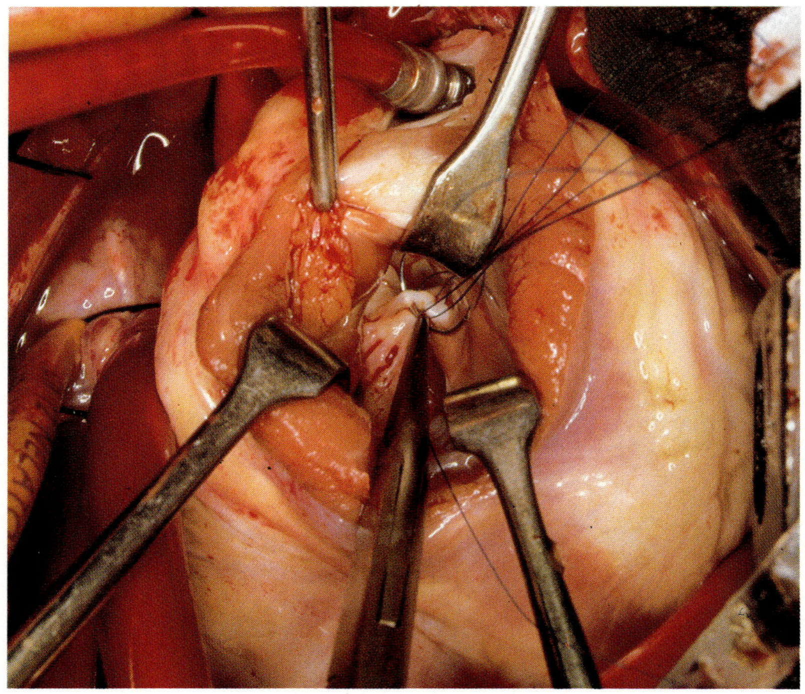

22 More stitches are placed along the lower margin of the defect, taking great care to keep them entirely on the right side of the septum, as they would endanger the conduction mechanism if placed through the whole lower rim of the defect.

23

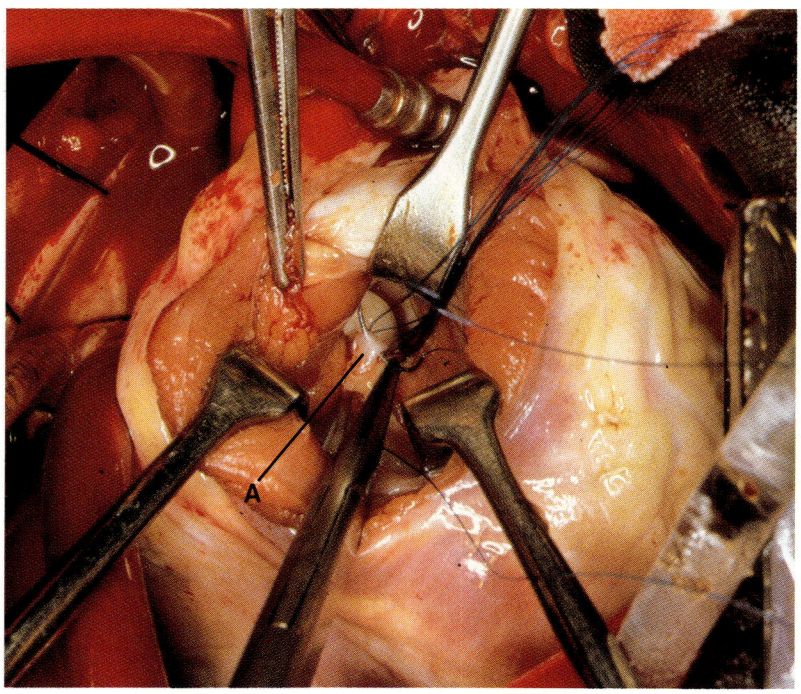

23 When working along the lower margin, the stitches are placed into the septal leaflet of the tricuspid valve (**A**) as soon as possible as this provides firm tissue to suture to but does not contain bundle tissue.

24

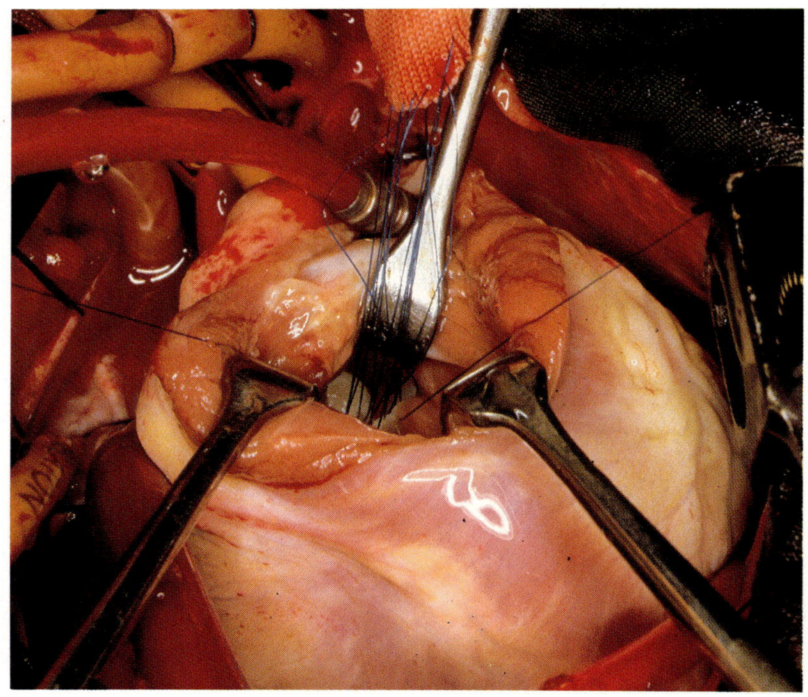

24 Seven stitches have now been placed and the patch is slid down carefully into position.

25

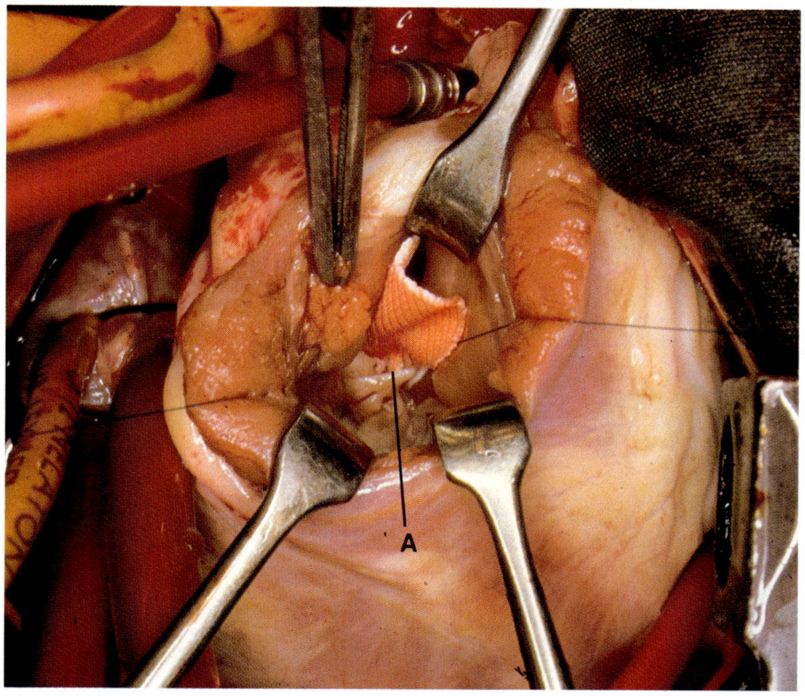

26

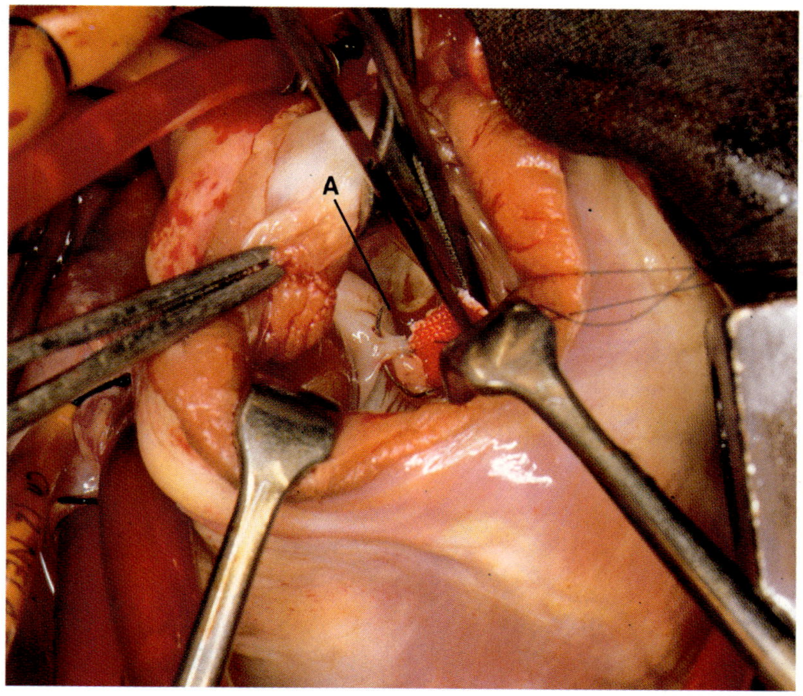

25 The patch is now down in position and all the sutures have been pulled tight. The septal leaflet of the tricuspid valve (**A**) is seen and its function should not be affected by the sutures placed in its base.

26 The suture is continued and here the uppermost attachment of the tricuspid valve is used for a last firm bite before the sutures have to be placed in muscle. Care must be taken not to damage a cusp of the aortic valve (**A**), which can be quite close.

27

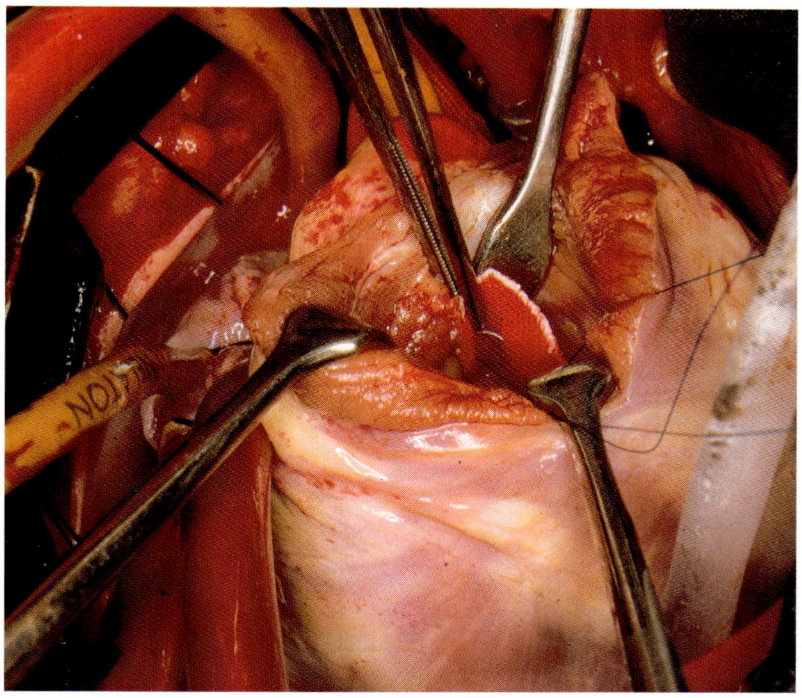

28

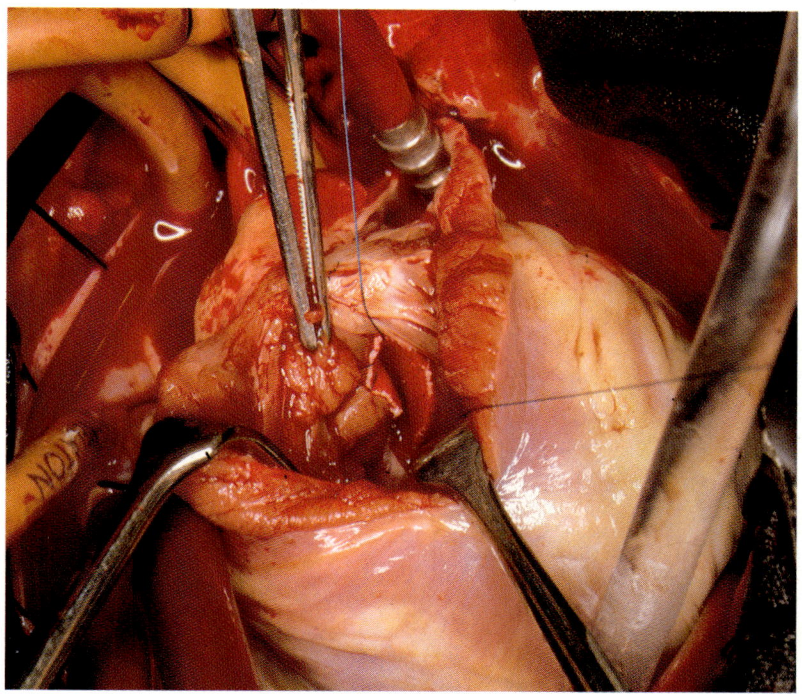

27 and 28 The remaining sutures are placed up the right side of the defect and large bites are taken of both muscle and patch.

29

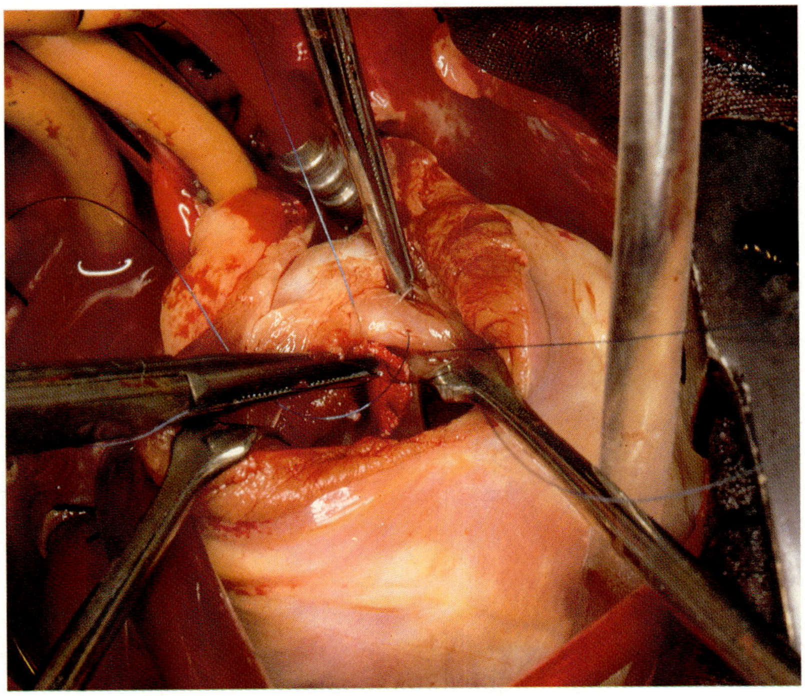

30

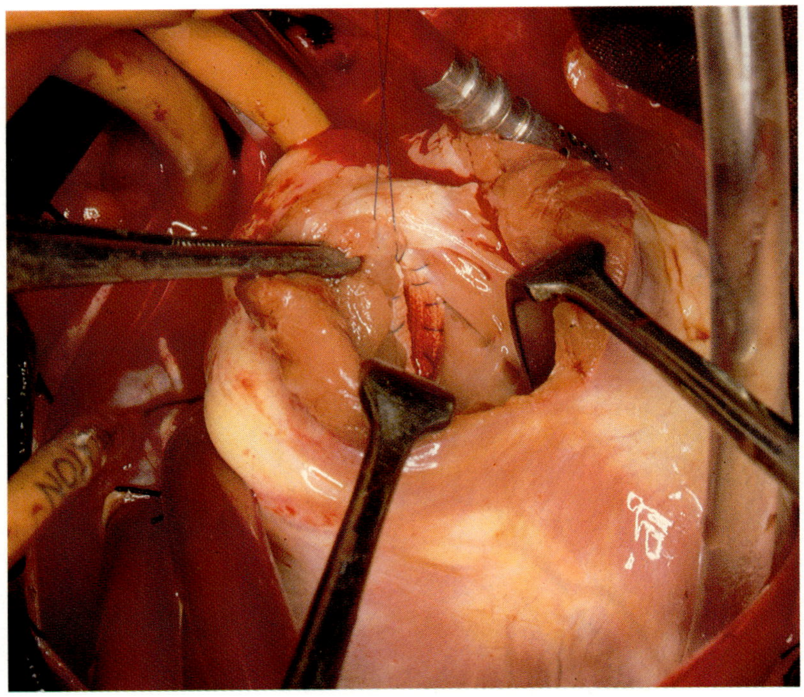

29 and 30 The suture is then held and the other end of the suture used to finish the left hand side of the patch up to the top of the defect.

31

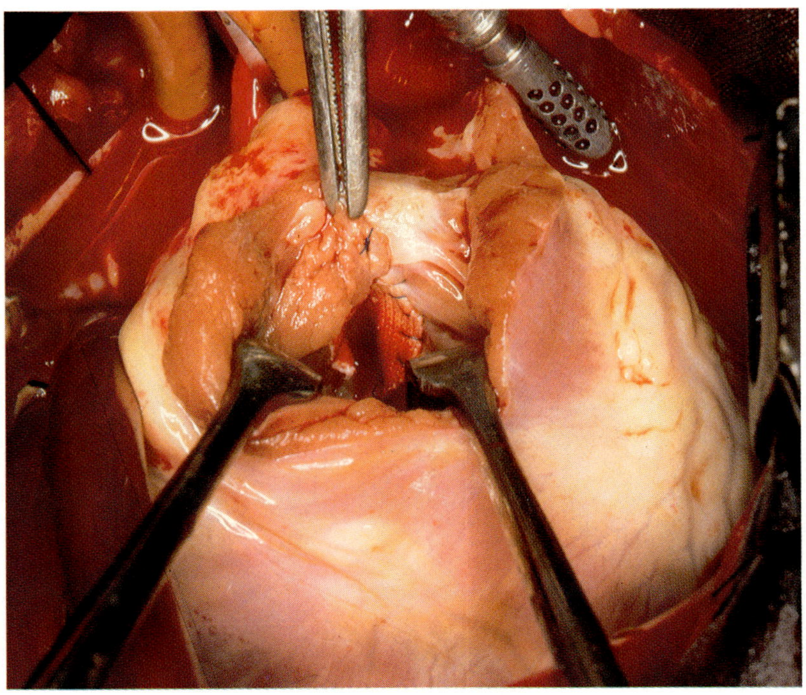

31 The two suture ends are then tied and the defect closed completely.

32

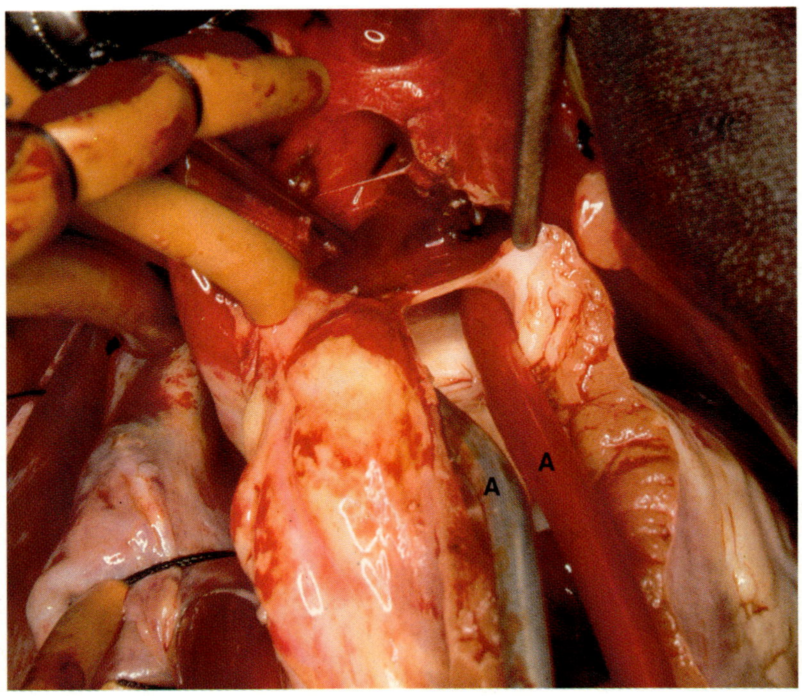

32 Attention is turned again to the pulmonary artery and suckers (**A**) have been used to remove blood from the right and left pulmonary arteries.

33

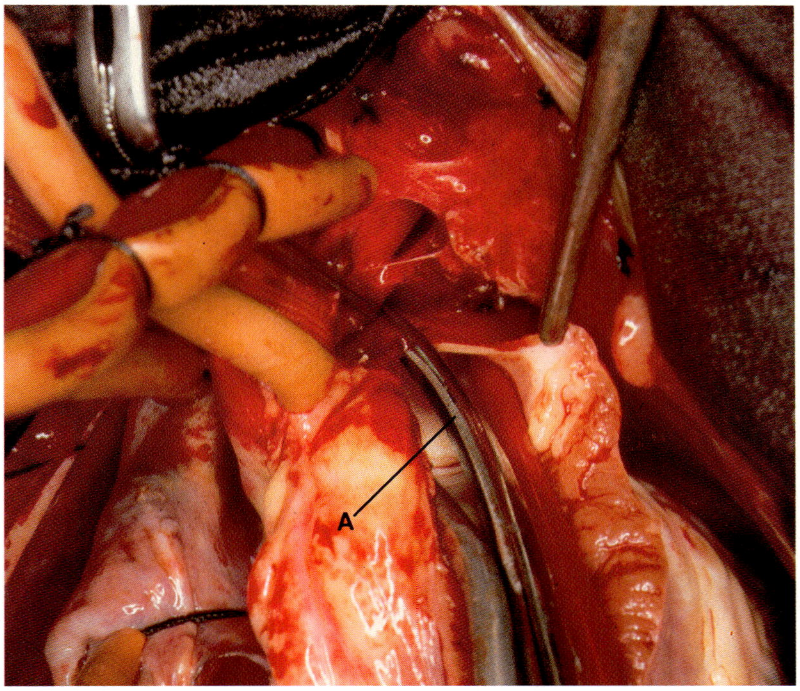

33 The incision in the main pulmonary artery is extended with scissors (**A**) up to the bifurcation.

34

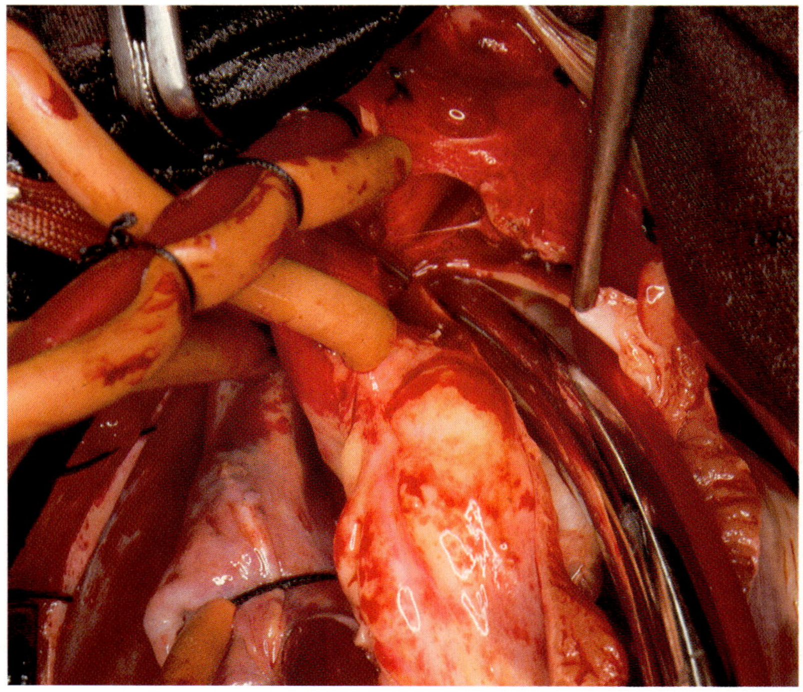

34 A Hegar dilator has been passed into the right pulmonary artery.

35

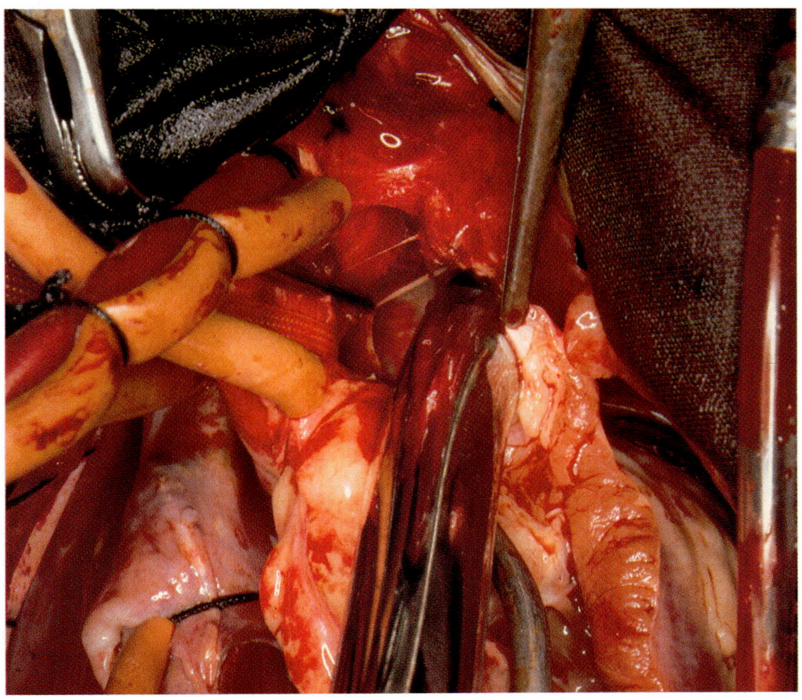

35 A Hegar dilator has been passed into the left pulmonary artery. It can be seen that, despite the small size of the main pulmonary artery, the size of the branches is very satisfactory.

36

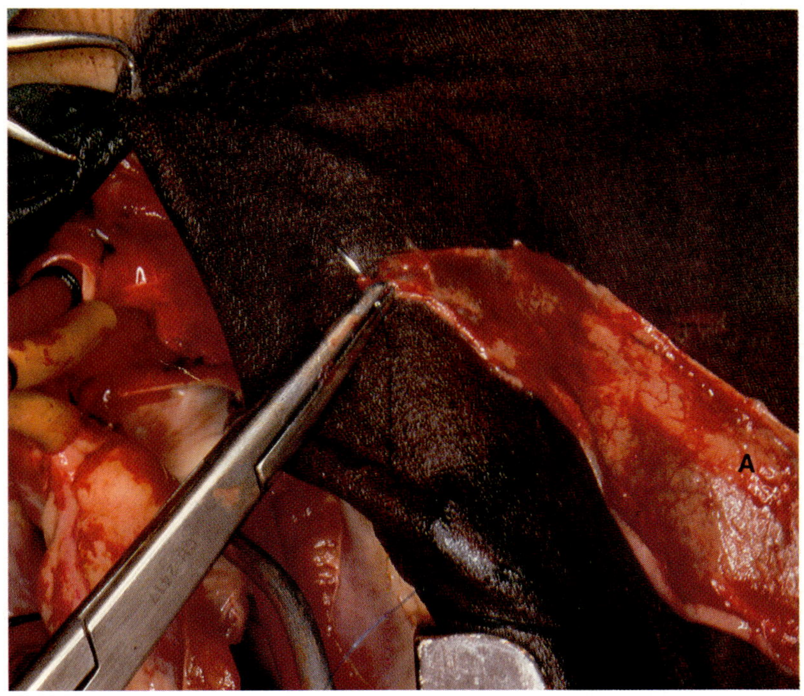

36 A piece of pericardium (**A**), which was taken when the pericardium was first opened, is to be used as the patch to enlarge the outflow tract. The first stitch of a continuous Prolene suture is being placed in the patch.

37

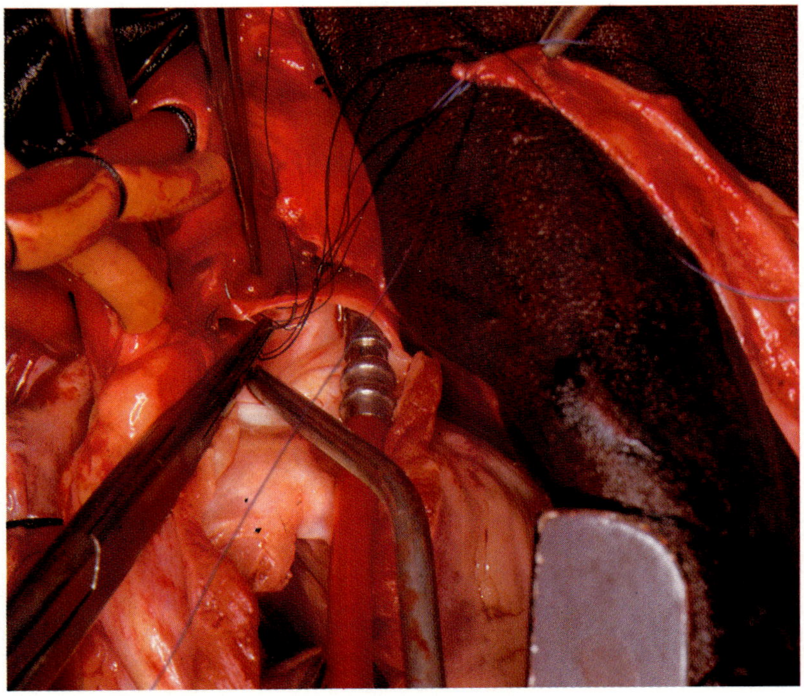

37 Several sutures are placed through the patch and pulmonary artery before sliding down the patch into position.

38

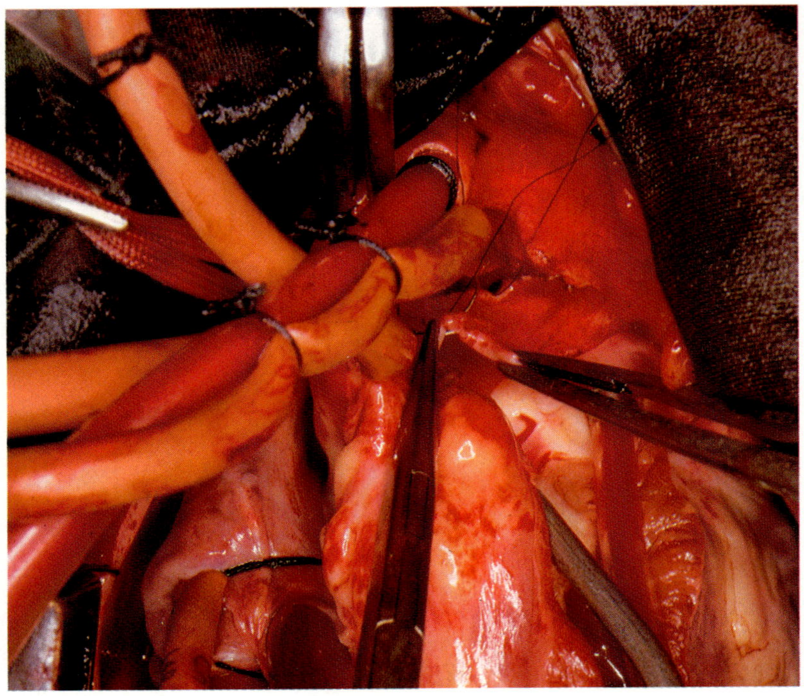

38 The right side of the patch is sutured in with one end of the suture.

39

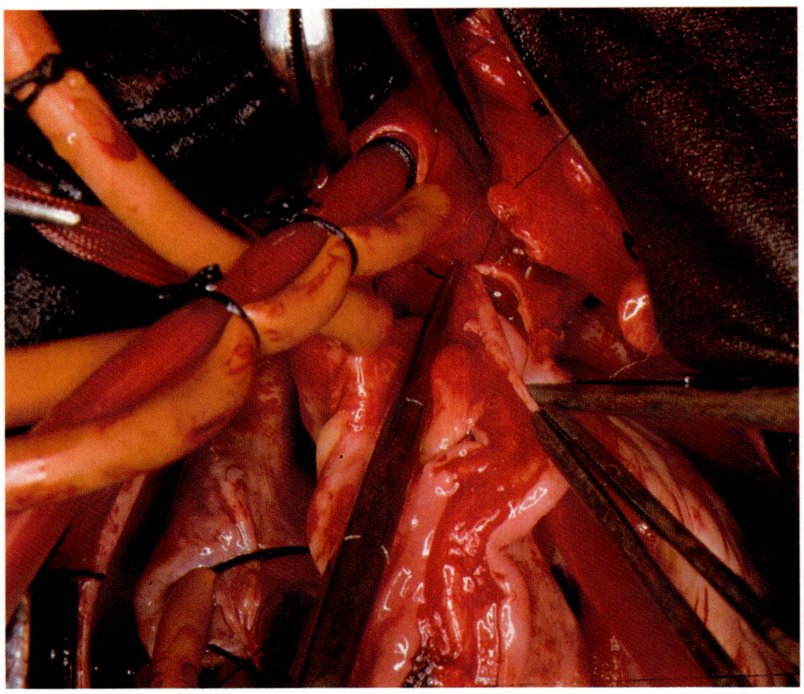

39 The other end of the suture is then used to suture the left side of the patch.

40

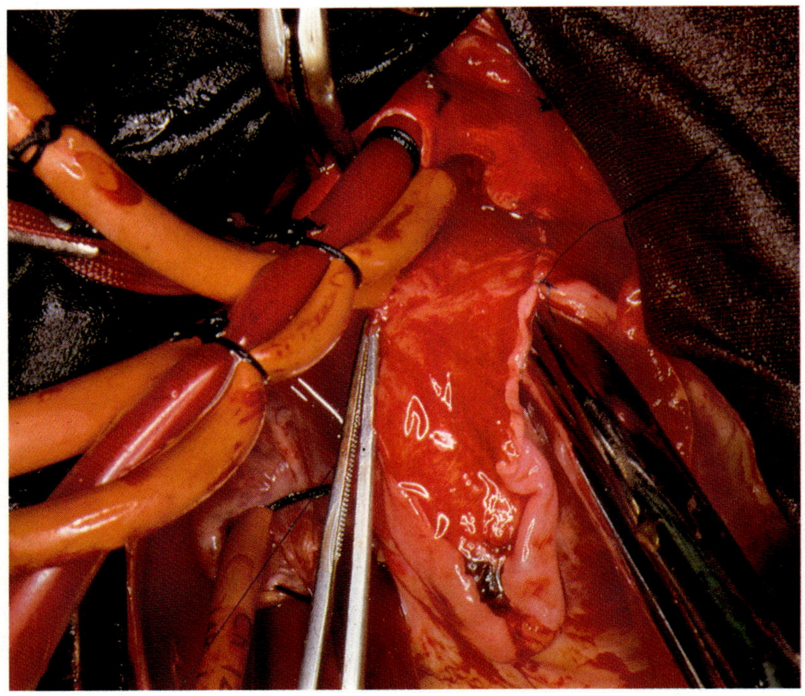

40 The continuous suture has been locked and a Hegar dilator (**A**) is used to check that the pulmonary arteries have not been narrowed.

41

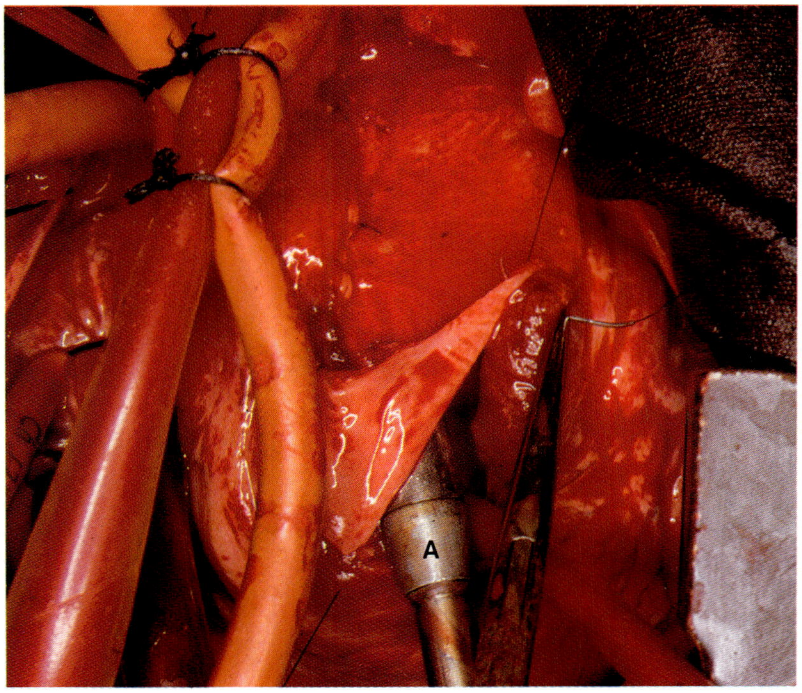

41 The remainder of the patch is sutured in and, after removing air from the heart, the aortic clamp has been released. A sucker (**A**) returns blood to the bypass machine.

42

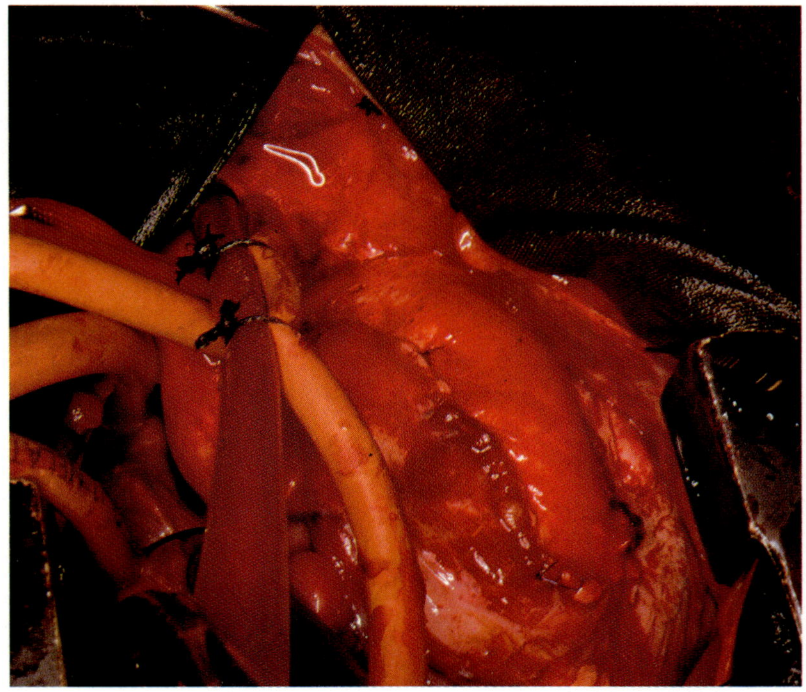

42 The insertion of the pericardial patch into the right ventricular outflow tract is now complete and cardiopulmonary bypass can be discontinued and the left ventricular vent removed.

43

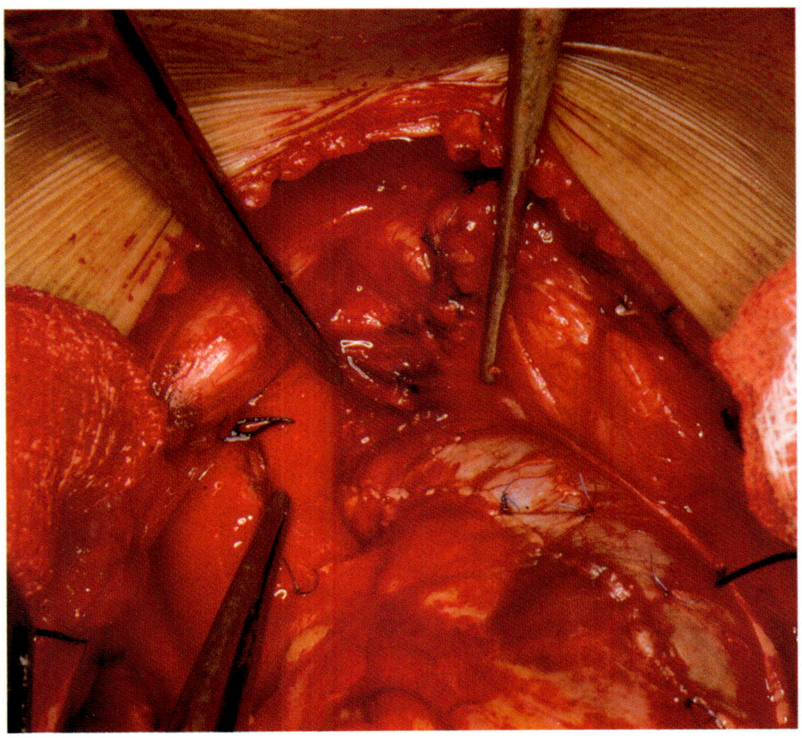

43 The arterial and venous cannulae have been removed and, with forceps retracting the aorta, the full extent of the patch can be seen.

Correction with unicusp homograft patch to outflow tract

44
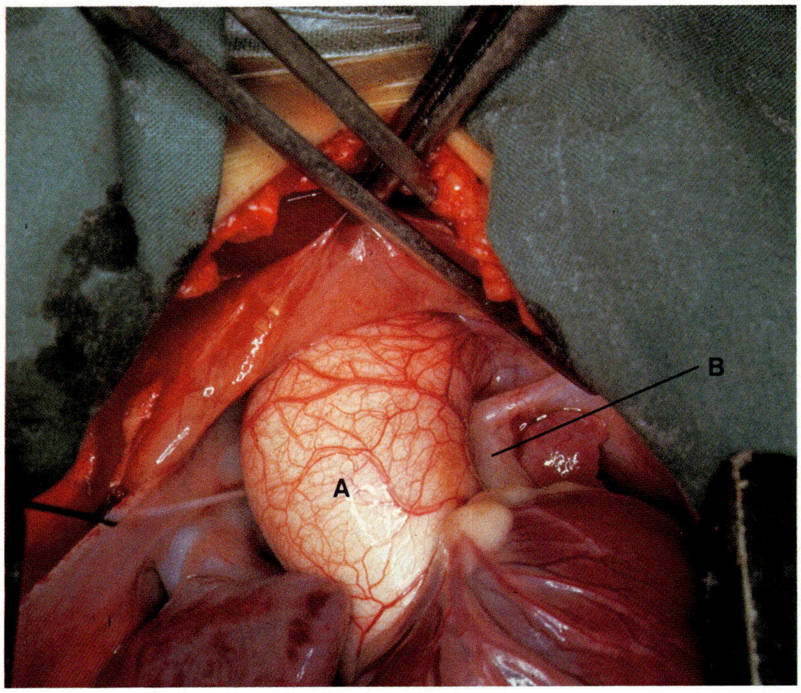

45
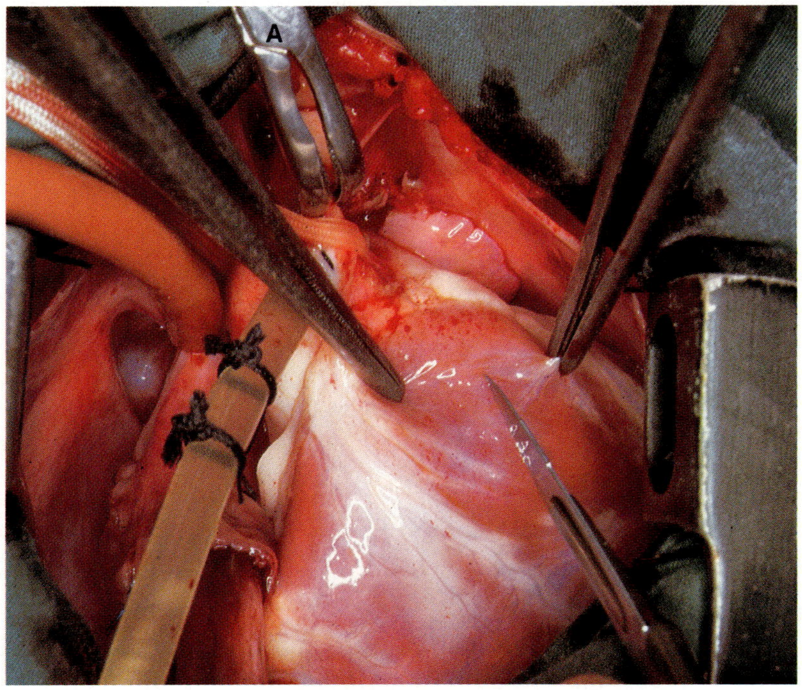

44 This infant with a large aorta (**A**) has a markedly underdeveloped pulmonary artery (**B**).

45 Hypothermia has been used and the circulation arrested. A clamp (**A**) has been placed across the ascending aorta distal to the aortic cannula which contains clear fluid because it has been used for the introduction of cardioplegic fluid (see Chapter 1). As the pulmonary artery is so small, an outflow patch is certain to be needed and therefore a longitudinal right ventriculotomy is made.

46
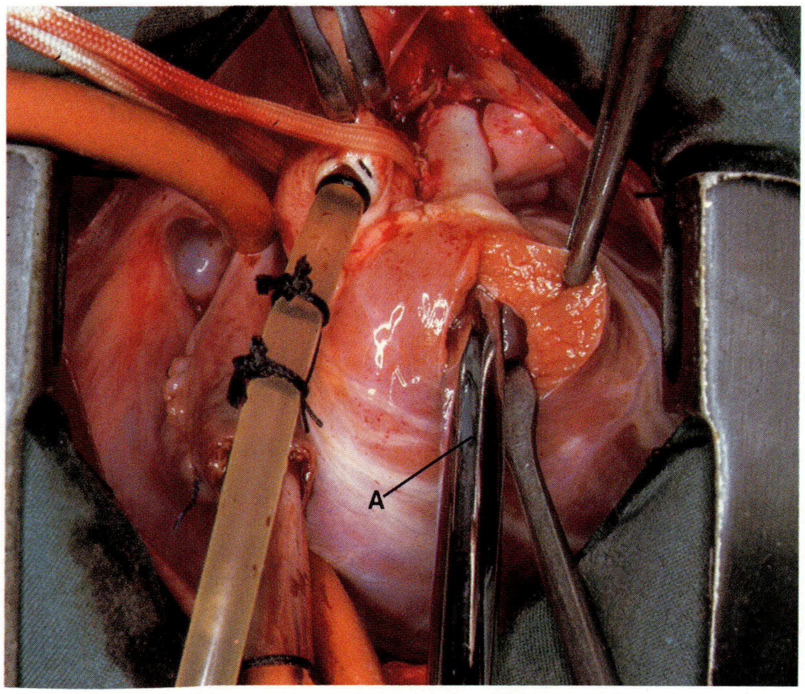

47
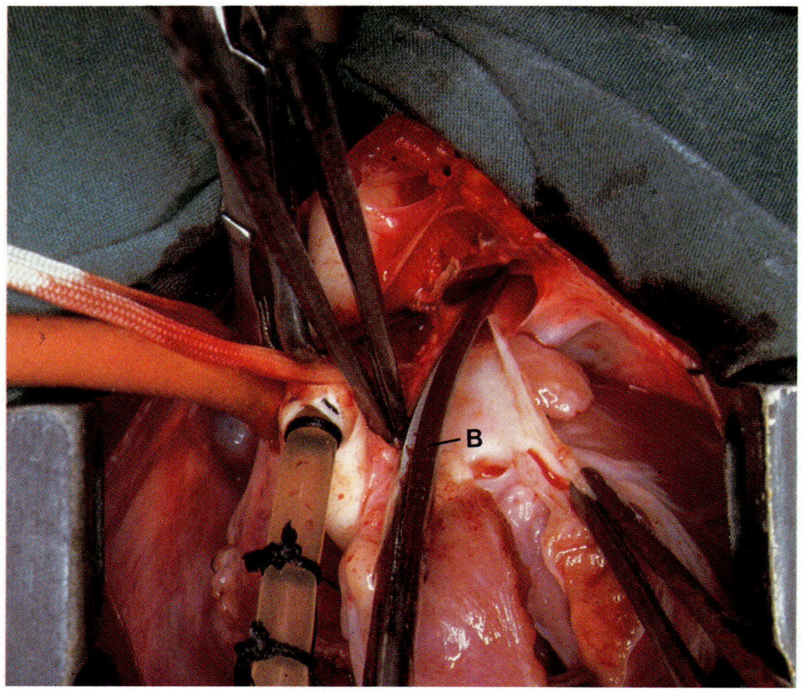

46 and 47 The small size of the pulmonary valve ring is confirmed with a Hegar dilator (**A**) and the pulmonary artery is opened up longitudinally with scissors (**B**).

48

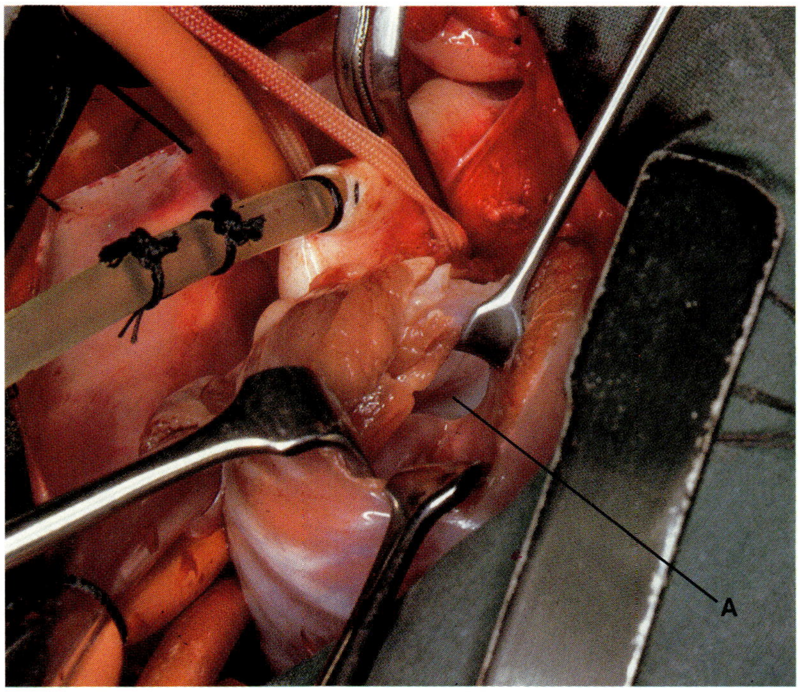

49

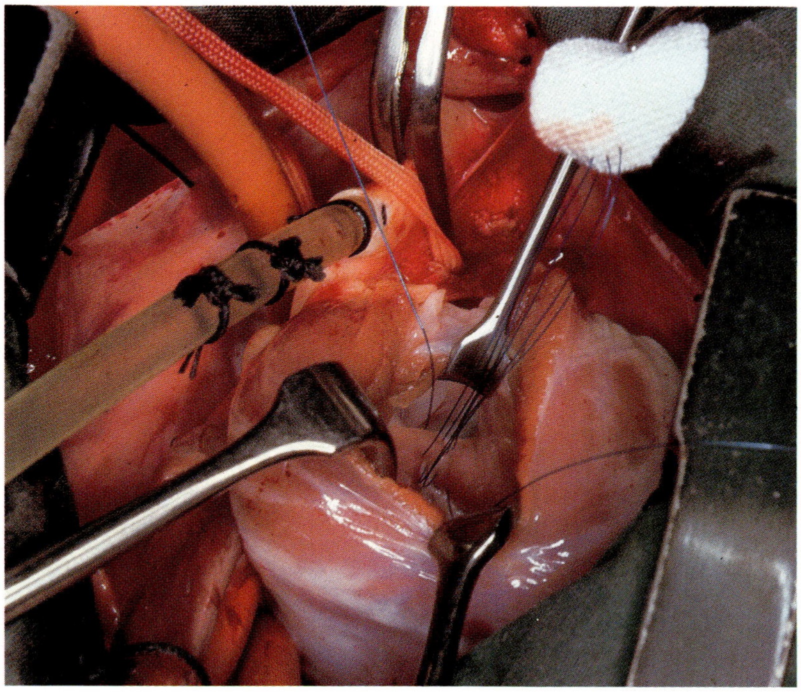

48 to 50 The ventricular septal defect (**A**) has been exposed with retraction and is closed with a dacron cloth patch using continuous Prolene suture.

50

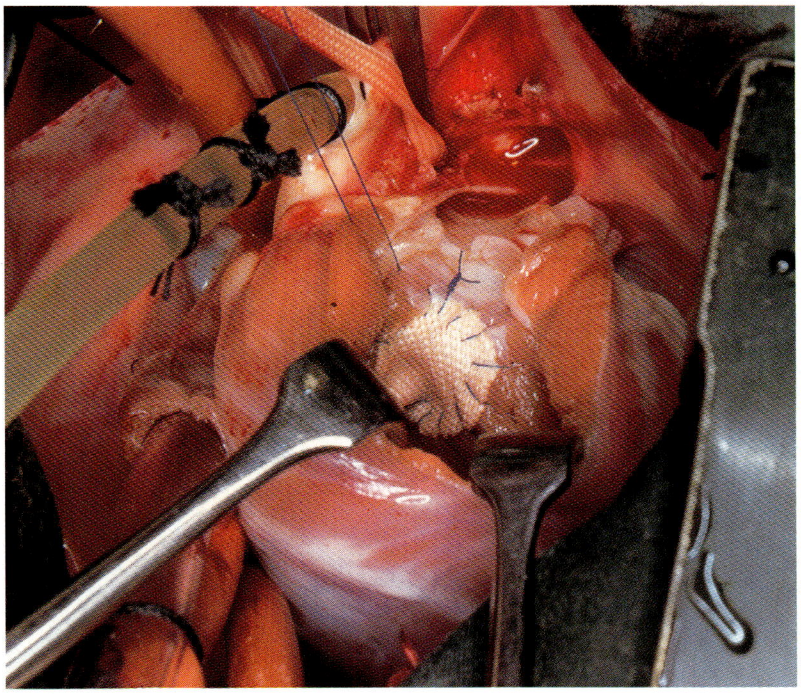

51

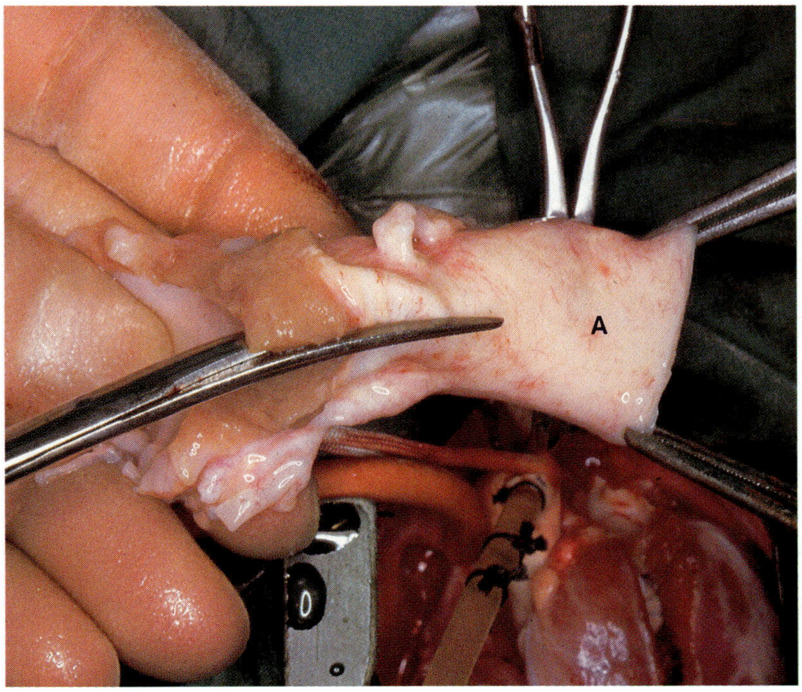

51 It has been decided to use part of a homograft aortic valve for the patch as this will prevent, or greatly reduce, pulmonary regurgitation after correction. That piece of aorta bearing the non-coronary cusp is used and the homograft (**A**) is opened longitudinally opposite this.

52

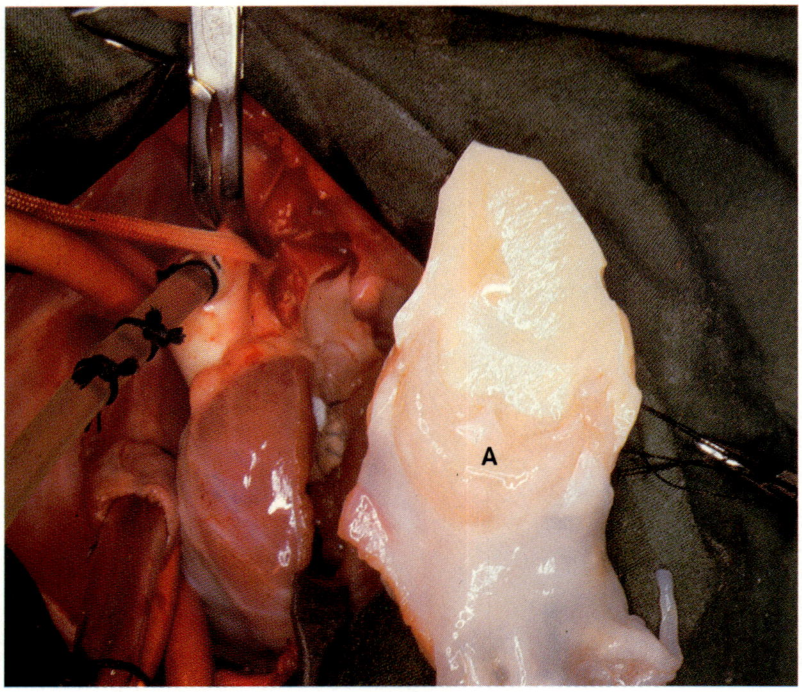

53

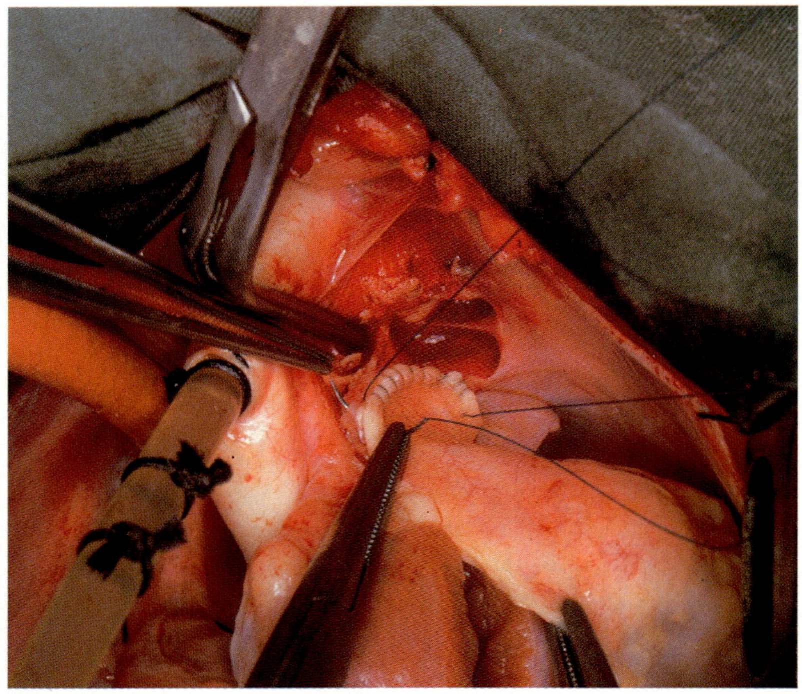

52 The unicusp patch is seen from the inside with part of the anterior leaflet of the mitral valve left attached as this closes the ventriculotomy conveniently. The length of aortic wall left above the cusp matches the length of incision in the pulmonary artery so that the cusp (**A**) lies at the same level as the patient's pulmonary valve.

53 to 55 The homograft patch is now sutured into position with continuous Prolene sutures.

54

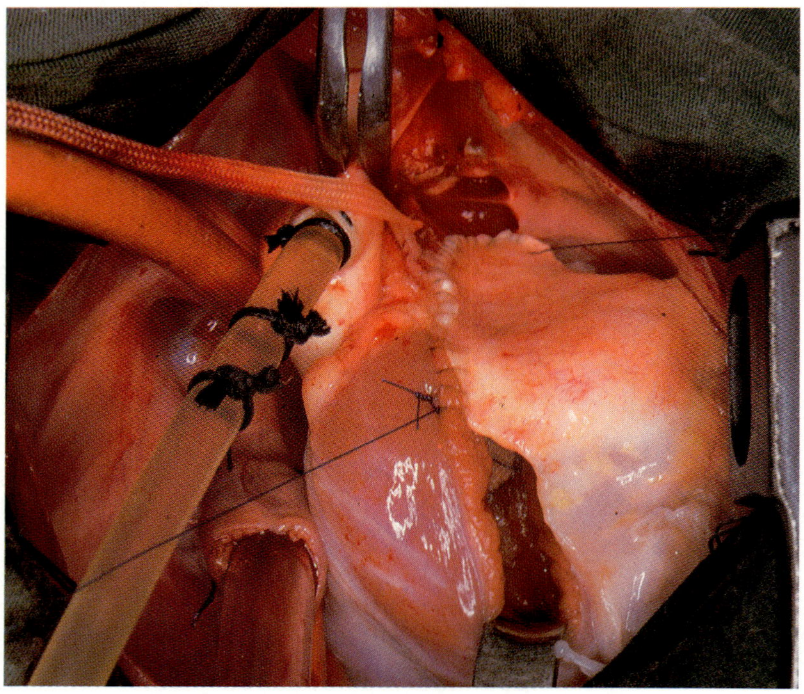

55

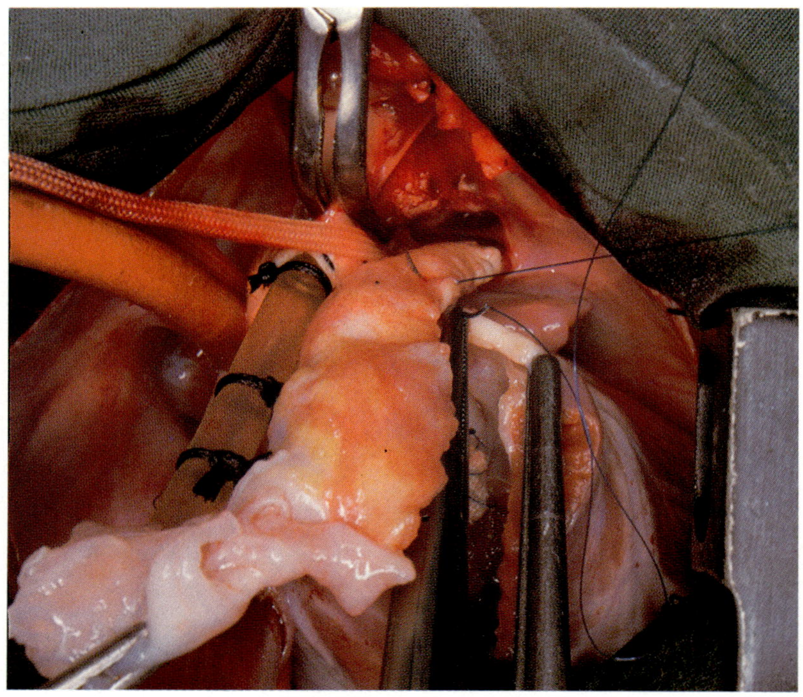

56

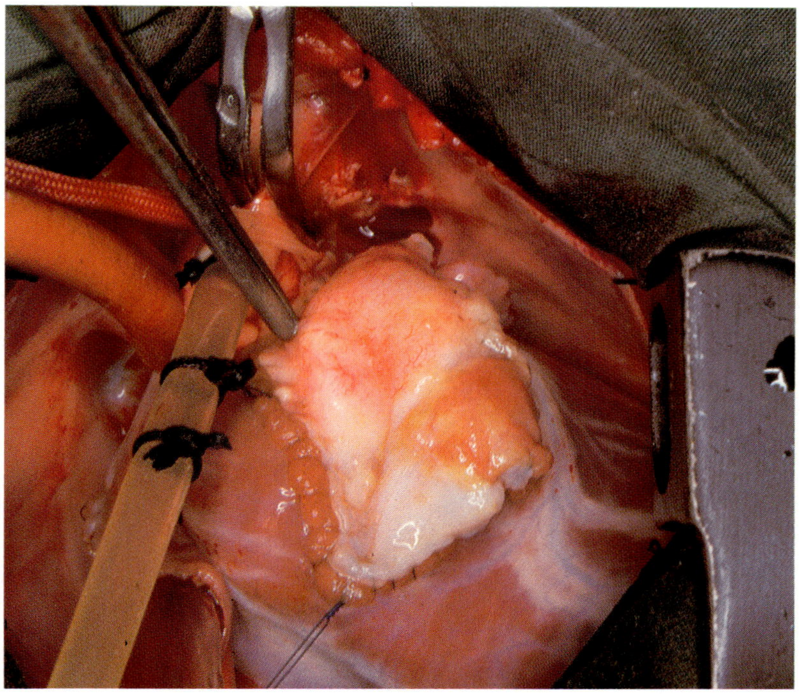

56 The homograft patch is now sutured in completely and the patient is ready for cardiopulmonary bypass to be recommenced.

57

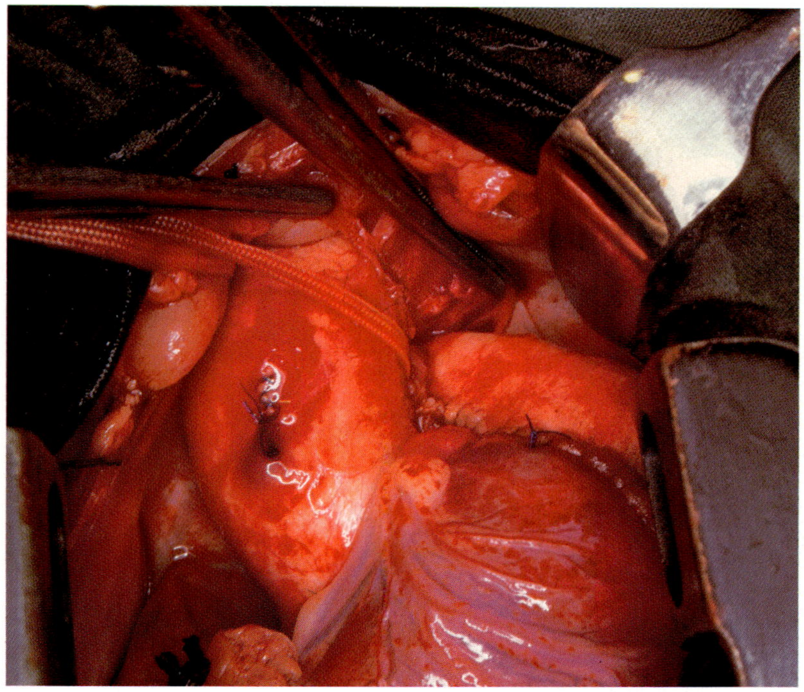

57 The final appearance of the patch is seen once bypass has been discontinued and the cannulae removed.

Correction through a transverse right ventriculotomy

58

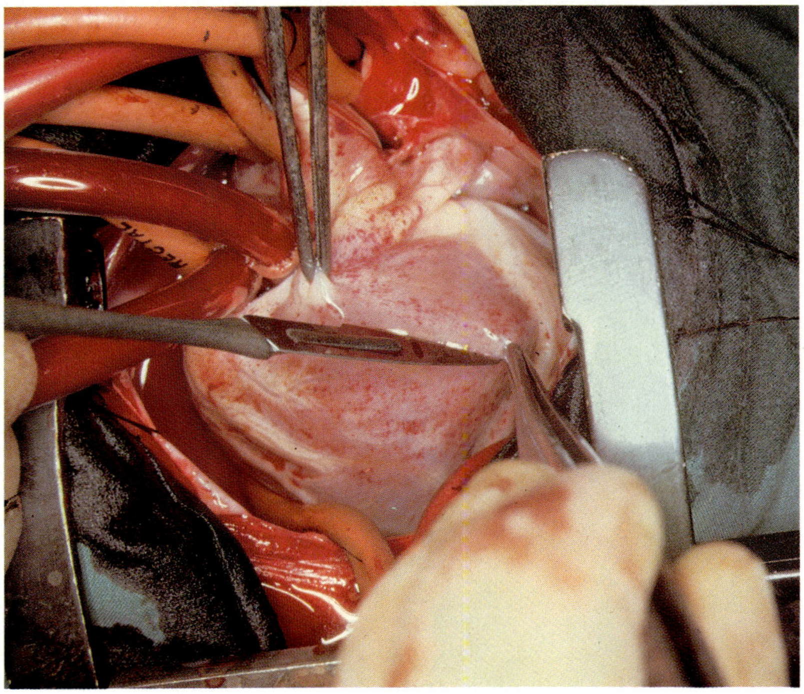

59

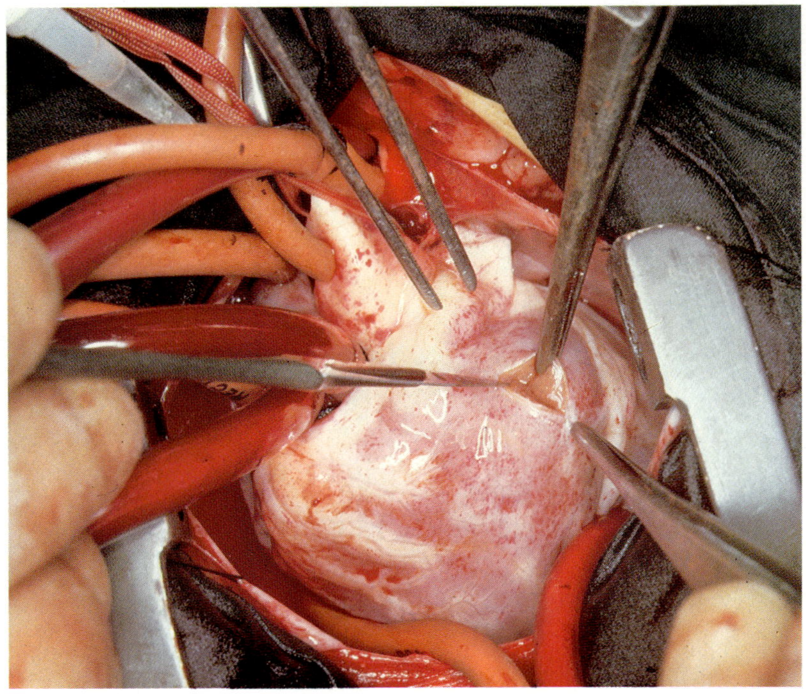

58 and 59 Pre-operative studies have shown this patient to have an adequate sized pulmonary artery and valve ring, and the obstruction is entirely infundibular. A transverse right ventriculotomy is therefore made and this avoids the need for any patch to be inserted.

60

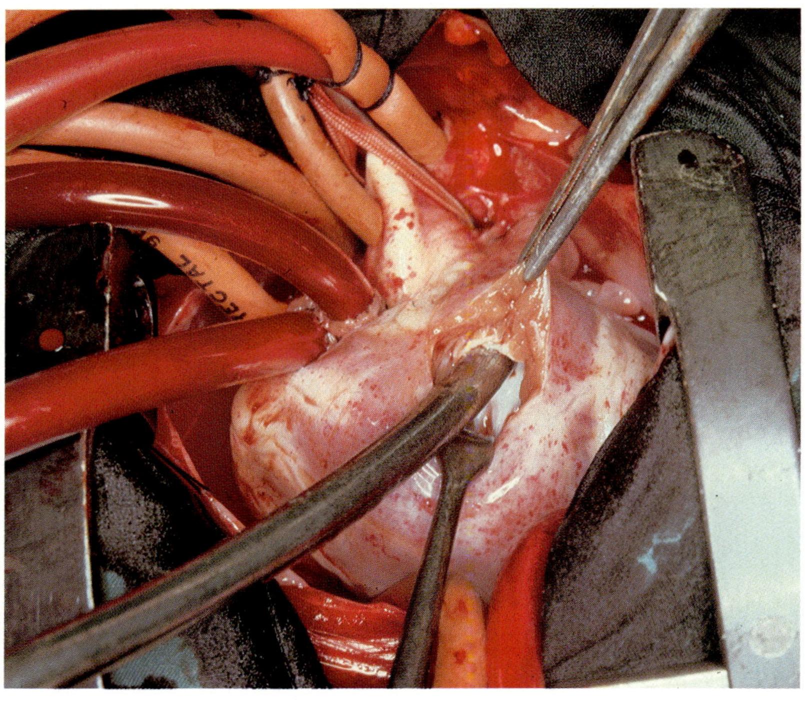

61

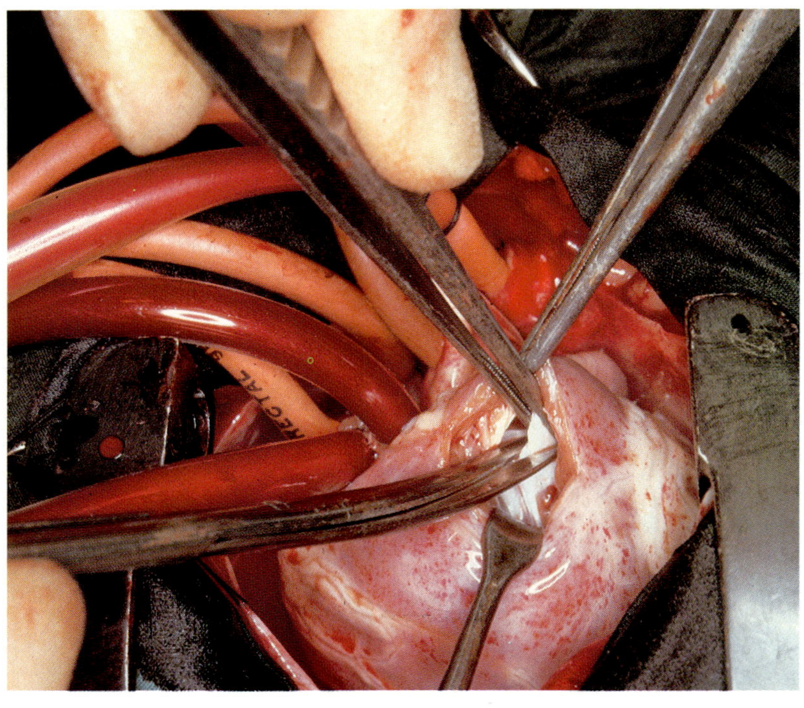

60 Initially only a small Hegar dilator will pass through into the pulmonary valve.

61 Obstructing fibrous tissue and muscle are removed.

62

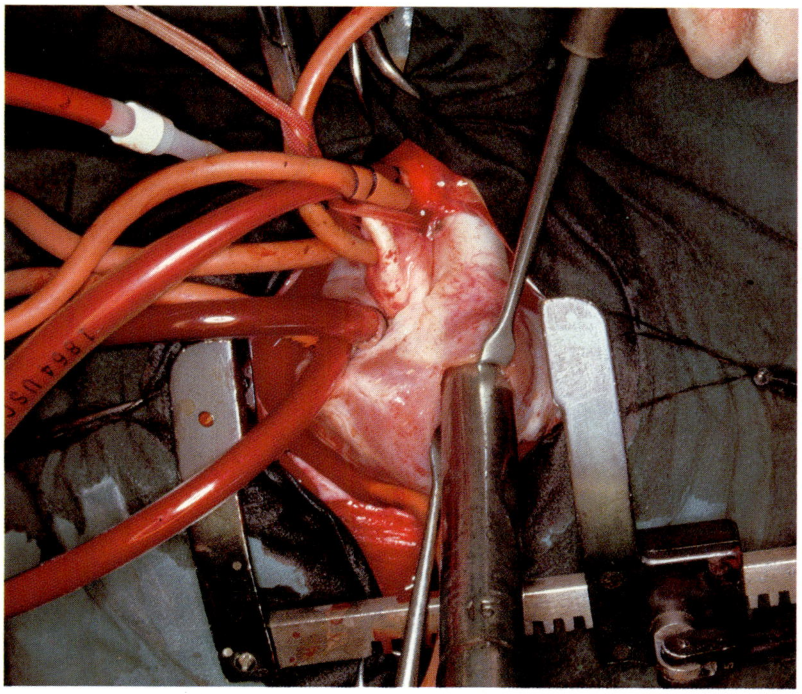

62 After the infundibular resection, a size 15 Hegar dilator can pass into the pulmonary artery.

63

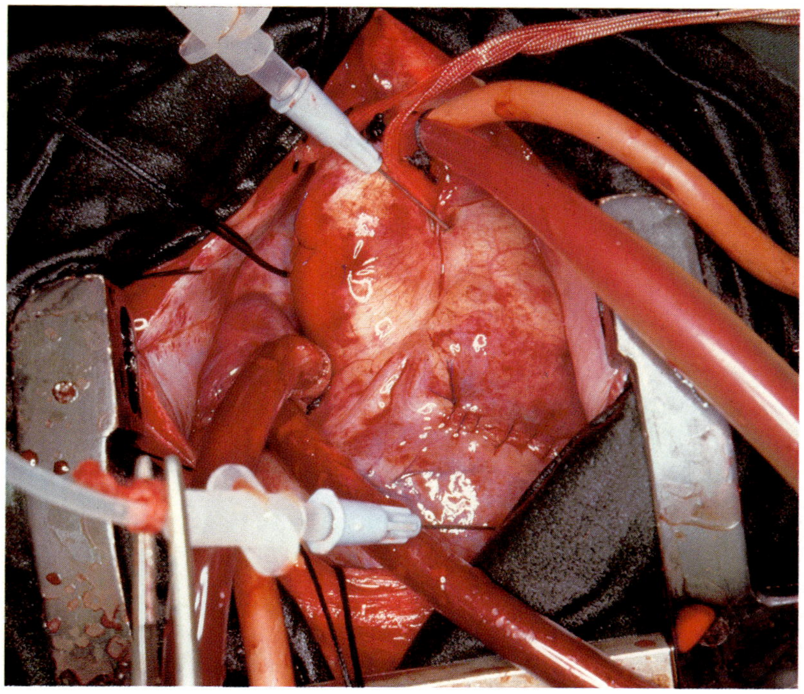

63 Correction is now complete and simultaneous pressures are measured by needles placed in the right ventricle and pulmonary artery. This should show no significant obstruction between the two and right ventricular pressure can be compared with the systemic pressure.

Dura mater patch to right ventricle

64 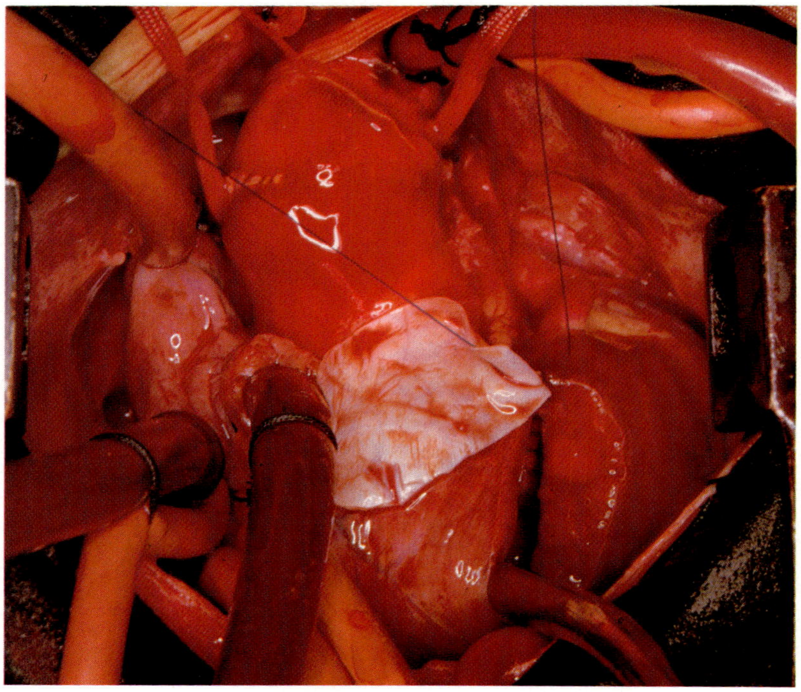

64 to 66 When there is doubt as to whether a patch will be needed across the valve ring, a vertical ventriculotomy is recommended[4]. This should stop short of the valve ring and obstructing infundibular muscle and fibrous tissue is resected. If there is any stenosis of the pulmonary valve, this can be dealt with from below or, if necessary, through a separate pulmonary arteriotomy, but leaving the valve ring intact. Then the valve ring can be measured with Hegar dilators to assess whether it is of adequate size. If not, the incision can be carried through the valve ring and a transannular patch inserted, but if it is adequate, then the pulmonary valve competence can be preserved. However, unlike a transverse ventriculotomy, if a vertical ventriculotomy is closed directly, it might narrow the infundibulum. Therefore it is recommended that the vertical ventriculotomy should be closed with a small patch of pericardium, dacron cloth or, as illustrated here, dura mater.

65 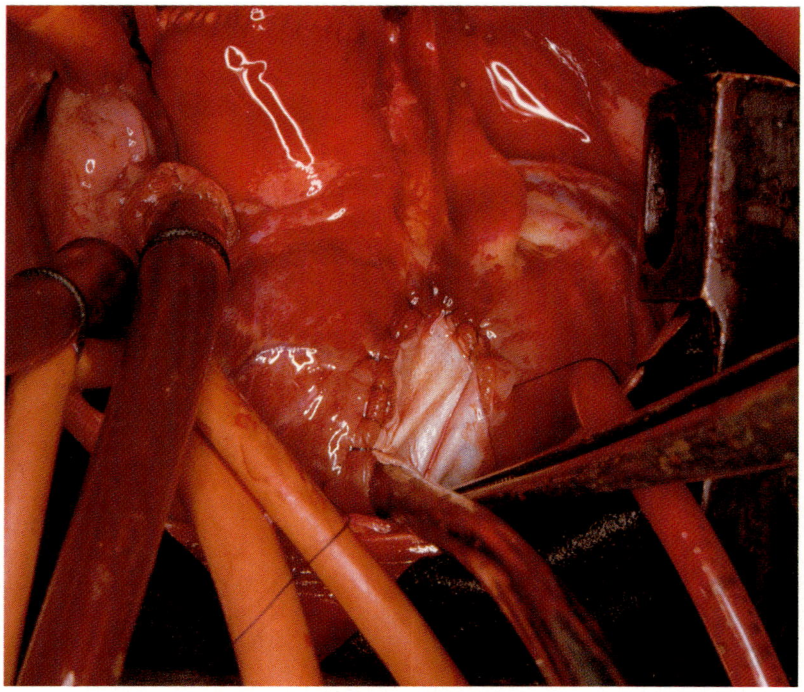

66 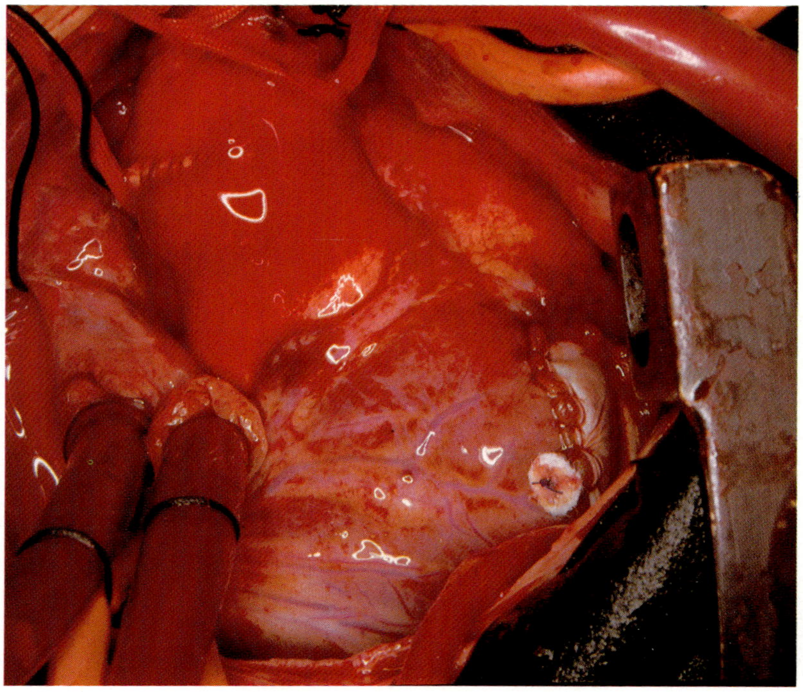

13: Repair of transposition of the great arteries

The anatomy in transposition of the great arteries is represented in diagram **A**. The aorta (**A**) arises from the right ventricle (**B**) and the pulmonary artery (**C**) from the left ventricle (**D**). This results in two parallel circulations: the blue desaturated blood returning from the body is pumped by the right ventricle to the aorta and the red saturated blood returning to the left atrium is pumped by the left ventricle to the lungs. Fortunately, mixing occurs at the foramen ovale (**E**) and ductus arteriosus but, soon after birth if the duct closes, this mixing is inadequate and the baby becomes very blue.

The introduction of balloon septostomy by Rashkind in 1966[1] revolutionised the management of this condition. Previously, in these very blue neonates usually presenting in the first day or so of life, the only procedure available was the surgical creation of an atrial septal defect (Blalock-Hanlon)[2] to improve mixing. This procedure is hardly ever performed now and therefore is not described in this chapter. However, after a balloon septostomy, these babies usually do very well and an elective 'correction' can usually be planned between about six to twelve months of age.

The most frequently used definitive operation, and that described in this chapter, is the Mustard procedure[3]. This operation involves the removal of the remaining atrial septum and the insertion of a baffle to redirect blue blood to the left ventricle and thence to the lungs, and the red blood to the right ventricle and on to the aorta. Occasional problems have been associated with the Mustard procedure, such as arrhythmias and baffle obstruction and possible long-term problems such as right ventricular failure and tricuspid regurgitation remain a worry for the future.

With the hope of reducing some of these problems, many surgeons have changed to using the Senning procedure[4], which was, in fact, originally introduced before the Mustard procedure.

The logical method of treating this condition is by switching the great arteries to their rightful positions. This, however, is not very easy because of the need to reposition the coronary arteries at the same time. When the left ventricle has been prepared to maintain the systemic pressure, as when a large ventricular septal defect is present, this would seem to be a sensible approach[5,6].

Cardiopulmonary bypass is needed and, as it is usual to perform the Mustard procedure in infancy, the profound hypothermia technique is particularly appropriate as it allows removal of the venous cannula and an unobstructed view of the atrium.

Diagram A

A – Aorta
B – Right ventricle
C – Main pulmonary artery
D – Left ventricle
E – Foramen ovale
F – Coronary sinus
G – Tricuspid valve
H – Inferior vena cava
J – Superior vena cava
K – Right atrium
L – Mitral valve

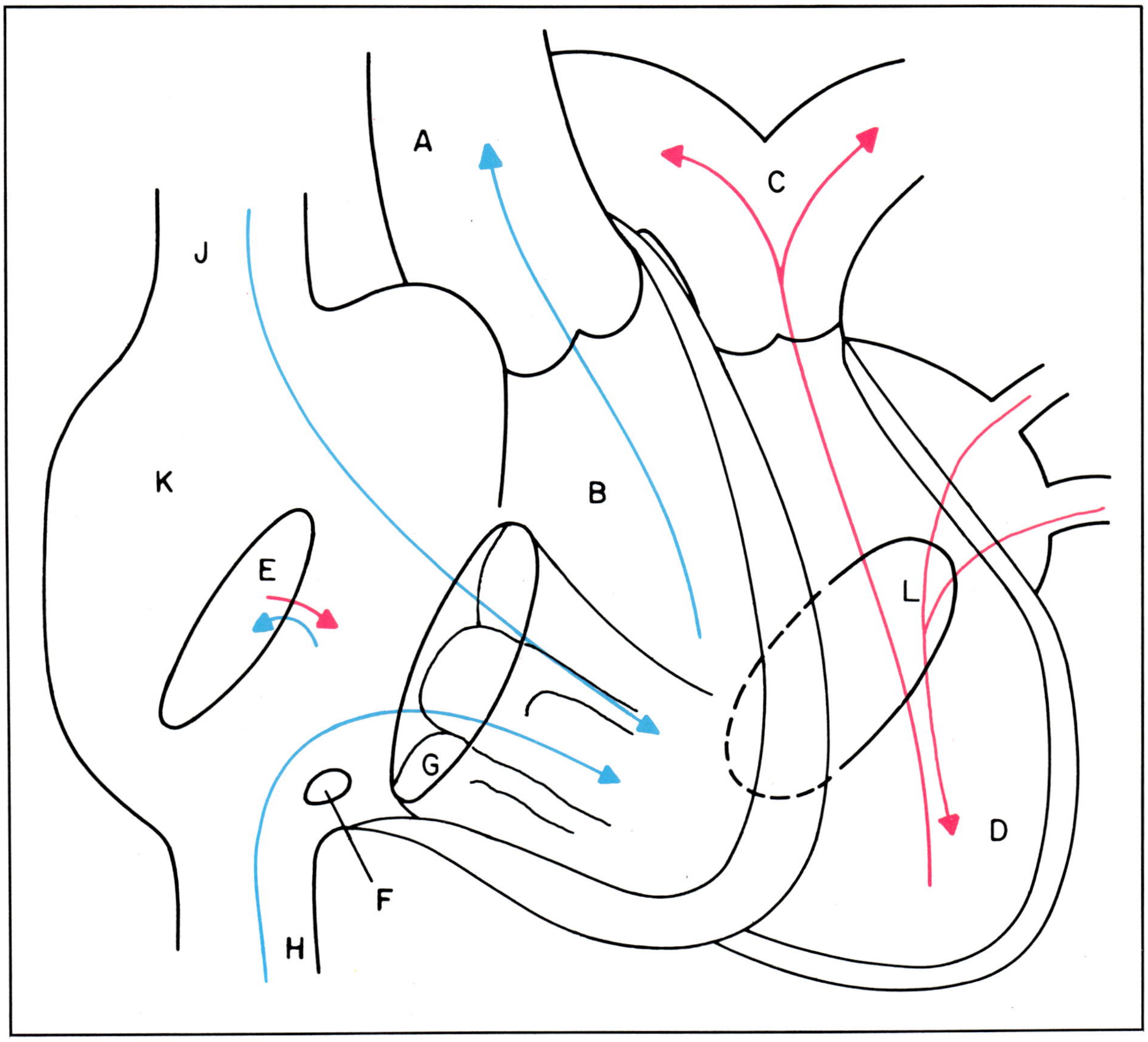

The Mustard procedure

Diagram **B** shows the effect of performing the Mustard procedure. The blue, desaturated blood returning from the superior vena cava (**J**) and inferior vena cava (**H**) passes behind the pericardial baffle (**E**), through the mitral valve (**L**), into the left ventricle (**D**) and then to the pulmonary arteries. The red, saturated blood returning from the pulmonary veins (**K**) passes over the baffle (**E**), through the tricuspid valve (**G**), into the right ventricle (**B**) and into the aorta.

The coronary sinus (**F**) is shown draining behind the baffle with the other blue blood. However, if it is felt that suturing around the lip of the coronary sinus would endanger the atrioventricular node (**N**), the suture line can be taken behind the coronary sinus, which would therefore drain with the red blood, but this is unimportant.

Diagram B

- **A** – Aorta
- **B** – Right ventricle
- **C** – Main pulmonary artery
- **D** – Left ventricle
- **E** – Pericardial baffle
- **F** – Coronary sinus
- **G** – Tricuspid valve
- **H** – Inferior vena cava
- **J** – Superior vena cava
- **K** – Pulmonary veins
- **L** – Mitral valve
- **M** – Posterior wall of left atrium
- **N** – Atrio ventricular node

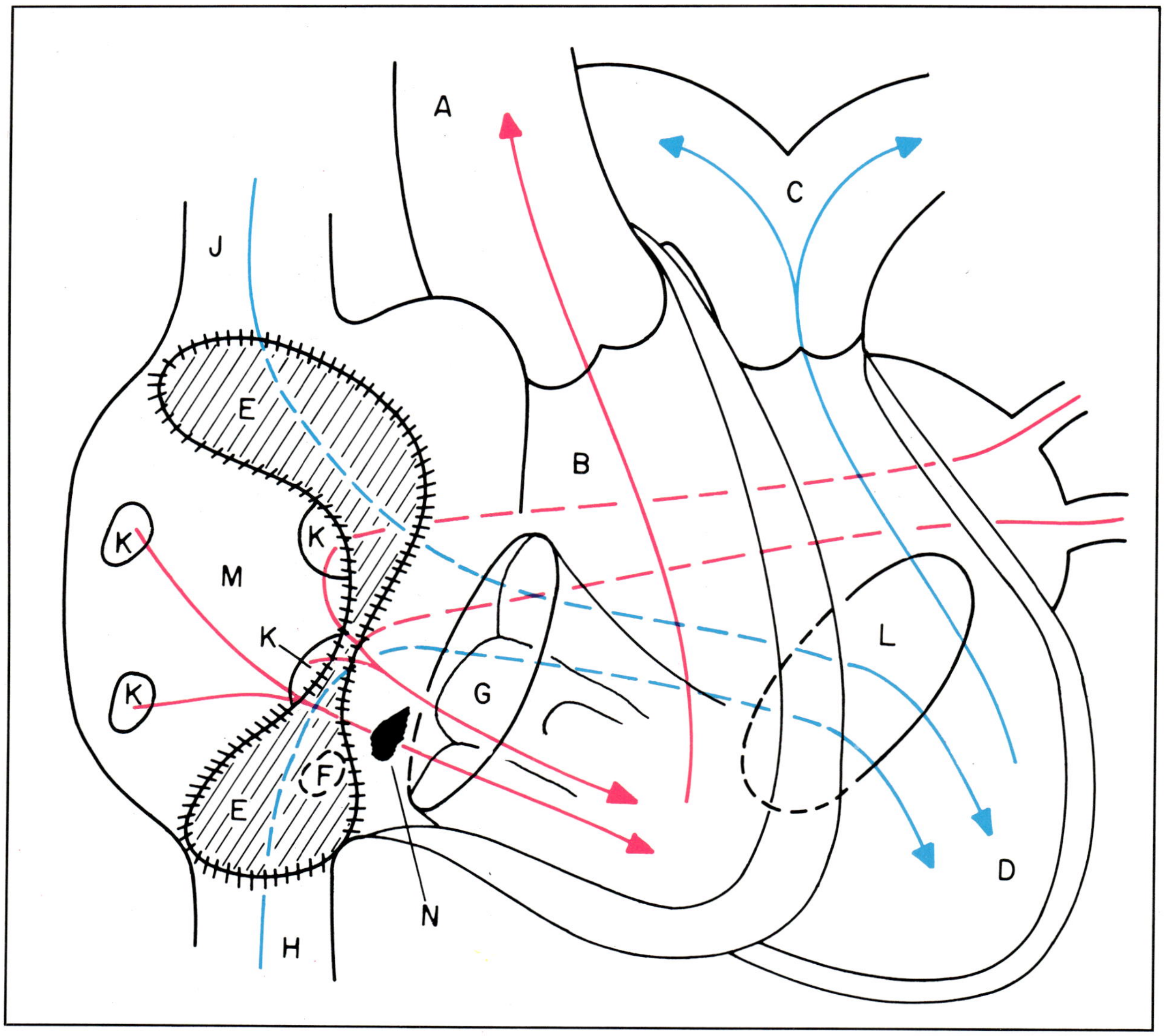

1

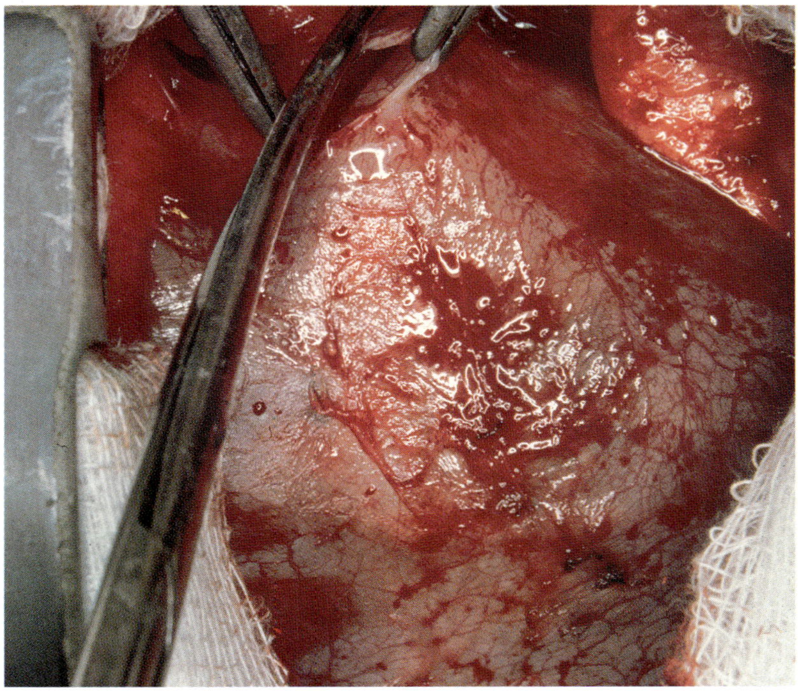

1 After dividing the sternum, the pericardium is exposed and the pleura dissected carefully back on each side.

2

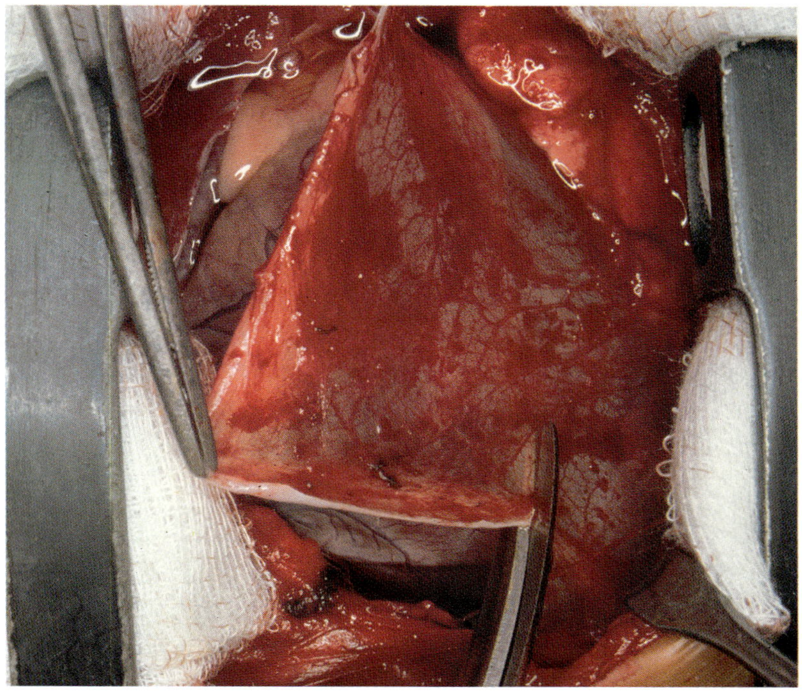

2 Most of the anterior part of the pericardium is cut out to be used for the baffle. Care should be taken to avoid opening the pleura.

3

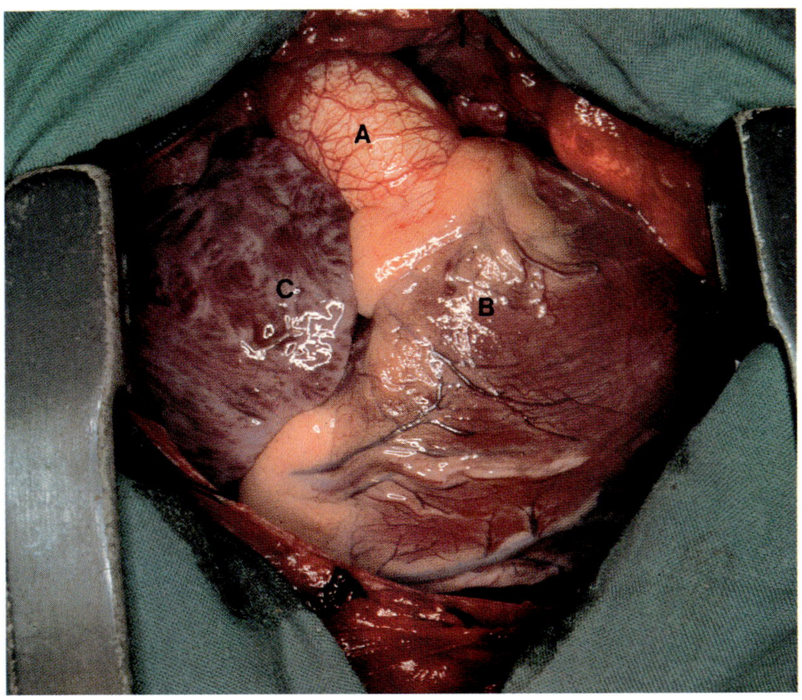

3 The typical transposition anatomy is seen, with the anterior aorta (**A**) coming off the right ventricle (**B**). The right atrium (**C**) is large.

4

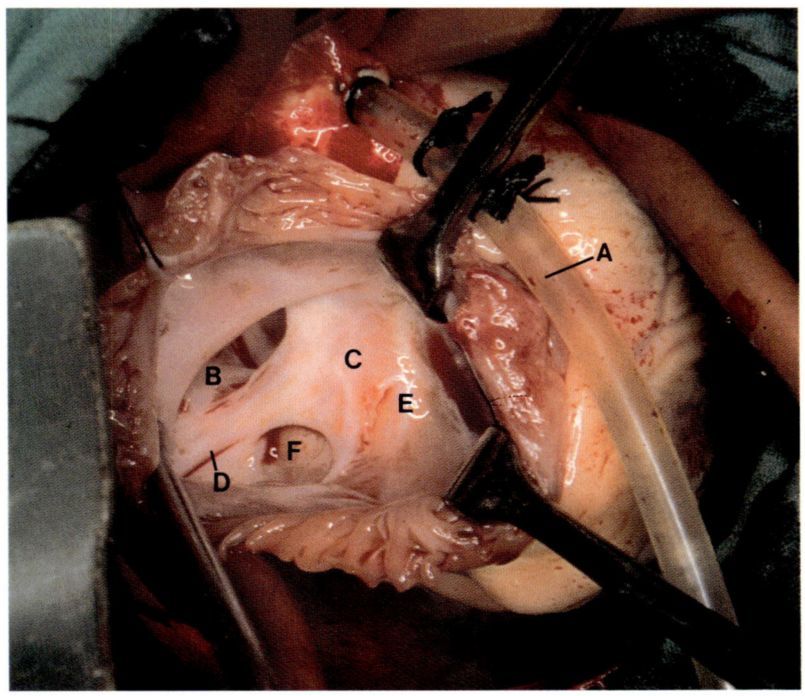

4 Profound hypothermia has been used (see Chapter 1) and the aortic cannula (**A**) has been used to infuse cardioplegic solution into the ascending aorta. The right atrium has been opened widely and the venous cannula removed. The atrial septal defect (**B**), formed as a result of a previous Rashkind procedure, is large and has provided good mixing. The atrioventricular node (**C**) is at the apex of the triangle of Koch, formed by the tendon of Todaro (**D**) and the tricuspid valve ring (**E**), and just clear of the coronary sinus (**F**).

5

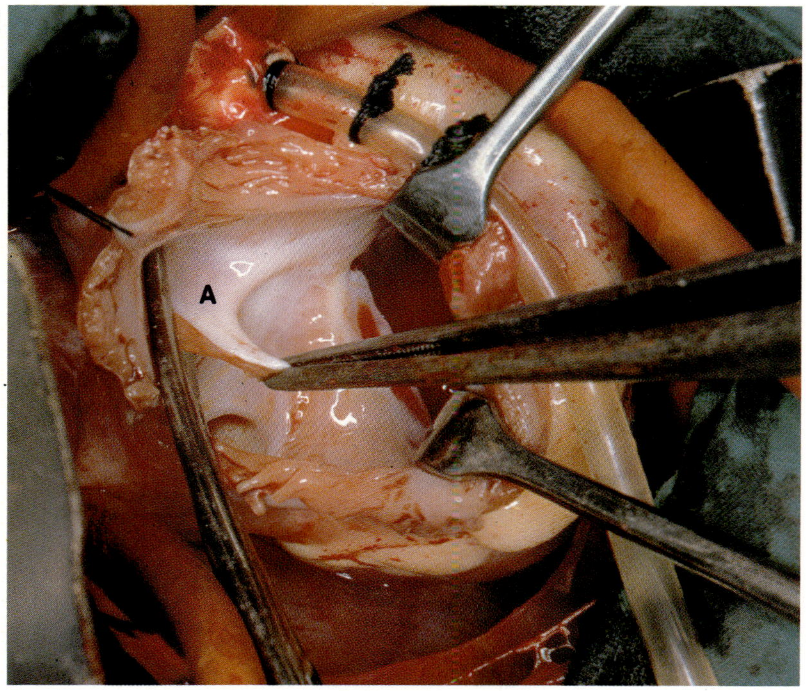

5 The first step is to remove the remainder of the atrial septum (**A**). In doing so care must be taken not to cut outside the atrium, particularly above, where it is also possible to damage the artery to the sinoauricular node.

6

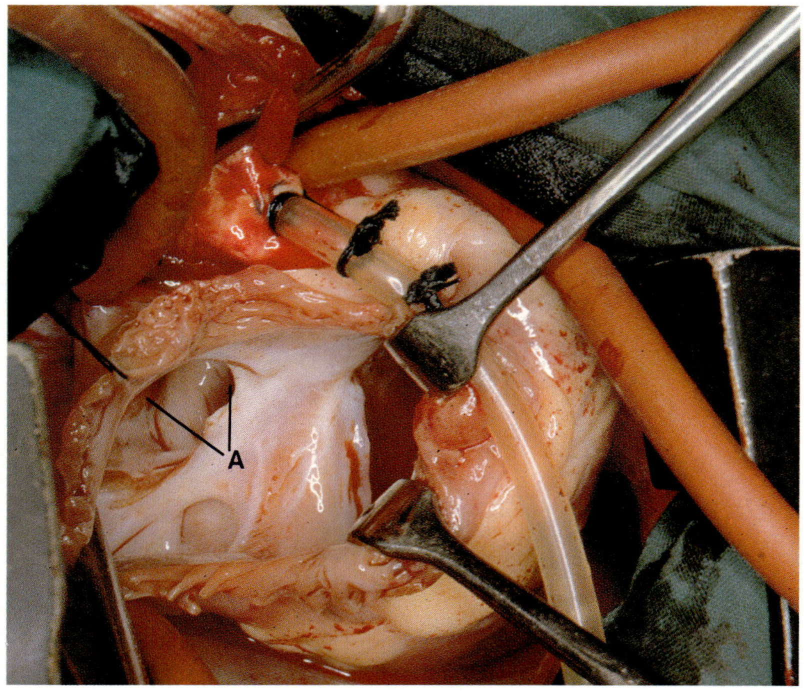

6 The atrial septum has been removed, producing, in effect, a common atrium. Pulmonary veins (**A**) can just be seen entering the back of the left atrium.

7

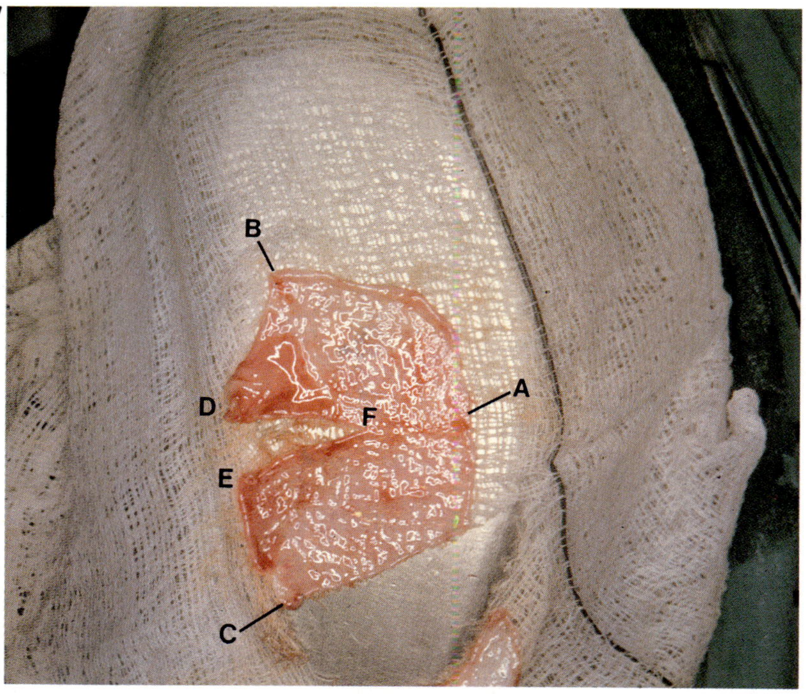

7 The baffle is prepared by cutting the piece of pericardium into a suitably sized trouser shape. (The lettering is referred to in the following description of the operation.)

8

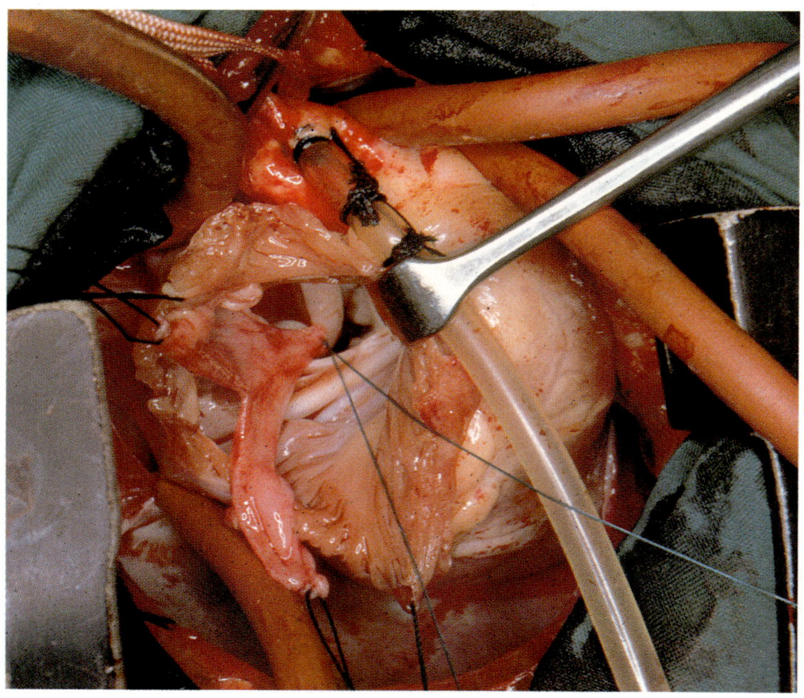

8 The first suture is placed at point **A** on the baffle and into the posterior wall of the left atrium just above the middle of the mitral valve. The retractor has been placed through the mitral valve to retract it forward and help with exposure.

9

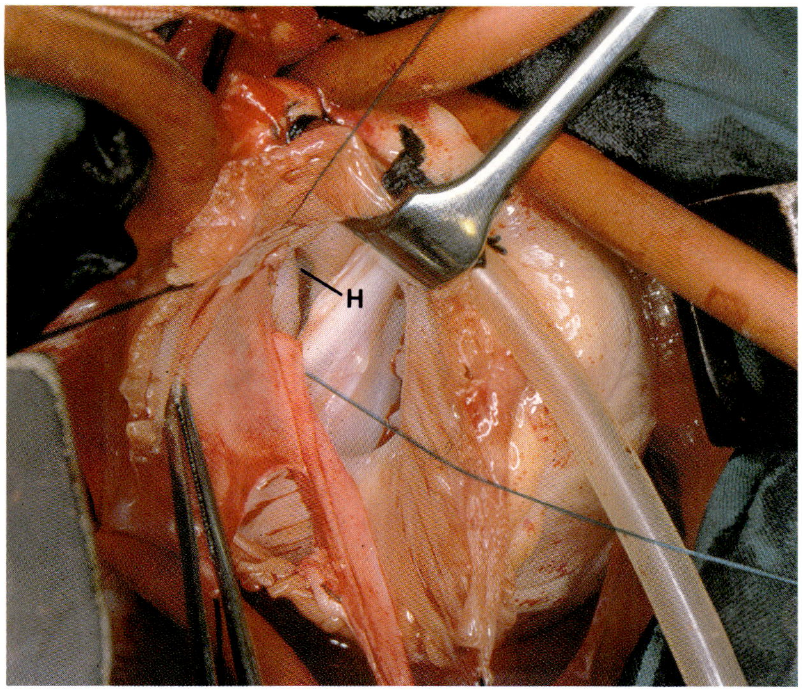

10

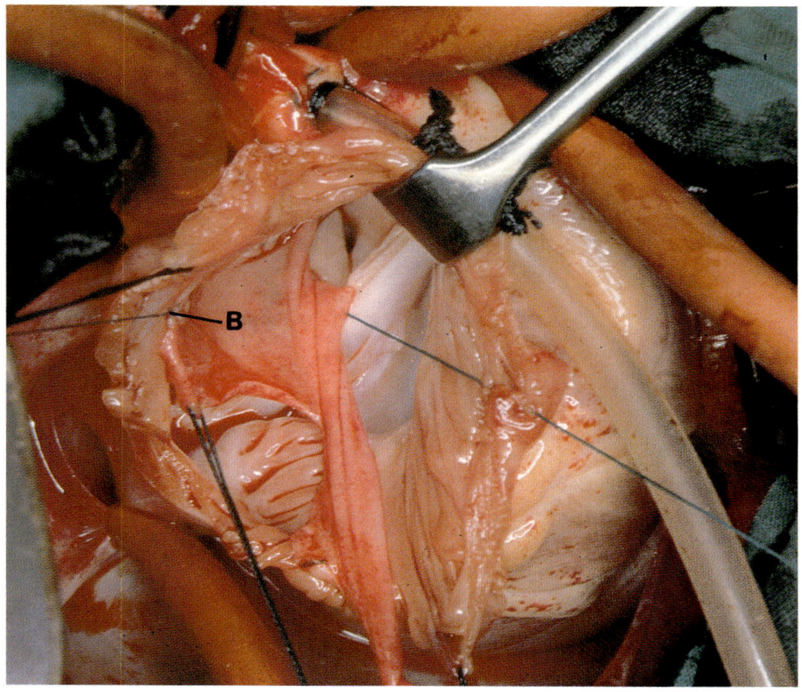

9 The continuous suture is taken superiorly posterior to the left atrial appendage (**H**), but anterior to the pulmonary veins.

10 The suture has been continued to point **B** on the baffle and the suture is locked and held.

11

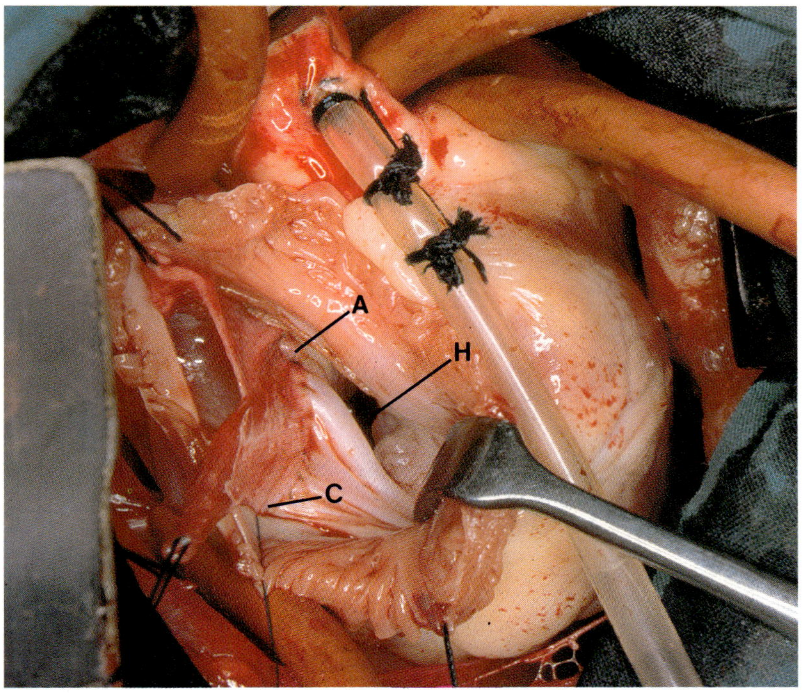

12

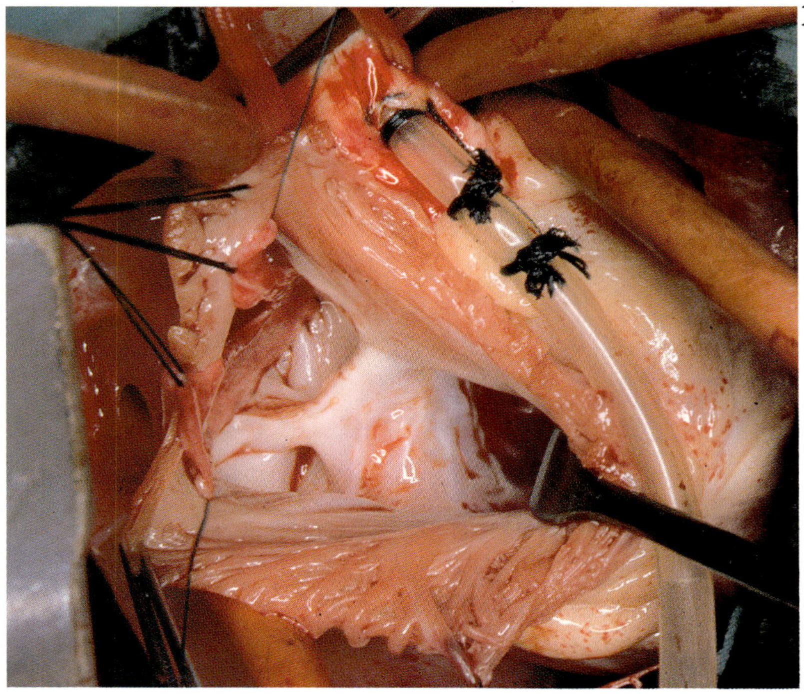

11 Starting again at point **A** with the other end of the suture, the continuous suture is taken behind the mitral valve (**H**), across the inferior surface of the left atrium well away from the coronary sinus but anterior to the pulmonary veins, until point **C** on the baffle is fixed just lateral to and above the entrance of the inferior vena cava.

12 The retractor has now been moved from the mitral to the tricuspid valve and, starting with the suture that was held at point **B**, the suture line continued across to the left anterior to and around the entrance of the superior vena cava to point **D**.

13

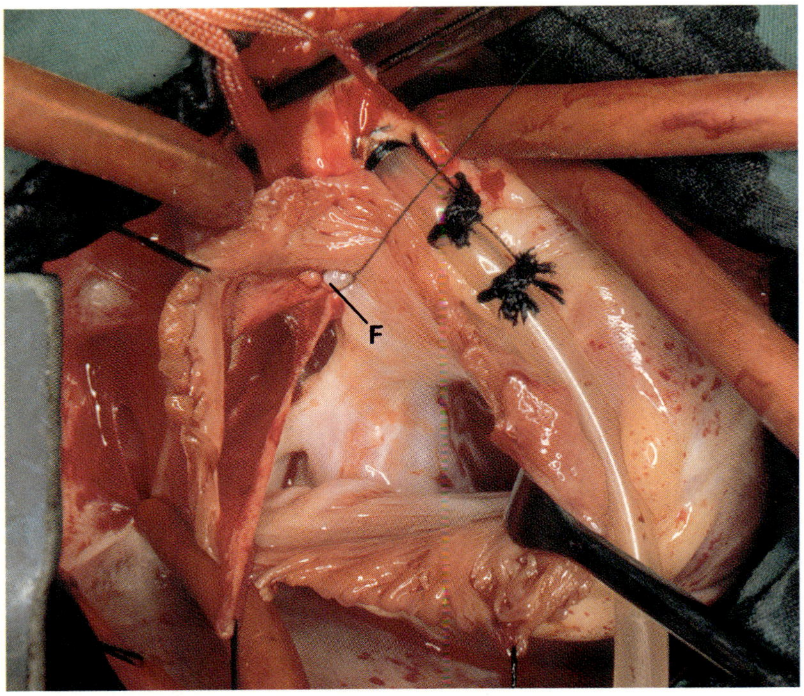

13 By continuing the same suture down to point **F**, the baffle is folded forward by completing the upper half of the baffle insertion.

14

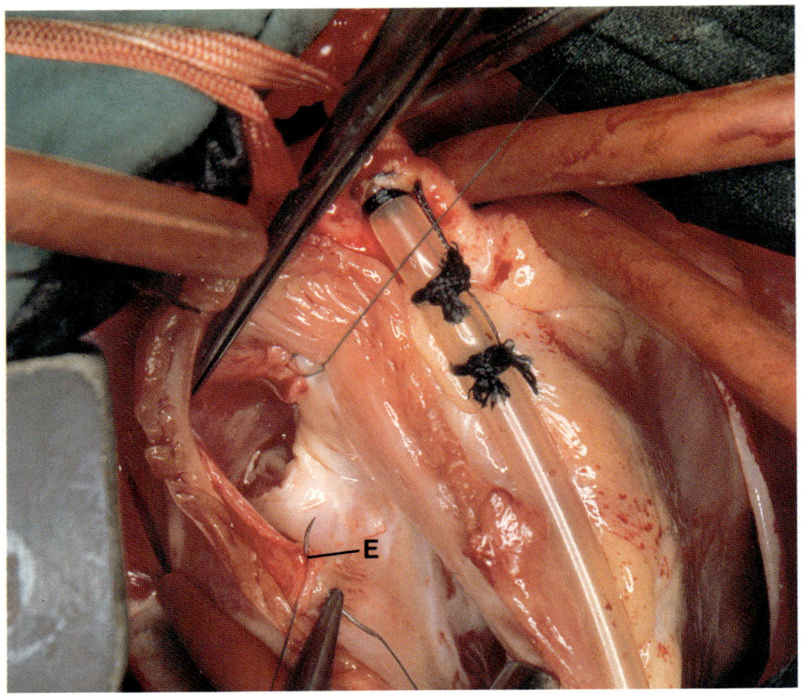

14 The suture held at point **C** is now continued around the entrance of the inferior vena cava inferiorly to point **E**, leaving the coronary sinus behind the baffle.

15

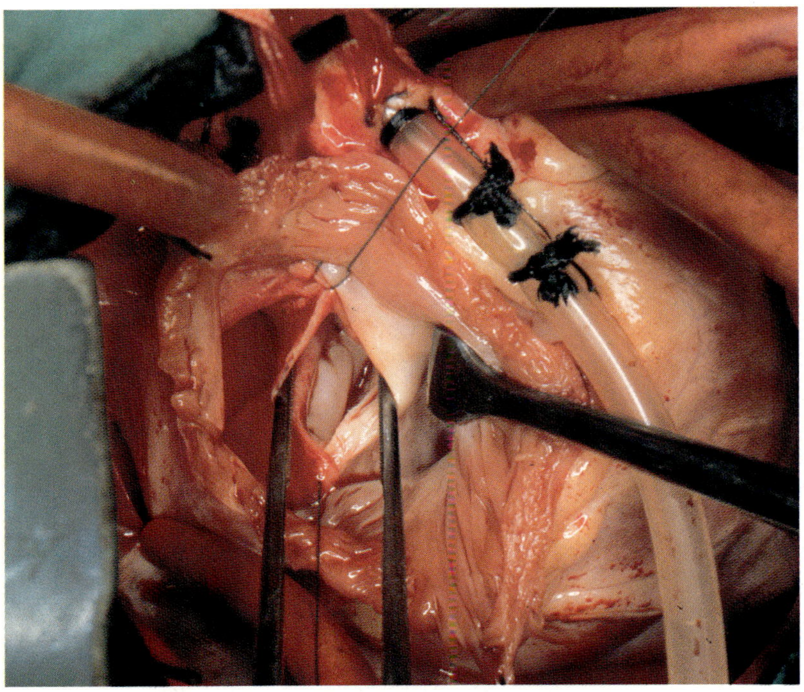

15 The suture is continued until only a fairly small part of the inferior limit of the baffle needs to be completed. This is a good point at which to insert the venous cannula through the left atrial appendage and, with the baffle not completed, the cannula can be seen and positioned.

16

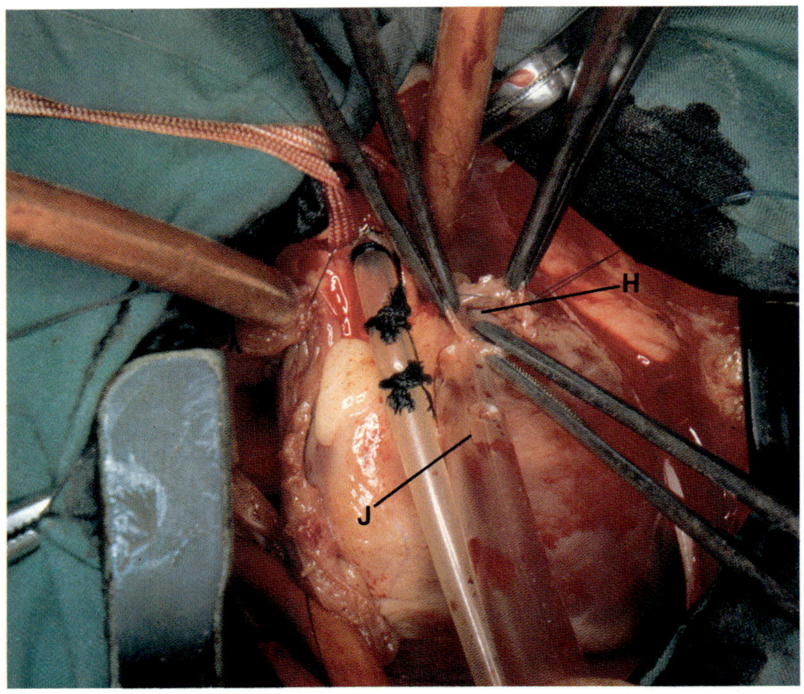

16 The left atrial appendage (**H**) has been opened and a purse-string suture placed around it. The venous cannula (**J**) is about to be inserted.

17

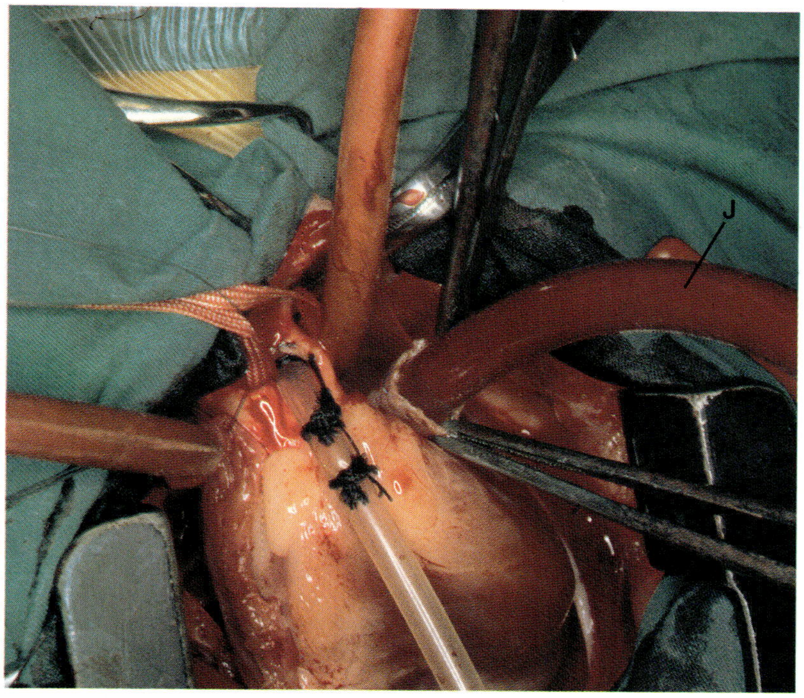

18

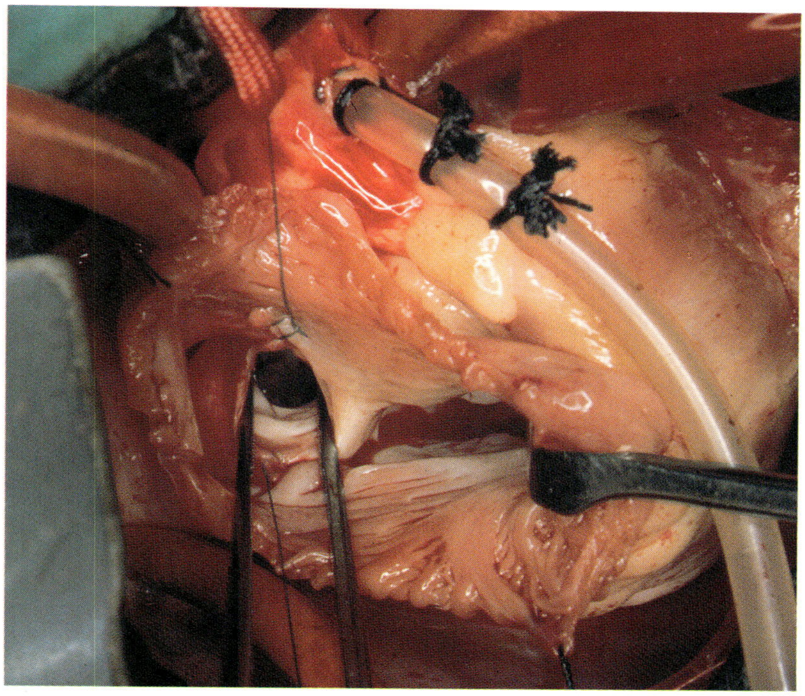

17 and 18 The venous cannula (**J**) has been inserted into the left atrial appendage and is being guided into position to lie behind the baffle.

19

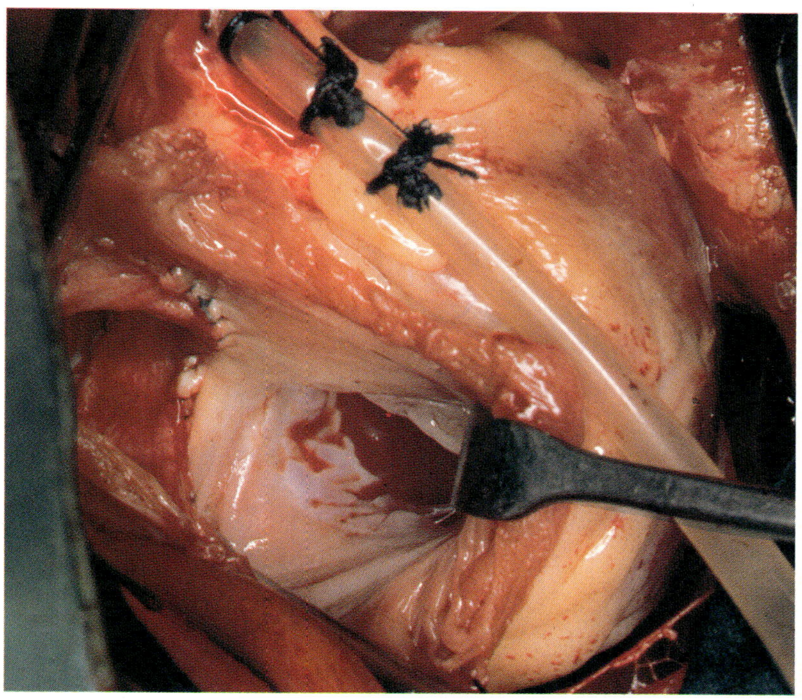

19 The suture line of the baffle is now complete. The retractor is holding the tricuspid valve wide open.

20

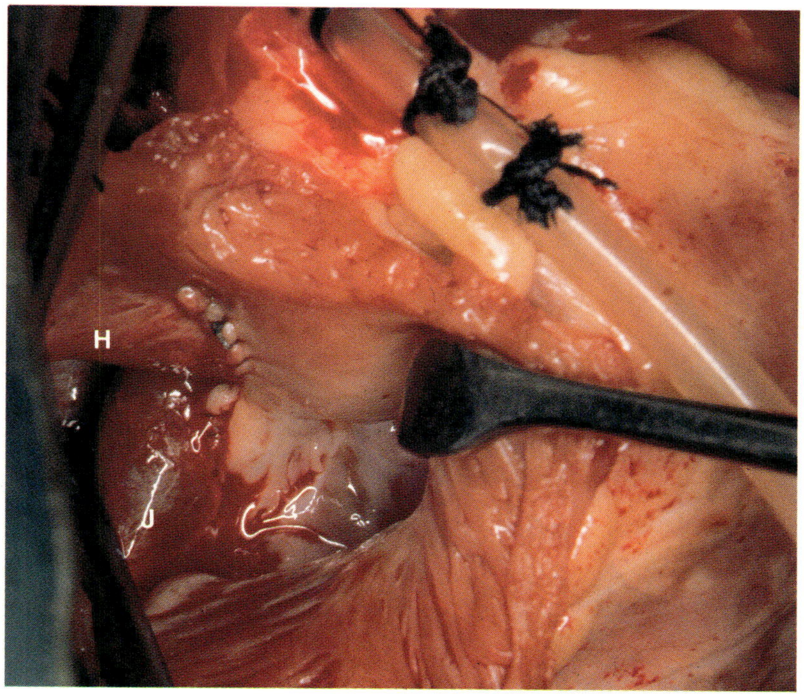

20 The vena caval snares have been released and blood fills out the superior (**H**) and inferior (**J**) limbs of the baffle. The right atrial incision is closed directly or with an extra widening patch if necessary. Air is removed from the heart and bypass recommenced and the patient rewarmed.

14: Correction of persistent truncus arteriosus

This condition results from a failure of septation of the truncus arteriosus, so that a single large vessel arises from both ventricles, astride the interventricular septum. There is therefore a ventricular septal defect and the truncal valve may have from two to six cusps. The pulmonary artery arises from the single large vessel usually on the left side and rather posterior. If there is a definite main pulmonary artery coming off, this is Type 1. If the two pulmonary arteries come off separately but at virtually the same place, this is Type 2 and if the two pulmonary arteries come off at opposite sides of the ascending aorta, this is Type 3. Type 1 is the commonest and is illustrated in this chapter.

The anatomy is illustrated in diagram **A** which shows the blue, desaturated blood returning via the right atrium (**A**) to the right ventricle (**B**). However, this blue blood mixes with the red saturated blood coming from the left ventricle (**C**) and passes through the truncal valve (**D**), from where this mixed blood passes to the aorta (**E**) and pulmonary artery (**F**). As the pulmonary vascular resistance is considerably less than the systemic resistance, more blood flows around the lungs than around the body, and this large left-to-right shunt results in early heart failure and failure to thrive. Therefore, most of these patients present in early infancy. There may be some response to anti-failure therapy, but most need an operation in early infancy or they would die. Although pulmonary artery banding (see Chapter 8) is possible, this is not a satisfactory solution and correction is preferable.

The first successful report of correction of this condition was by McGoon in 1968[1] and he used a homograft conduit. It is basically the same operation described in this chapter. Cardiopulmonary bypass is used and the profound hypothermia technique (see Chapter 1) is appropriate in infants. After cross-clamping the aorta and pulmonary artery, cardioplegic solution is given to protect the myocardium. The pulmonary artery is then divided from the truncus arteriosus and the resulting defect in the aorta closed directly. A right ventriculotomy is then made and the high ventricular septal defect closed through it with a dacron cloth patch. The distal end of the conduit is then anastomosed to the pulmonary artery and the proximal end to the right ventriculotomy. As can be seen in diagram **B**, this results in a remarkably normal final anatomy and physiology. The truncal valve can occasionally be regurgitant and care must be taken not to let the left ventricle distend when the aortic clamp is released.

Diagram A

A – Right atrium
B – Right ventricle
C – Left ventricle
D – Truncal valve
E – Ascending aorta
F – Pulmonary artery
G – Left atrium
H – Ventricular septal defect

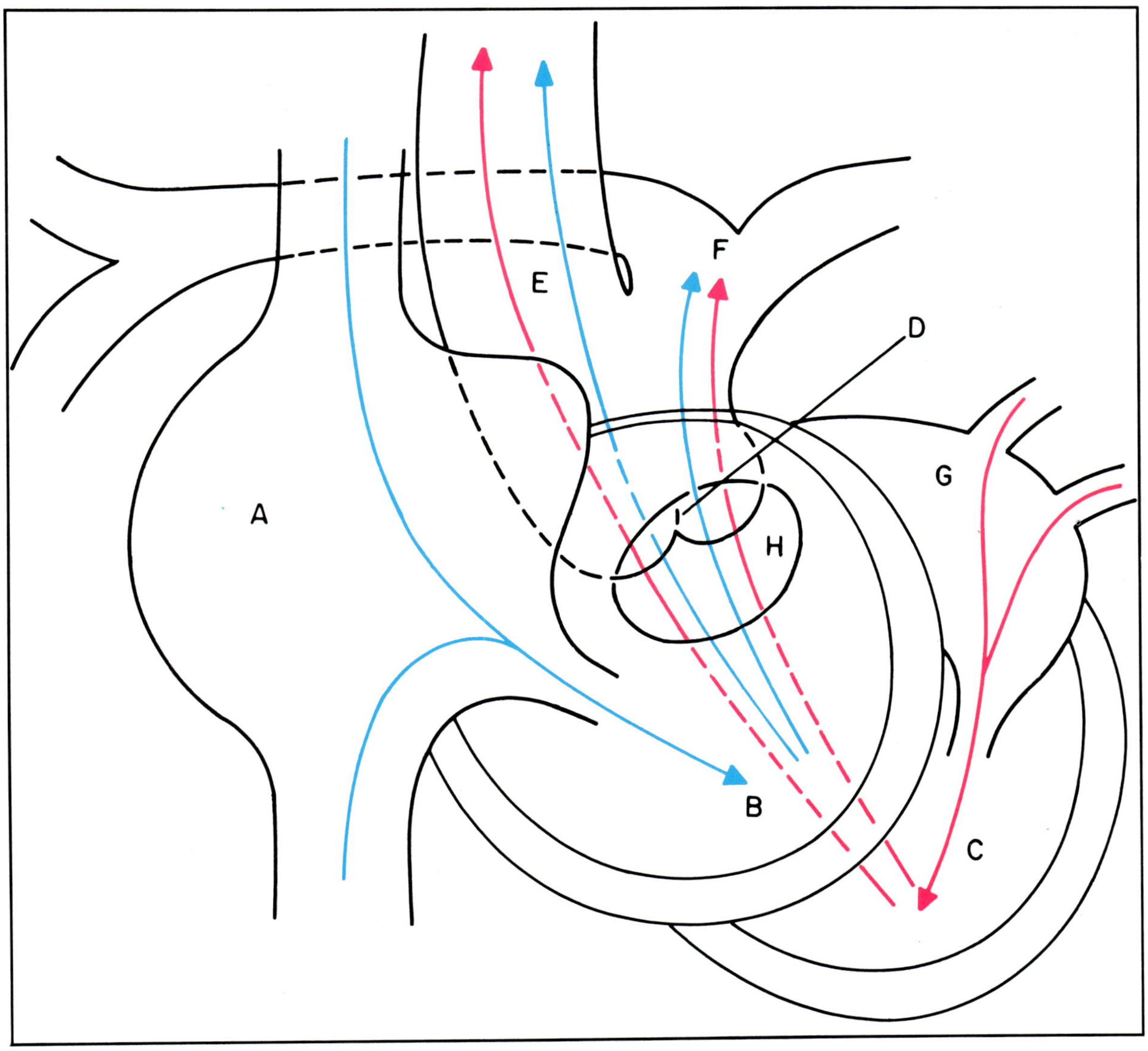

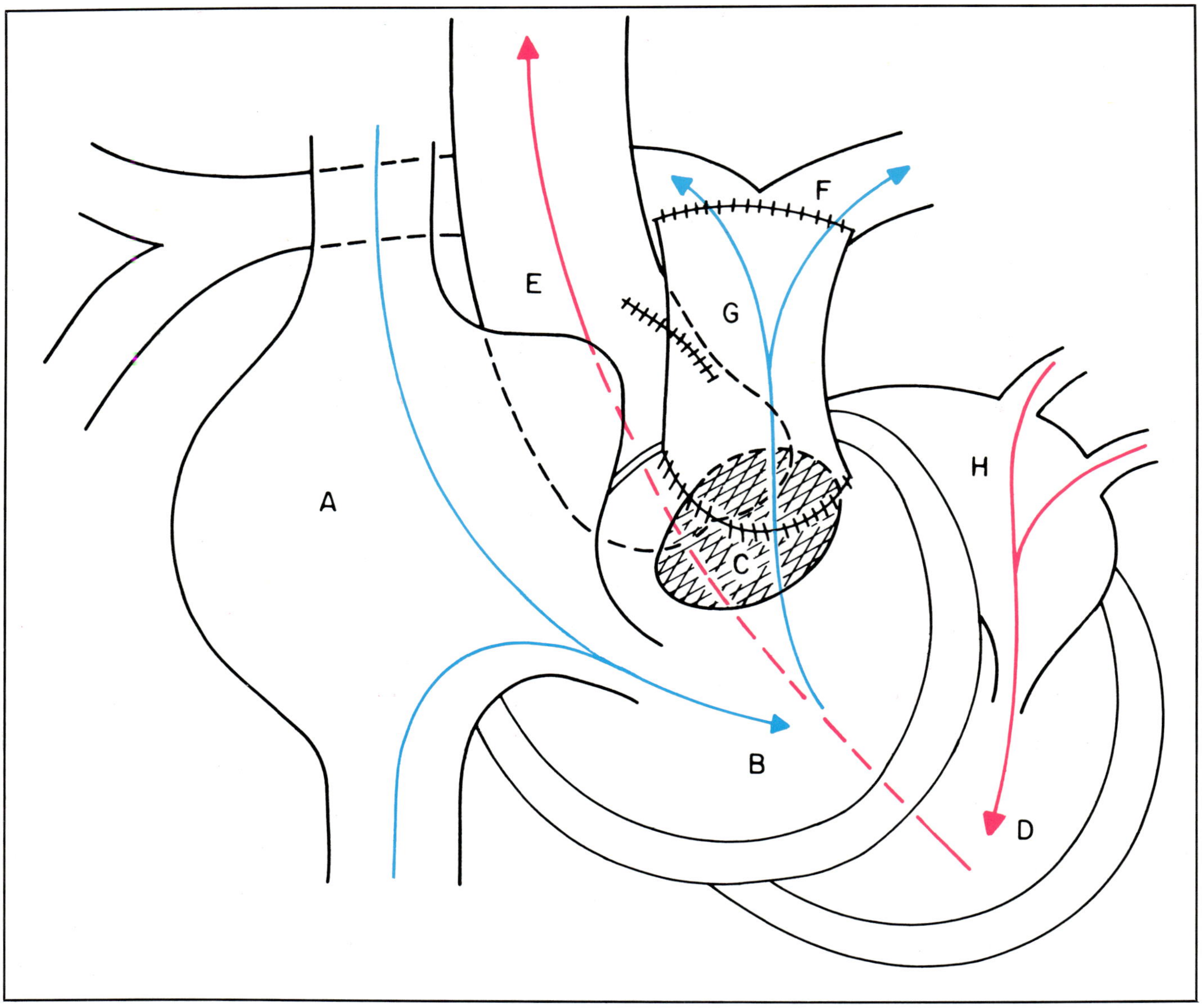

Diagram B

A – Right atrium

B – Right ventricle

C – Ventricular septal defect — closed with dacron patch

D – Left ventricle

E – Ascending aorta

F – Pulmonary artery

G – Homograft conduit

H – Left atrium

1

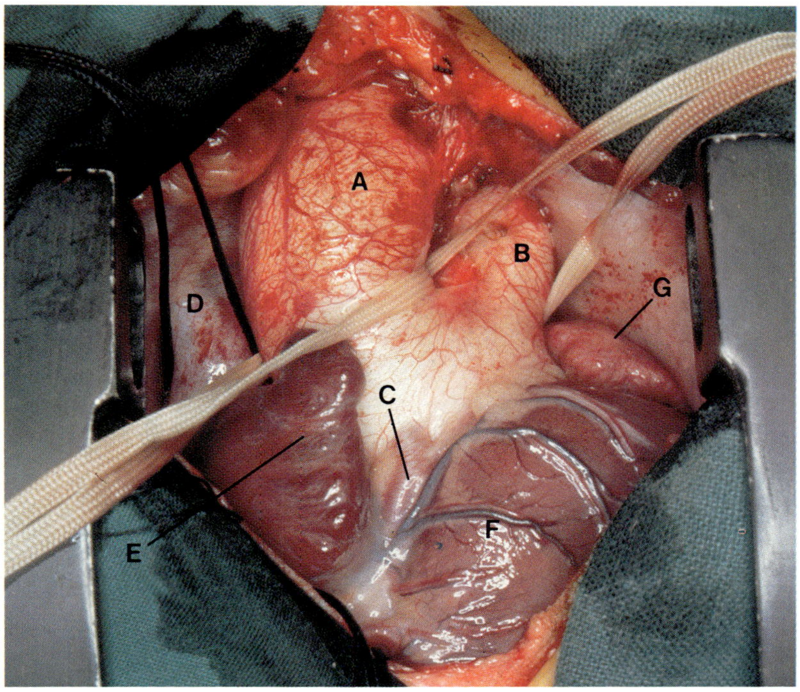

1 This shows the ascending aorta (**A**) and main pulmonary artery (**B**) coming off the common truncus arteriosus. The right coronary artery (**C**) is also seen coming off anteriorly. The superior vena cava (**D**), right atrial appendage (**E**), right ventricle (**F**) and left atrial appendage (**G**) are also seen. Tapes have been placed around the aorta and pulmonary artery to make it easier to clamp them.

2

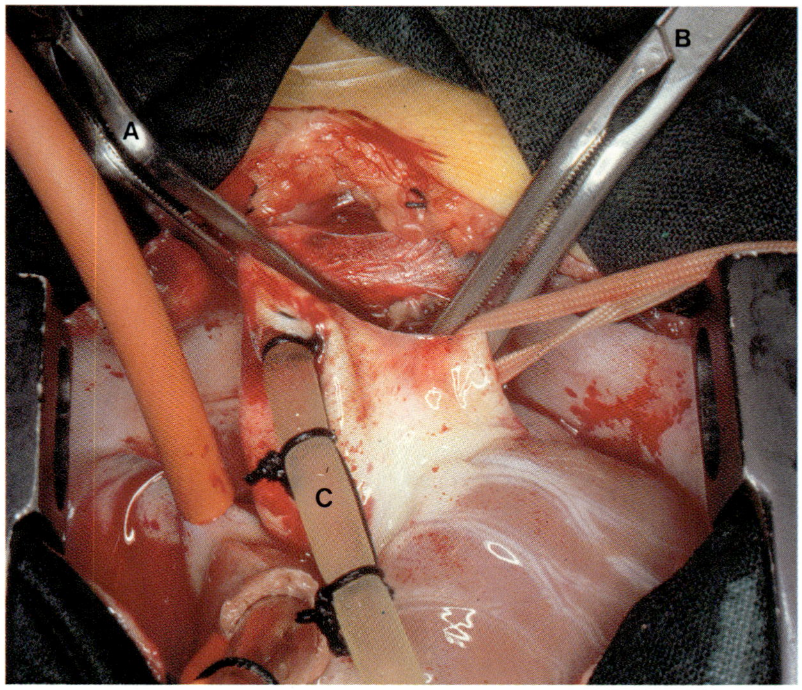

2 The patient has been cooled on cardiopulmonary bypass and the circulation stopped. A clamp (**A**) has been placed on the ascending aorta and another clamp (**B**) on the main pulmonary artery. Cardioplegic solution has been infused through the aortic cannula (**C**) to help preserve the myocardium.

3

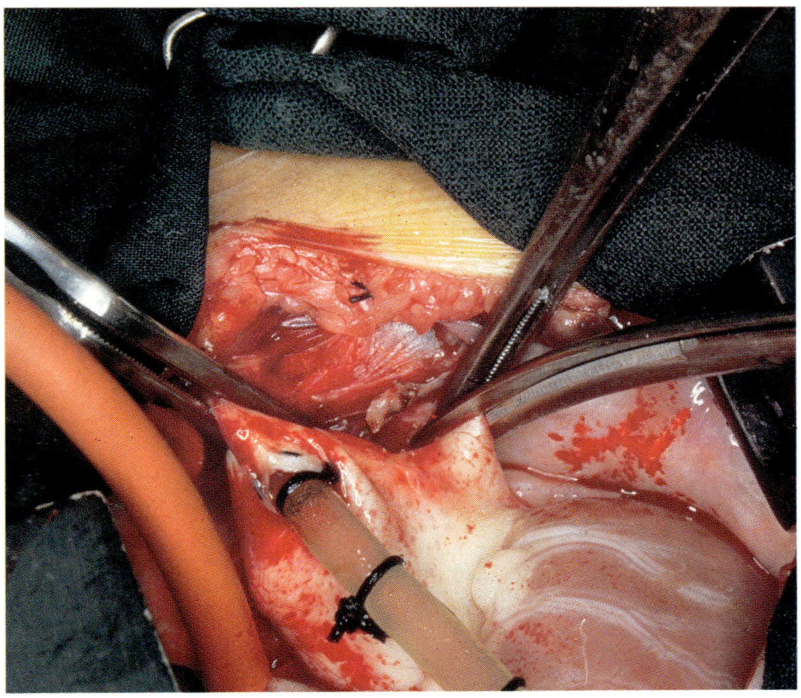

4

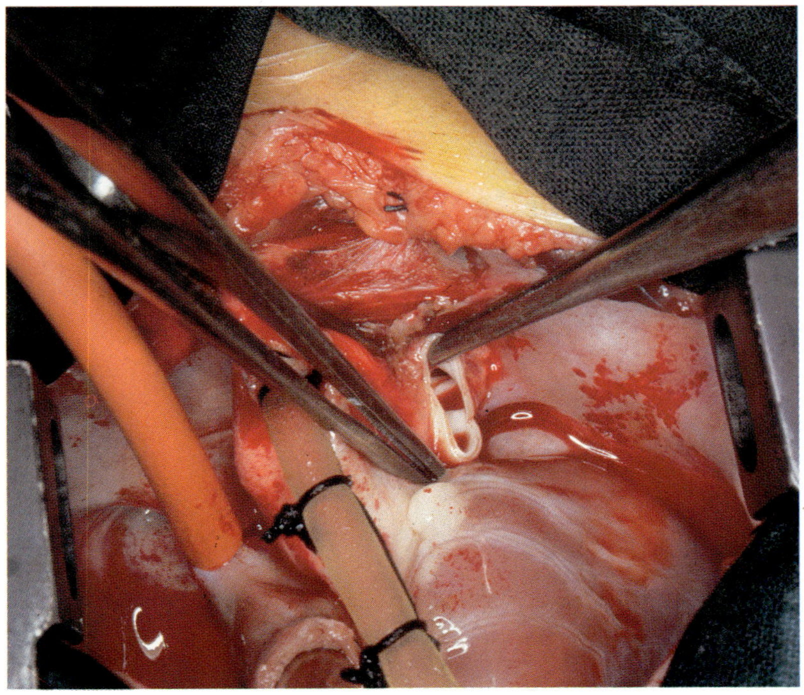

3 and 4 The main pulmonary artery is cut from the truncus arteriosus with scissors. Great care must be taken not to damage the left coronary artery, and to leave a sufficient amount of aortic wall above it, to allow direct closure of the defect left by the removal of the pulmonary artery.

5
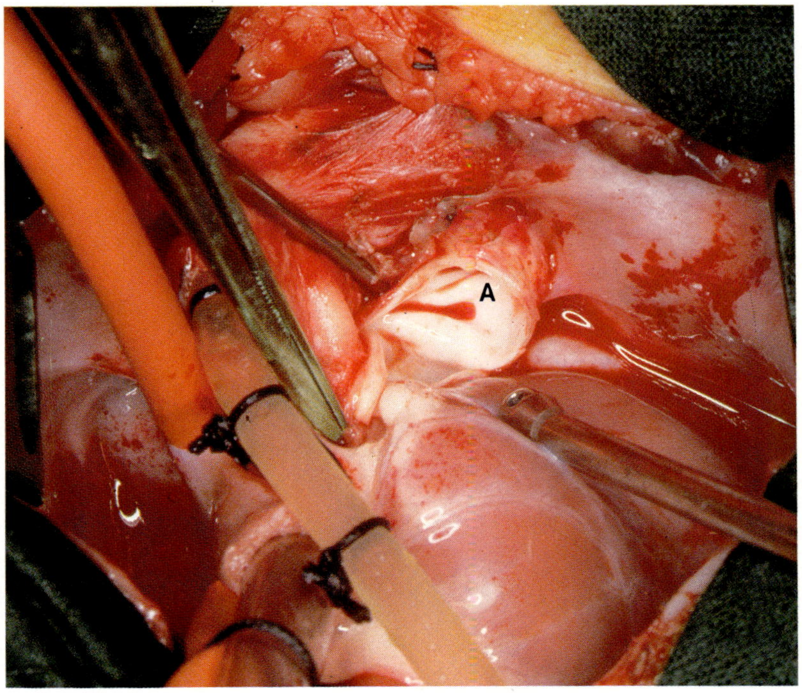

5 The opened pulmonary artery (**A**) is shown and the correct size of homograft can be selected to fit it.

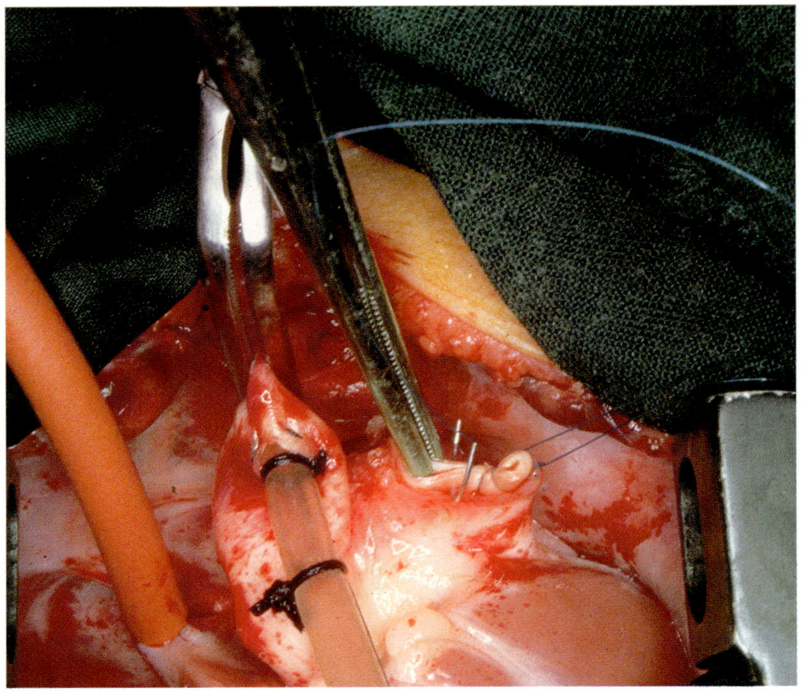
6

6 The defect remaining in the aorta, where the pulmonary artery was removed, is now sutured with a double layer of continuous Prolene.

7
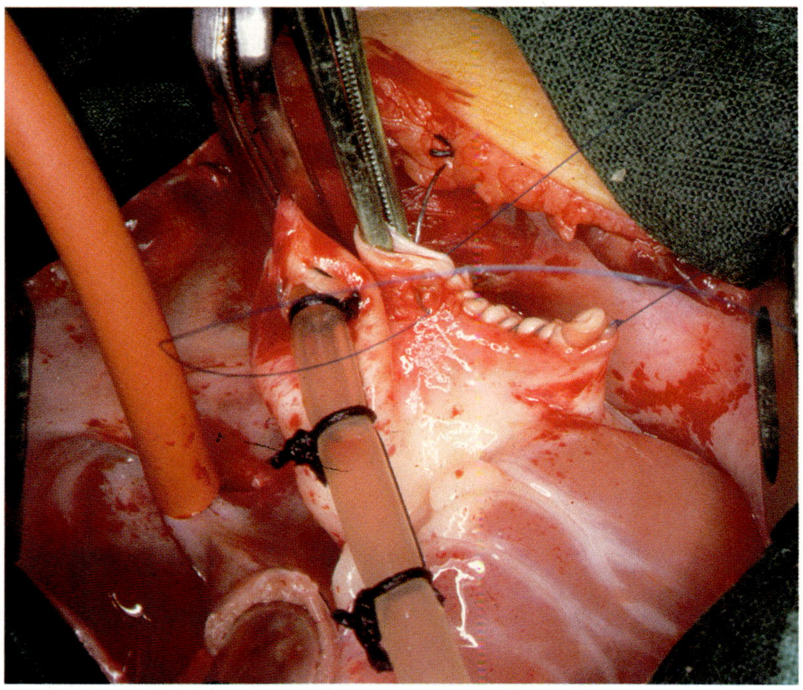

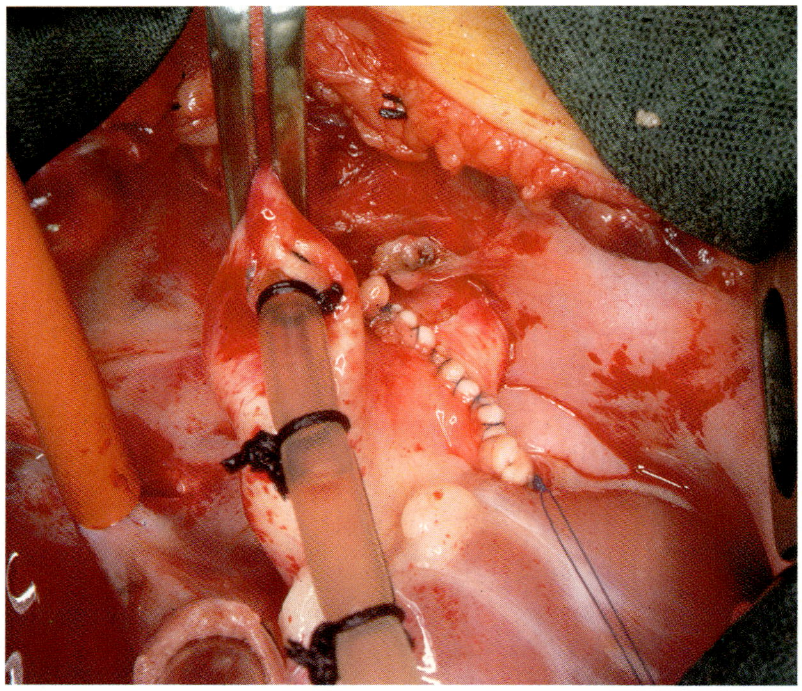
8

7 and 8 The double layer closure of the aortotomy is completed.

9

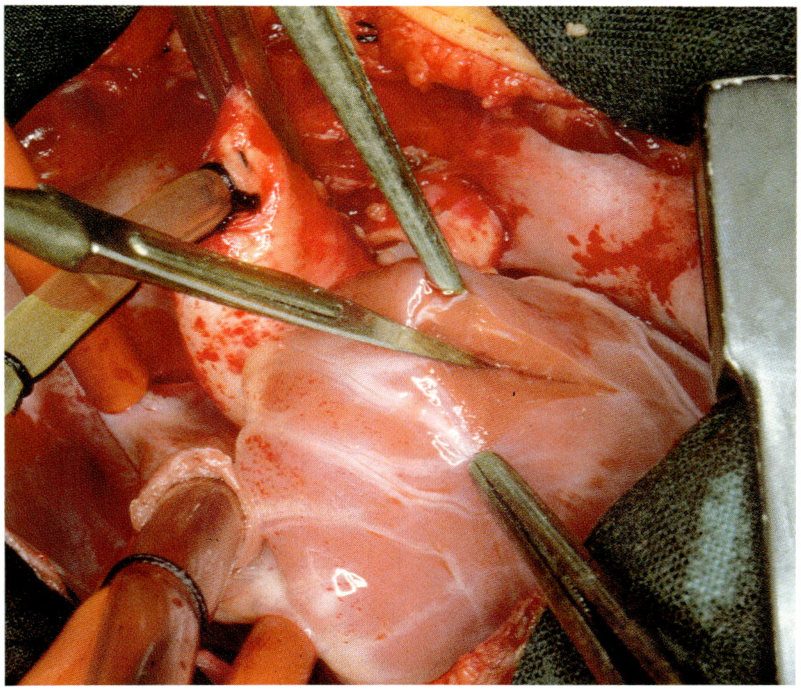

10

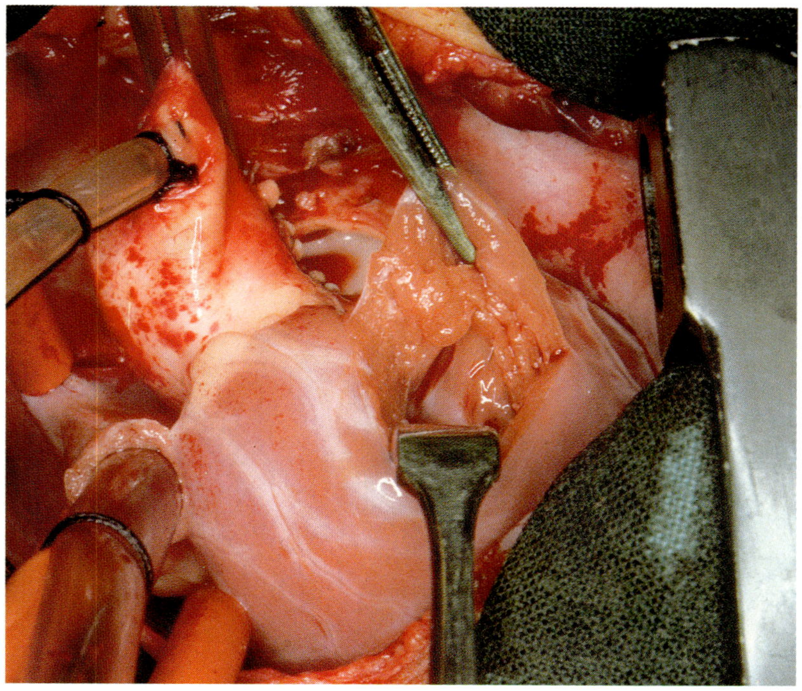

9 and 10 A transverse right ventriculotomy is made, avoiding coronary arteries. Retraction shows the markedly thickened right ventricular muscle.

11

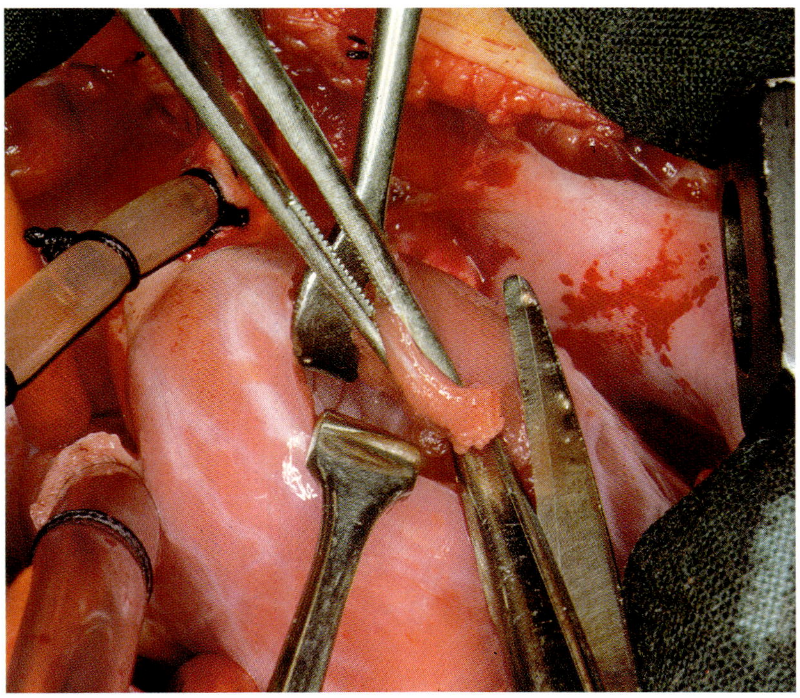

12

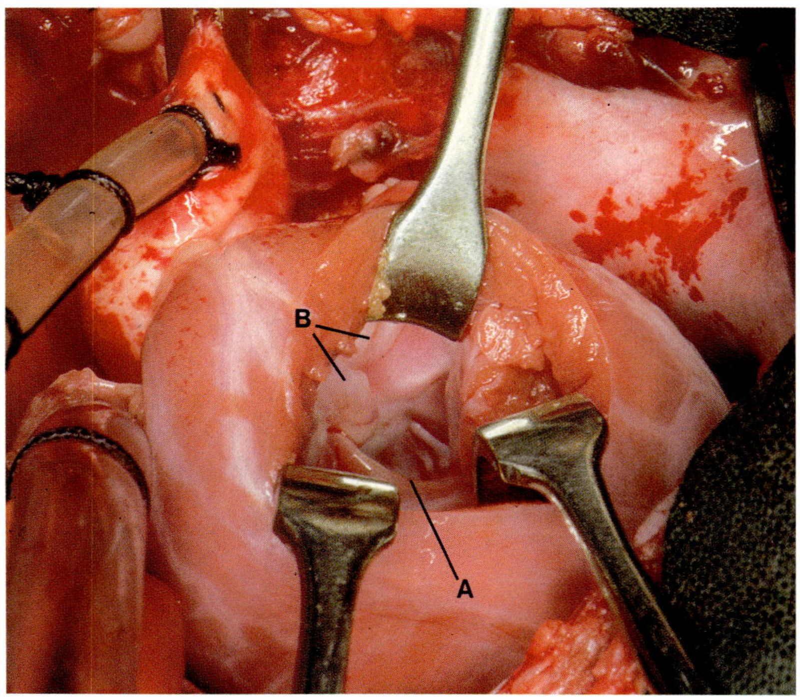

11 Some of the thickened right ventricular muscle is cut away superiorly to prevent it obstructing the new outflow tract. However, great care must be taken not to damage the leaflets of the truncal valve or the left coronary artery.

12 Retraction of the ventriculotomy shows the lower margin of the ventricular septal defect (**A**) and the truncal valve cusps (**B**).

13
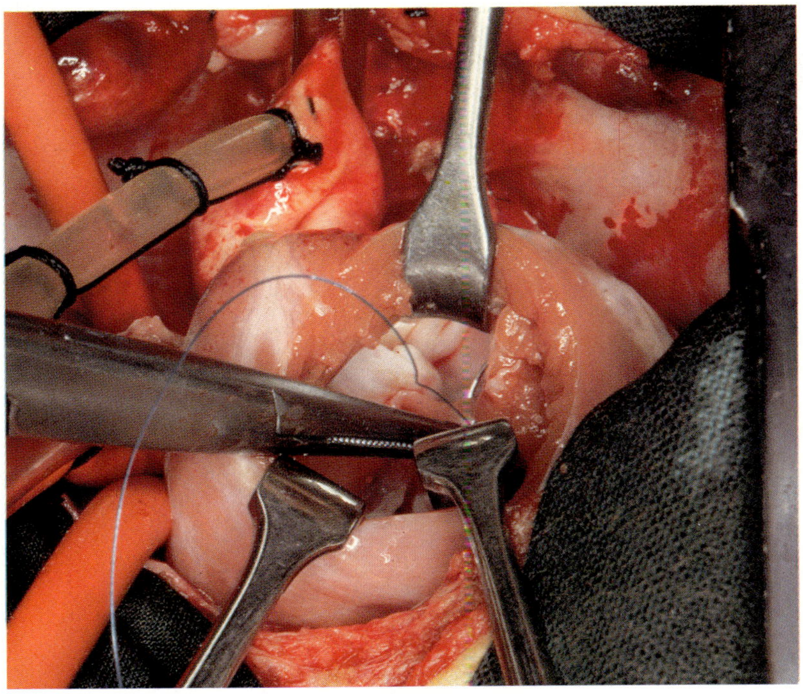

14
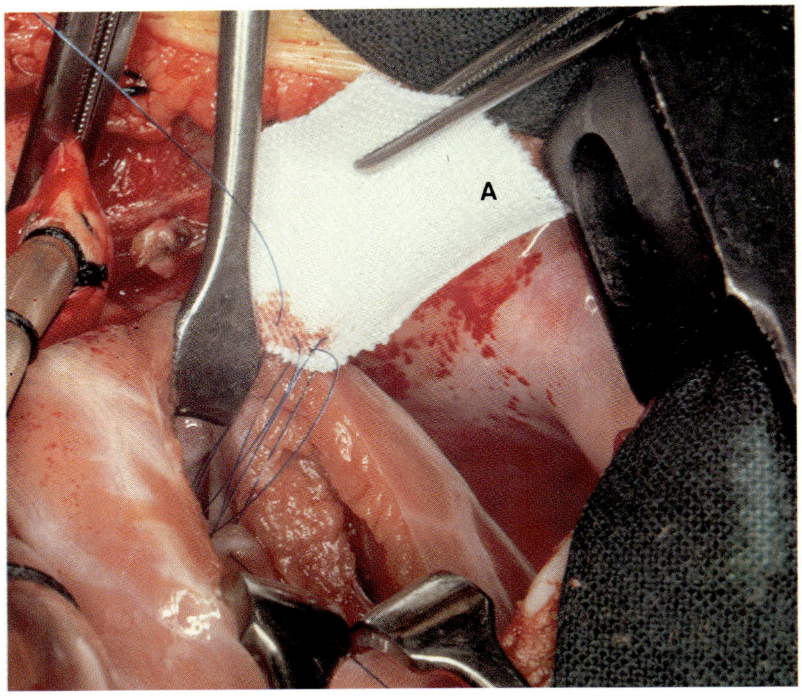

13 The ventricular septal defect must now be closed and a suture is being inserted at the left end of the lower margin of the defect. Although the defect in this condition is high and the conduction mechanism is well below the edge of the defect, it is usual to stay on the right-hand side of the septum when placing the sutures.

14 Several sutures are placed in the dacron cloth patch (**A**) before sliding it down in position.

15
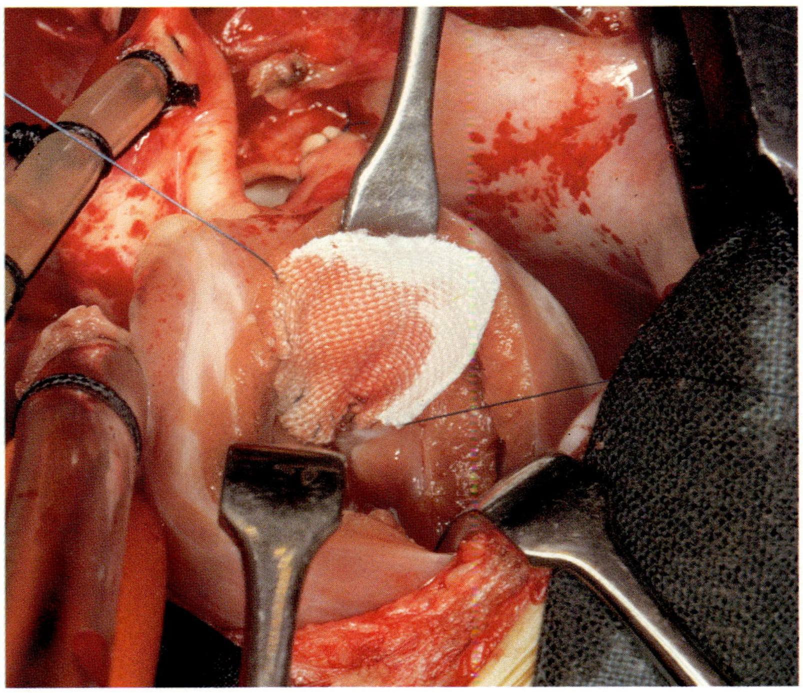

16
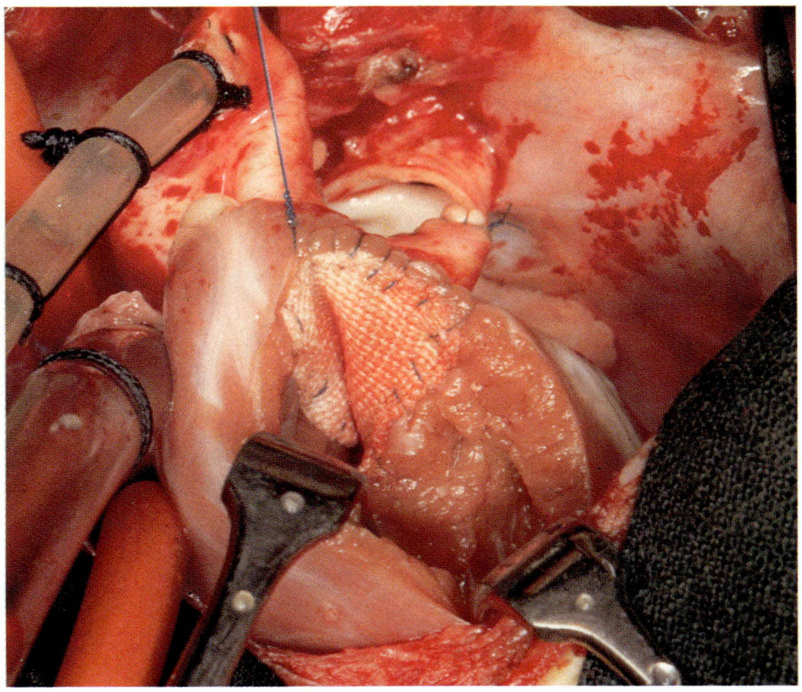

15 The patch has been slid down into position and the continuous Prolene suture taken up the right side of the patch, taking great care to avoid the truncal valve cusps.

16 The patch is now sutured securely into position and it can be seen to come right to the top of the ventriculotomy. This gives a firm hold for the posterior sutures of the proximal anastomosis of the homograft.

17
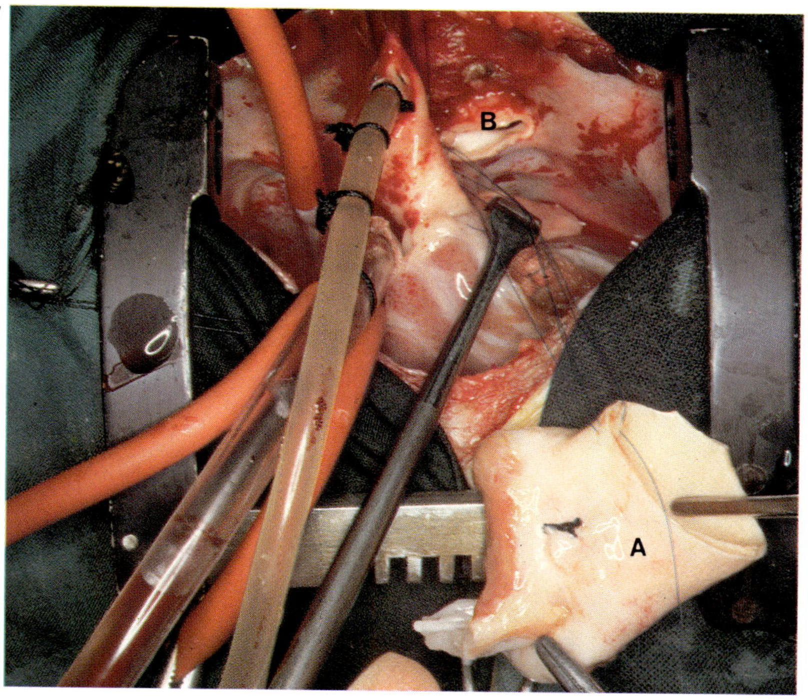

18
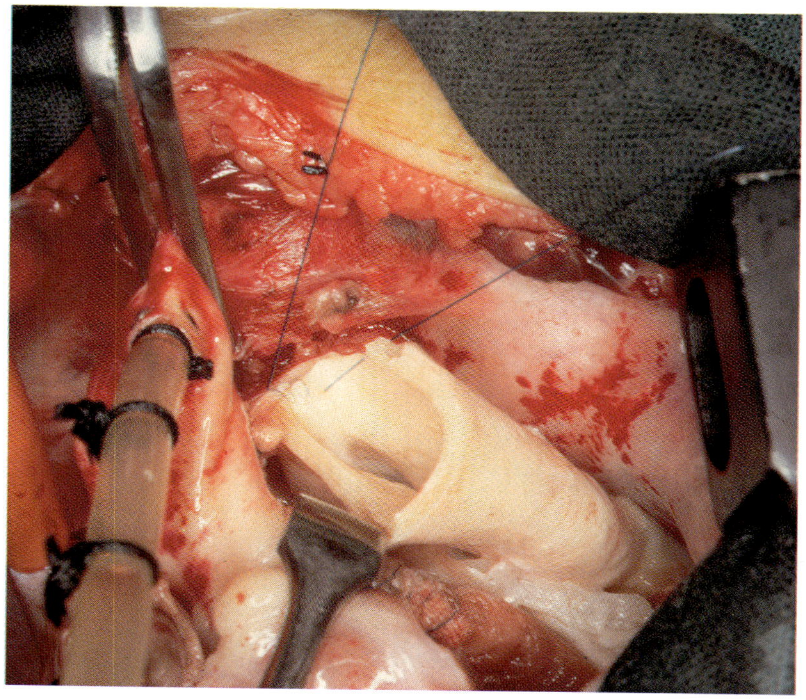

17 and 18 The homograft (**A**) is now anastomosed to the pulmonary artery (**B**) using continuous Prolene sutures. Several sutures have been placed before sliding down the homograft into position and first suturing the posterior part of the anastomosis.

19
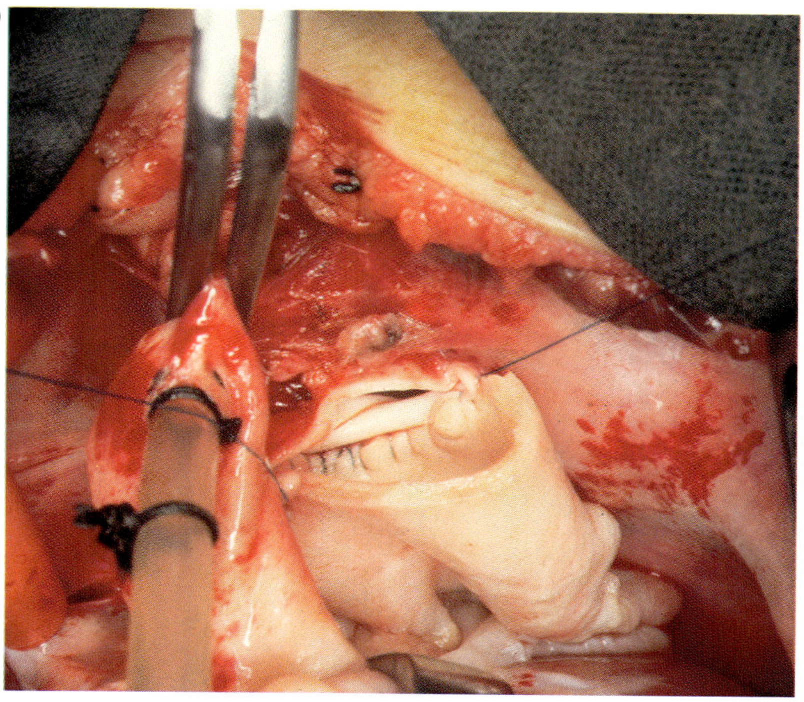

20
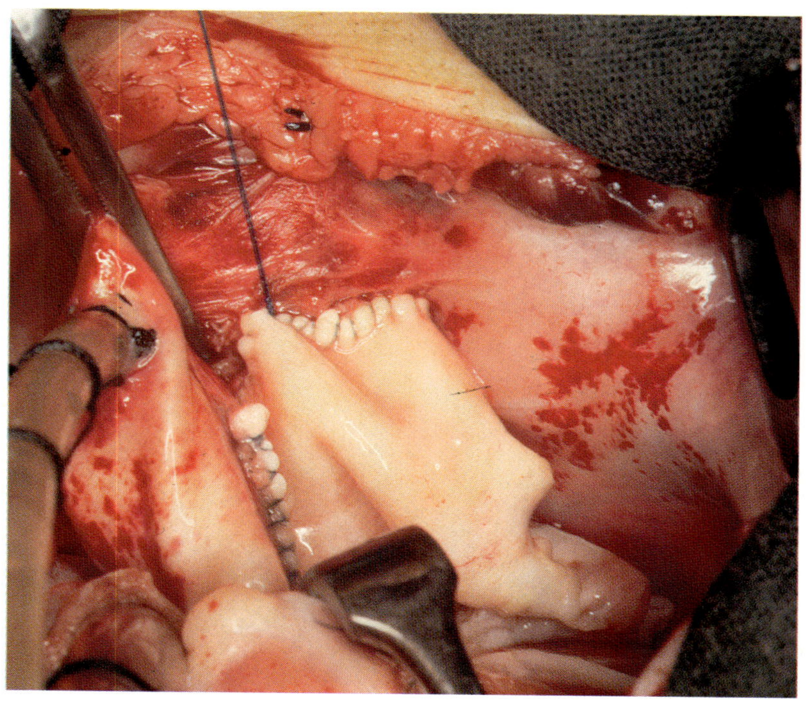

19 and 20 The remainder of the distal anastomosis between the homograft and pulmonary artery is completed with continuous Prolene.

21

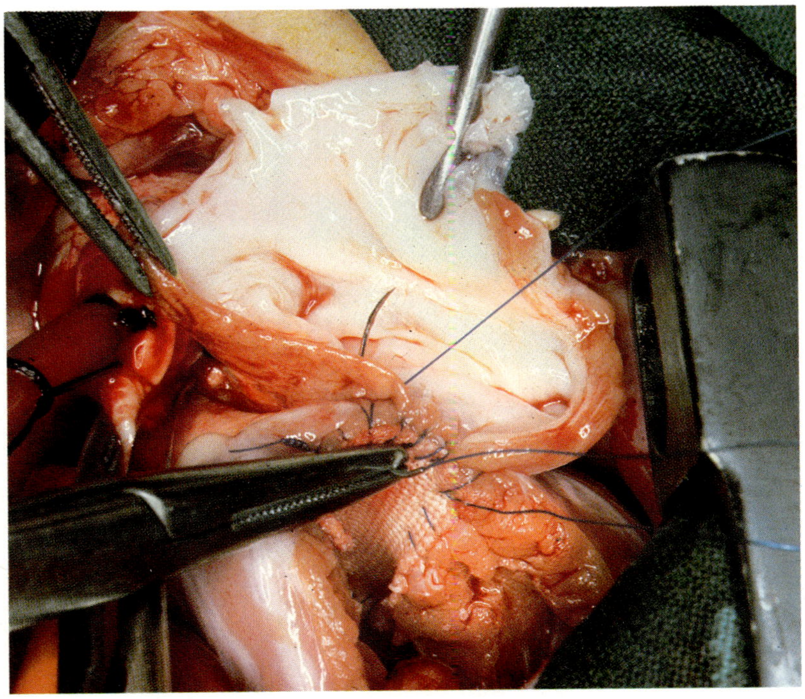

22

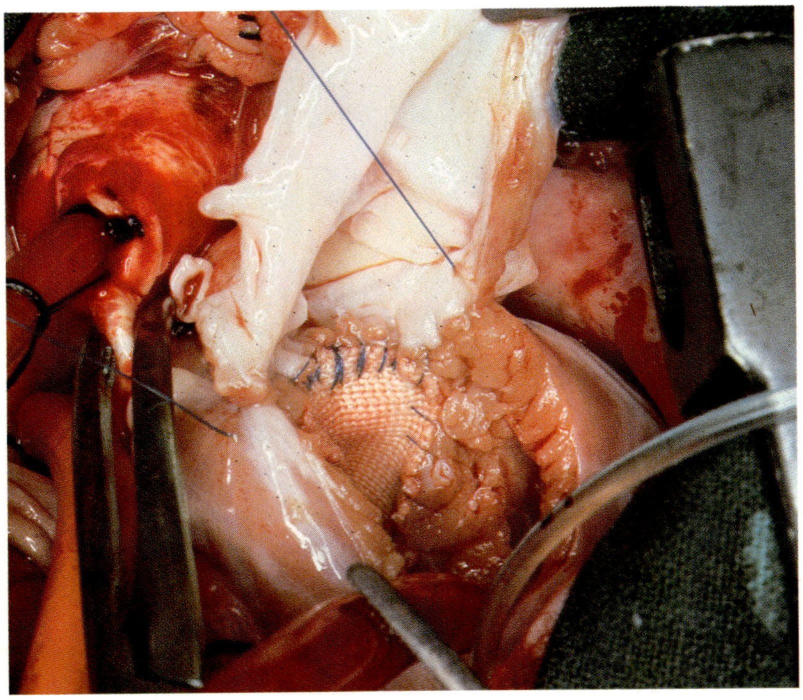

21 and 22 The posterior layer of the proximal anastomosis between the homograft and the right ventricle is performed using continuous Prolene. The suture passes through the dacron patch closing the ventricular septal defect, as well as the right ventricular muscle and homograft, for extra strength.

23

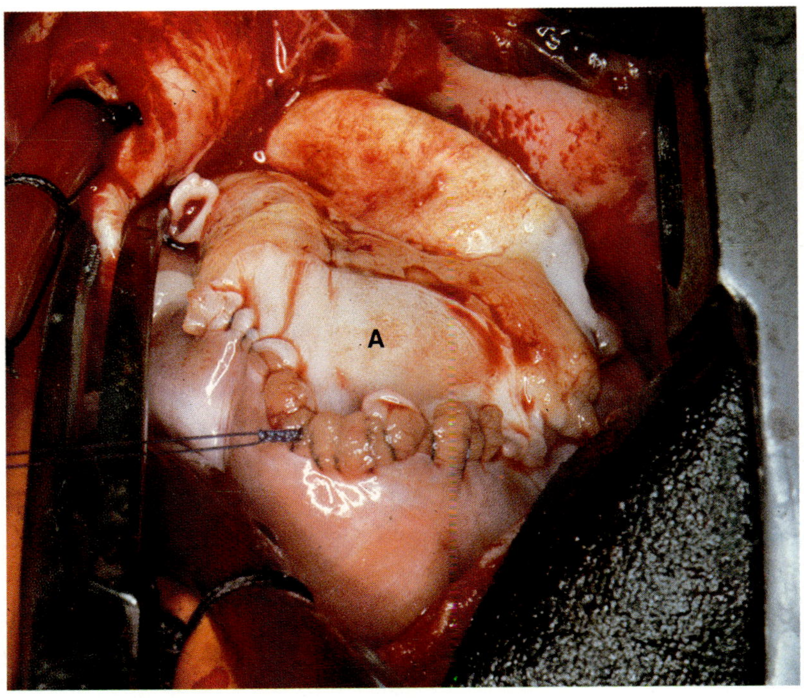

24

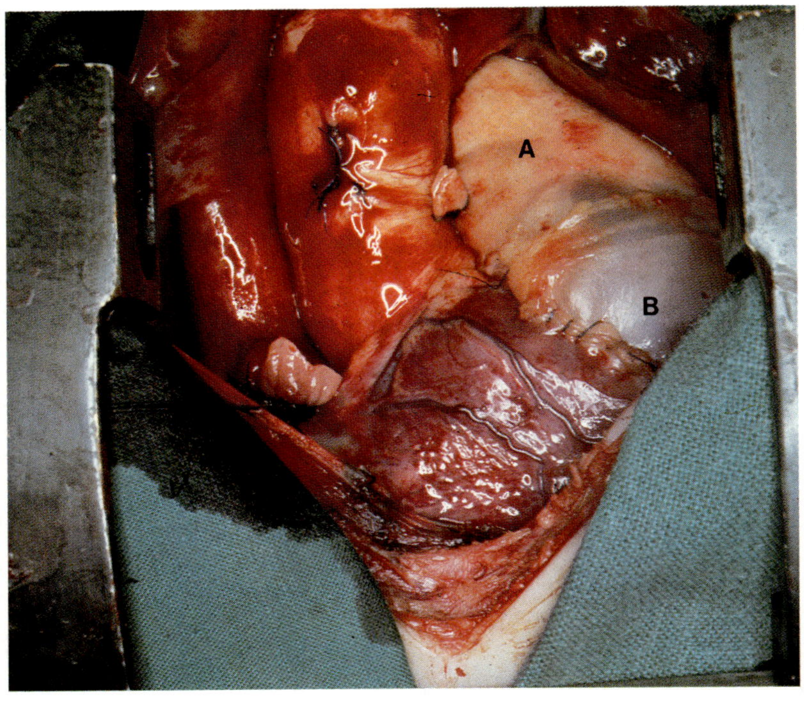

23 The remainder of the proximal anastomosis is performed and the anterior leaflet of the mitral valve of the homograft (**A**) nicely closes the ventriculotomy.

24 The final picture before closing the chest shows the position of the homograft (**A**) and its anterior leaflet of the mitral valve (**B**) forming the new right ventricular outflow tract and pulmonary artery.

15: Repair of total anomalous pulmonary venous drainage

In this condition the saturated blood returning from the lungs does not go directly to the left atrium, but passes to a common pulmonary venous trunk. The blood then passes by a supracardiac, intracardiac or infradiaphragmatic route to the right atrium (**A**), where it mixes with the desaturated blood returning from the superior (**B**) and inferior (**C**) vena cavae. Mixed blood passes through the tricuspid valve (**D**) to the right ventricle (**E**) and through the atrial septal defect (**F**) into the left atrium. The patient is therefore cyanosed, because mixed blood passes through the left side of the heart to the aorta, and also usually in heart failure as excess mixed blood passes through the right side of the heart to the lungs.

In the supracardiac type (see diagram **A**), the common pulmonary venous trunk (**G**) drains into a left superior vena cava (**H**) which runs up to join the left innominate vein (**J**) and thence via the superior vena cava to the right atrium. Correction involves connecting the common trunk via a wide anastomosis to the back or upper part of the left atrium, ligating the left superior vein and closing the atrial septal defect. The normal circulation of blood is then achieved.

As virtually all patients presenting with this condition are young infants, it is particularly appropriate to use deep hypothermia, and total circulatory arrest with removal of the venous cannula makes the operation much easier. In older patients, routine cardiopulmonary bypass with two venous cannulae is used.

Diagram A – Supracardiac type

- **A** – Right atrium
- **B** – Superior vena cava
- **C** – Inferior vena cava
- **D** – Tricuspid valve
- **E** – Right ventricle
- **F** – Atrial septal defect
- **G** – Common pulmonary venous trunk
- **H** – Left superior vena cava
- **J** – Left innominate vein

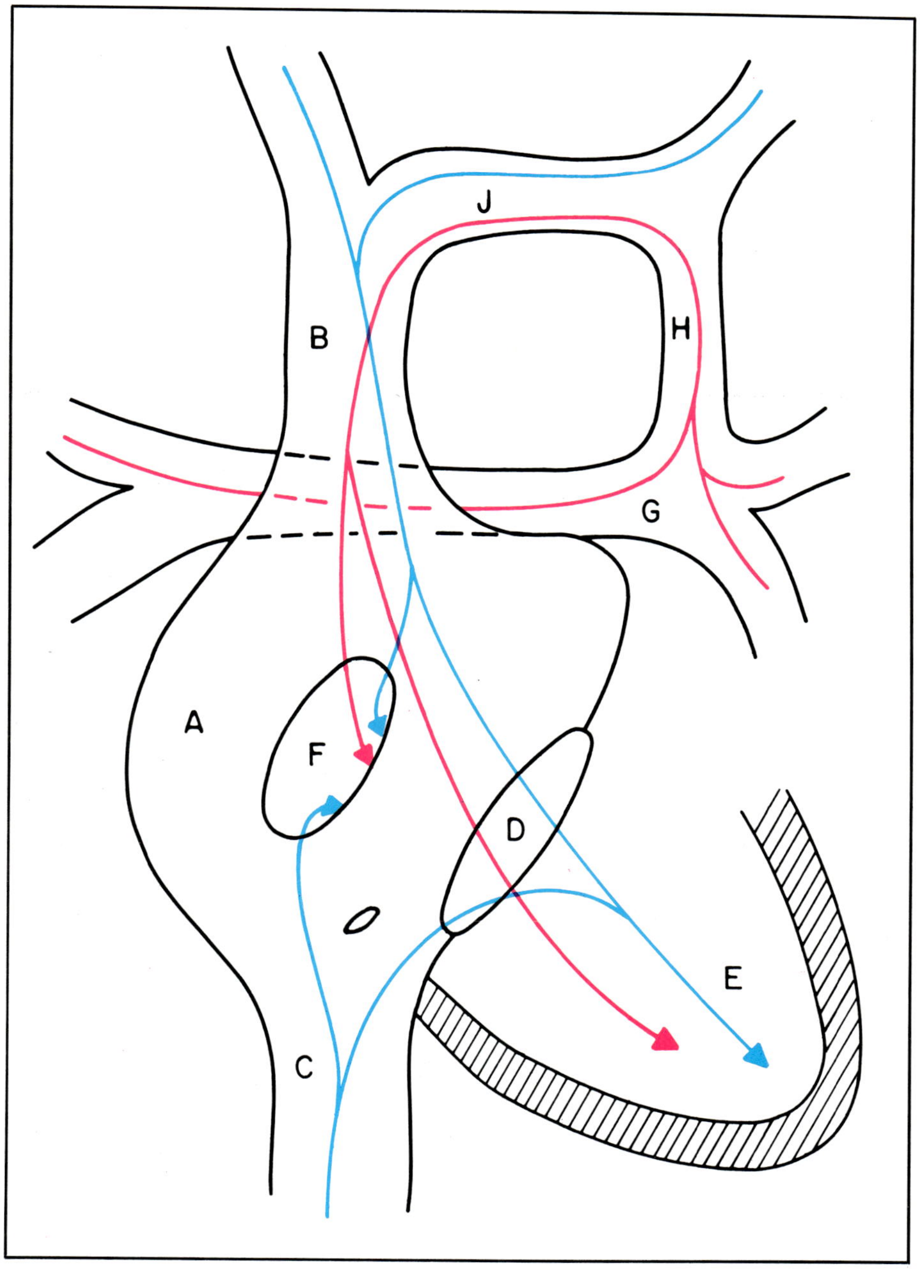

REPAIR OF TOTAL ANOMALOUS PULMONARY VENOUS DRAINAGE

In the intracardiac type (see diagram **B**), the common trunk (**G**) runs down to join the coronary sinus (**H**), which is therefore abnormally large, and reaches the right atrium. Correction is achieved by resecting the tissue separating the coronary sinus orifice and the atrial septal defect, and placing a patch over both to redirect the saturated blood returning via the coronary sinus, behind the patch and into the left atrium.

Diagram B – Intracardiac type

A – Right atrium

B – Superior vena cava

C – Inferior vena cava

D – Tricuspid valve

E – Right ventricle

F – Atrial septal defect

G – Common pulmonary venous trunk

H – Coronary sinus

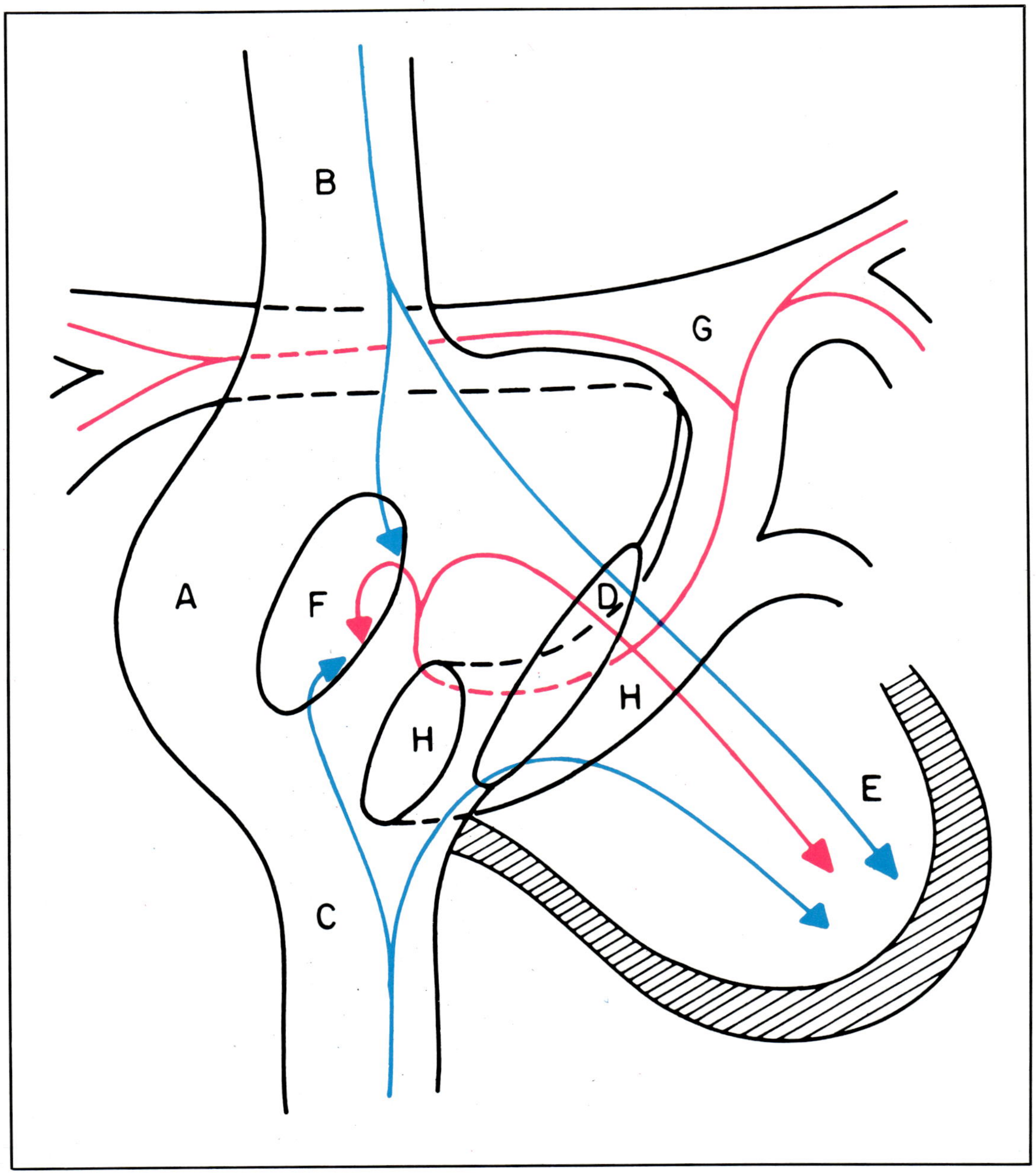

In the infradiaphragmatic type (see diagram **C**), the pulmonary veins drain to a vertically running common pulmonary venous trunk (**G**), which passes down in front of the oesophagus, through the diaphragm to enter the portal system. There is often a stenosis here and the blood also has to traverse the liver before passing via the hepatic veins into the inferior vena cava and thence to the right atrium. Again, correction requires an anastomosis between the common trunk and the back of the left atrium with ligation of the common trunk just above the diaphragm, and closure of the atrial septal defect.

Diagram C – Infradiaphragmatic type

A – Right atrium
B – Superior vena cava
C – Inferior vena cava
D – Tricuspid valve
E – Right atrium
F – Atrial septal defect
G – Common pulmonary venous trunk

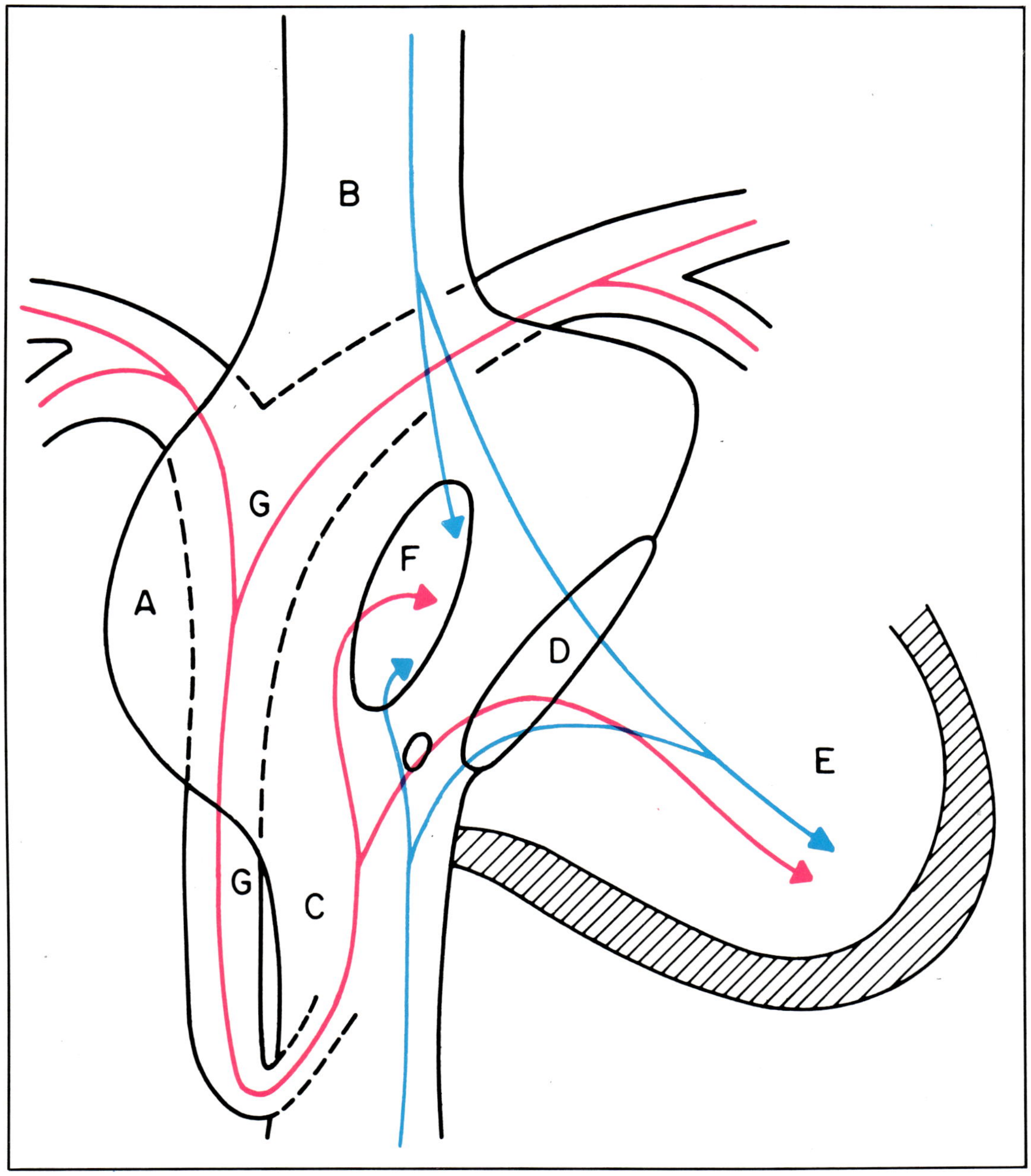

Supracardiac type (intra-atrial anastamosis)

1

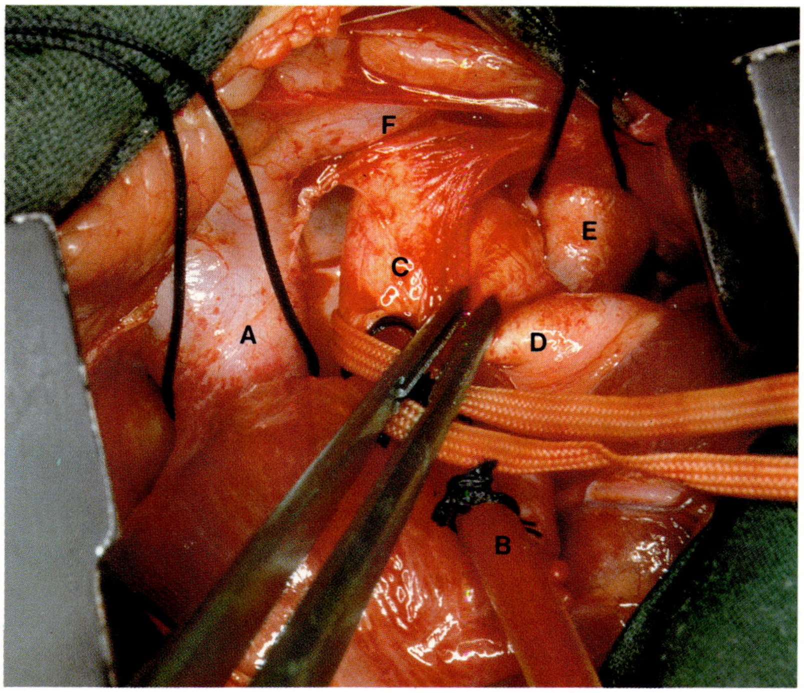

2

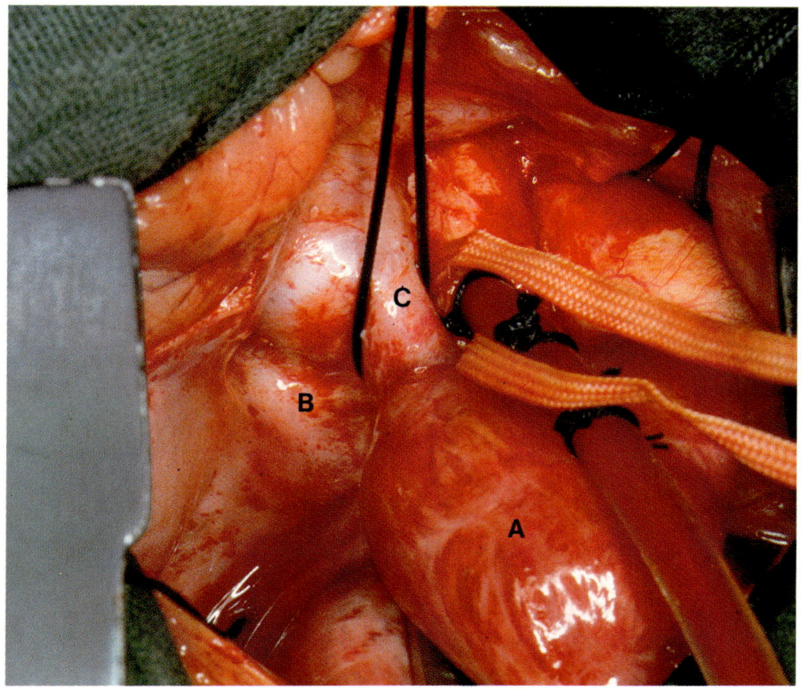

1 A tape has been placed around the superior vena cava (**A**) and a cannula (**B**) has been inserted into the ascending aorta (**C**). The main pulmonary artery (**D**) is being retracted to the right with forceps to reveal the left superior vena cava (**E**) which takes blood from the common pulmonary trunk to the left innominate vein (**F**).

2 The right atrium (**A**) has been pulled to the left to reveal the common pulmonary venous trunk (**B**) which lies behind the superior vena cava (**C**). It is because the pulmonary veins do not drain into the left atrium that the heart has such mobility.

3

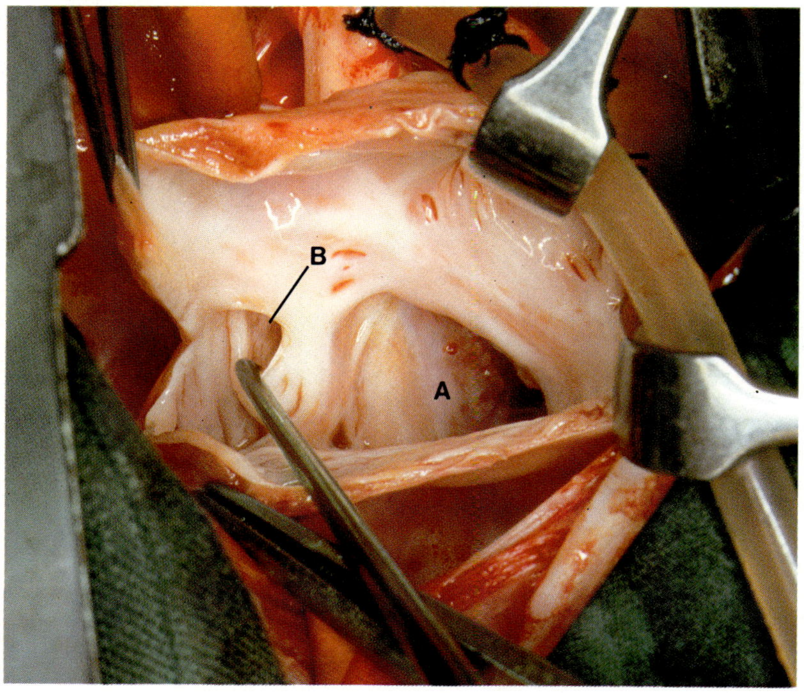

4

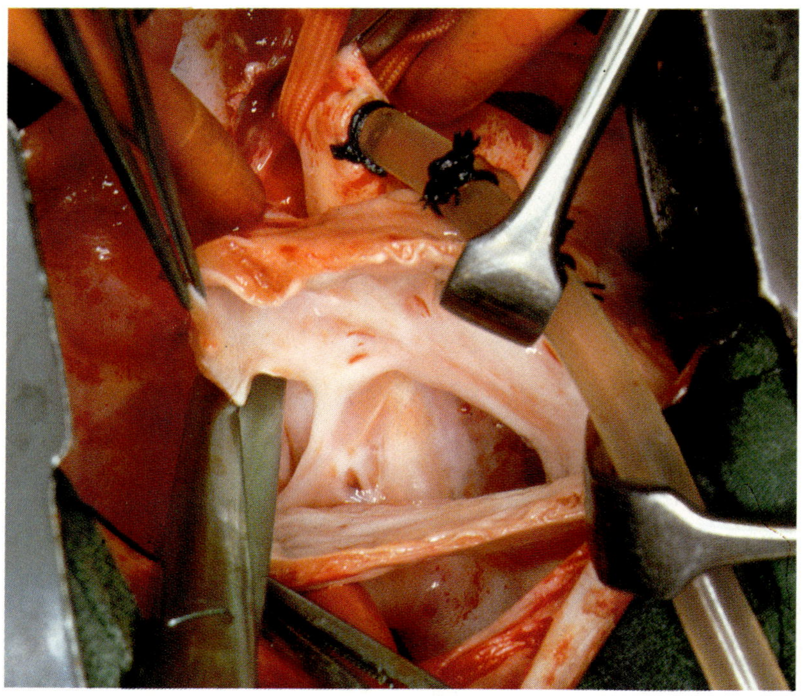

3 The right atrium has been widely incised, revealing the tricuspid valve (**A**) and atrial septal defect (**B**).

4 The atrial incision is continued with scissors, through the atrial septal defect and across the back of the left atrium, so as to produce an incision matching the common pulmonary venous trunk for anastomosis.

5

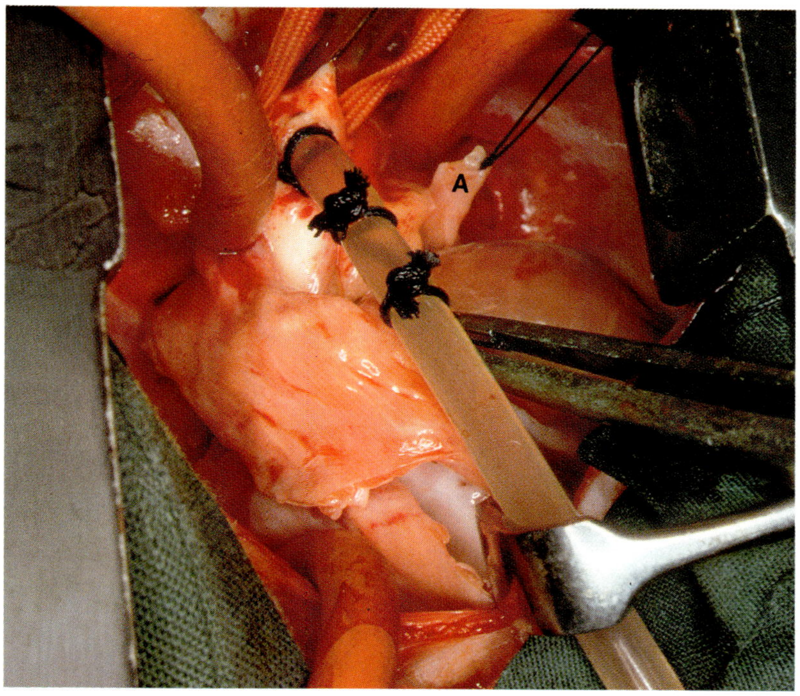

6

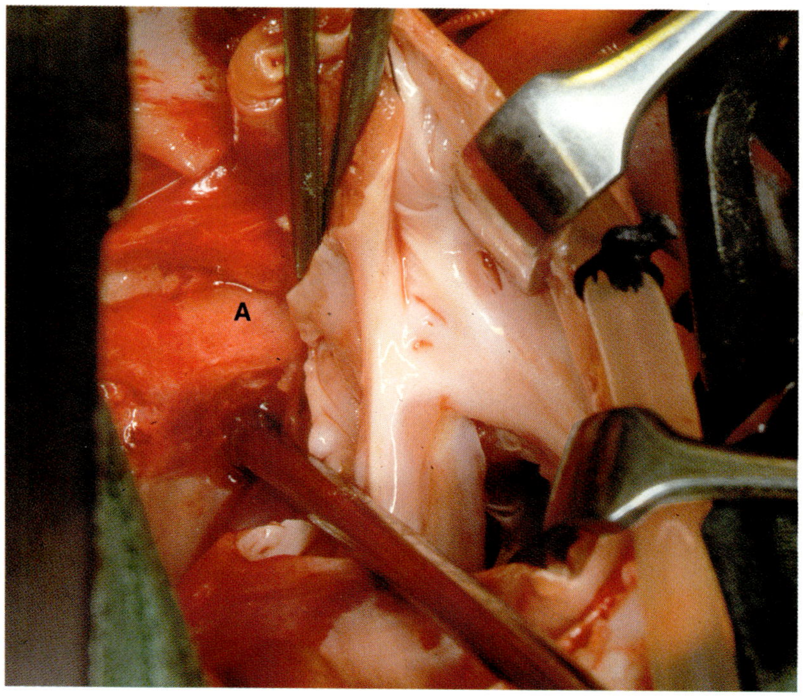

5 It is helpful to place a tie on the left atrial appendage (**A**) to prevent it being pulled too far to the right and making too long an incision in the back of the left atrium.

6 Having made the transverse incision in the back of the left atrium, the common pulmonary venous trunk (**A**) is assessed to see where the matching incision in it should be.

7

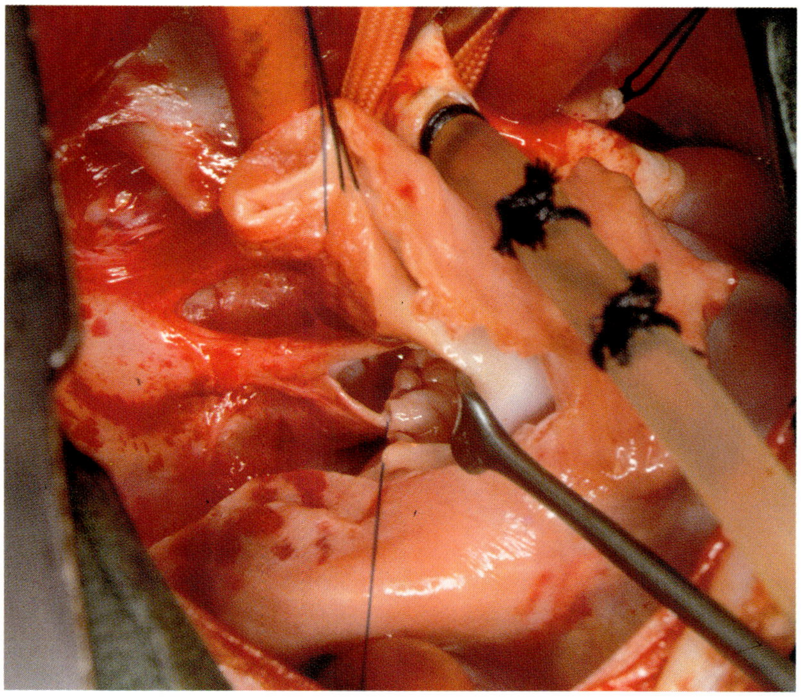

8

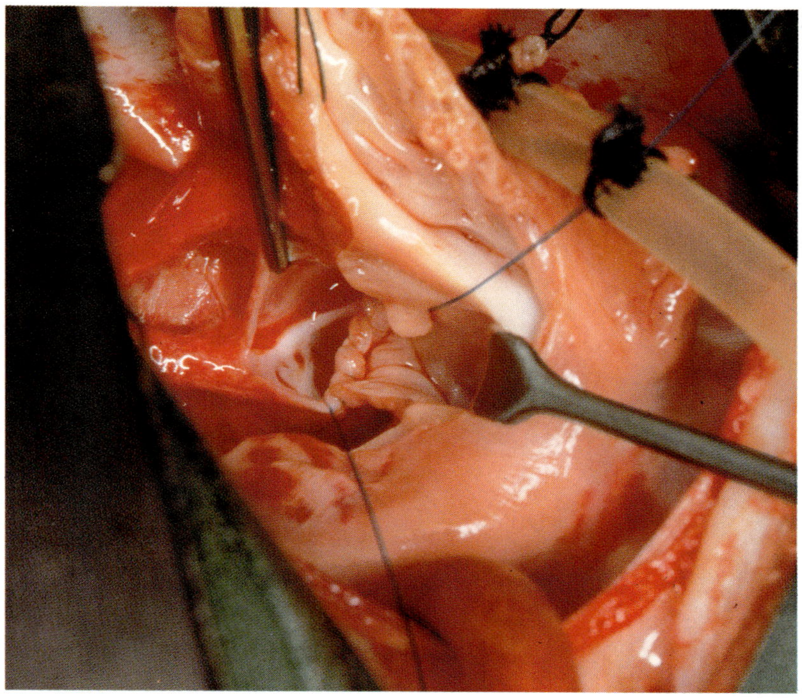

7 and 8 Starting at the left-hand end, a continuous Prolene suture is brought forward on both sides of the incision in the common pulmonary venous trunk, so as to bring down the left atrial wall onto it and create a large communication between the two. It may help future growth of the anastomosis if some interrupted sutures are used.

9

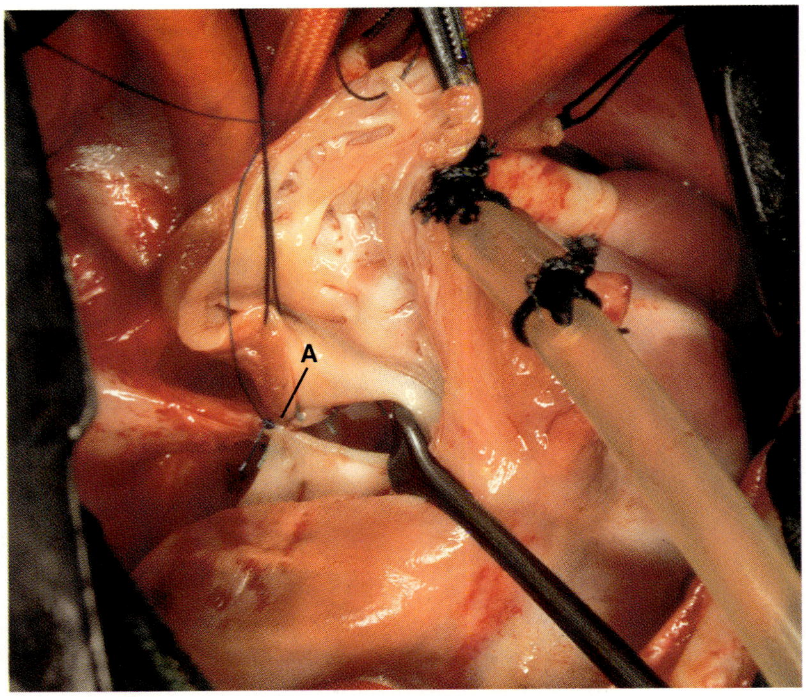

9 The anastomosis is now complete and the common pulmonary venous trunk, atrial wall and atrial septal defect all meet at point **A.**

10

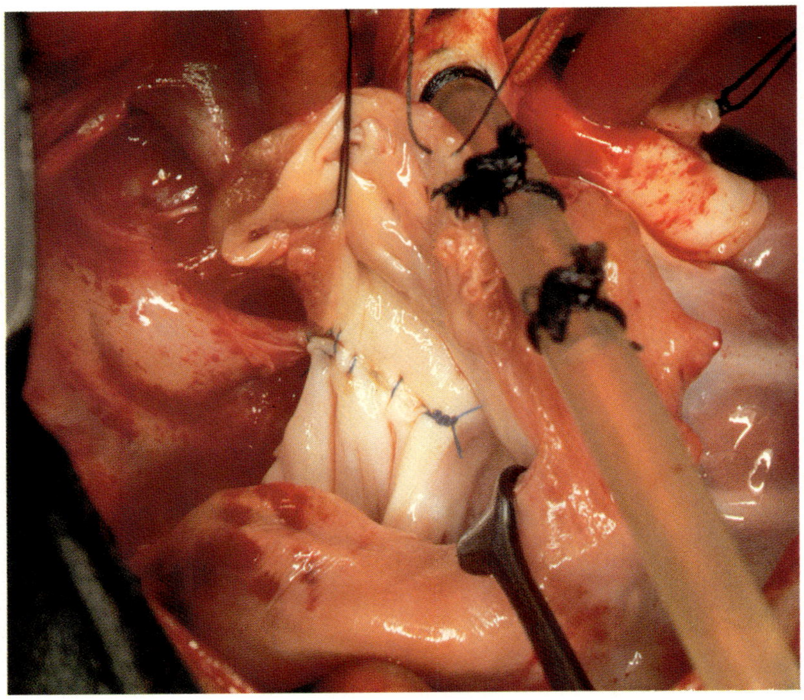

10 The atrial septal defect is closed with continuous Prolene.

11

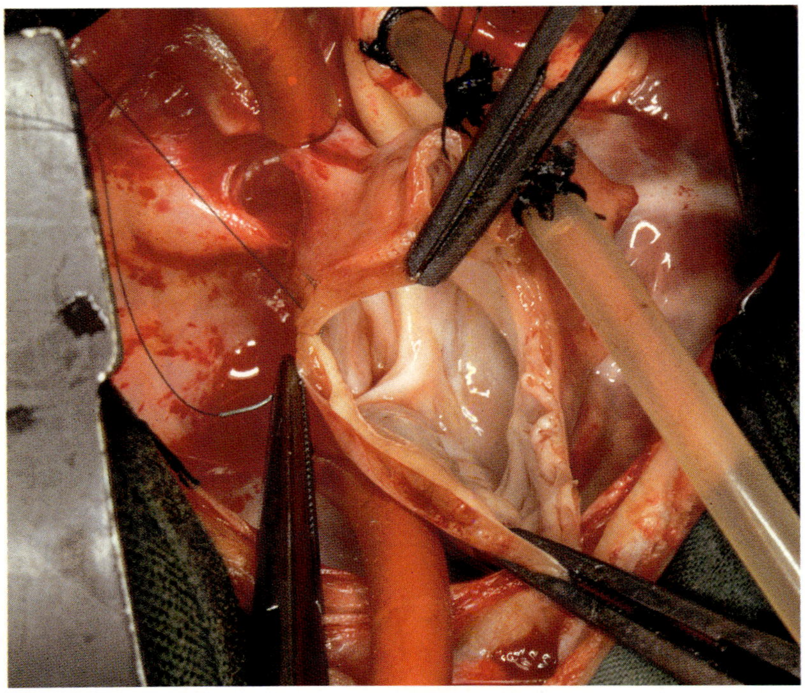

11 The right atrium is also closed with continuous Prolene and in fact the incision is larger than necessary and could have been started more laterally.

Supracardiac type (extra-atrial anastamosis)

12
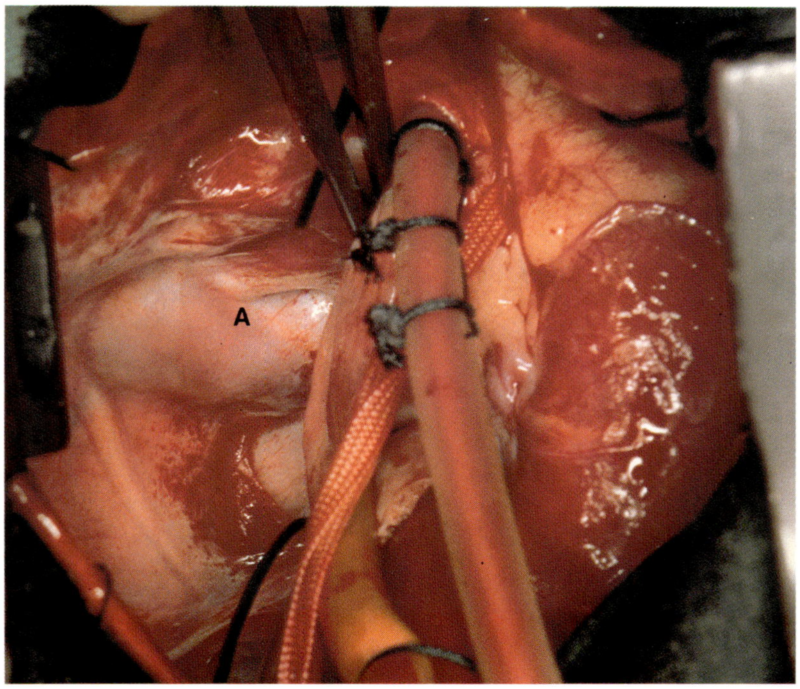

12 In a different patient with a supracardiac defect, retraction of the heart to the left reveals a large distended common pulmonary venous trunk (**A**).

13
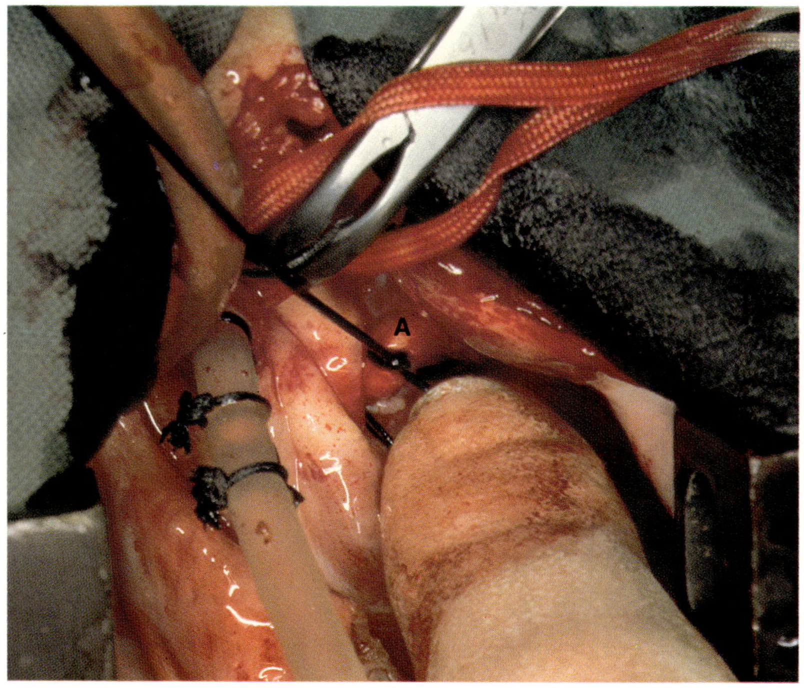

13 After circulatory arrest has been established, the left superior vena cava (**A**) has been ligated.

14
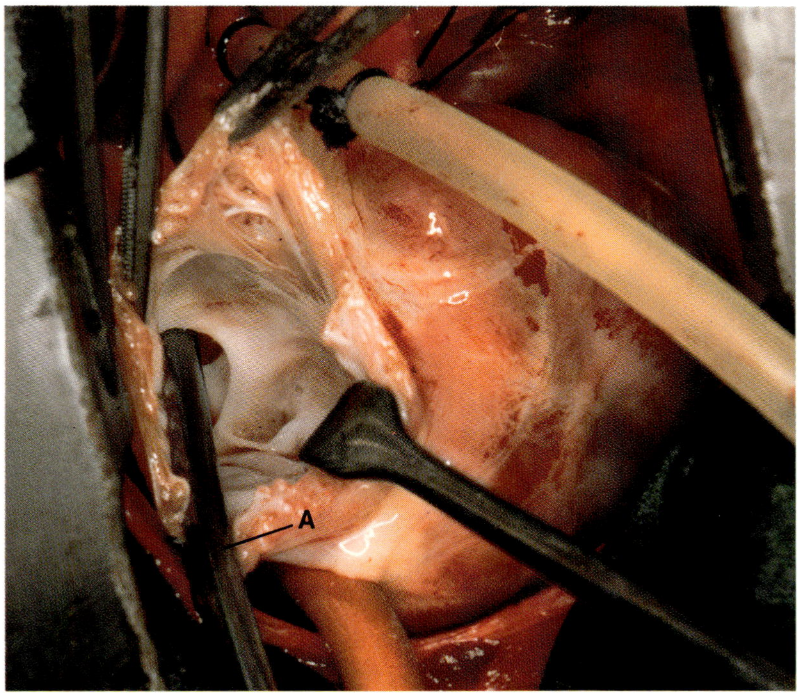

14 The right atrium has been opened and the venous cannula removed. A sucker (**A**) has been passed through the atrial septal defect into the left atrium.

15
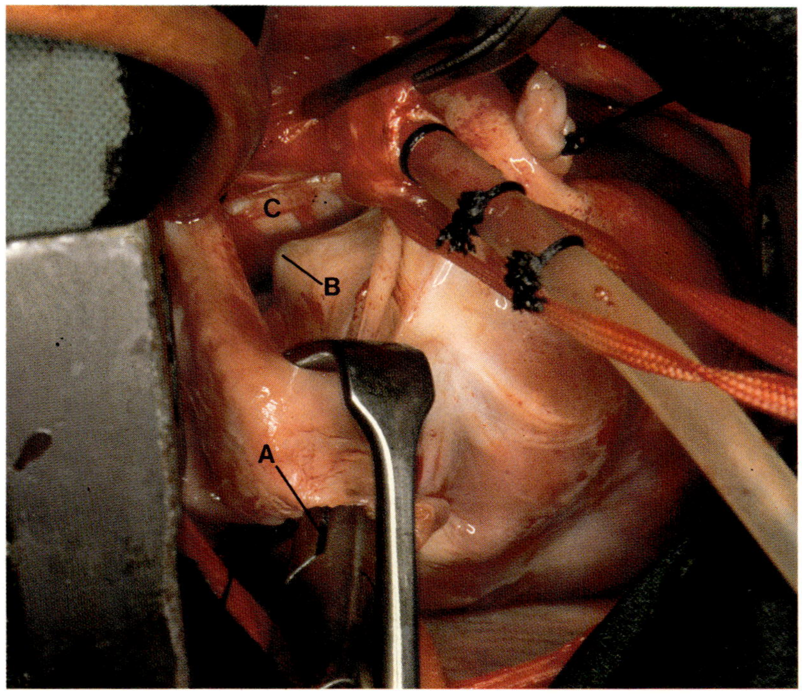

15 Because of the rather high position of this large pulmonary venous trunk, it was felt that it would be easier to anastomose the trunk to the upper surface of the left atrium from outside. A pair of forceps (**A**) has been passed into the right atrium, through the atrial septal defect and is tenting up the left atrium (**B**) in close proximity to the common pulmonary venous trunk (**C**).

16
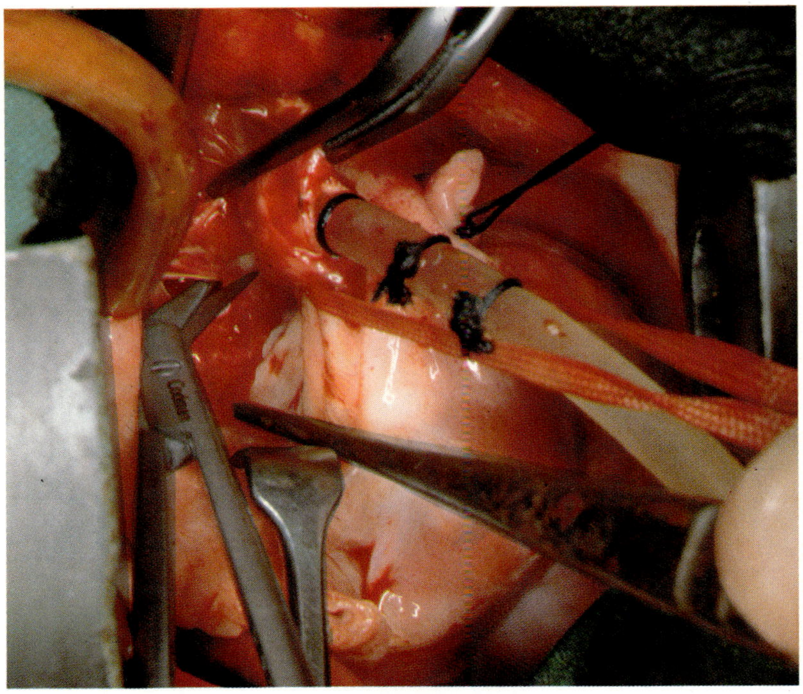

17
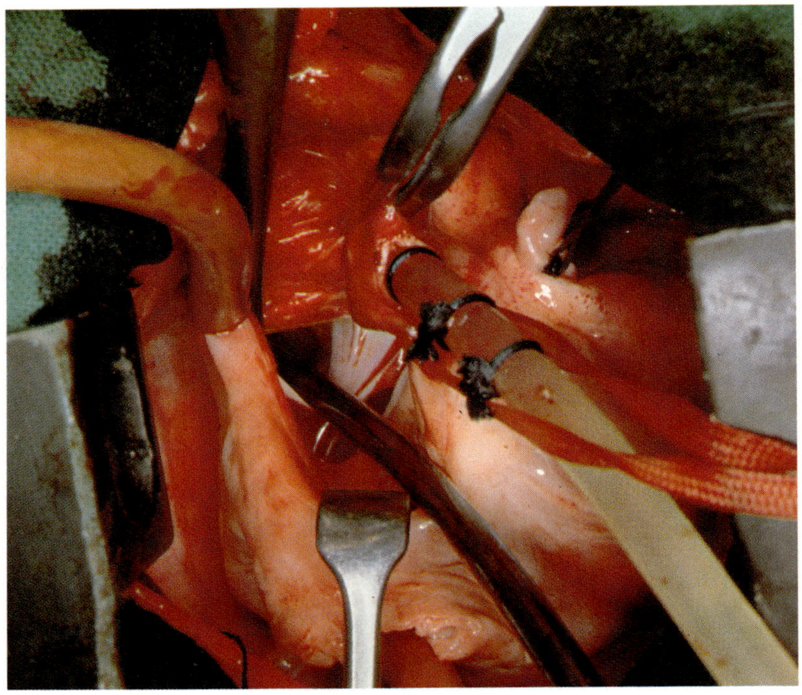

16 and 17 An incision is made with fine scissors in the common pulmonary venous trunk.

18
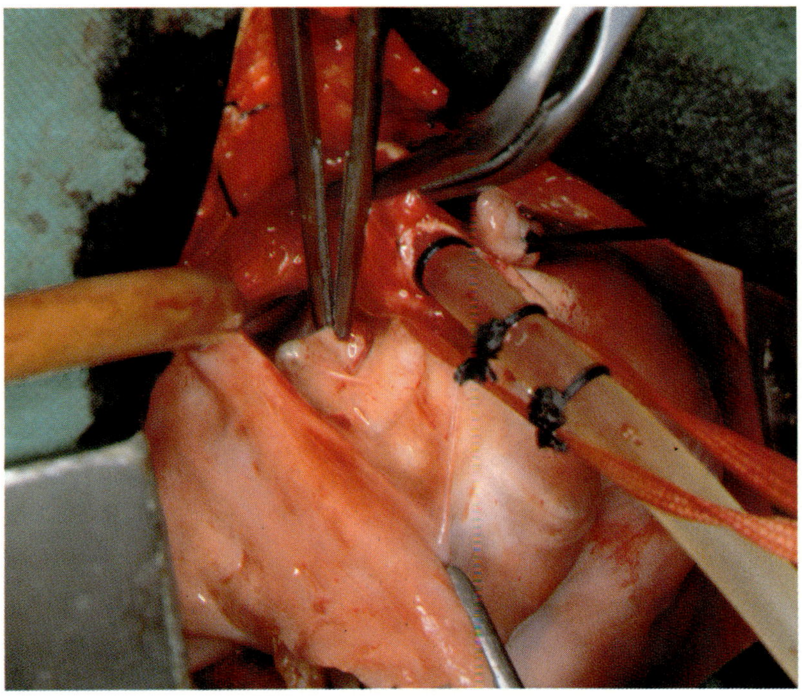

19
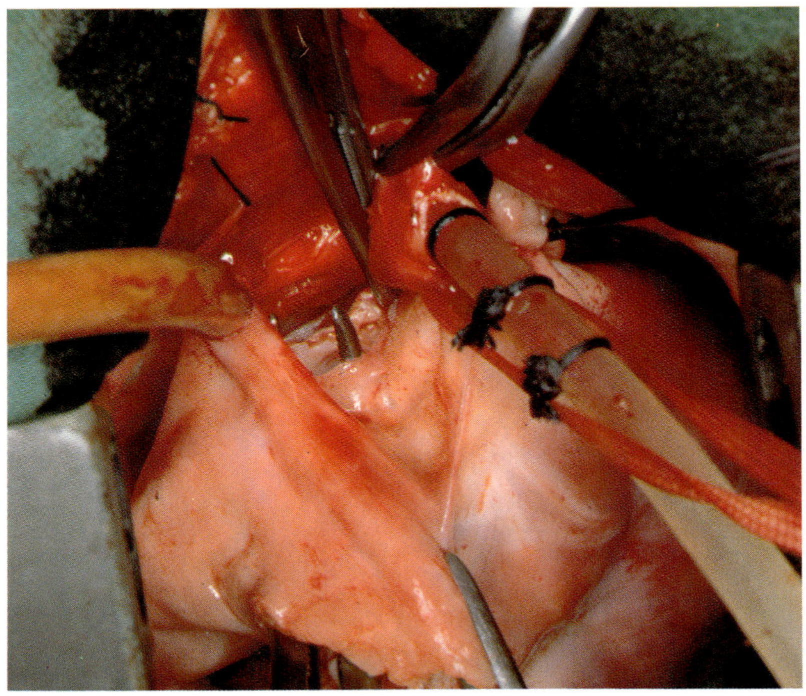

18 and 19 A matching incision is then made in the upper posterior wall of the left atrium and the forceps can be pushed through.

20

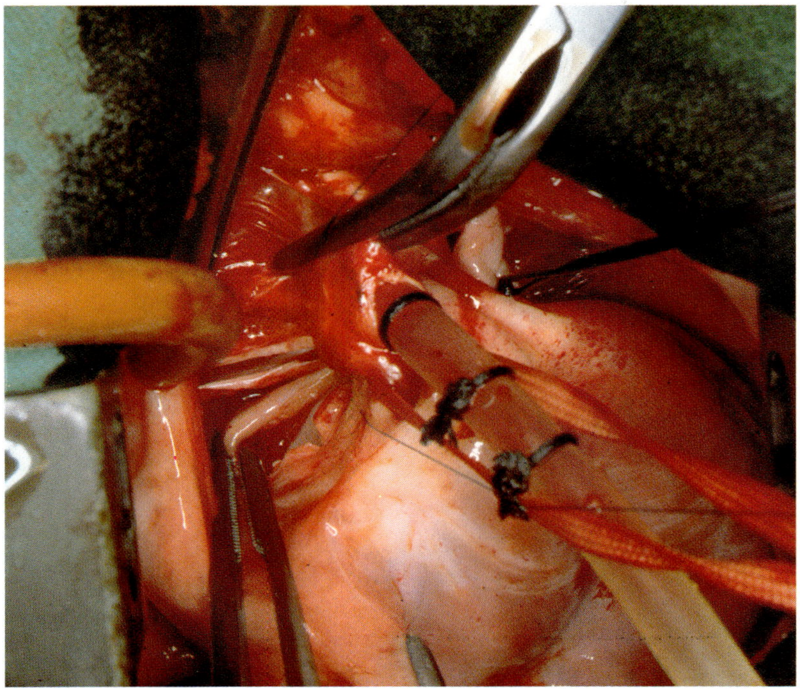

21

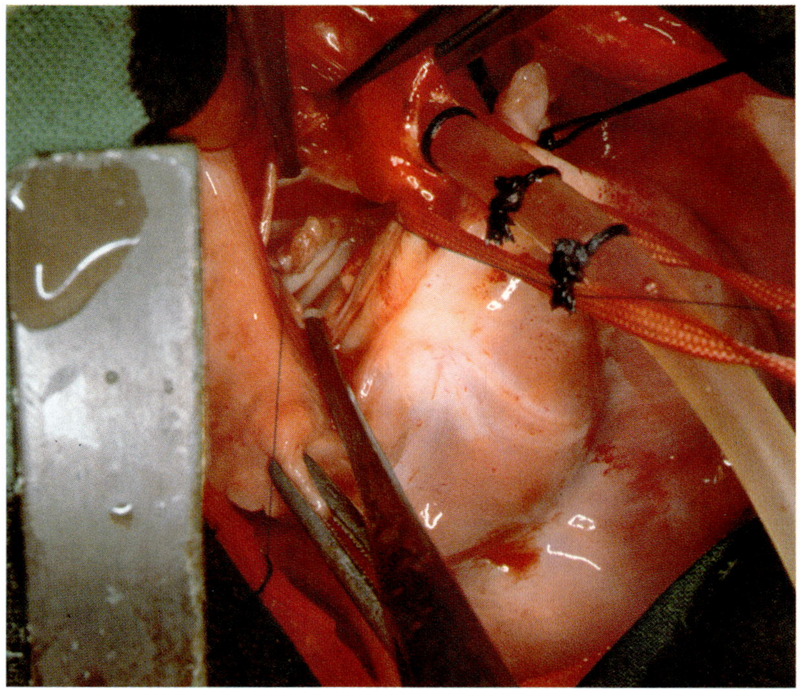

20 and 21 The posterior layer of the anastomosis is then performed with continuous Prolene.

22

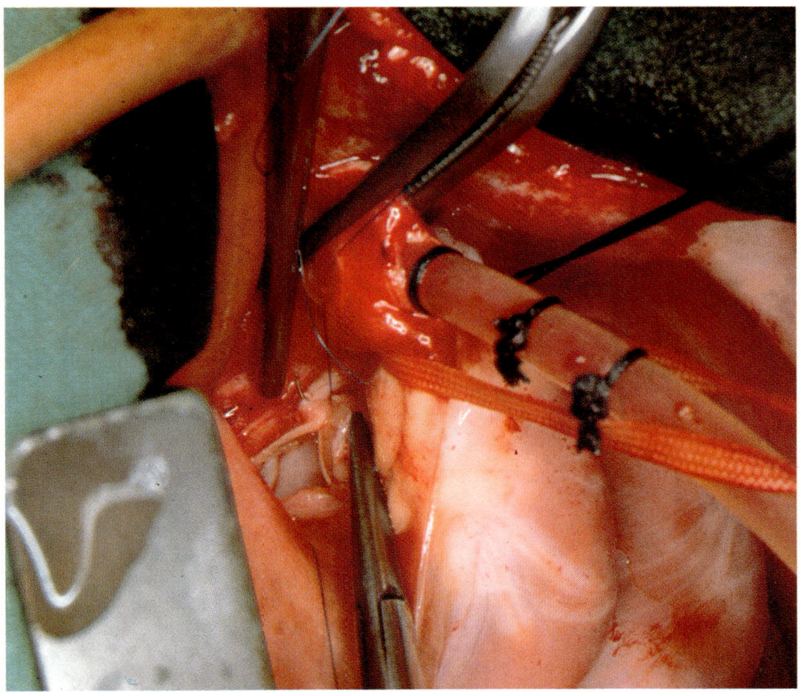

23

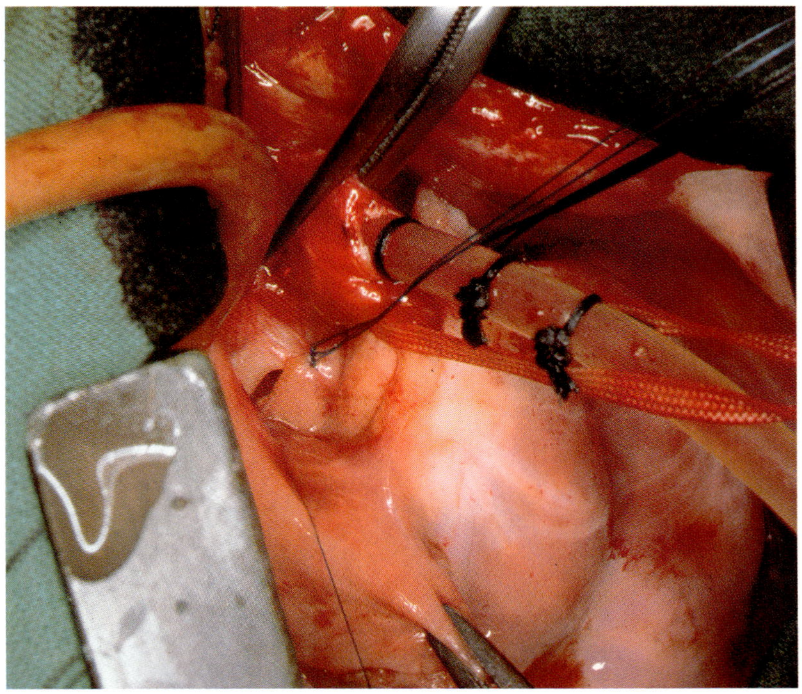

22 and 23 The anterior layer is completed, initially with continuous Prolene, but then with interrupted sutures to allow for growth.

24

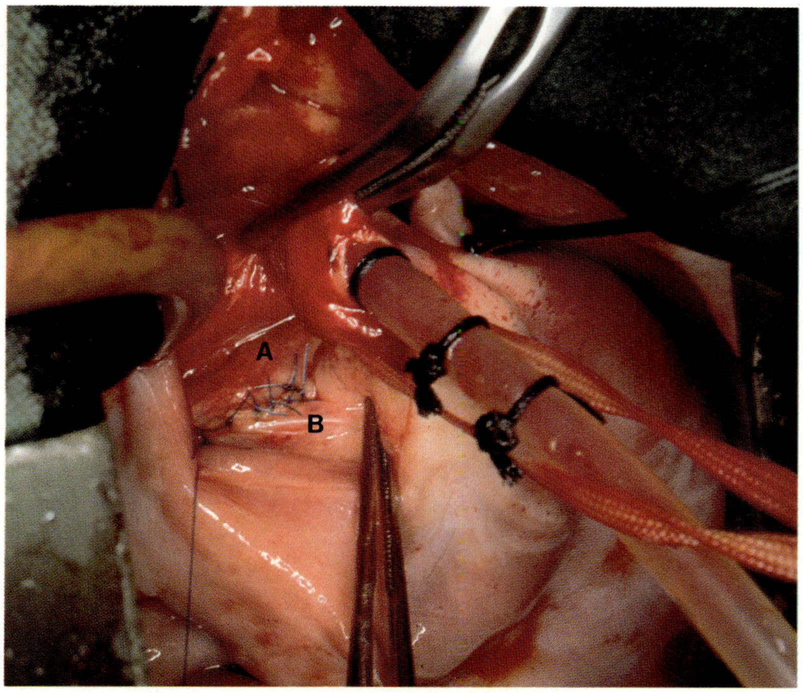

24 The interrupted sutures completely close the anterior part of the anastomosis between the common pulmonary venous trunk (**A**) above and posteriorly, and the left atrium (**B**) below and anteriorly.

25

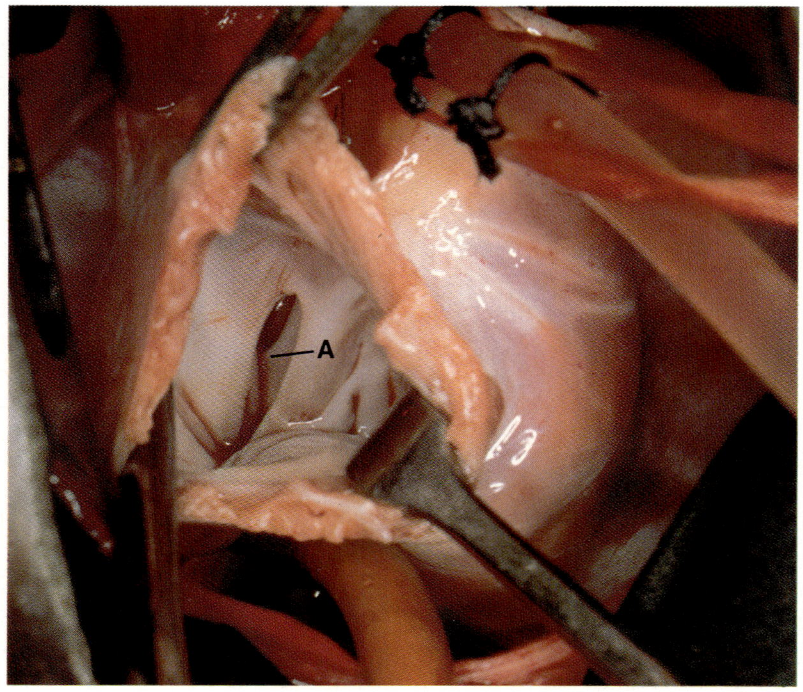

25 Returning to the atrium, the atrial septal defect (**A**) must be closed.

26

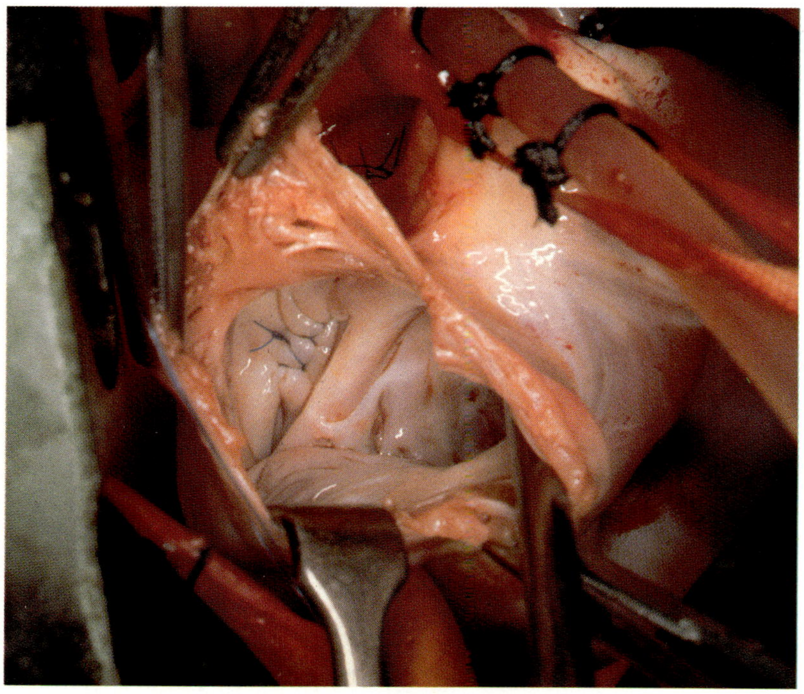

26 The atrial septal defect has been closed with continuous Prolene and the atrium must be closed.

Intracardiac type

27

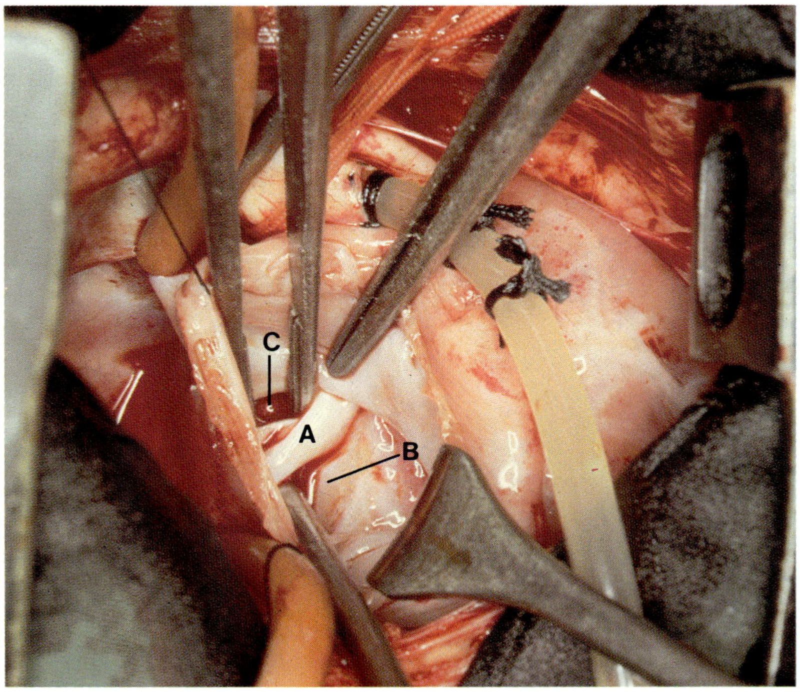

28

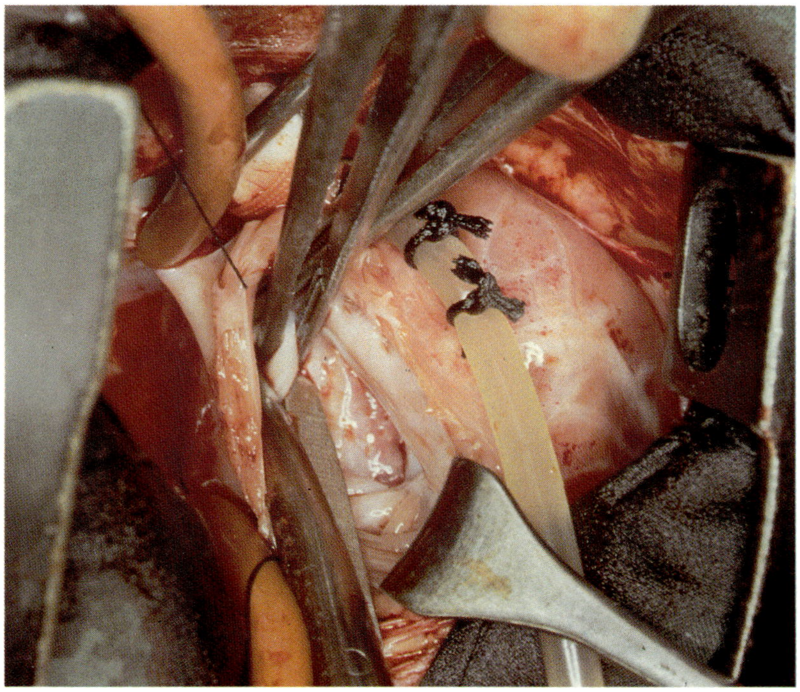

27 The right atrium has been opened to demonstrate the ridge of tissue (**A**) separating the large coronary sinus (**B**), through which all the pulmonary venous blood returns, and the atrial septal defect (**C**), held open by forceps.

28 The ridge of tissue is incised with scissors and a wedge removed, taking great care not to cut outside the left atrium posteriorly, but to leave a wide passage from the coronary sinus into the left atrium.

29

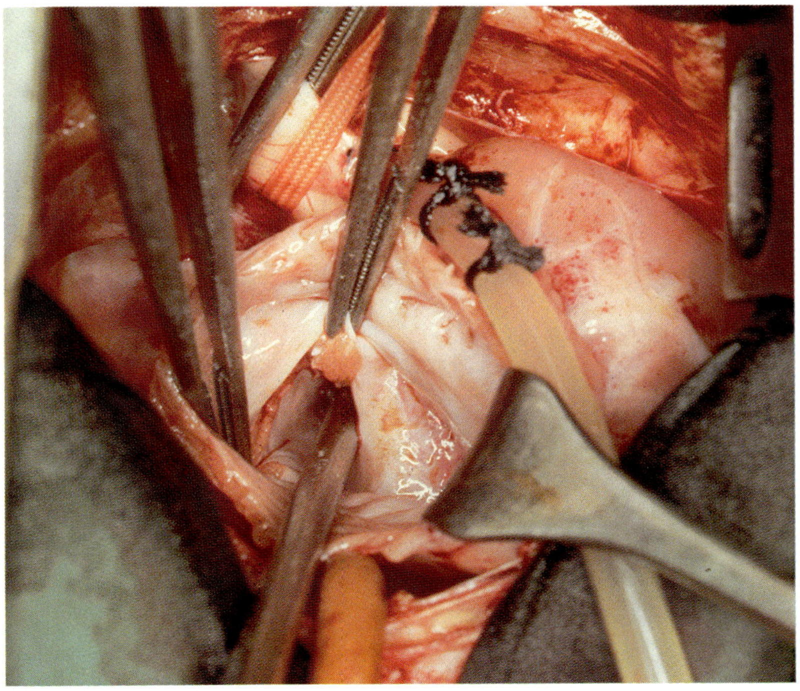

30

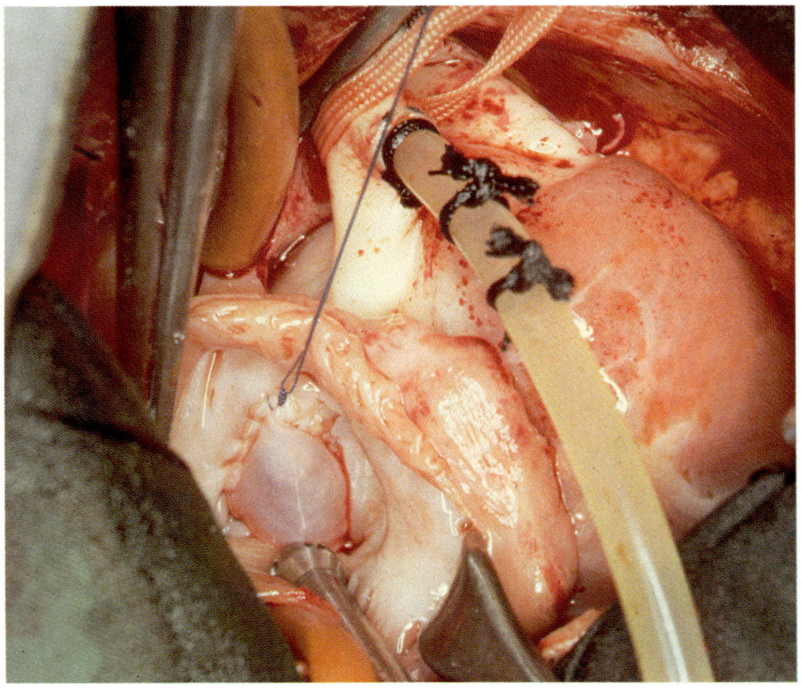

29 and 30 A wide communication is revealed and a patch of pericardium sutured over the resulting single defect completes the repair.

Infradiaphragmatic type

31

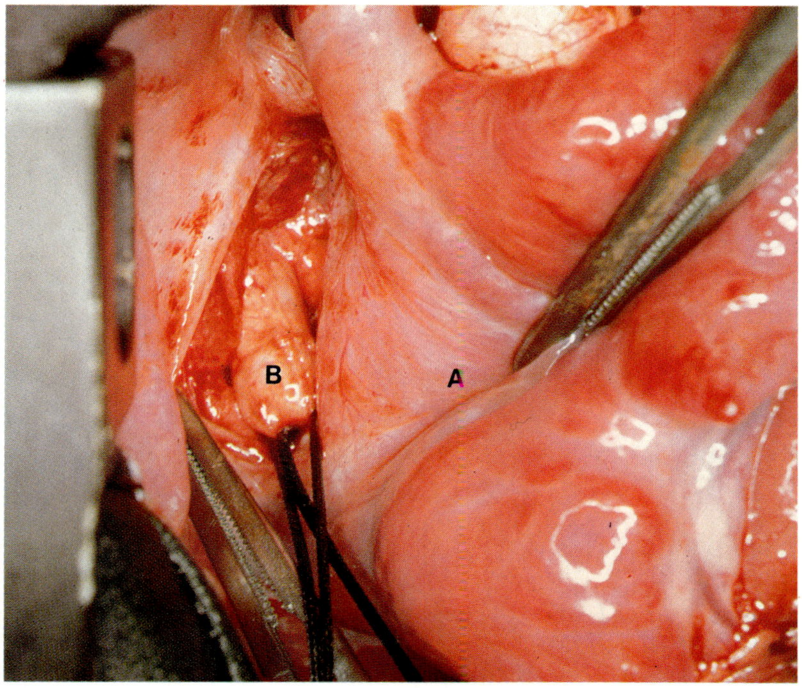

31 The right atrium (**A**) has been pulled to the left to reveal the common pulmonary venous trunk (**B**) running down towards the diaphragm. Ligatures have been placed around it before tying it off.

32

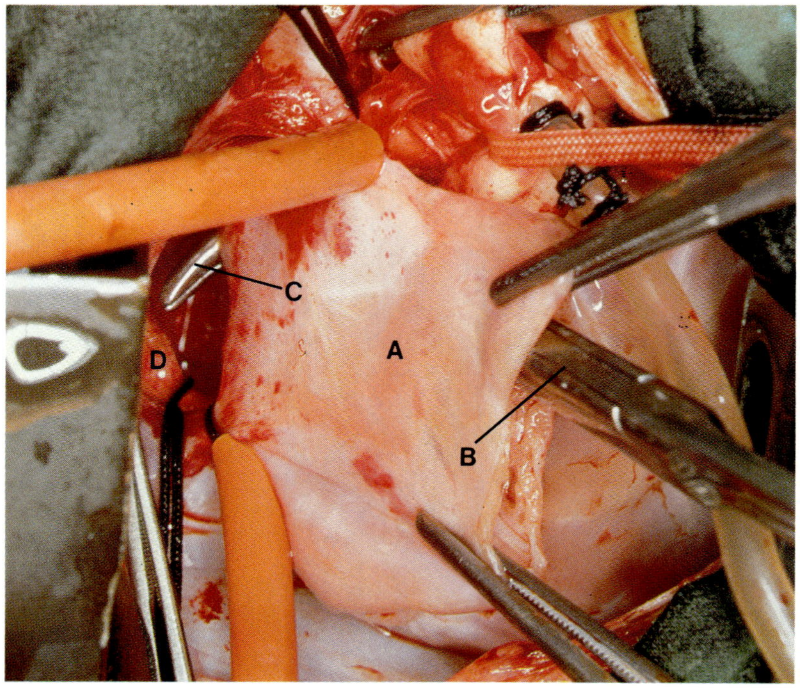

32 After circulatory arrest has been established, the right atrium (**A**) has been opened, and a pair of forceps (**B**) passed into the right atrium, through the atrial septal defect and out (**C**) through an incision in the left atrium opposite the common pulmonary venous trunk (**D**).

33

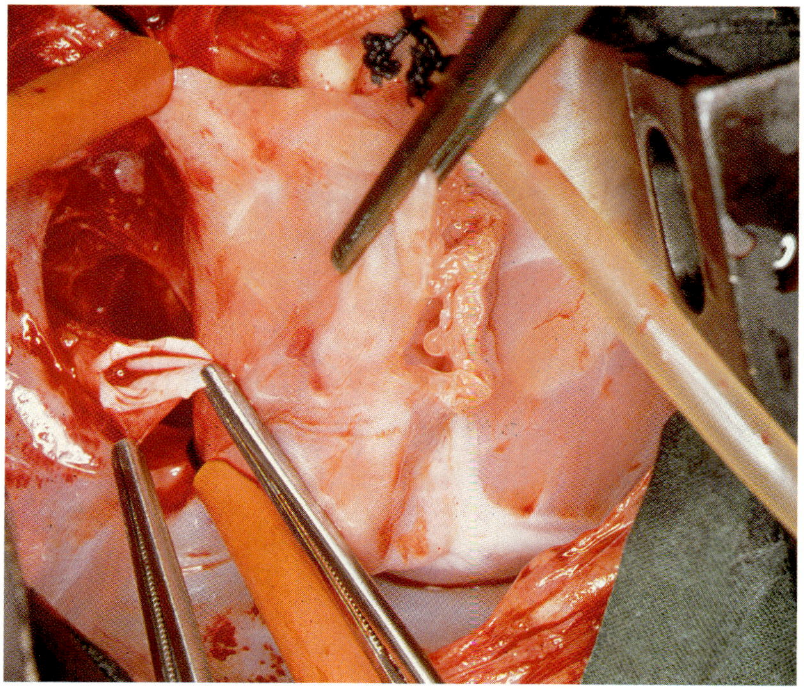

34

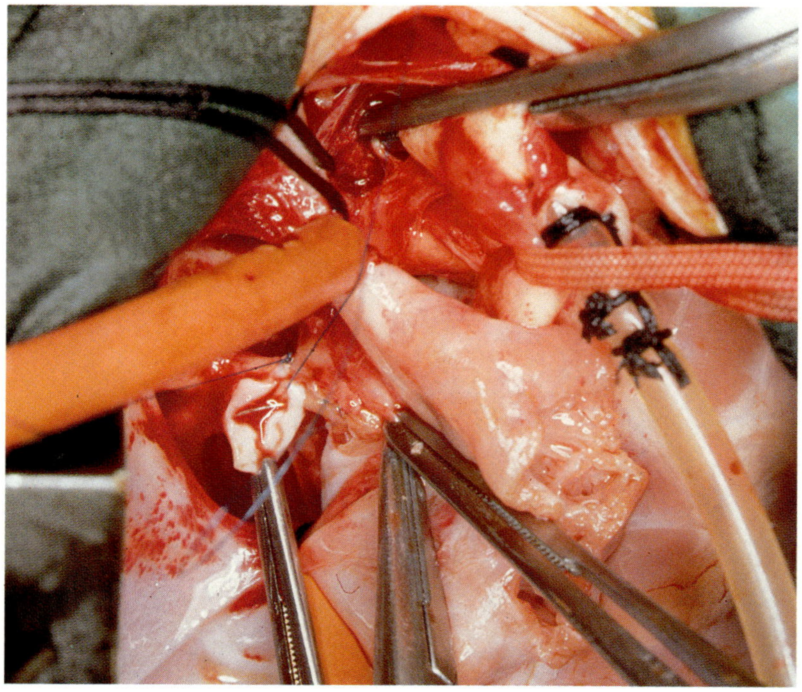

33 and 34 The common pulmonary venous trunk has been ligated and divided and the upper end is being anastomosed to the incision in the left atrium.

35
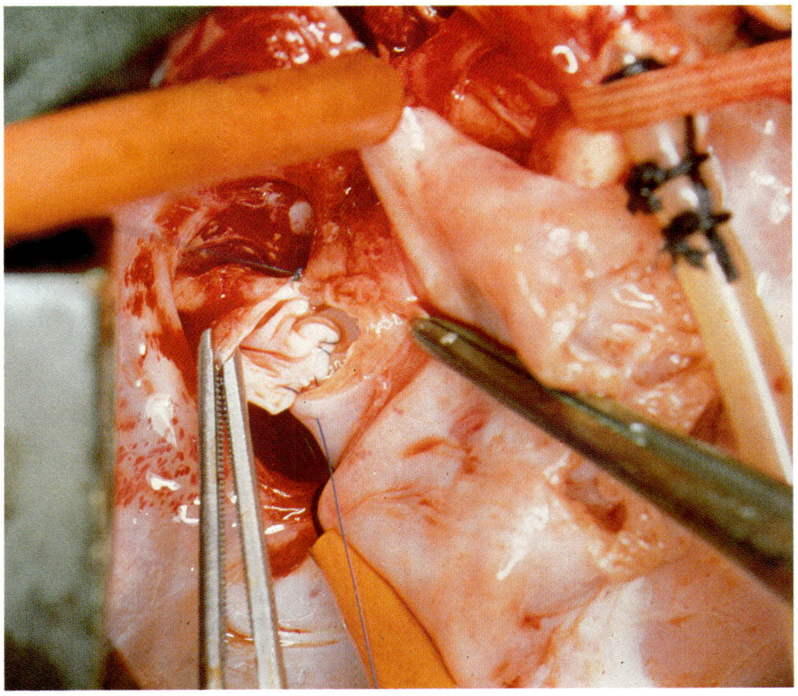

36
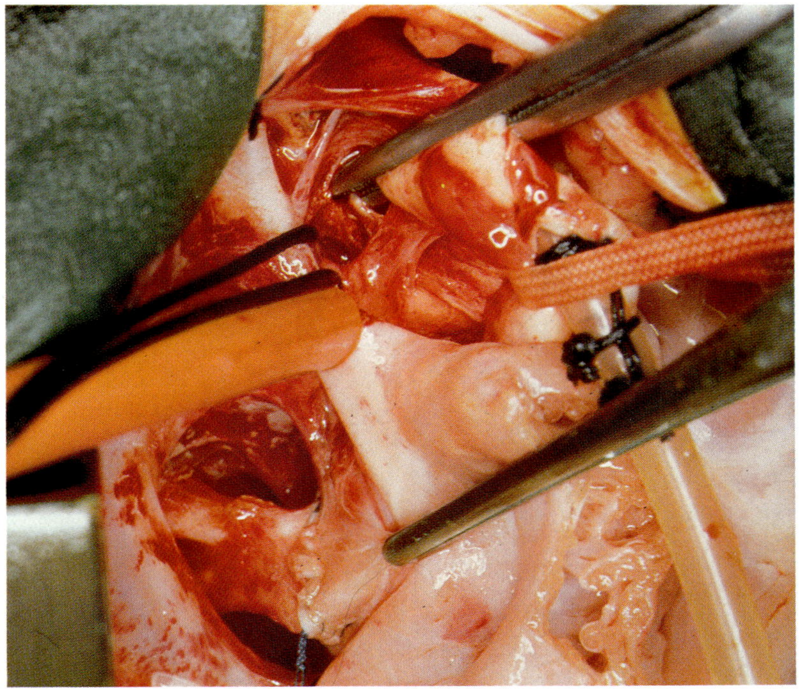

35 and 36 The anterior part of the anastomosis is completed. In this infant, in fact only the right lung drained inferiorly, the left lung drained superiorly and it was therefore easy to detach the trunk and turn it forward. Often, however, the trunk may be small and the anastomosis quite difficult and it may not be necessary or desirable to divide the trunk.

37
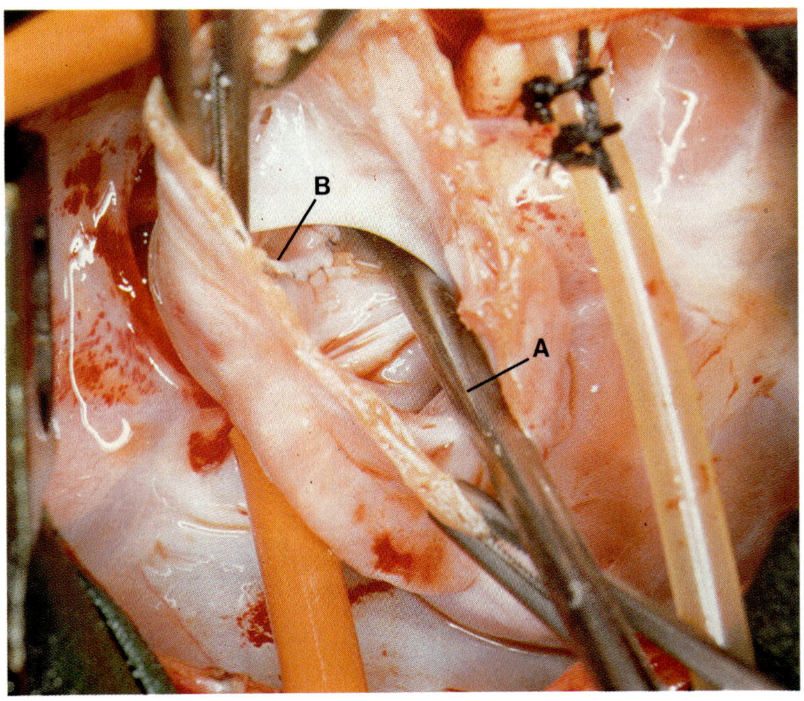

37 Looking into the right atrium and through the atrial septal defect, which is retracted with a sucker (**A**), the anastomosis can be seen from inside (**B**).

38
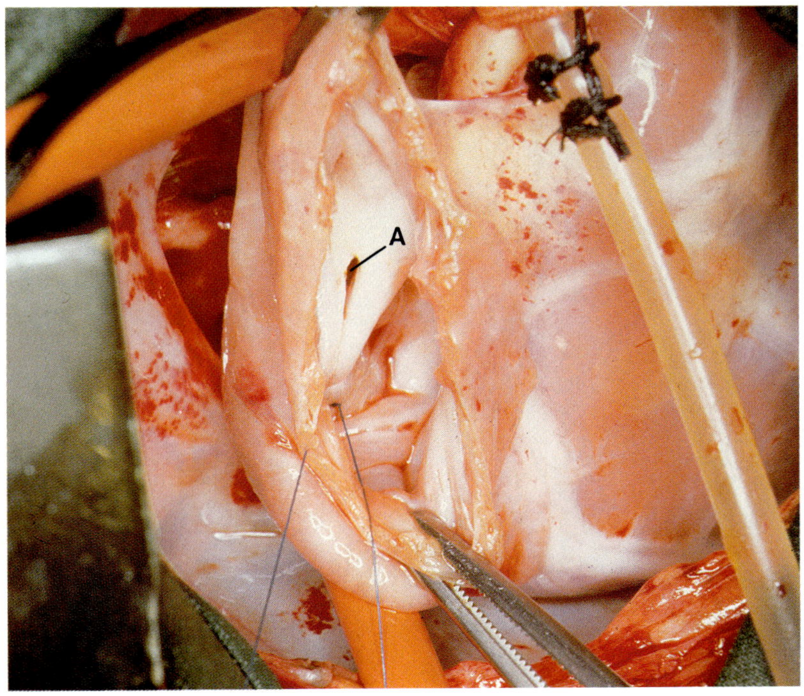

38 The atrial septal defect (**A**) is being closed with continuous Prolene.

Repair of partial anomalous pulmonary venous drainage

39

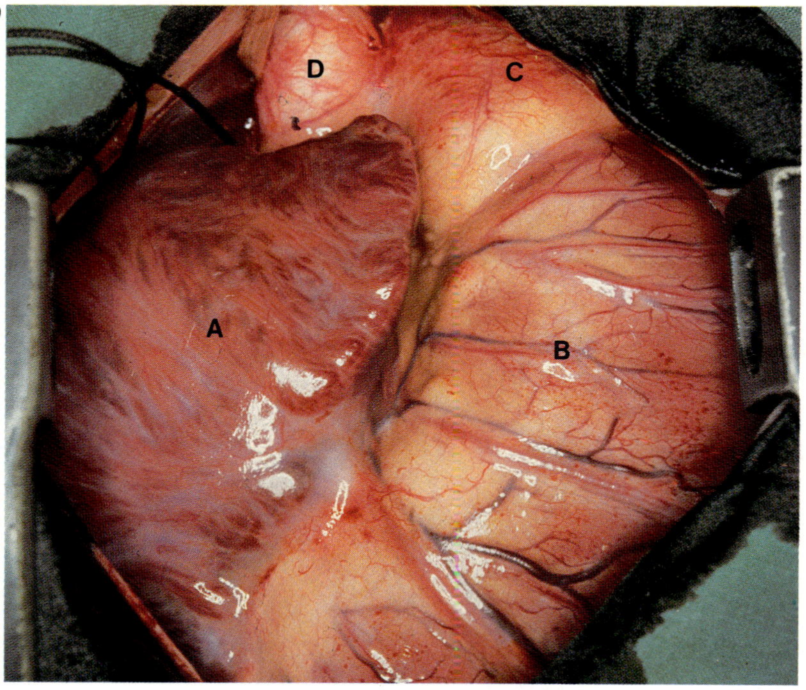

40

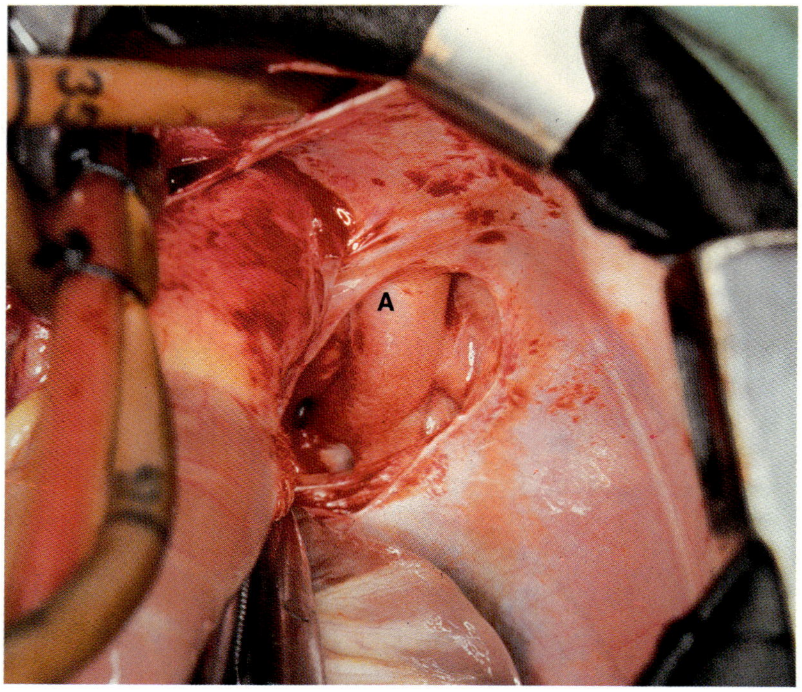

39 This is the heart of an older child with supracardiac anomalous venous drainage from the left lung only. Note the very large right atrium (**A**), right ventricle (**B**) and pulmonary artery (**C**), compared to the ascending aorta (**D**), as evidence of a large left-to-right shunt.

40 The left superior vena cava (**A**) is fed by several left pulmonary veins.

41

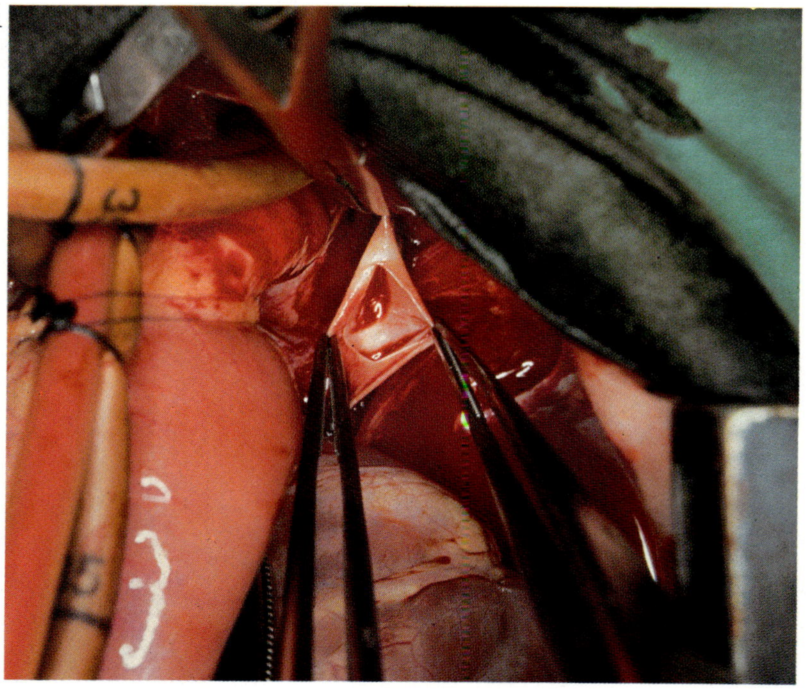

42

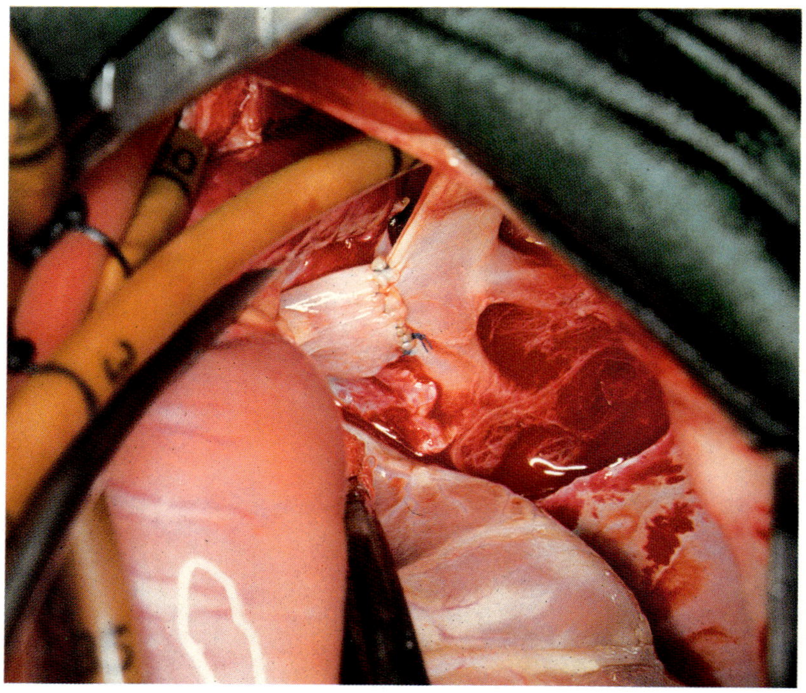

41 and 42 A longitudinal incision has been made in the left superior vena cava which is then anastomosed to the left atrial appendage. Having established a normal drainage to the left atrium, ligation of the left superior vena cava and closure of the atrial septal defect complete the repair. This illustrates another way of making the anastomosis with the left atrium by using the adjacent left atrial appendage.

16: The Fontan procedure

The Fontan procedure was first used successfully for the repair of tricuspid atresia in 1968[1]. The concept of using the right atrium to pump blood to the lungs has also been used in the repair of other conditions such as single ventricle[2]. Various modifications of Fontan's original procedure have been developed. Kreutzer[3] detached the pulmonary artery and valve from the ventricle and anastomosed it directly to the right atrial appendage and Bjork[4] anastomosed the right atrial appendage directly to the outlet chamber with an additional pericardial patch.

Most commonly in tricuspid atresia, patients have ventriculoarterial concordance and this is illustrated in diagram **A.** The desaturated blood returns to the right atrium (**A**) and, because the tricuspid valve is atretic, passes through an atrial septal defect (**B**) and into the left atrium (**C**), where it mixes with saturated blood returning from the lungs, and on to the left ventricle (**D**). The mixed blood being pumped from the left ventricle passes mainly into the ascending aorta (**E**) but some passes through the ventricular septal defect (bulboventricular foramen) (**F**), into the outlet chamber (**G**) and on into the pulmonary artery (**H**). The size of the ventricular septal defect and the presence of pulmonary stenosis, or even atresia, determine how much blood reaches the lungs.

Because the results of the Fontan procedure are not so good before four years of age[5], most patients will need a palliative operation before this age. If there is a diminished blood flow to the lungs, a Blalock, or modified Blalock shunt, is recommended (see Chapter 6) and if too much blood is flowing to the lungs, pulmonary artery banding will be needed (see Chapter 8). If a Fontan procedure is to be successful in later years, it is very important to prevent the development of pulmonary vascular disease.

If the Fontan procedure can be delayed until at least four years of age, an adult-size valve can be inserted. Homograft valves would seem to be the conduit of choice for this operation and give superior

Diagram A

A – Right atrium
B – Atrial septal defect
C – Left atrium
D – Left ventricle
E – Ascending aorta
F – Ventricular septal defect (bulboventricular foramen)
G – Outlet chamber
H – Pulmonary artery

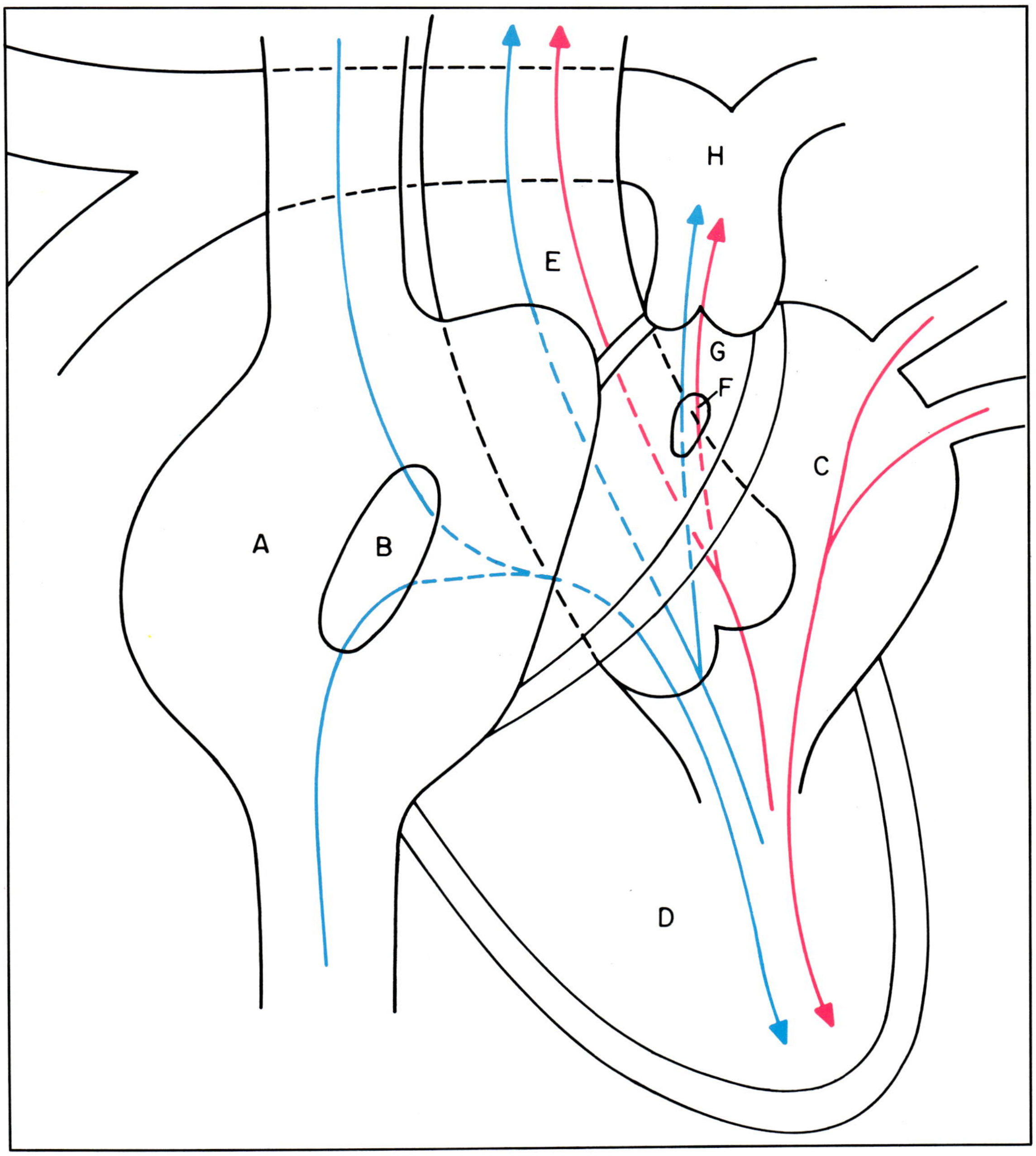

results to pig valves mounted in dacron tubes.

When present, an outlet chamber should be incorporated in the repair if possible, because it can help considerably with pushing blood to the lungs, provided a valved conduit is used. Diagram **B** illustrates the Fontan procedure for tricuspid atresia with an outlet chamber. Cardiopulmonary bypass is used and it is helpful to place the venous cannulae directly into the cavae as it is important to restrict the incision in the right atrium so as to preserve its function. The right atrium (**A**) is therefore opened through an incision in the tip of the atrial appendage which can be enlarged if necessary for the anastomosis with the proximal end of the homograft later. The atrial septal defect is closed and it is usually advisable to use a patch (**B**). The outlet chamber (**C**) is then opened, taking care to avoid the coronary arteries which delineate it, and the pulmonary valve is inspected. The pulmonary valve and ring must not form any obstruction as even a small pressure gradient between the right atrium and pulmonary artery will jeopardise the procedure. The ventricular septal defect (bulboventricular foramen) (**D**) is then closed and the distal end of the homograft (**E**) sutured to the outlet chamber. The proximal end of the homograft is then sutured to the atrial appendage, trimming off part of the appendage as necessary.

This procedure is illustrated in the following pictures, but if there is no outlet chamber, it is necessary to anastomose the conduit direct from the right atrial appendage to the pulmonary artery – usually to the right of the aorta, as illustrated on page 164.

Cardiopulmonary bypass is needed and it is helpful to insert the two venous cannulae directly into the vena cavae, rather than through the atrial appendage, where they would be in the way.

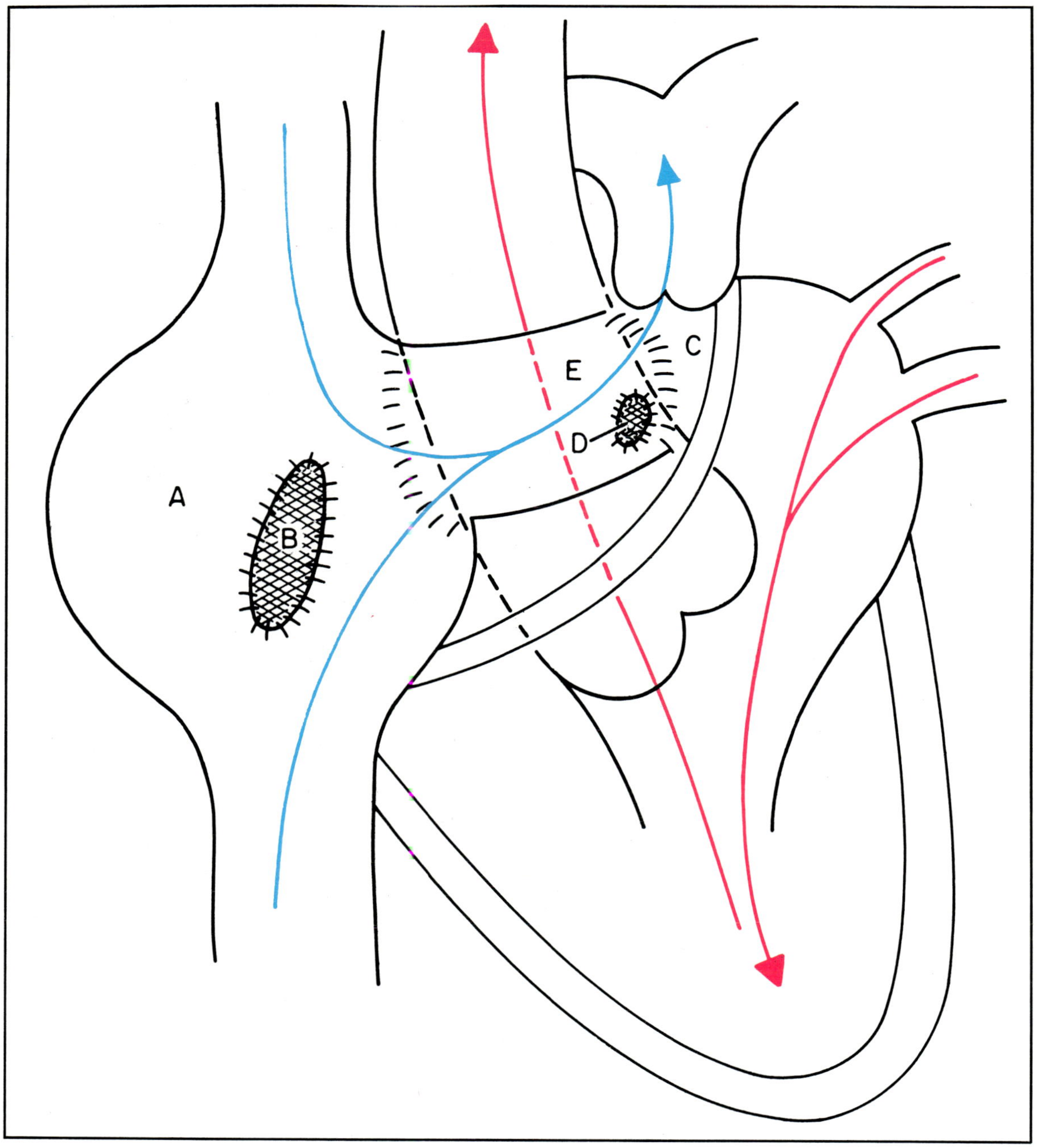

Diagram B

A – Right atrium

B – Patch closing atrial septal defect

C – Outlet chamber

D – Patch closing ventricular septal defect

E – Aortic homograft conduit

1

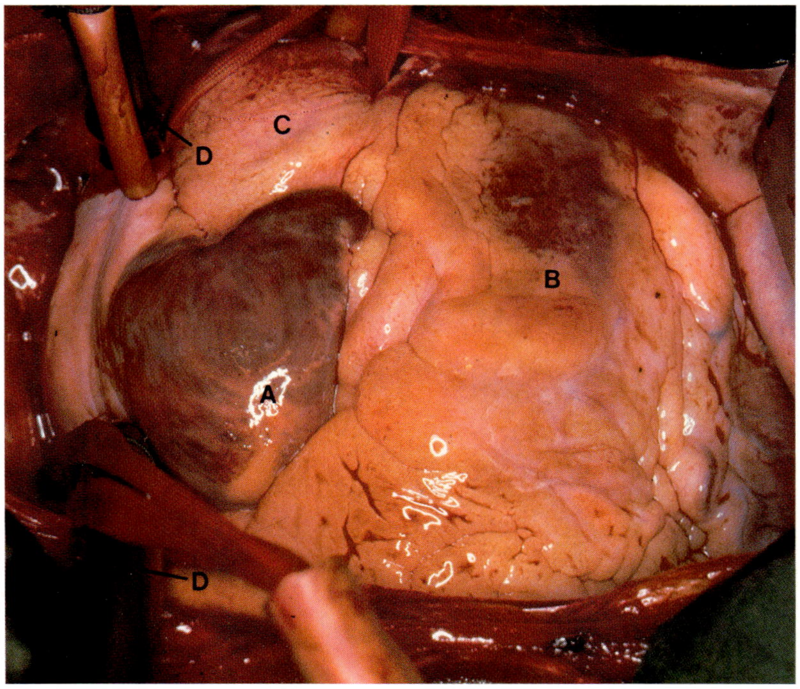

2

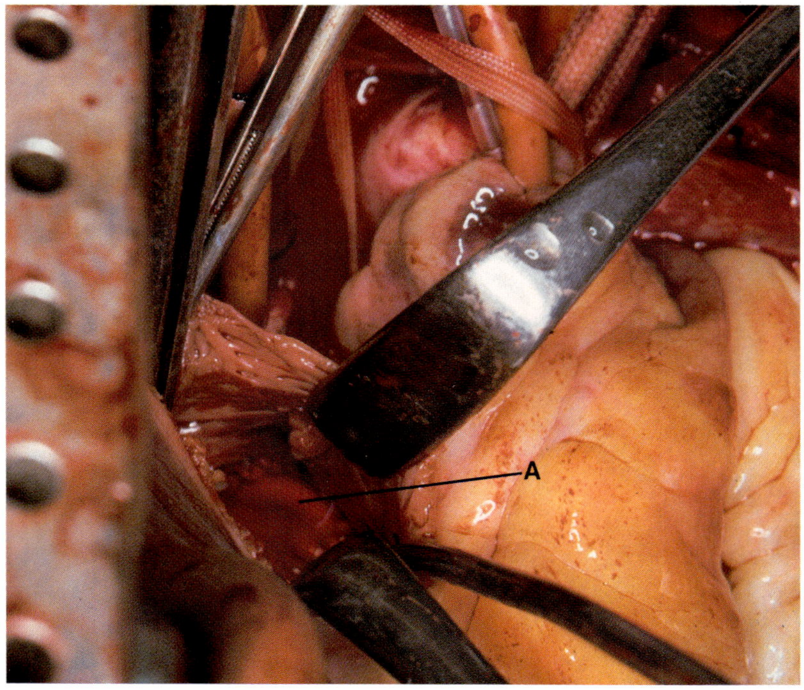

1 This view of the heart of a patient with tricuspid atresia shows the tense right atrium (**A**), outlet chamber (**B**), ascending aorta (**C**) and separate venous cannulae (**D**) in the cavae.

2 A limited incision has been made in the right atrial appendage and, with retraction, it can be seen that the atrial septal defect has been closed with a dacron patch (**A**).

3

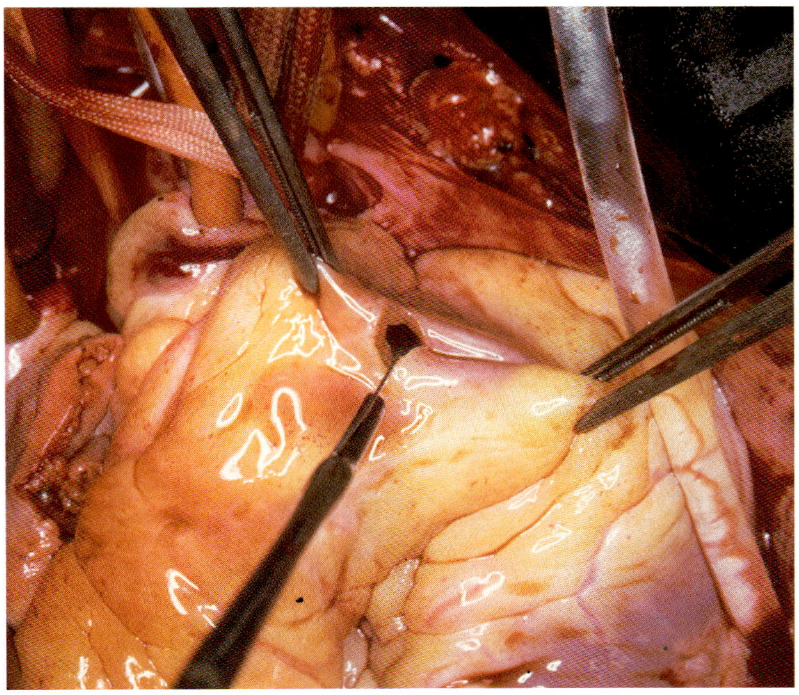

4

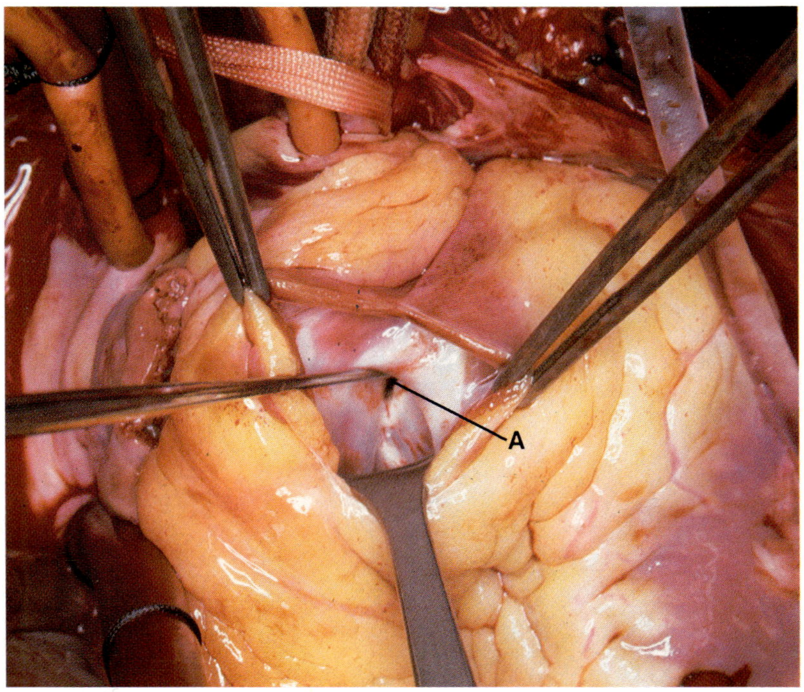

3 and 4 The outlet chamber is incised longitudinally and the incision extended to fit the distal end of the homograft conduit. In this case, a very small ventricular septal defect (**A**) is being held open with a Blalock hook.

5

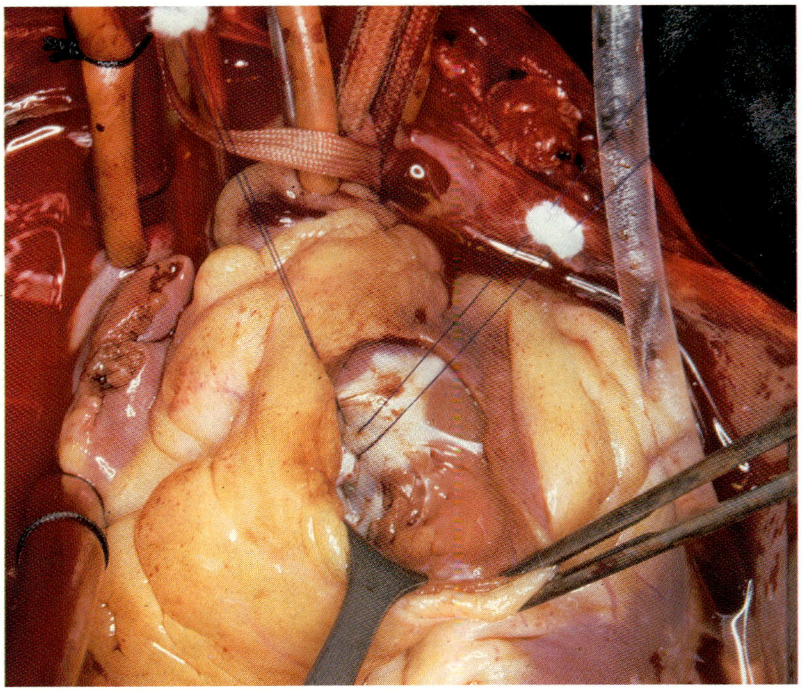

6

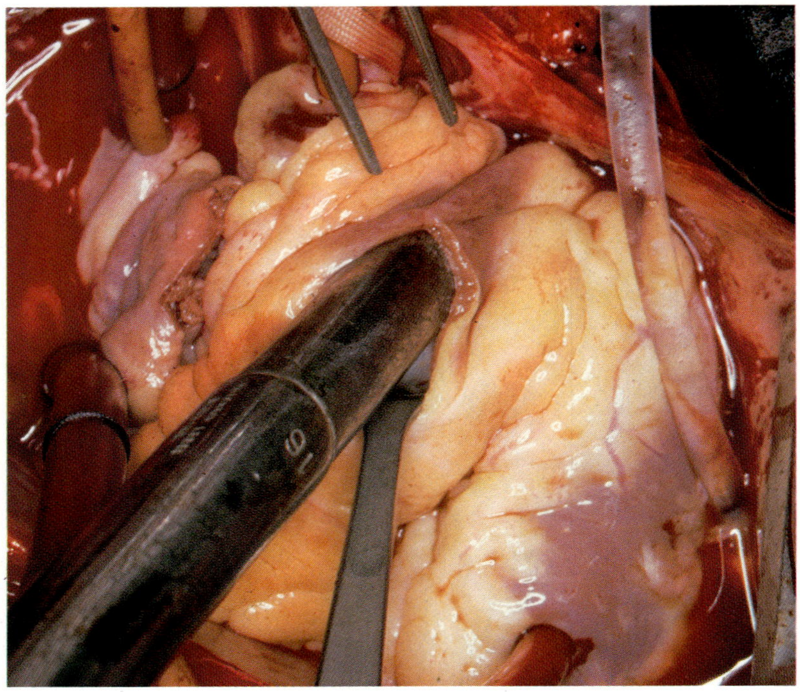

5 The ventricular septal defect is closed with two mattress sutures buttressed on pledgets of teflon felt.

6 The pulmonary valve ring is being measured and, in this case, takes a size 16 Hegar dilator.

7

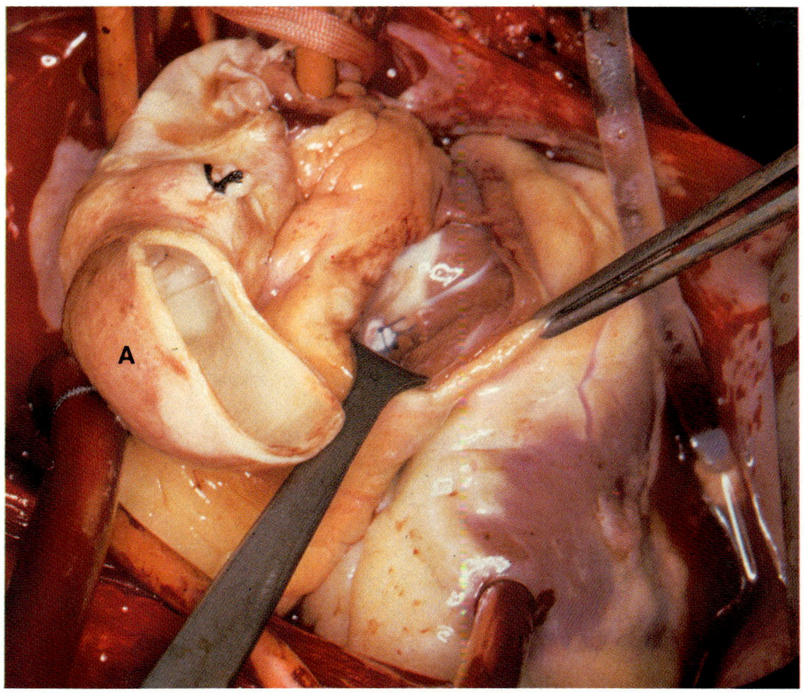

8

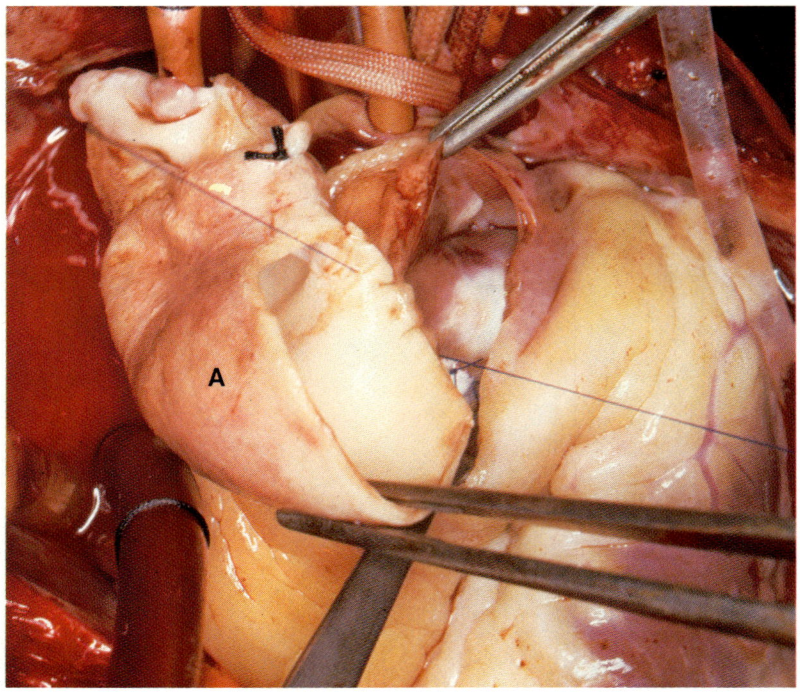

7 and 8 The distal end of the homograft (**A**) is anastomosed to the incision in the outlet chamber using continuous Prolene.

9

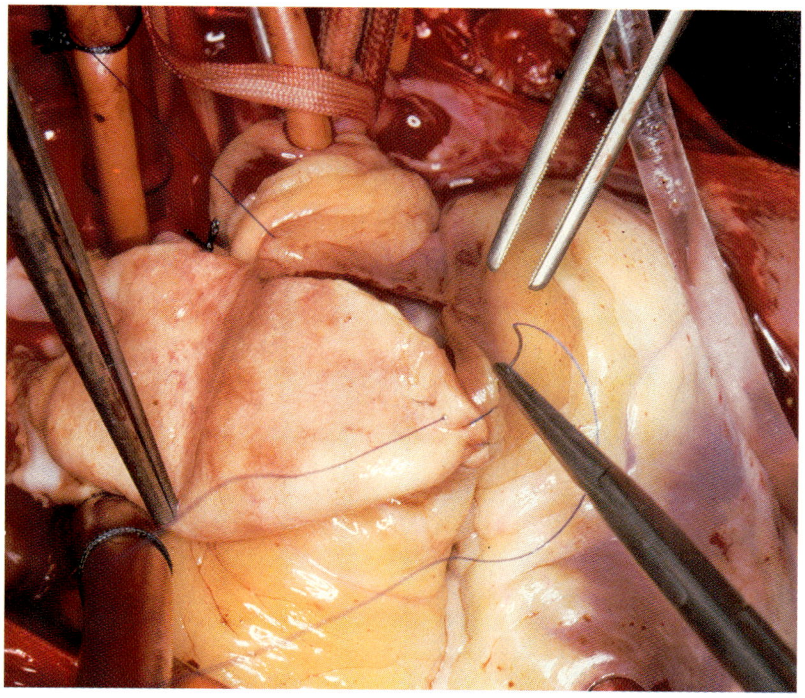

10

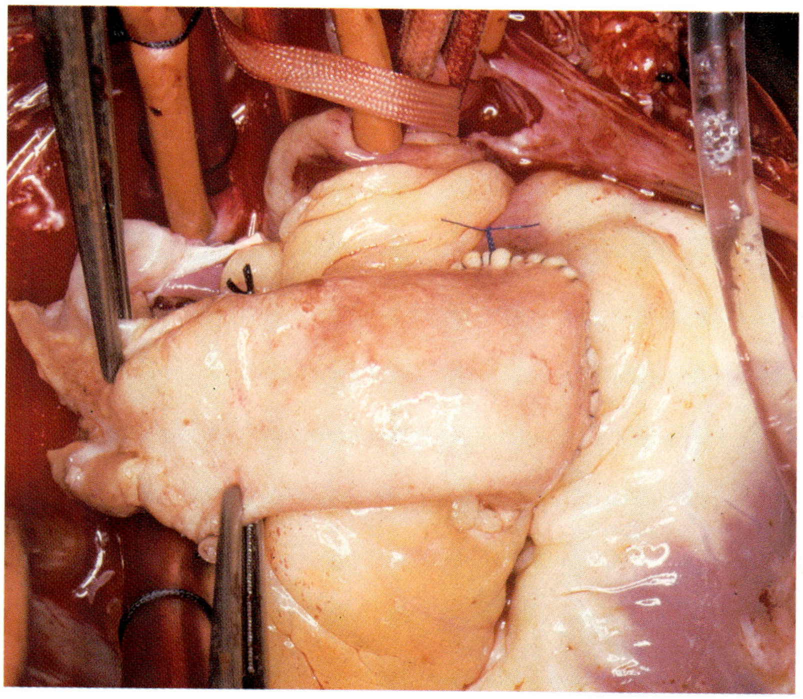

9 and 10 The distal anastamosis is completed anteriorly.

11

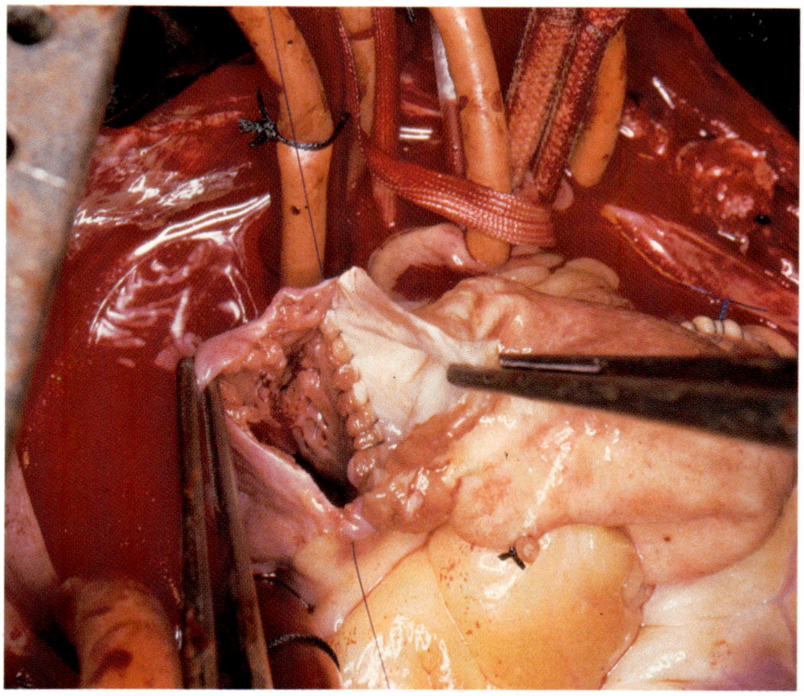

11 The proximal anastomosis is performed, again using continuous Prolene and starting posteriorly.

12

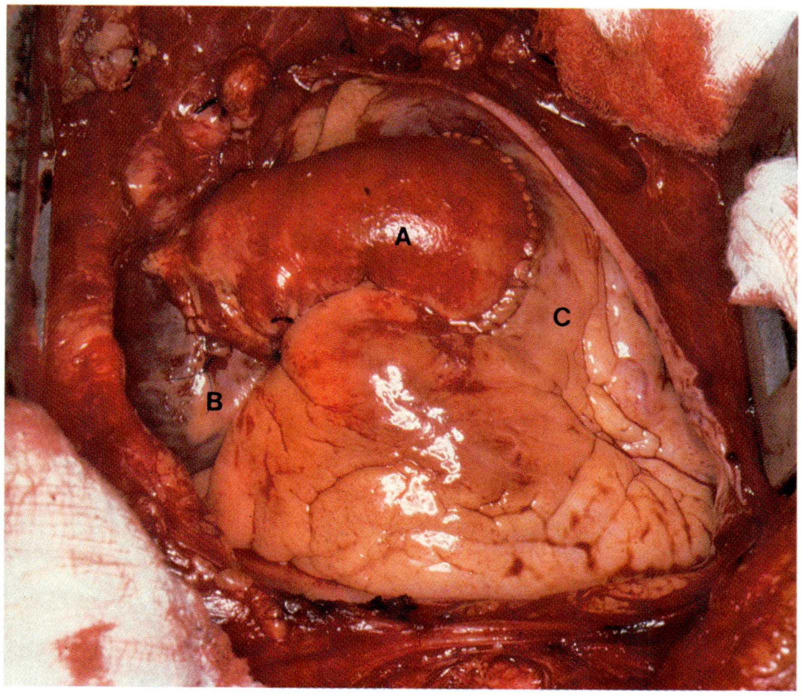

12 At the completion of the operation, the homograft conduit (**A**) can be seen linking the right atrium (**B**) to the outlet chamber (**C**).

13

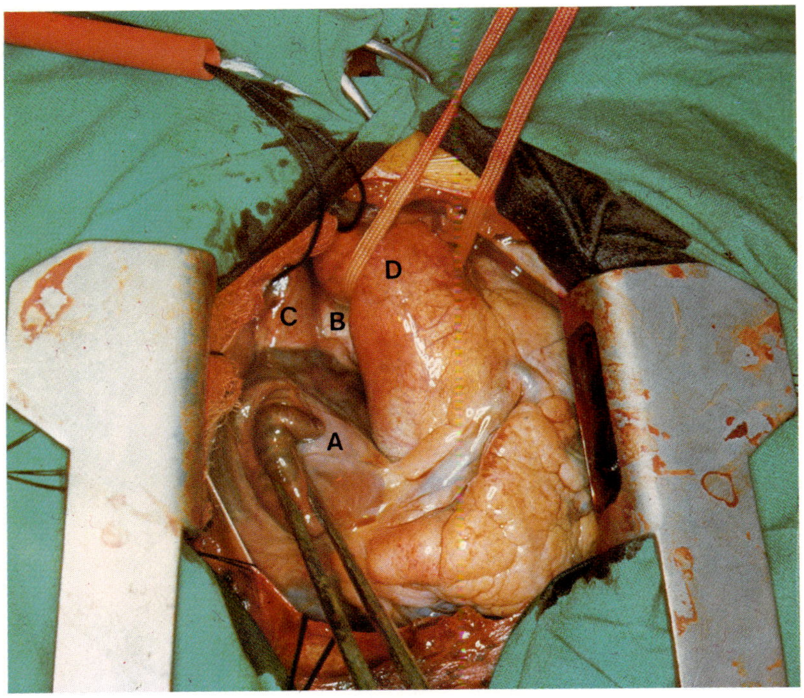

13 In a patient with no usable outlet chamber, a conduit must be placed between the right atrial appendage (**A**) (being retracted with forceps) and the right pulmonary artery (**B**). It must lie between the superior vena cava (**C**) and the ascending aorta (**D**).

14

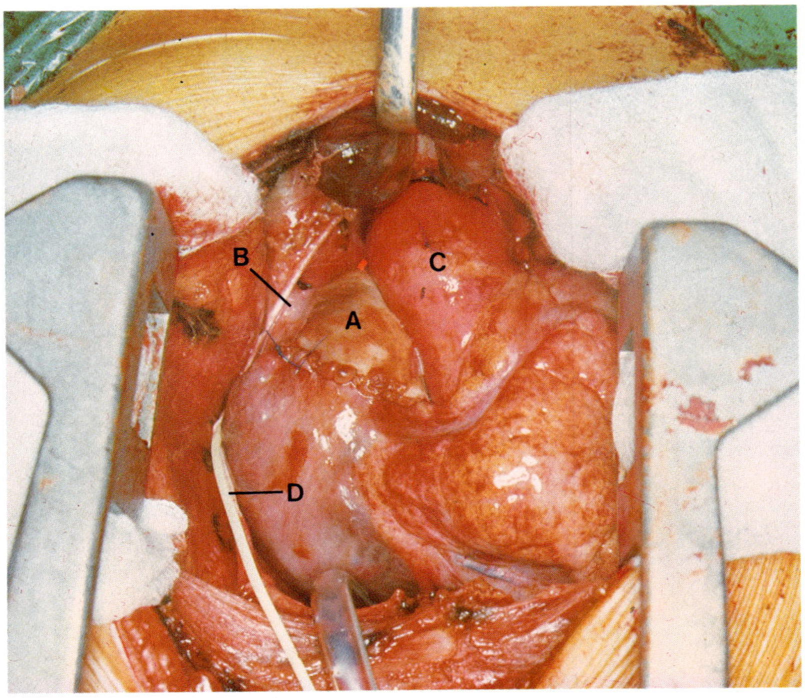

14 The final appearance is shown with the homograft (**A**) fitting between the superior vena cava (**B**) and the ascending aorta (**C**). A left atrial pressure line (**D**) has been inserted.

17: Correction of pulmonary atresia with ventricular septal defect

In this condition, there is no communication between the right ventricle and the pulmonary artery. The blue, desaturated blood returning to the heart, as illustrated in diagram **A**, passes through the right atrium (**A**), to the right ventricle (**B**) but the only exit is through the large ventricular septal defect (**C**) where it mixes with the red, saturated blood leaving the left ventricle (**D**), to pass into the ascending aorta (**E**). The only way into the pulmonary artery (**F**) is through the persistent ductus arteriosus (**G**).

As the amount of blood reaching the lungs is usually less than adequate, patients with this condition usually present early in infancy. Although it is possible to correct this condition in infancy, it is usual to perform initial palliation at this stage using either a Blalock-Taussig shunt (see Chapter 6) or a Waterston shunt (see Chapter 7). Correction can then be performed later at about five years of age.

Unfortunately the pulmonary arteries in this condition are often of inadequate size and indeed may not even connect. In an attempt to achieve a better blood supply, collateral vessels frequently develop, usually from the descending aorta, and supply segments of the lungs, connecting with the true pulmonary arteries in the hila of the lungs. These collateral vessels are frequently severely stenosed. The collateral vessels may cause pulmonary oedema if not tied off at the same time as operation.

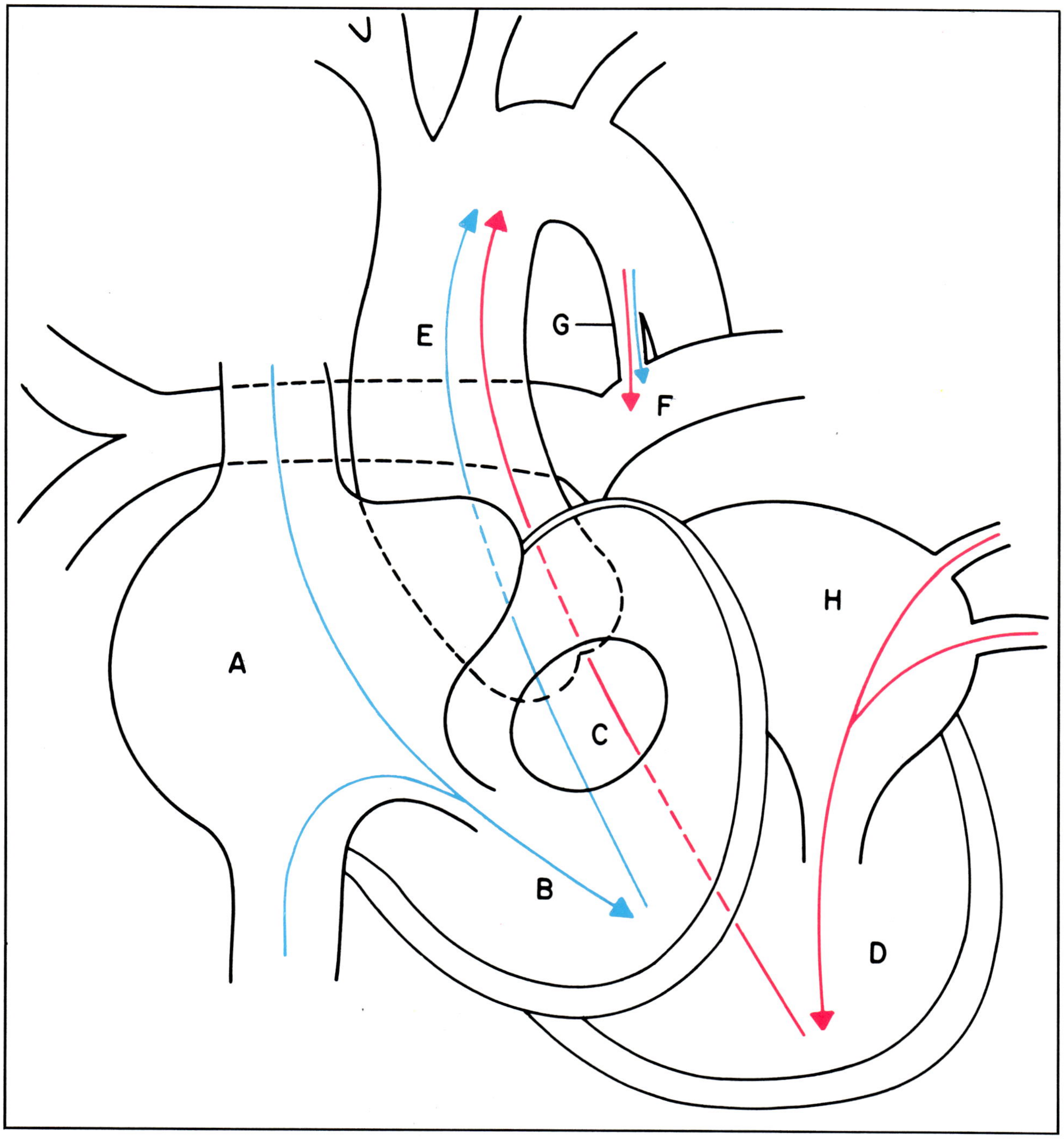

Diagram A

A – Right atrium

B – Right ventricle

C – Ventricular septal defect

D – Left ventricle

E – Ascending aorta

F – Pulmonary artery

G – Persistent ductus arteriosus

H – Left atrium

In this chapter, total correction is described, and this would only be suitable if the pulmonary arteries were of an adequate size to take the cardiac output. Cardiopulmonary bypass is used with two venous cannulae. If, as is usually the case, a previous shunt has been performed, this must be closed as a first step once cardiopulmonary bypass has been commenced. After cross-clamping the aorta and giving cardioplegic solution to protect the myocardium (see Chapter 1), a high right ventriculotomy is performed. Through this, the ventricular septal defect is closed with a dacron cloth patch. The pulmonary artery is opened and the distal end of the conduit sutured to it. The proximal end of the conduit is then sutured to the right ventriculotomy and, as can be seen in diagram **B**, blue desaturated blood then flows to the lungs and red, saturated blood around the body.

In this chapter, the conduit used is an antibiotic sterilised aortic homograft and this is extremely satisfactory. The first time this condition was successfully repaired using a homograft was by Ross in 1967[1]

Diagram B

A – Right atrium

B – Right ventricle

C – Ventricular septal defect—closed with dacron patch

D – Left ventricle

E – Ascending aorta

F – Pulmonary artery

G – Ligated ductus arteriosus

H – Left atrium

J – Homograft conduit

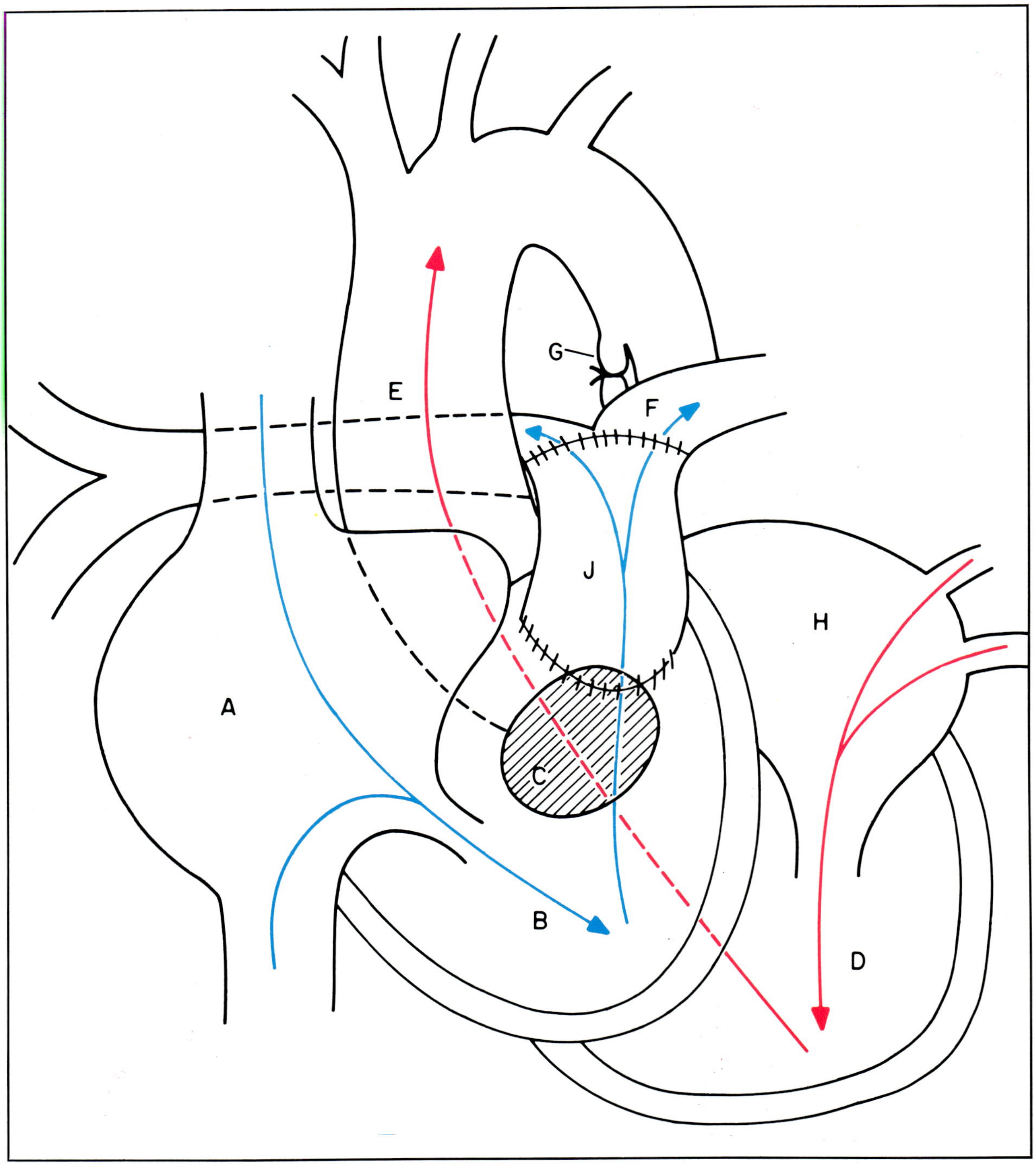

1

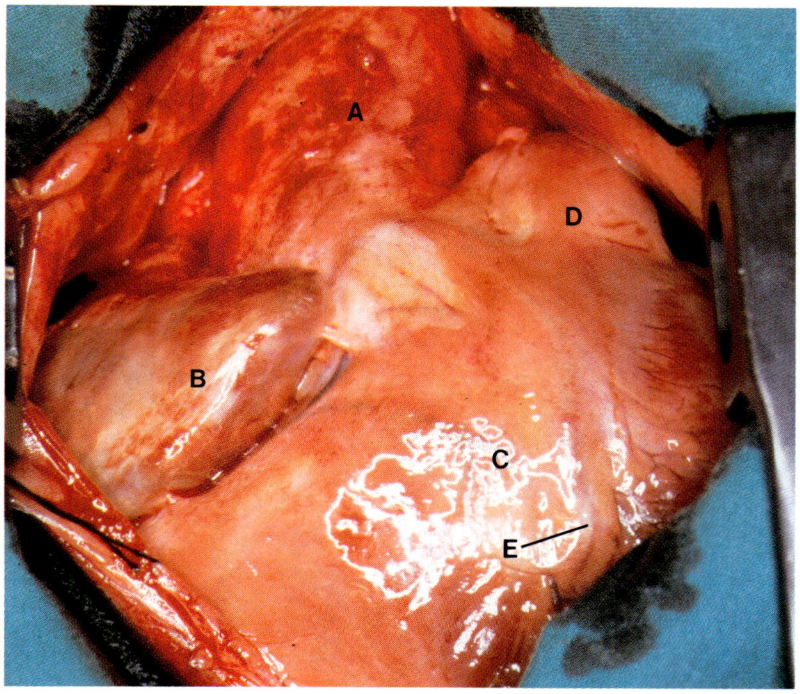

2

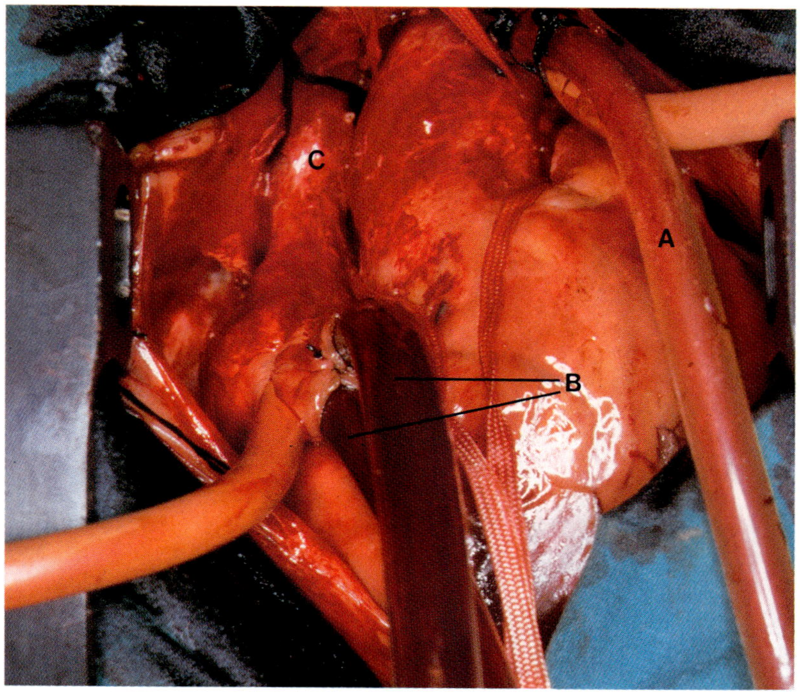

1 The large ascending aorta (**A**), right atrial appendage (**B**) and right ventricle (**C**) are shown. The main pulmonary artery (**D**) is small and does not communicate with the right ventricle. A fairly large right ventricular branch of the right coronary is seen (**E**) and must be guarded.

2 A cannula (**A**) has been inserted in the ascending aorta and two venous cannulae (**B**) have been inserted through the right atrial appendage into the superior vena cava (**C**) and inferior vena cava.

3

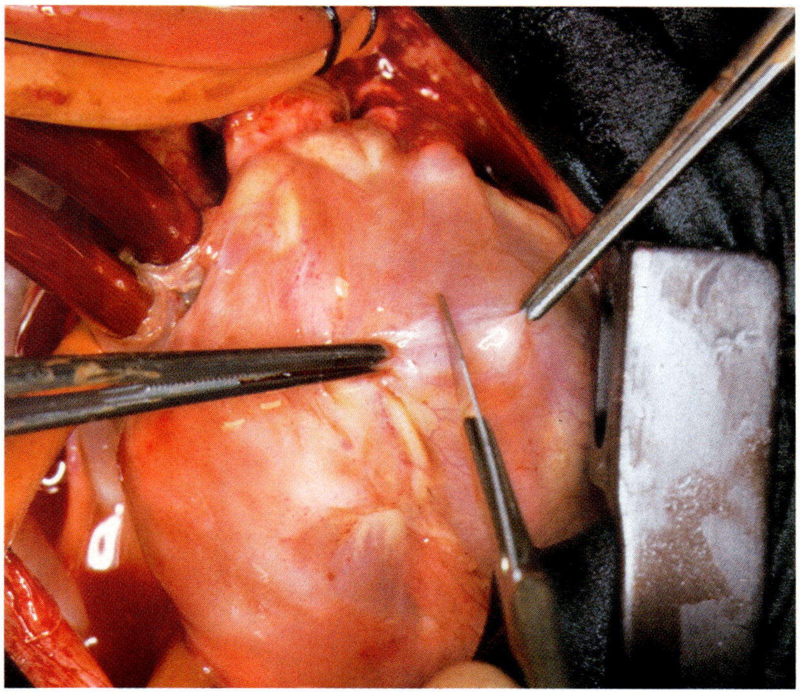

4

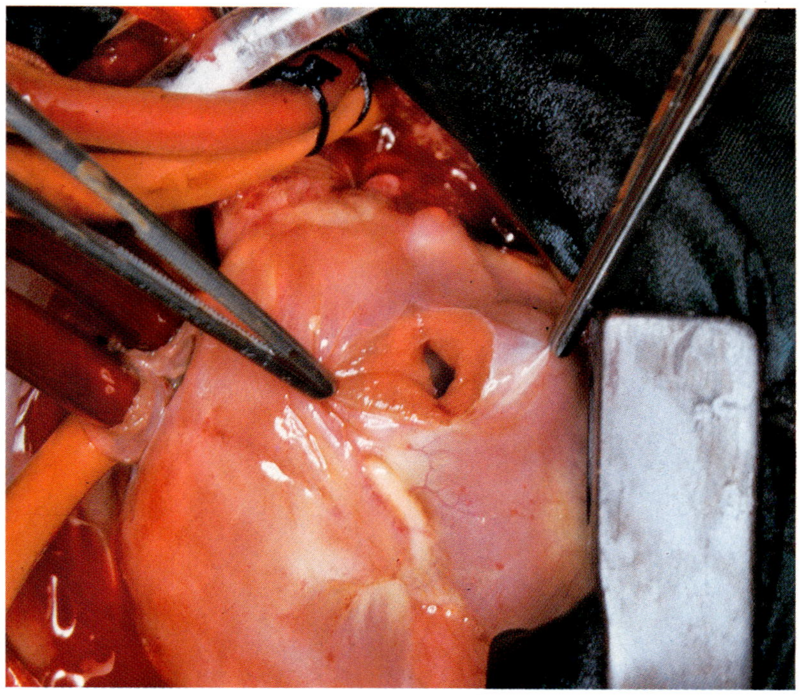

3 and 4 Cardiopulmonary bypass has been commenced, the aorta cross-clamped and the myocardium protected by infusing cardioplegic solution into the ascending aorta. A vertical incision is made in the right ventricle avoiding coronary arteries.

5

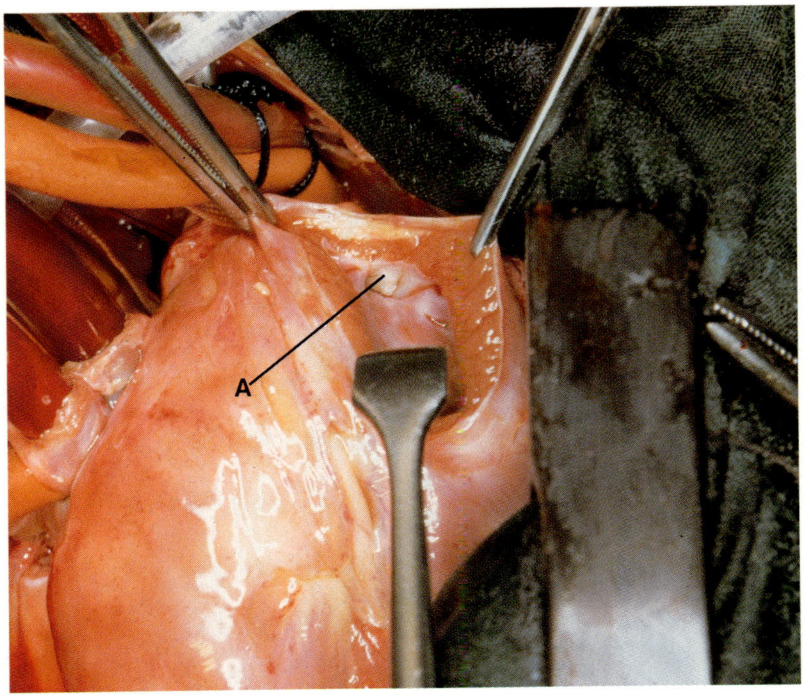

5 Retraction demonstrates atresia of the pulmonary valve (**A**) which is, however, in this patient still seen as a thin, fibrous remnant.

6

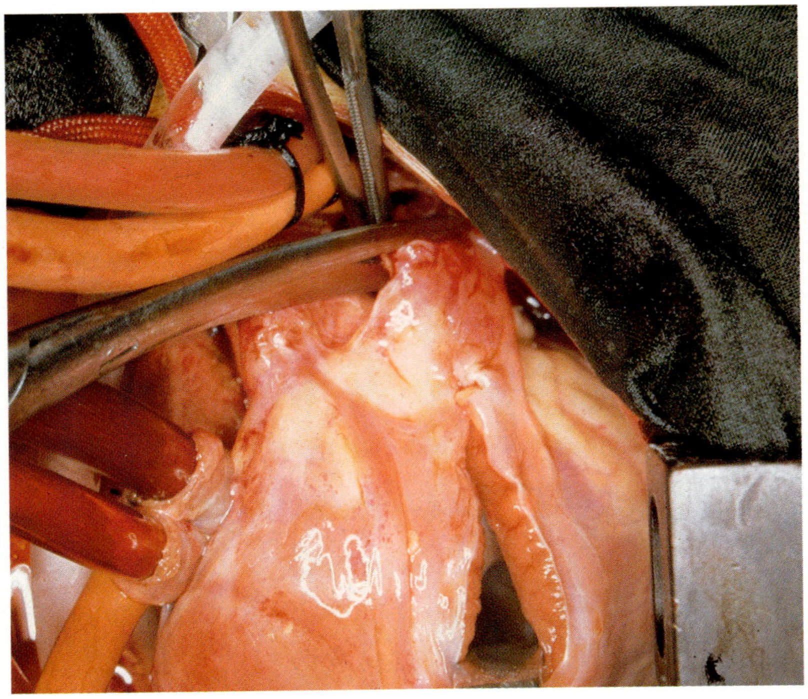

6 The main pulmonary artery is transected.

7

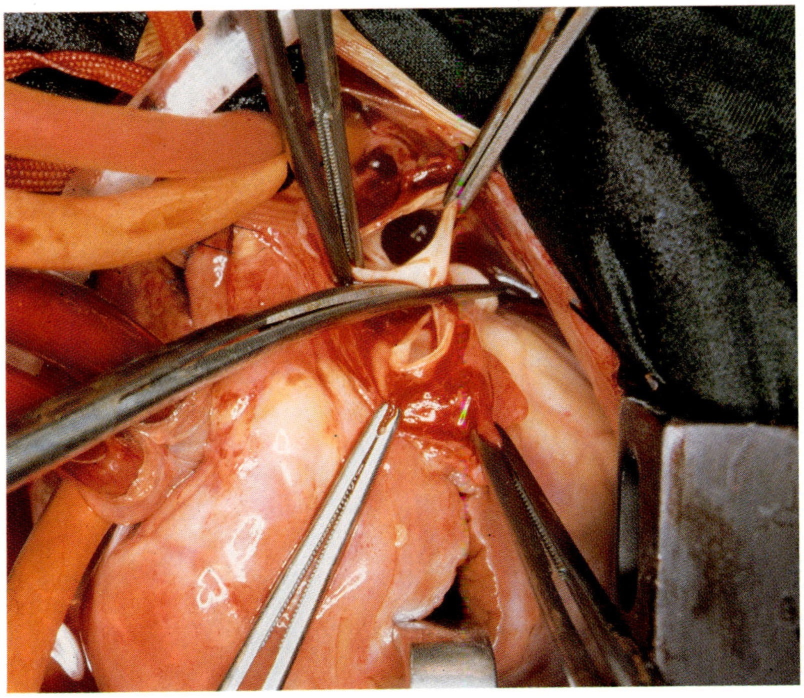

7 Transection of the main pulmonary artery reveals a reasonable size vessel, although it will be necessary to enlarge it by incising laterally to fit the homograft.

8

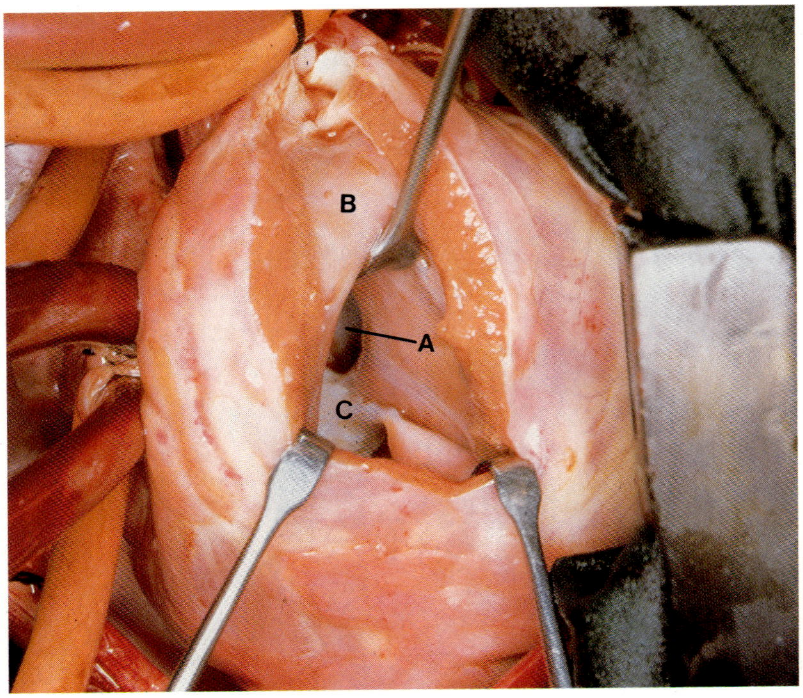

8 Attention is now turned to the ventricular septal defect (**A**) which is seen by gently retracting up on the conus septum (**B**). Part of the tricuspid valve is seen inferiorly (**C**).

9

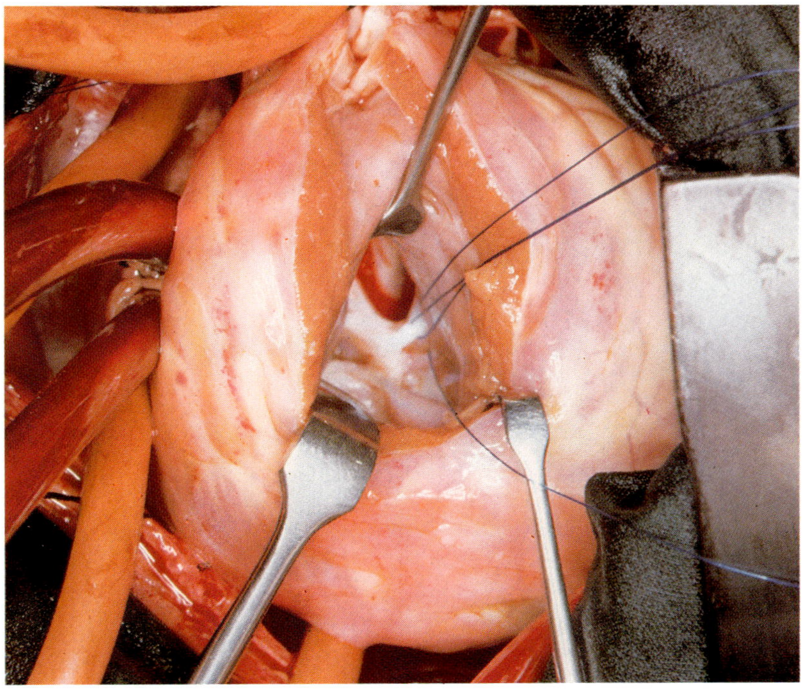

10

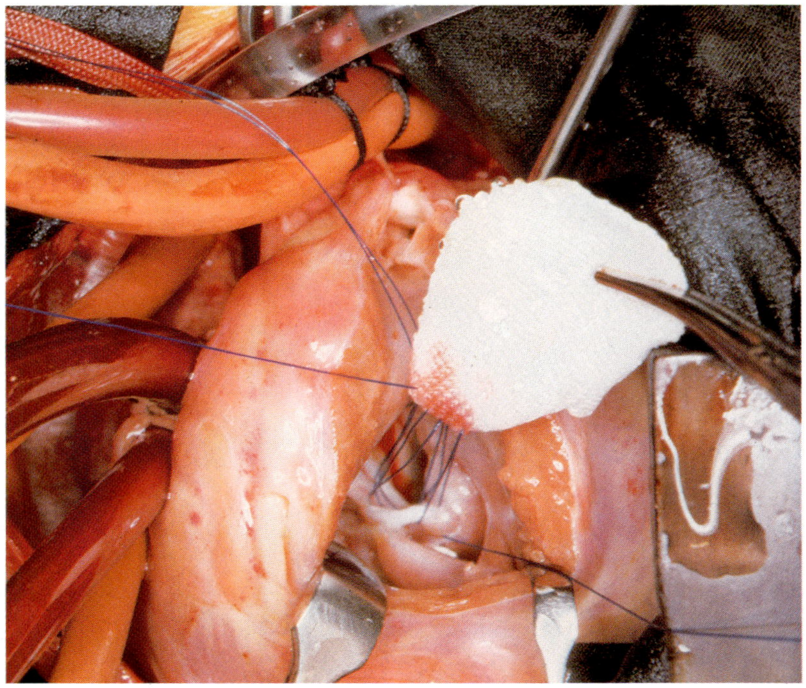

9 and 10 The ventricular septal defect is now closed with a dacron cloth patch using a continuous Prolene suture. It is helpful to place several sutures near the inferior margin of the defect before sliding the patch down. The sutures are placed on the right side of the septum and then into the septal leaflet of the tricuspid valve.

11

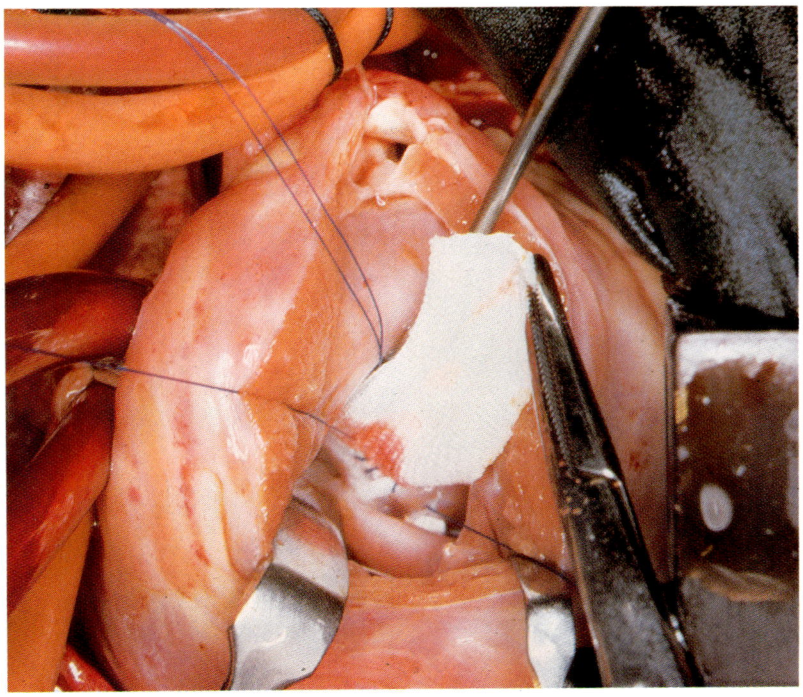

12

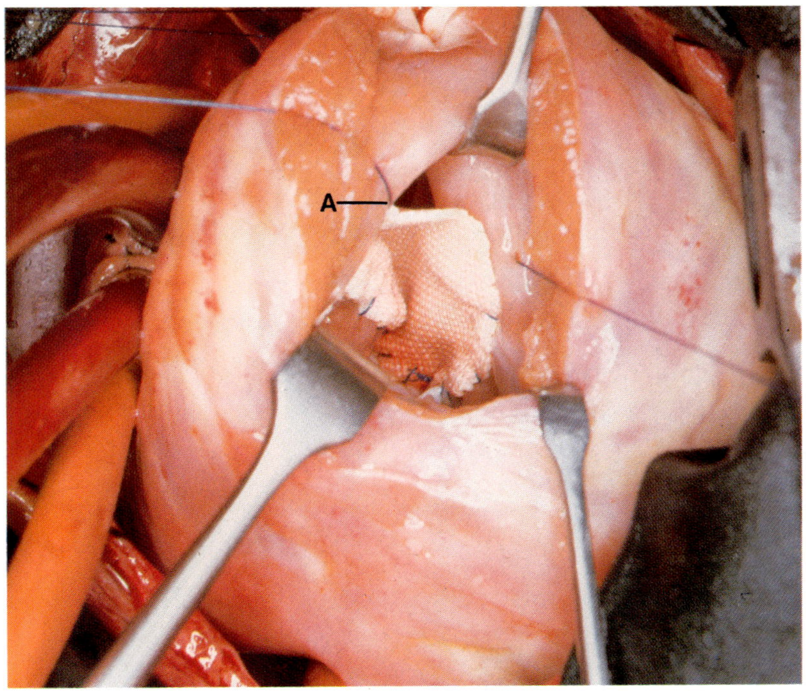

11 and 12 The patch has been slid down into position and the suture continued in a clockwise direction to point **A.** The other end of the suture is then continued in an anticlockwise direction.

13

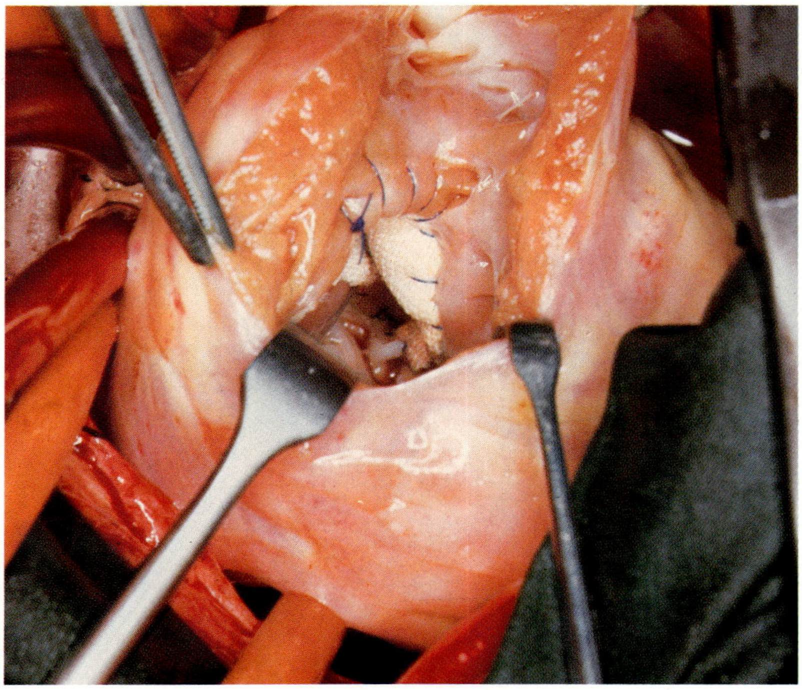

13 The patch suture is completed and the ventricular septal defect is closed completely.

14

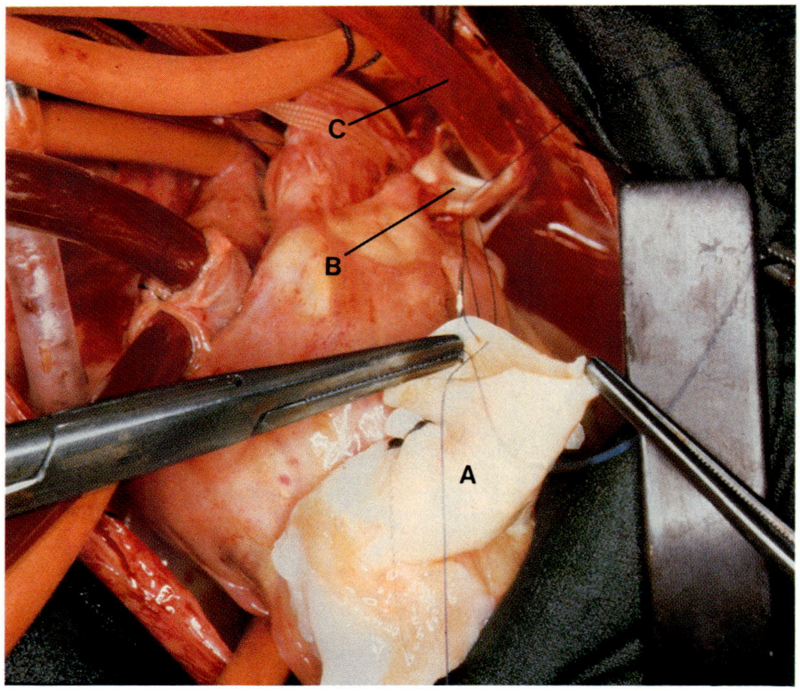

14 The distal anastomosis of the homograft (**A**) to the pulmonary artery (**B**) is now started at the centre of the posterior rim of the pulmonary artery. It is helpful to place several sutures before sliding the homograft into position. A sucker (**C**) placed in the left pulmonary artery sucks away collateral flow returning from the lungs.

15

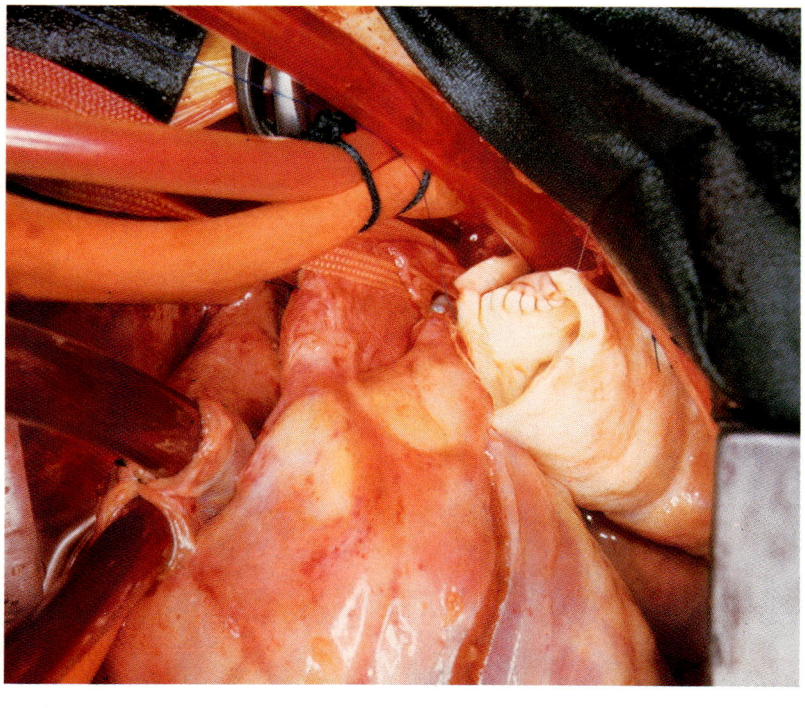

16

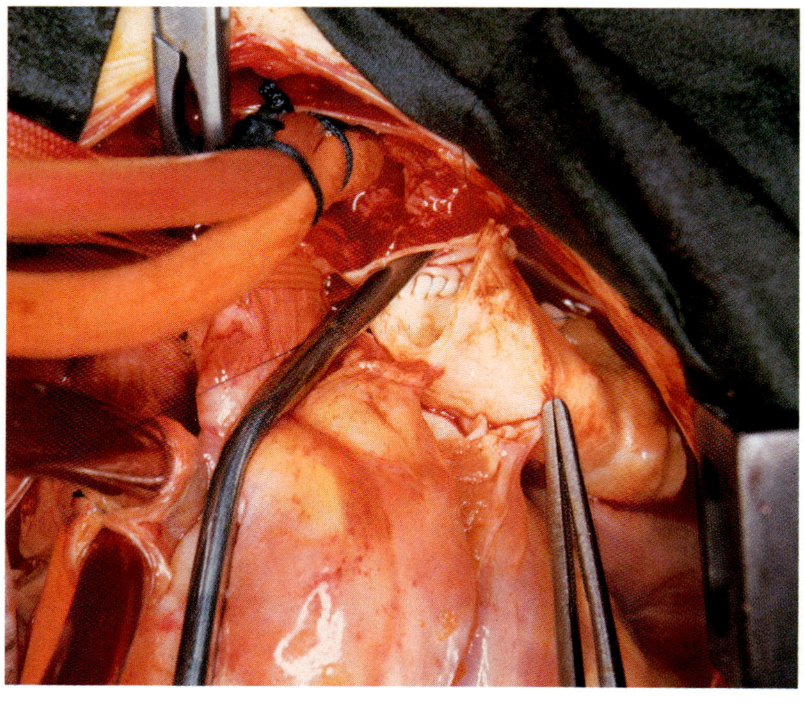

15 and 16 The posterior suture line is completed and the suture line continued around anteriorly.

17

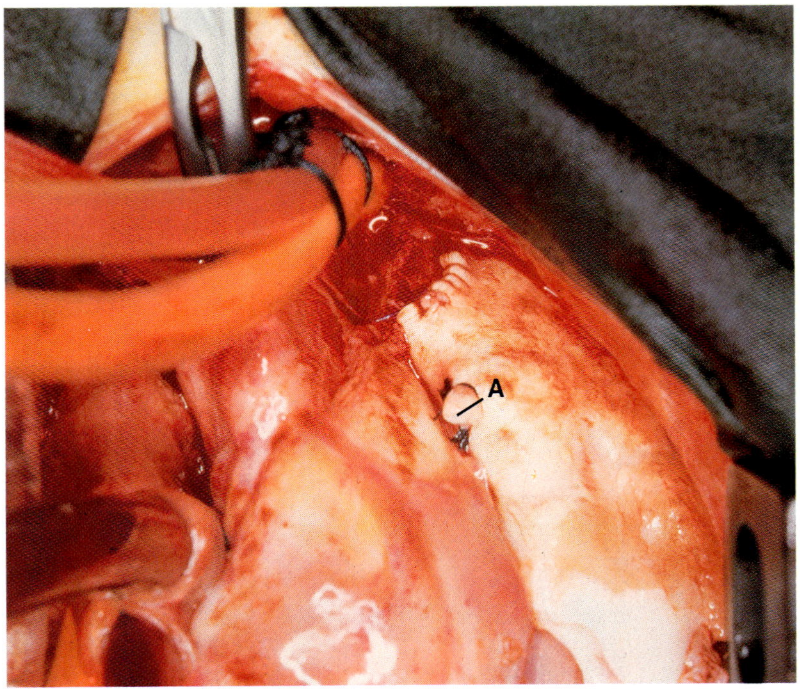

17 The upper anastomosis is now complete. It is obviously important to tie off the coronary arteries on the homograft and one can be seen here (**A**).

18

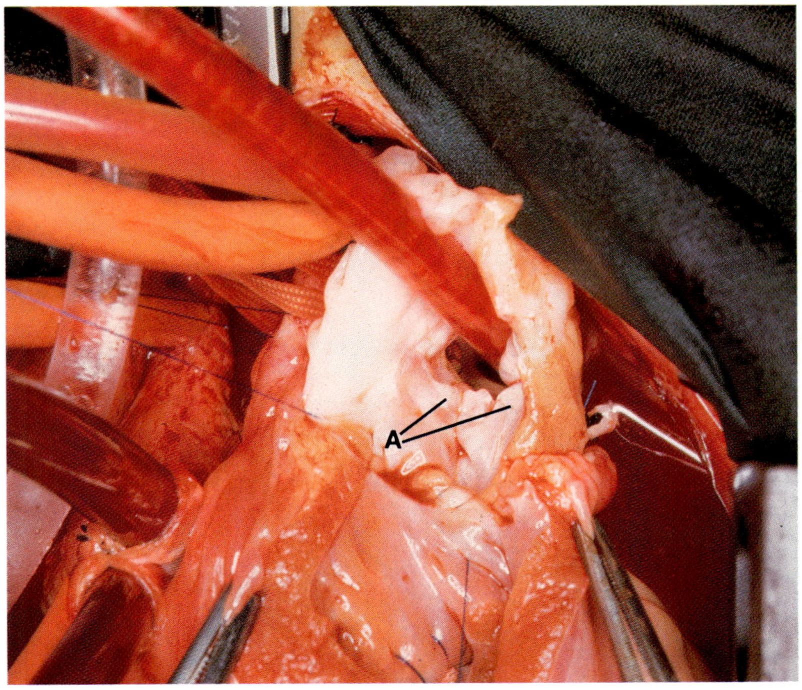

18 The posterior part of the proximal anastomosis of the homograft to the right ventriculotomy has been completed. The valve cusps of the homograft can be seen (**A**).

19

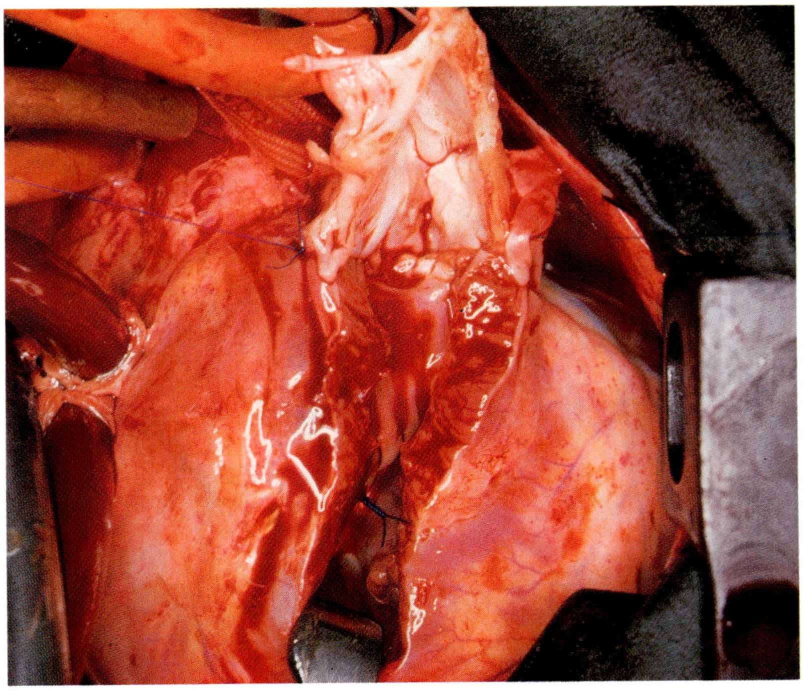

19 The aortic clamp has been released so that the remainder of the anastomosis can be completed with the myocardium perfused.

20

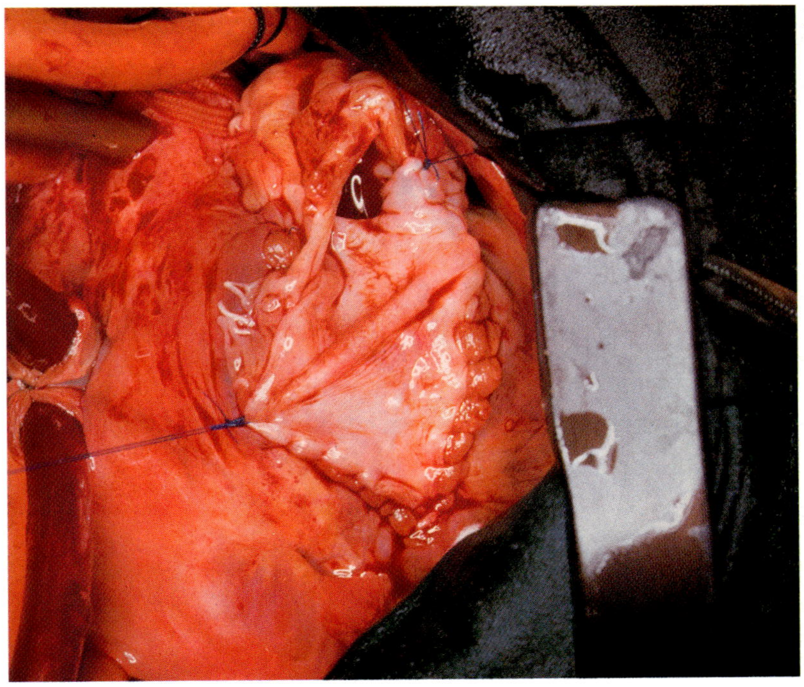

20 In this particular patient a longitudinal ventriculotomy had to be made to avoid damaging the coronary arteries. The homograft will not stretch to the lower end of the ventriculotomy and therefore a patch is necessary to close the lower part of the ventriculotomy. In this case, pericardium has been used.

21

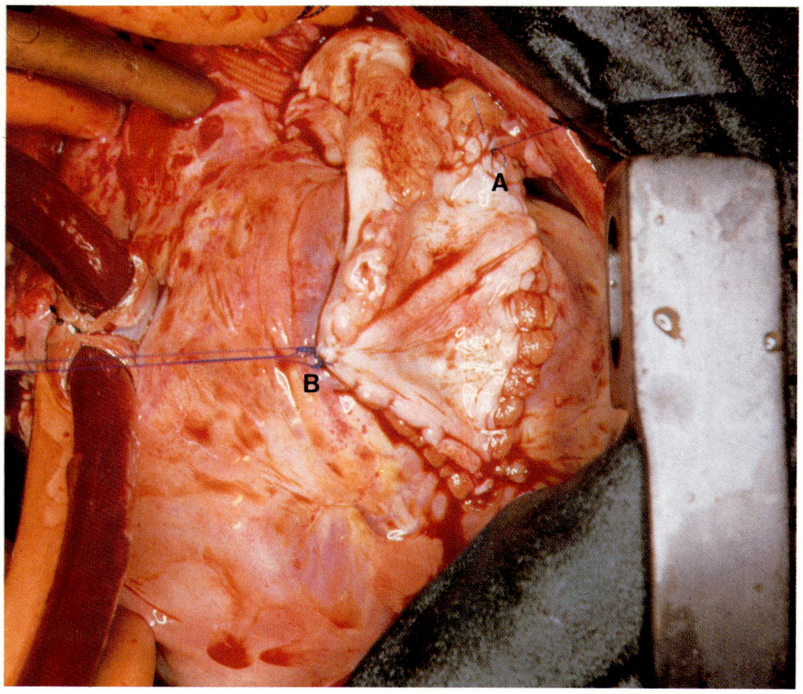

21 The pericardial patch has been sutured to the ventriculotomy and all that remains to be done is completion of the suture line between **A** and **B**.

22

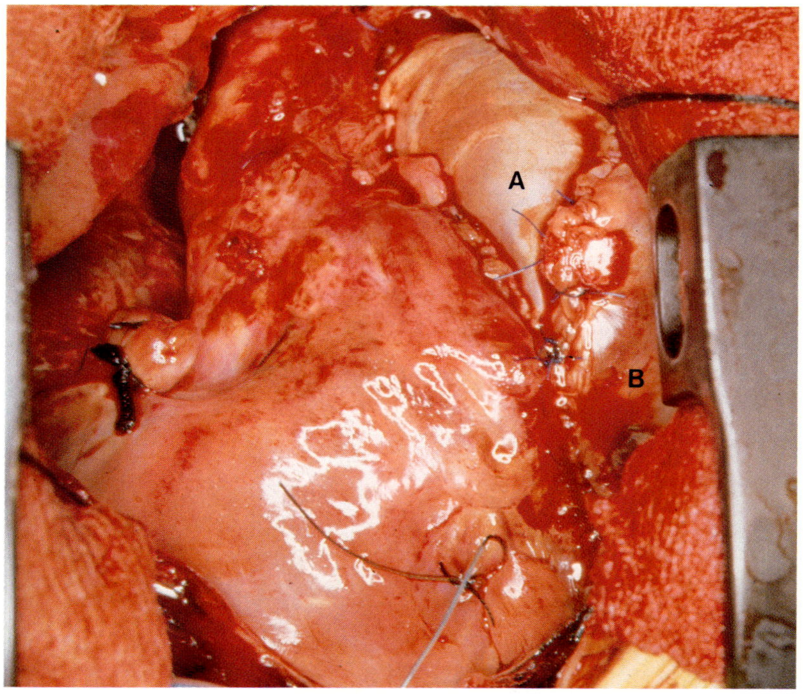

22 At the end of the operation, the homograft (**A**) and pericardial patch (**B**) can be seen to have formed a new main pulmonary artery and outflow tract very much of normal size and shape.

18: Pulmonary valvotomy

Stenosis of the pulmonary valve may be an isolated lesion or it may occur with other conditions. Frequently the valve may be bicuspid and it is often thickened and considerably distorted with fusion of the cusps. If the valve ring itself is narrowed, it may be necessary to widen the valve ring with a patch of, for instance, pericardium. If the valve cusps are very dysplastic, it may be better to excise them.

It is advisable to inspect the atrial septum and close any patent foramen ovale as otherwise this could be a source of air embolus during the procedure. Obviously, other conditions such as Fallot's tetralogy, of which the pulmonary stenosis is a part, will be corrected at the same time. Cardiopulmonary bypass is used for open pulmonary valvotomy with the use of two caval cannulae. It is usual to make an anterior longitudinal pulmonary arteriotomy and approach the valve from above. The fused cusps can then be separated carefully with a knife. When the right ventricle is being opened, for instance with correction of Fallot's tetralogy, it is possible to perform the valvotomy from below and save a pulmonary arteriotomy.

It is possible to perform a quick pulmonary valvotomy with the use of caval in-flow occlusion, but this does not allow the same precision. Also closed pulmonary valvotomy can be performed; again this does not allow precise valvotomy or patching of the valve if necessary.

1

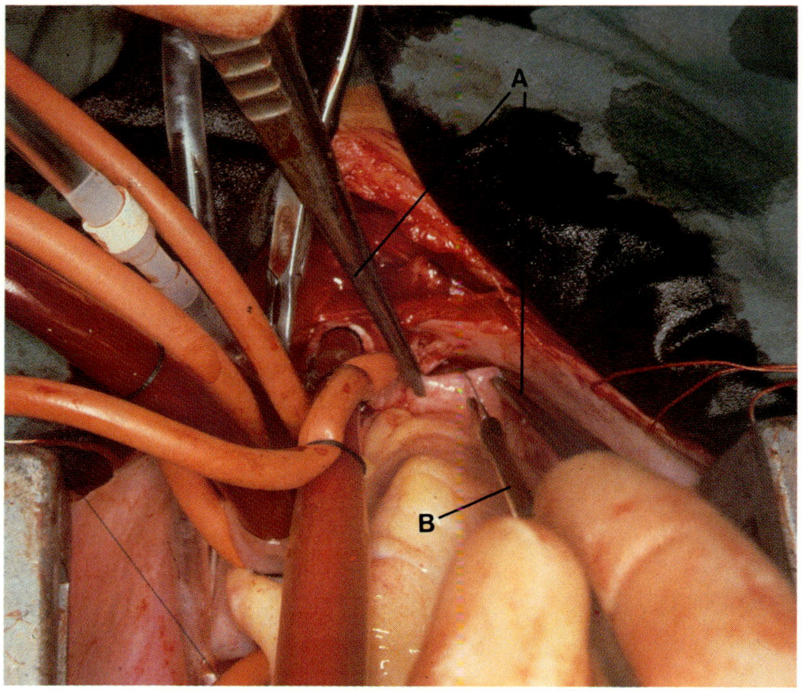

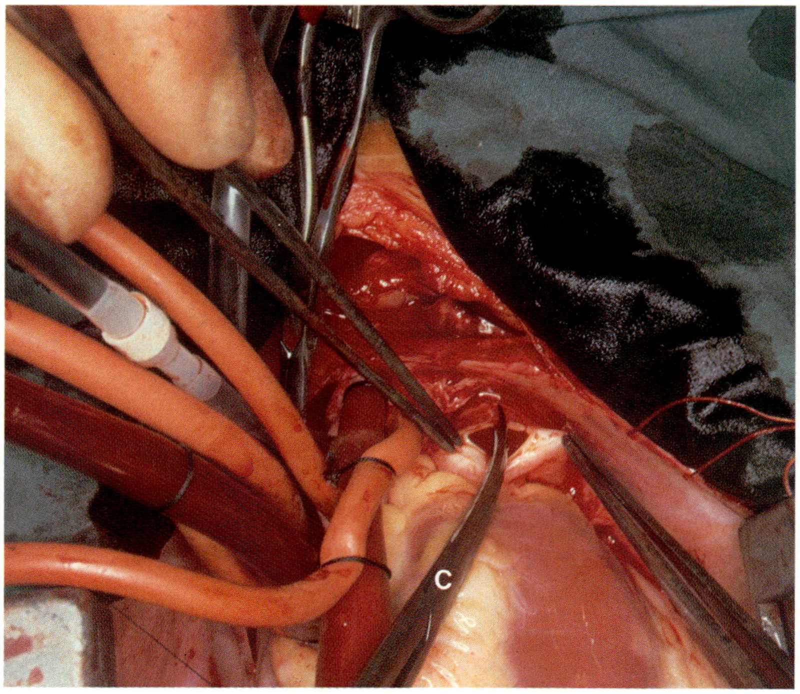

2

1 and 2 Cardiopulmonary bypass has been commenced and the pulmonary artery has been picked up between forceps (**A**). The pulmonary artery is incised with a knife (**B**) and the incision extended with scissors (**C**).

3

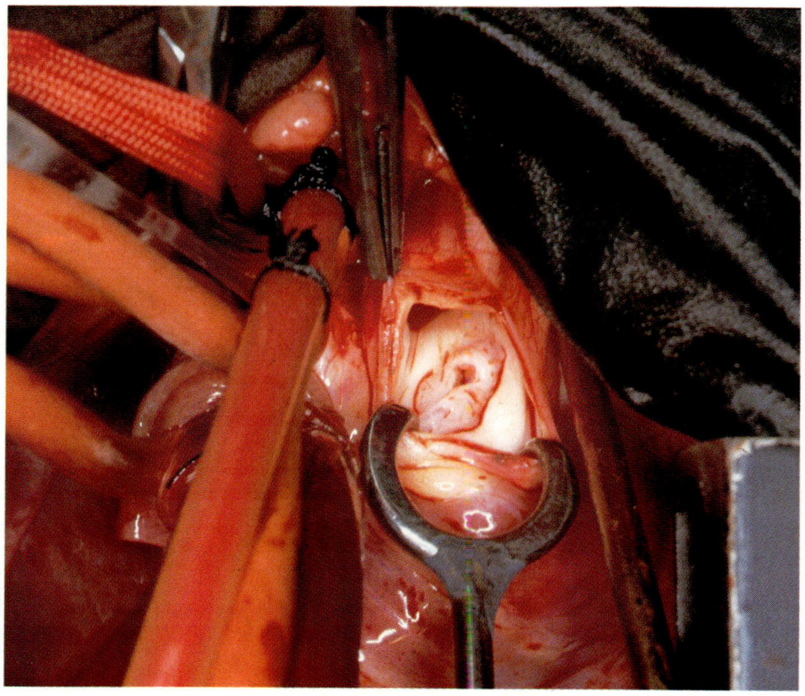

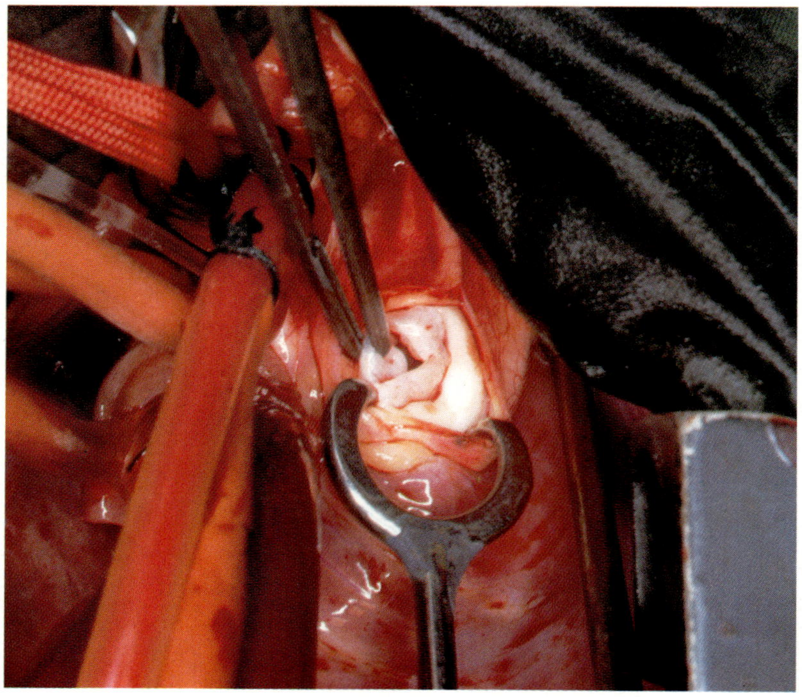

4

3 and 4 The pulmonary artery is held open with a retractor and a good view obtained of the thickened and fused valve cusps.

5

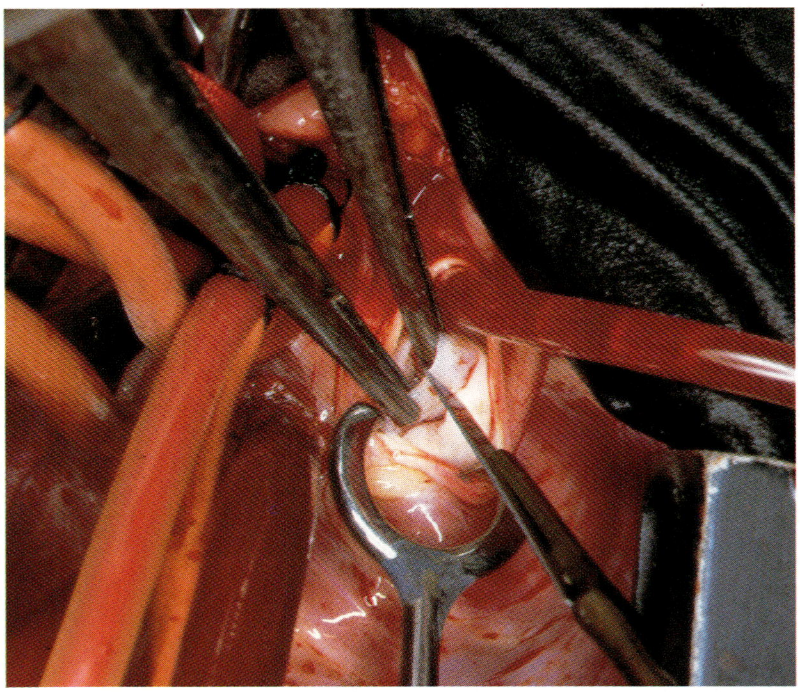

6

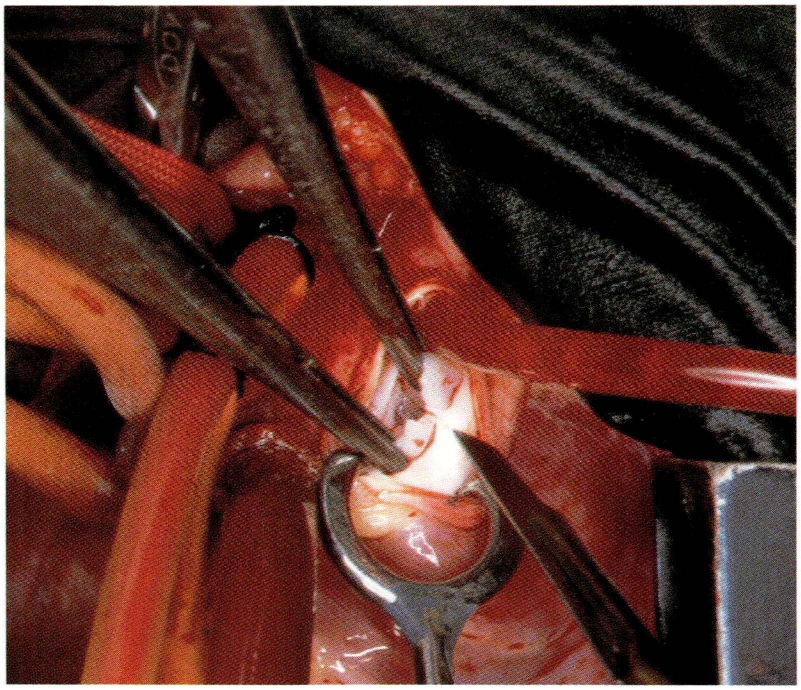

5 and 6 The commissure between the left anterior and posterior cusps is divided with a knife.

7

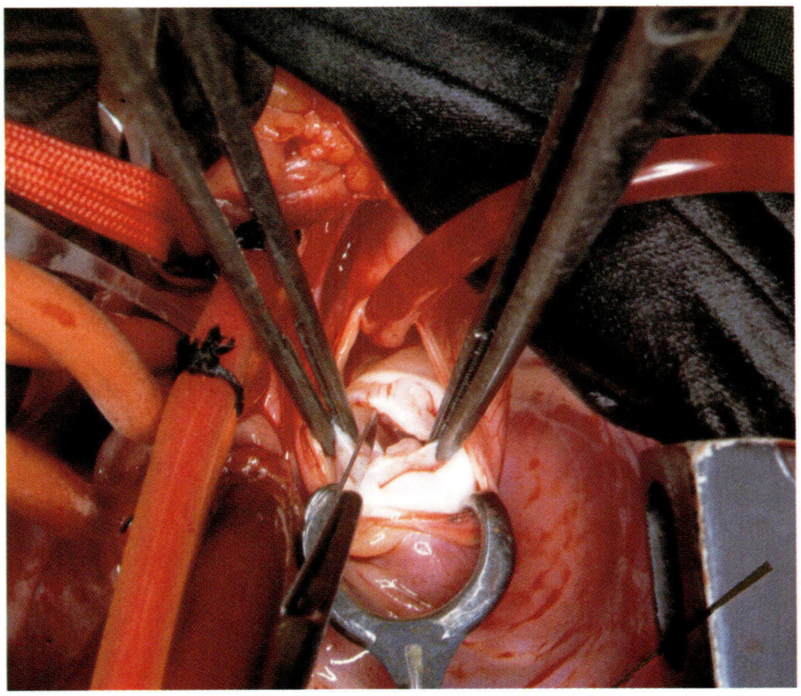

8

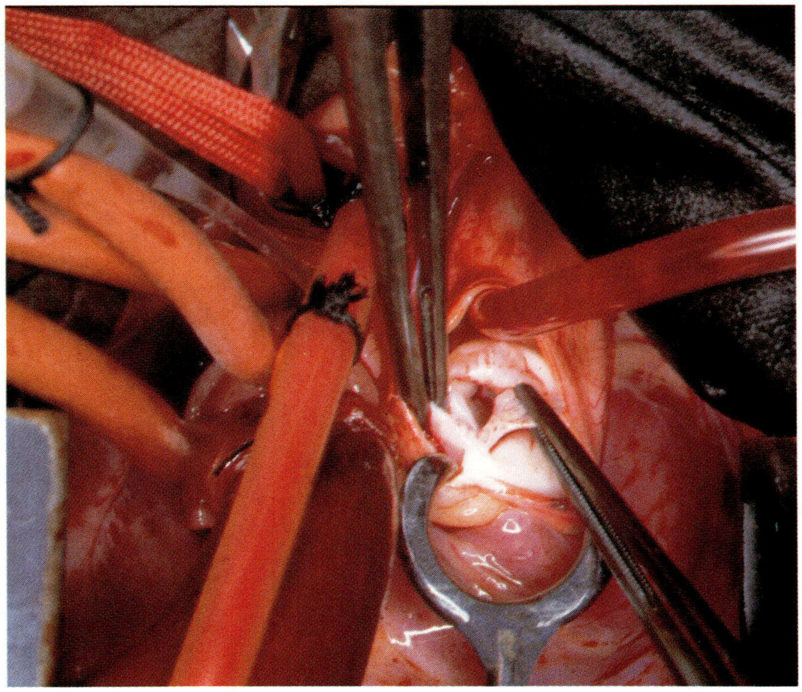

7 and 8 The commissure between the two anterior cusps is divided.

9

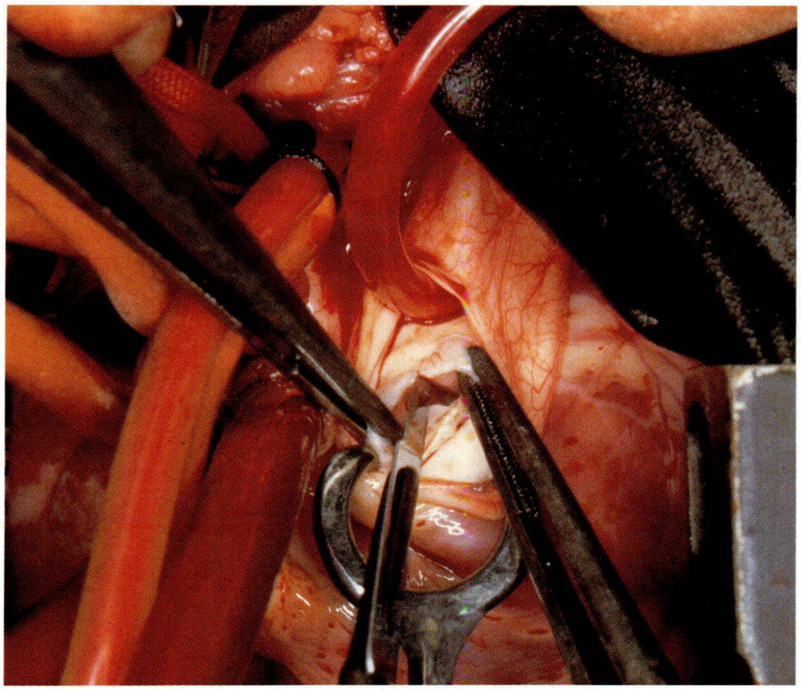

10

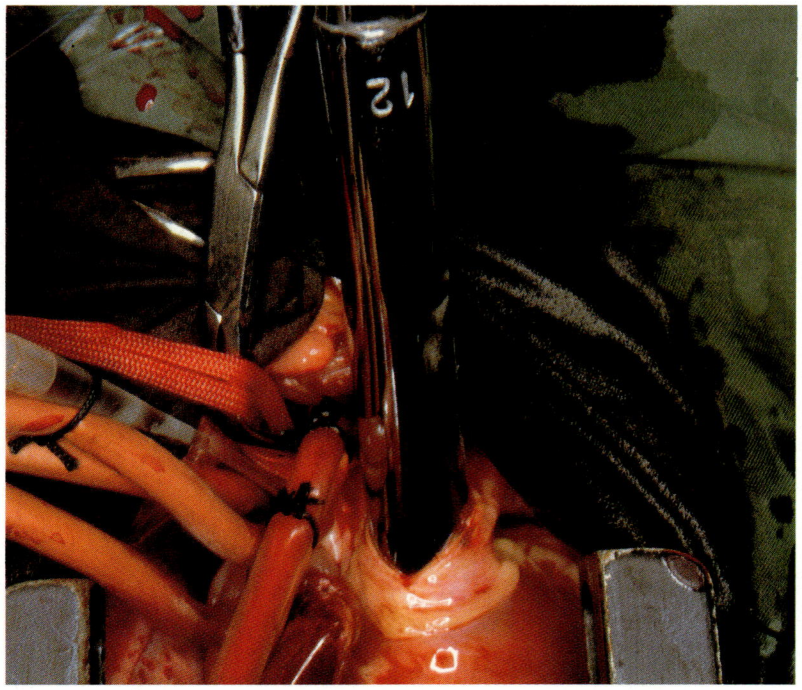

9 The commissure between the right anterior and posterior cusps is divided.

10 The size of the valve following valvotomy is measured and this helps to assess whether the pulmonary valve ring is of adequate size.

11

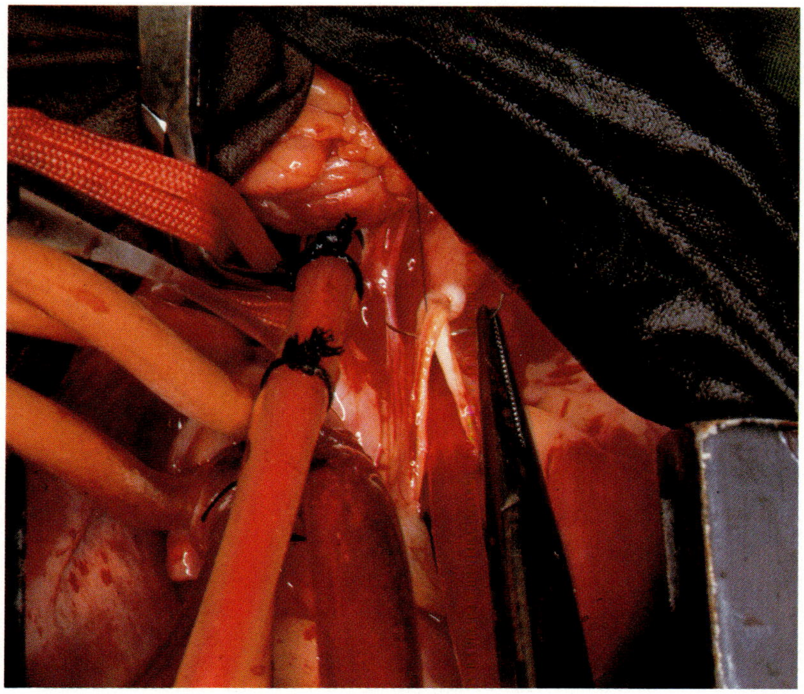

12

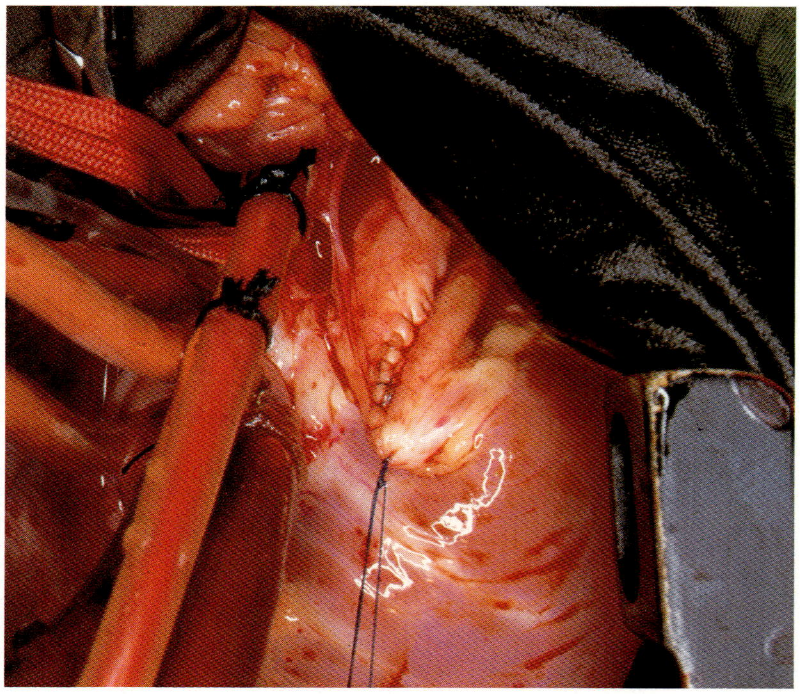

11 and 12 The pulmonary arteriotomy is closed with a continuous Prolene suture.

13

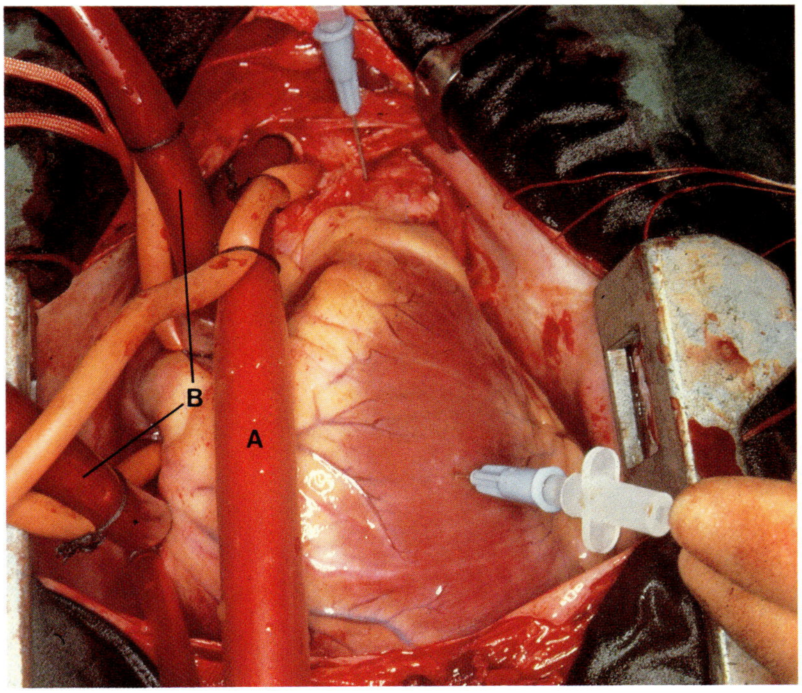

14

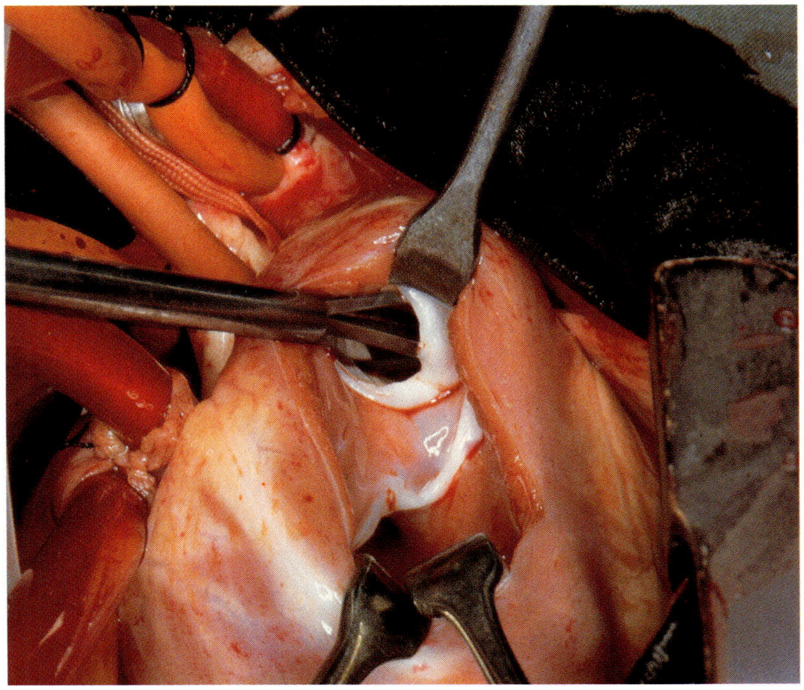

13 After bypass has been discontinued the pressure in the right ventricle and main pulmonary artery are measured to ensure relief of the stenosis. If there is still a marked gradient, it may be necessary to recommence cardiopulmonary bypass and insert a transannular patch. It not, the aortic (**A**) and venous (**B**) cannulae can be removed.

14 to 16 The right ventricle has been opened in this patient for the closure of a ventricular septal defect. It is therefore simpler to perform the pulmonary valvotomy from below with the help of a Potts-Riker retractor, with which the pulmonary valve can be pulled down and the fused commissures divided with a knife.

15

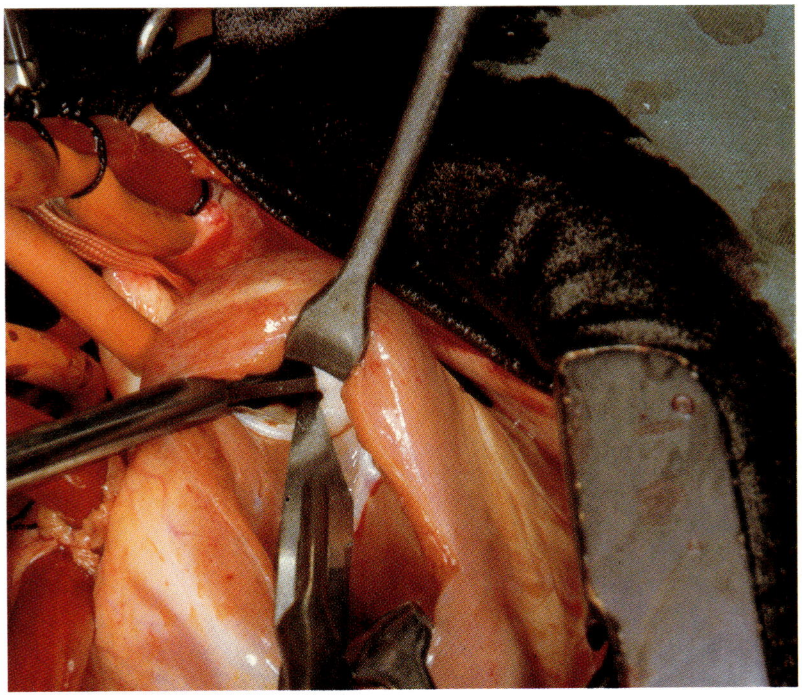

16

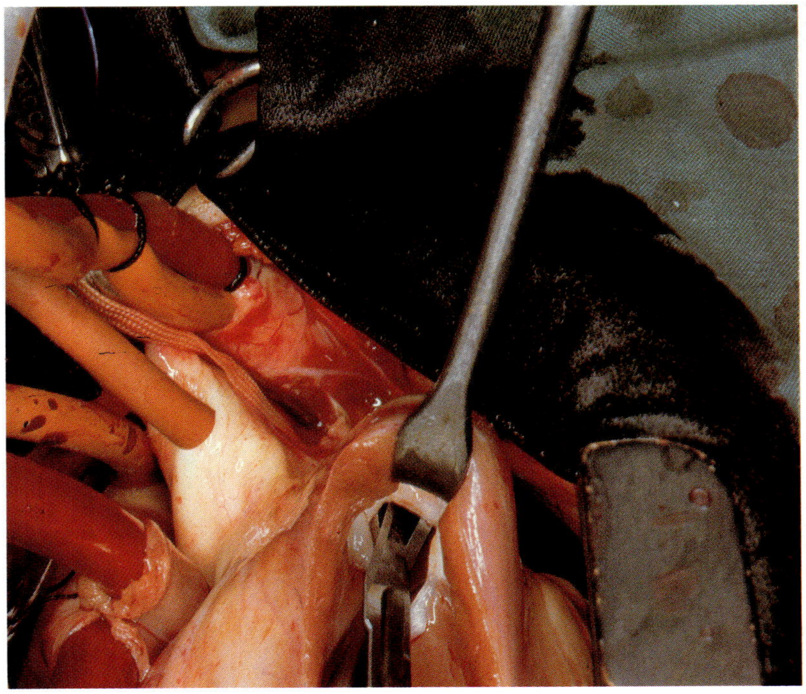

19: Relief of aortic stenosis

Aortic stenosis may be above the valve (supravalvar), at valve level (valvar) or below the valve (subvalvar). Valvar stenosis is much the commonest (see diagram **A**) and patients with this condition may present early in infancy, when they are usually in severe left heart failure. These patients may have very abnormal and thickened valve cusps with abnormalities of the left ventricle, such as endomyocardial fibrosis. The results of valvotomy on these dysplastic valves may be disappointing and it is important not to cause aortic regurgitation. Some valves may be only mildly stenosed or bicuspid and many patients remain asymptomatic until later life. However, in between these extremes there are the many children with valve stenosis whose symptoms may be quite mild, yet whose left ventricles may be under considerable strain and who require valvotomy.

Even if a satisfactory valvotomy is performed, it is extremely likely that all patients will need further surgery, probably valve replacement when they are older.

Supravalvar stenosis is quite rare and occurs above the level of the coronary arteries which are usually large (see diagram **B**). The obstruction is usually caused by a fibrous ridge which can jut out above the valve commissures and coronary arteries, making a shelf which, together with the cusp, allows only a small entrance into the sinus of Valsalva. In repairing this condition, it is usual to make a longitudinal incision down into the non-coronary sinus, cut out obstructing ridges and widen the aorta with a patch.

Subvalvar aortic stenosis (see diagram **C**) is also much less common than valvar stenosis and may be caused by a thin membrane just below the valve. In either case the operation to relieve the obstruction involves opening the aortic root and, with careful retraction of the aortic valve cusps, excising the obstructing membrane.

Cardiopulmonary bypass is needed to be able to expose the aortic valve but it is only necessary to use one venous cannula.

Diagram A – Valvar

A – Ascending aorta

B – Stenosed, bicuspid aortic valve

C – Hypertrophied left ventricle

D – Left coronary artery

E – Right coronary artery

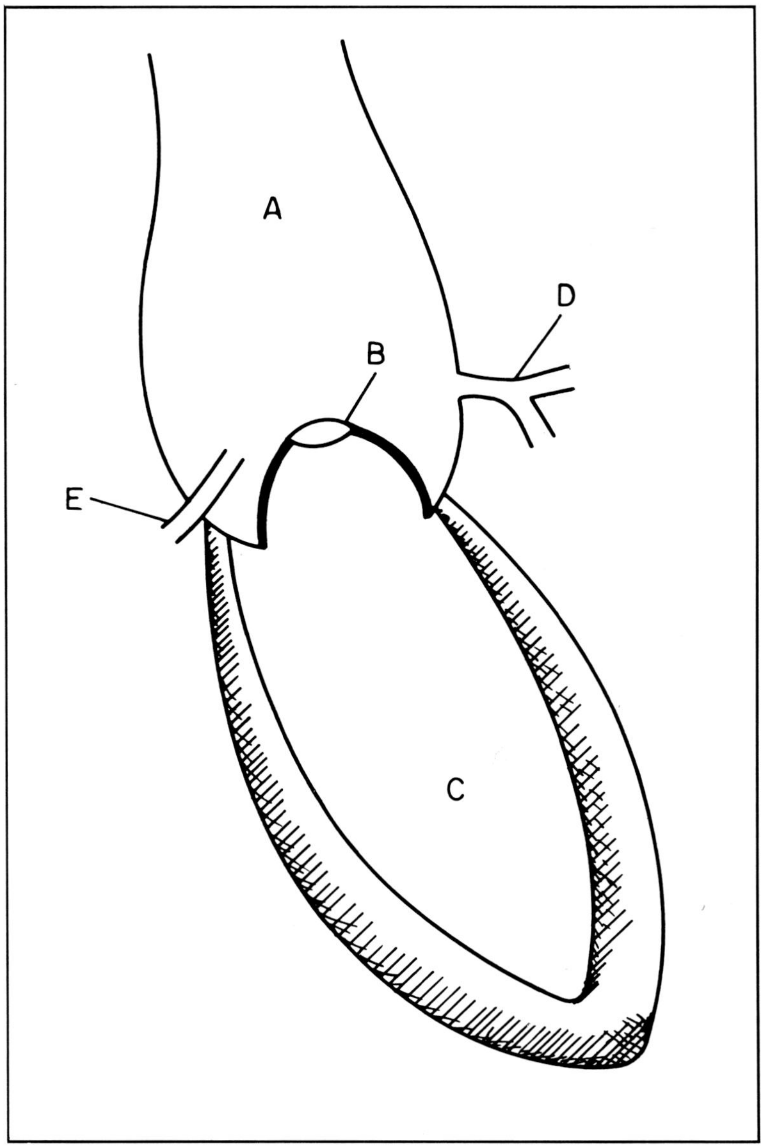

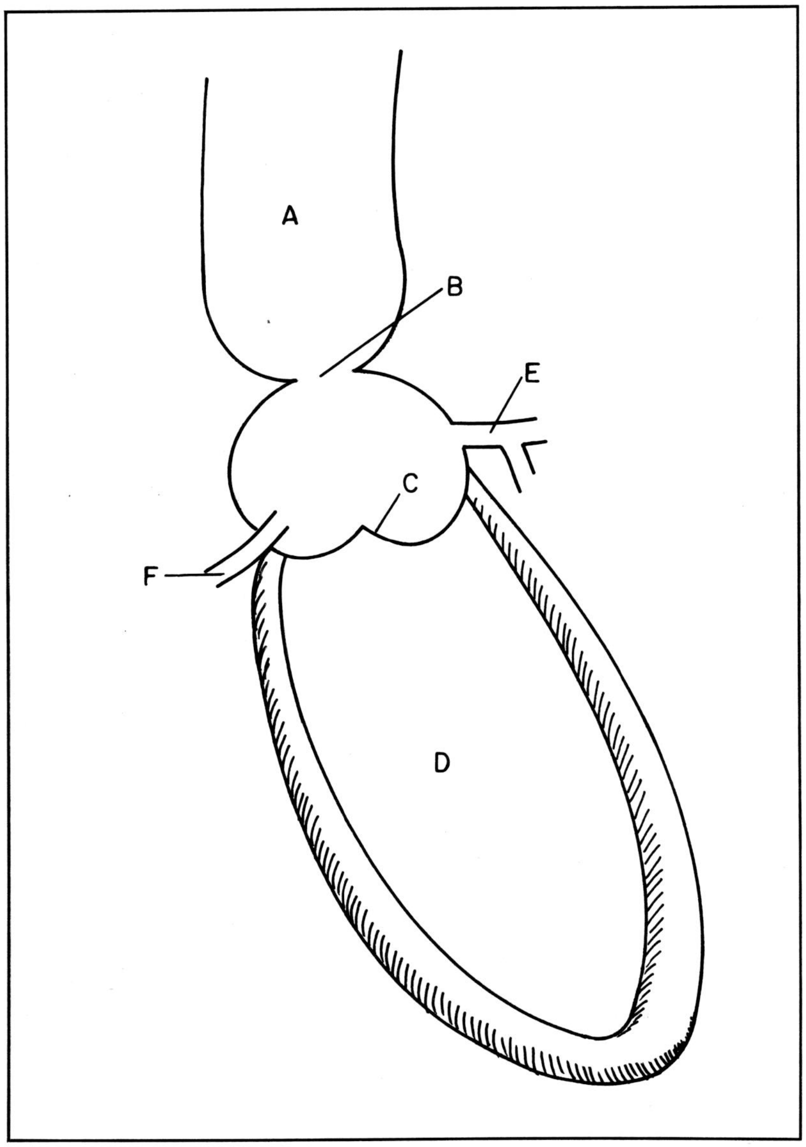

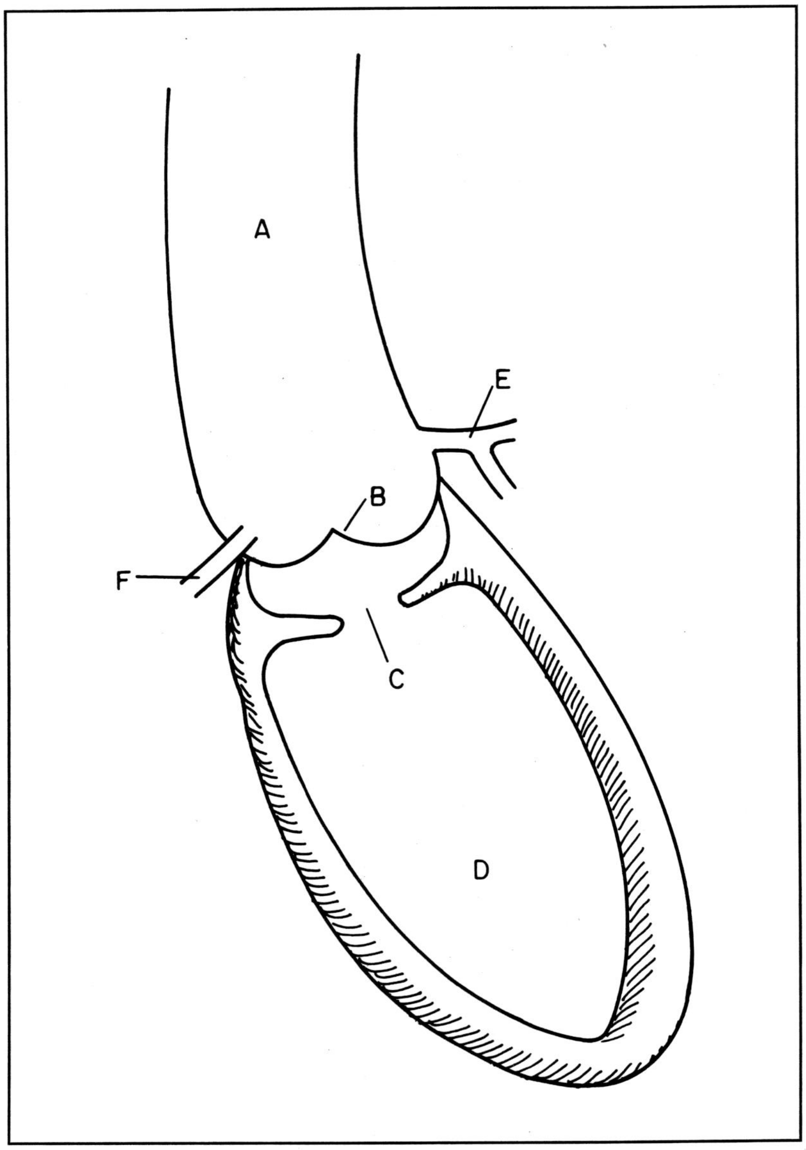

Diagram B – Supravalvar

A – Ascending aorta

B – Supravalvar aortic stenosis

C – Aortic valve

D – Left ventricle

E – Left coronary artery

F – Right coronary artery

Diagram C – Subvalvar

A – Ascending aorta

B – Aortic valve

C – Subvalvar obstruction

D – Left ventricle

E – Left coronary artery

F – Right coronary artery

1

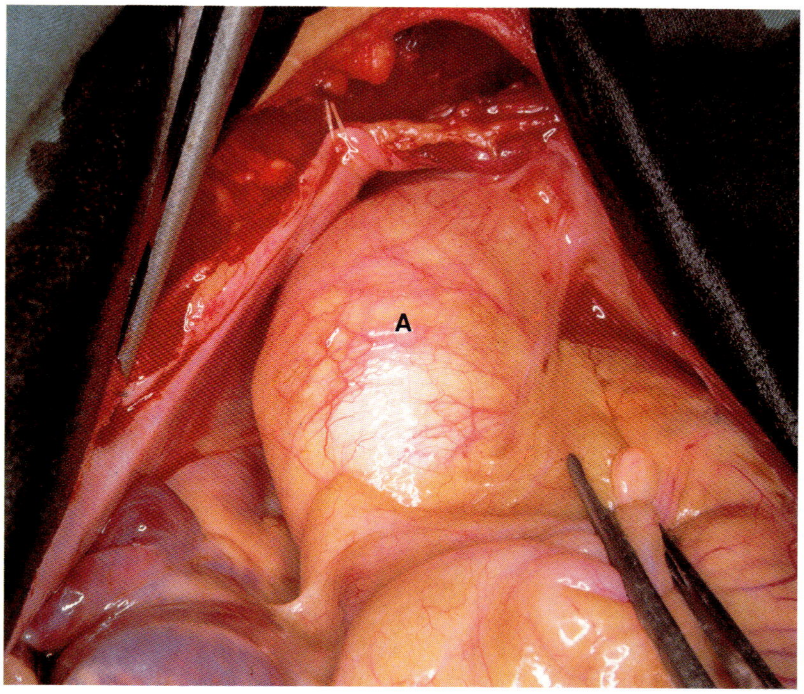

1 The ascending aorta (**A**) has a post-stenotic dilatation but the supra valvar stenosis is at a lower level and is obscured by fat.

2

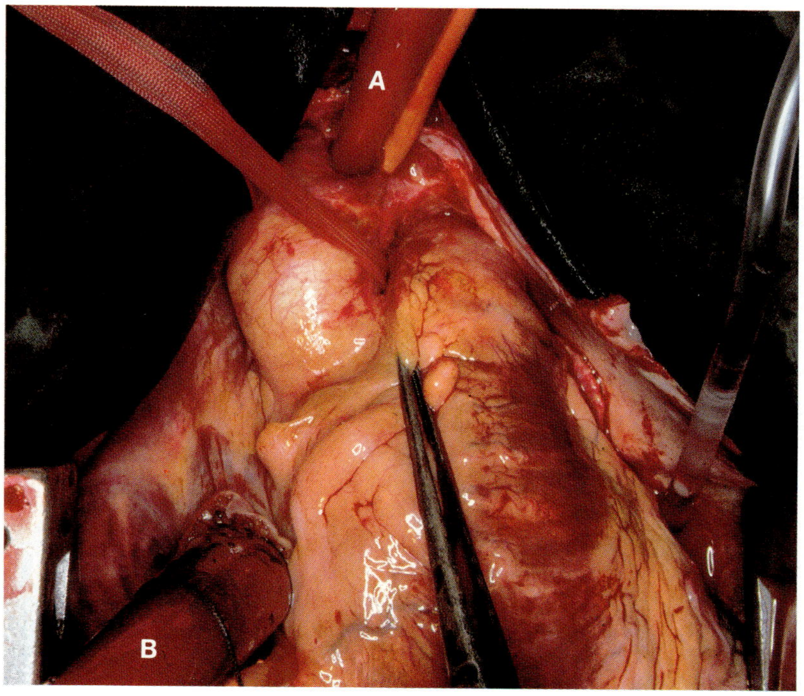

2 A cannula (**A**) has been inserted into the ascending aorta and a single venous cannula (**B**) has been inserted into the right atrial appendage.

3

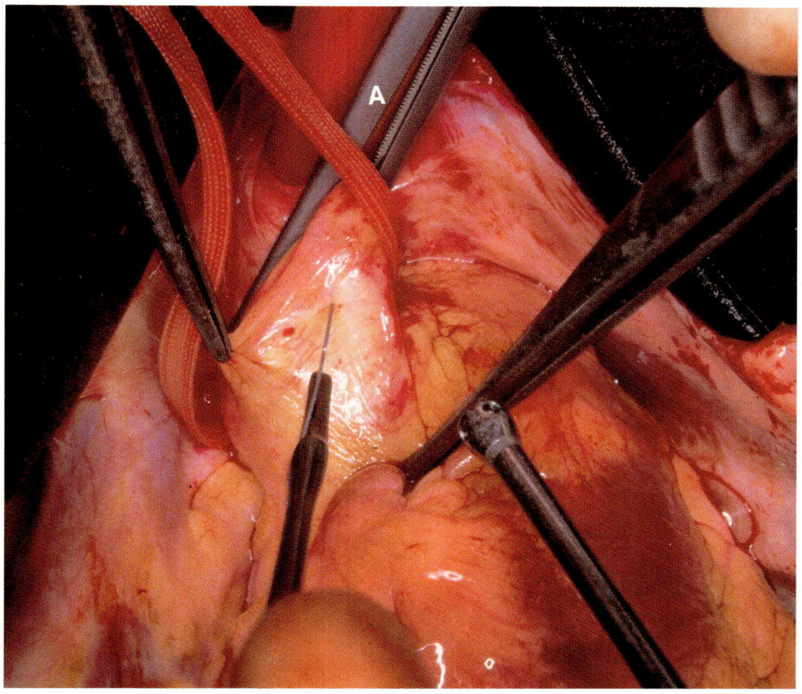

4

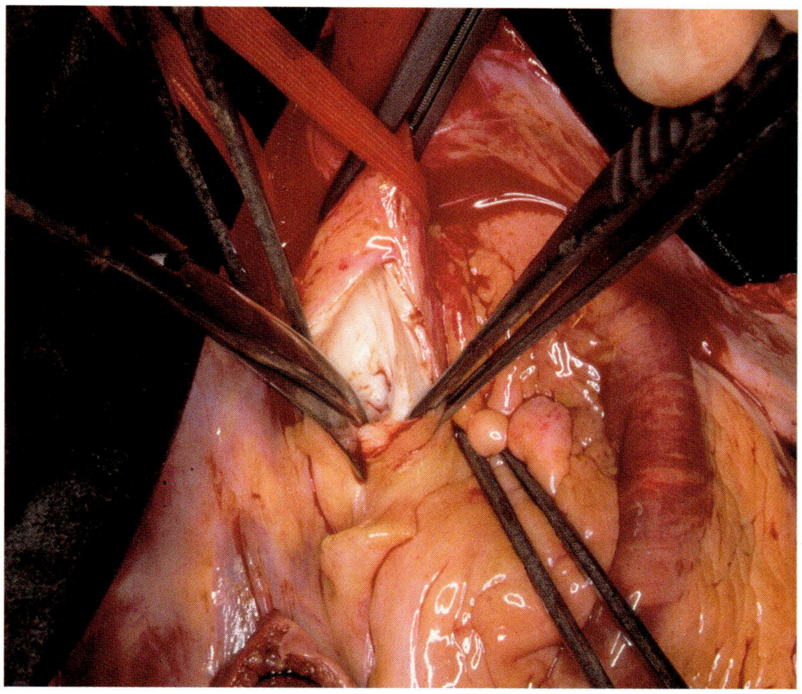

3 and 4 Once cardiopulmonary bypass has been established and an aortic cross-clamp (**A**) applied, the aorta is incised longitudinally.

5

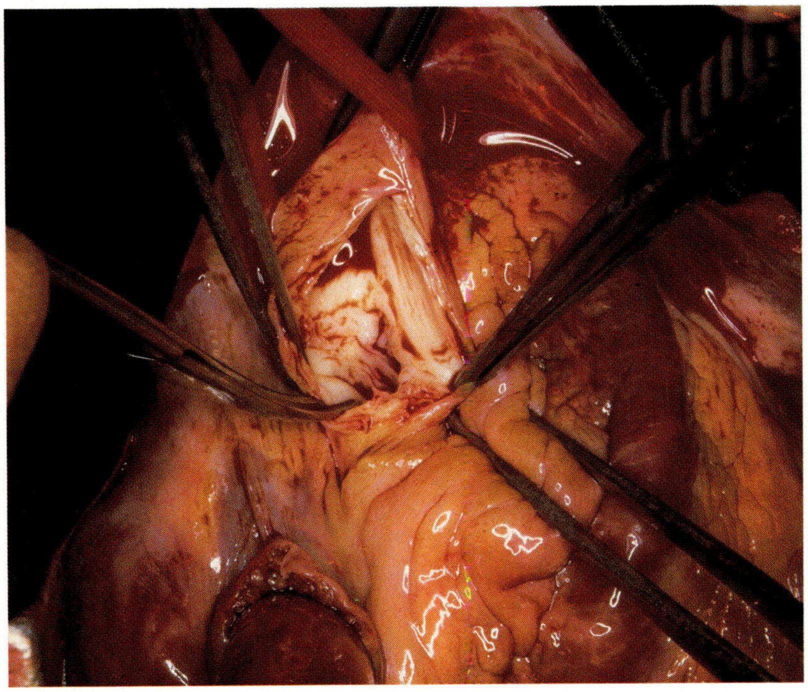

6

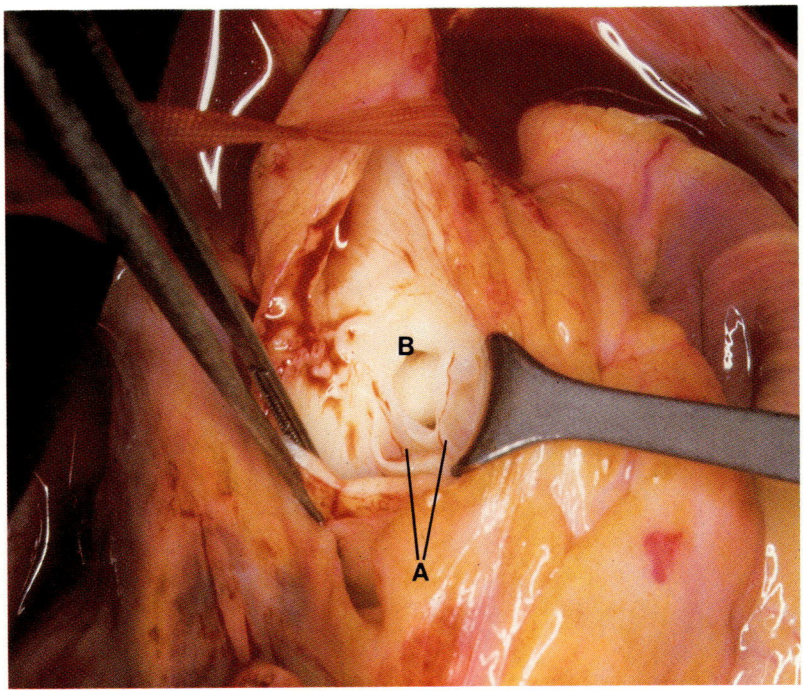

5 and 6 The incision is continued down through the stenosing fibrous obstruction and into the non-coronary sinus. The thin valve leaflets (**A**) are seen beneath the fibrous shelf (**B**) which overhangs the left sinus of Valsalva.

7

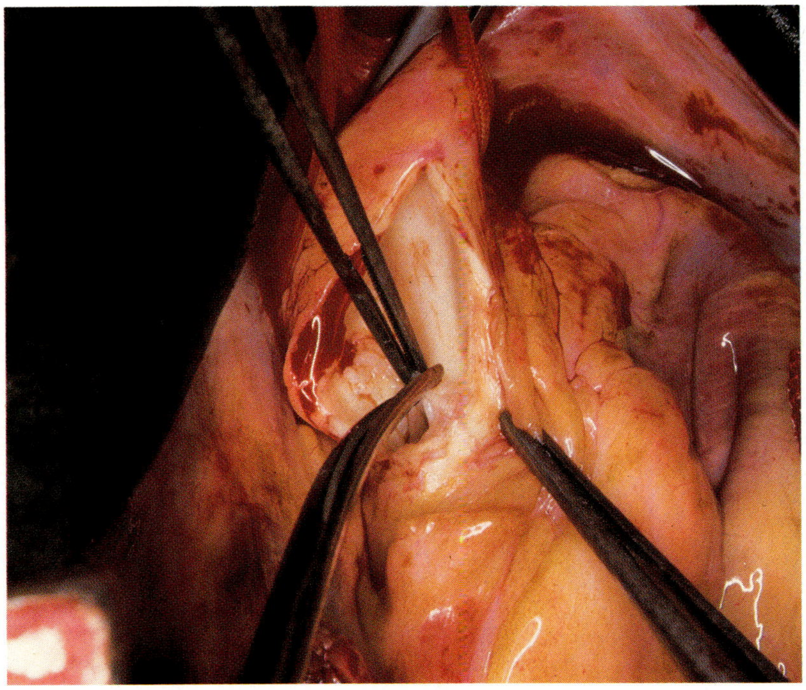

8

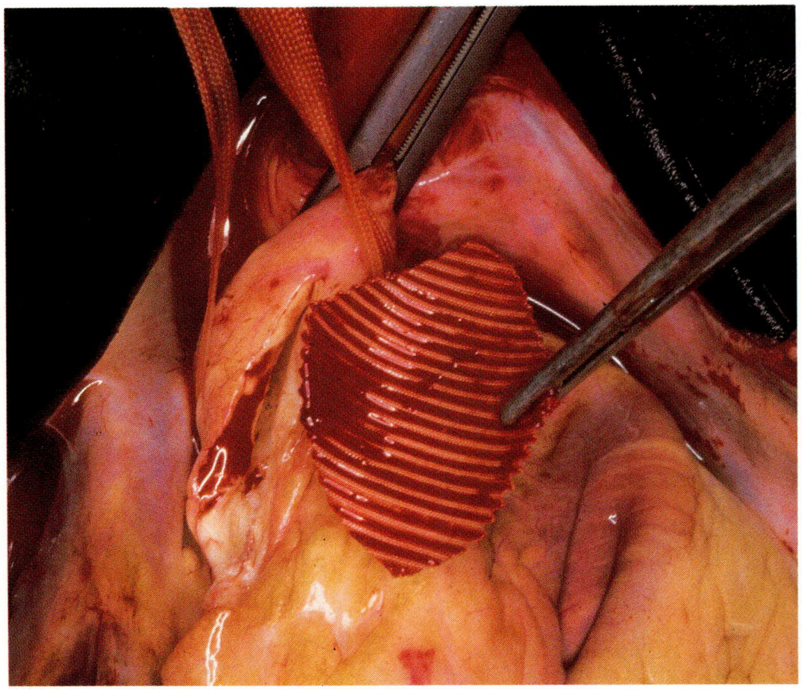

7 Part of the obstructing fibrous rim is excised, taking great care not to damage the valve.

8 The patch to be inserted is cut to the required shape and size and, in this case, is part of a pre-clotted woven dacron tube graft. If this material is used, it is helpful to turn it inside out so that the edges turn outwards making suturing easier. Other materials such as pericardium or dura mater can be used.

9

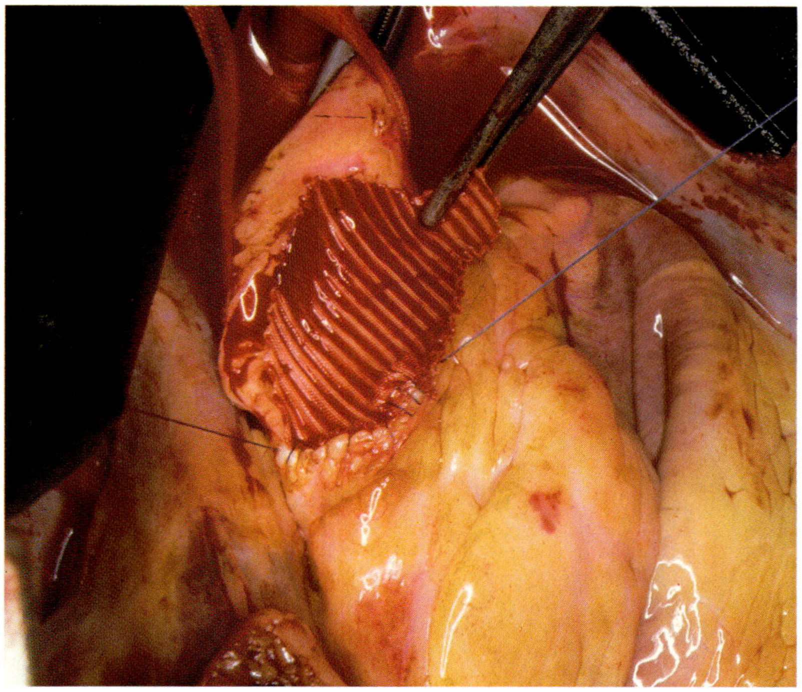

10

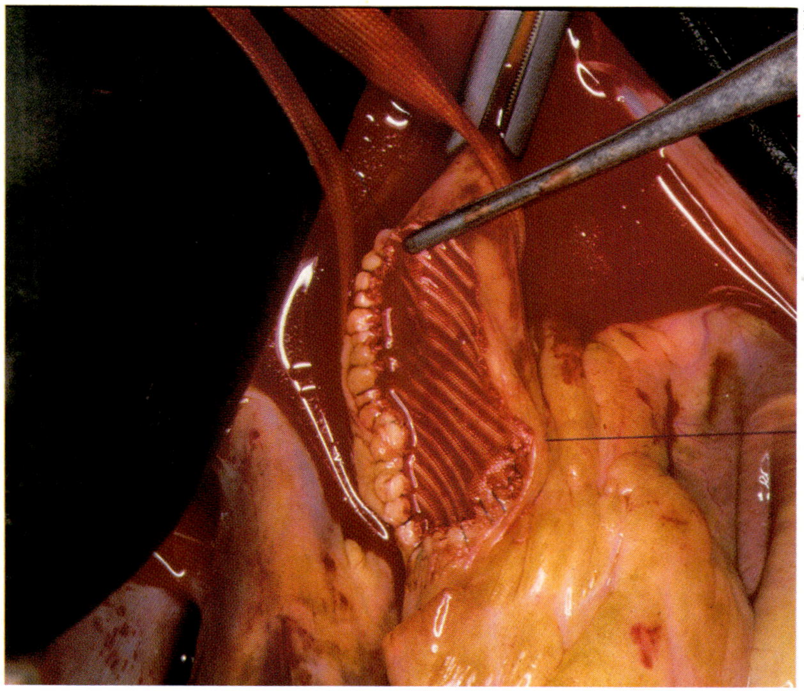

9 to 12 The dacron patch is sutured in with continuous Prolene and the aortic clamp released to show the wide relief of stenosis.

11

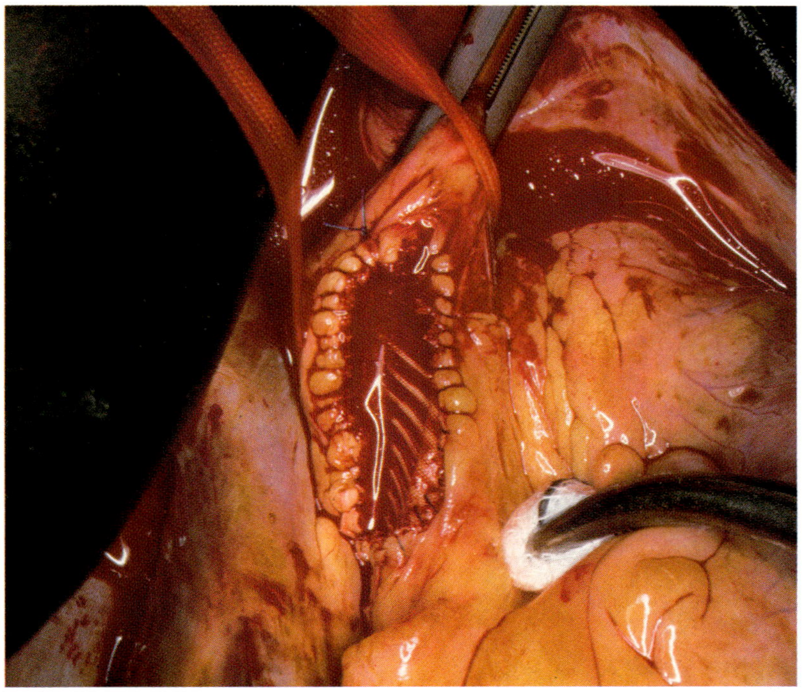

12

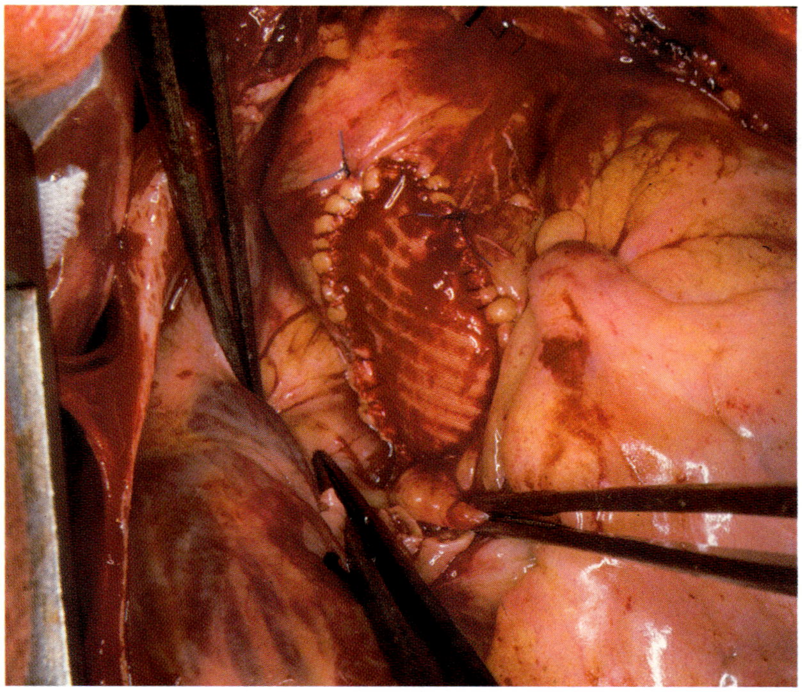

Aortic valvotomy

13

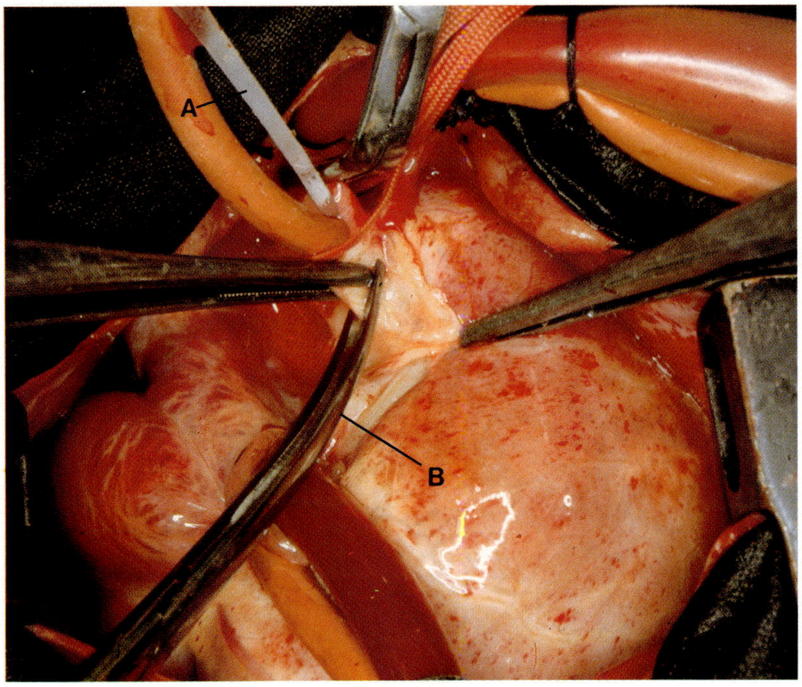

14

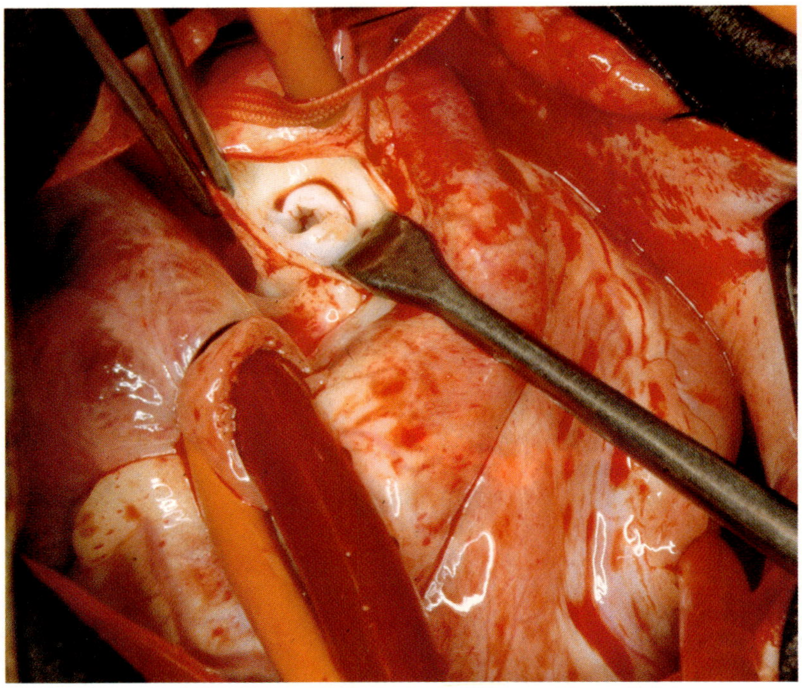

13 After the institution of cardiopulmonary bypass, cardioplegic solution has been given down the cannula (**A**). The ascending aorta is being opened with scissors (**B**).

14. Once the aorta has been opened and retracted the stenosed aortic valve is revealed. It is bicuspid with thickened cusps and the more anterior and leftward commissure is fused.

15

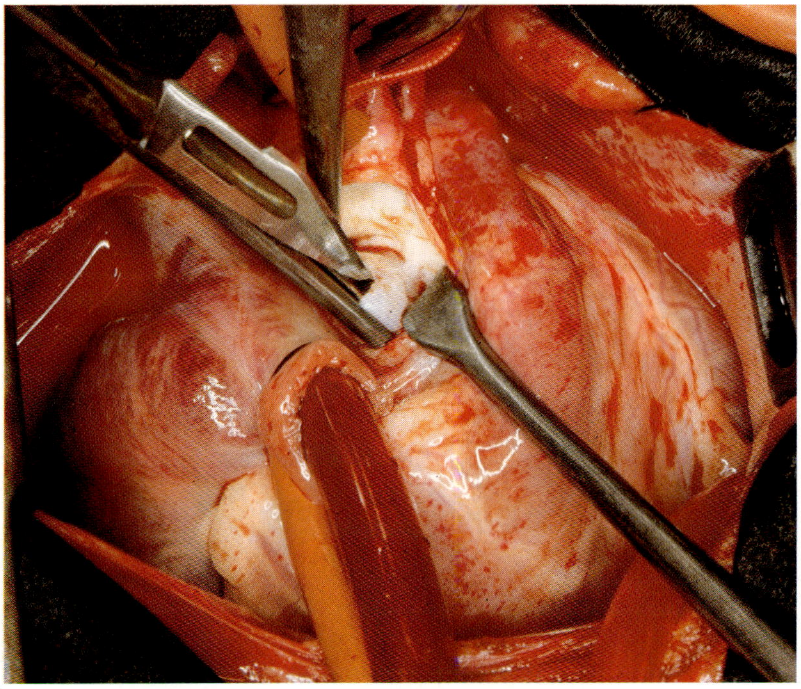

16

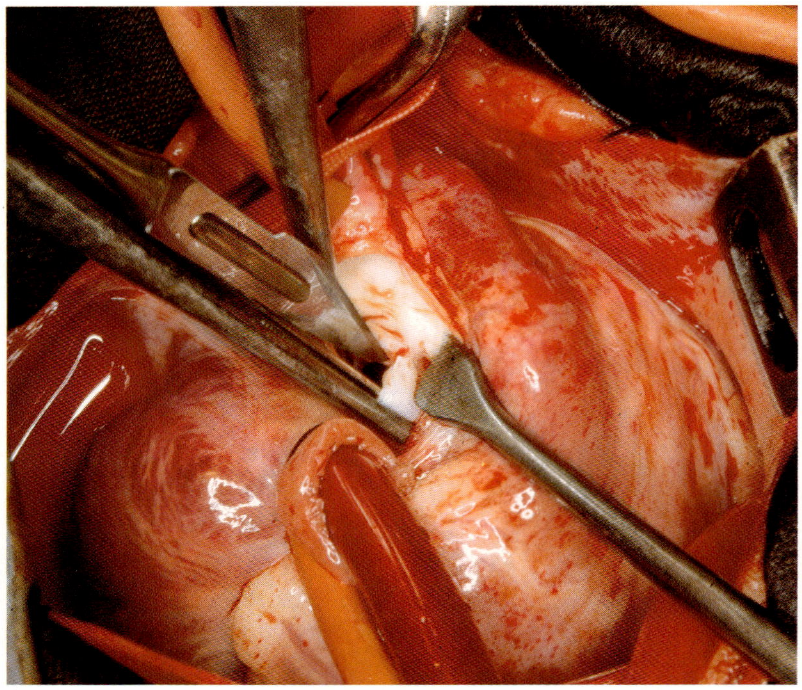

15 and 16 The fused commissure is divided with a knife as far towards the valve ring as possible, without weakening the cusp support. Although only a small incision is required, this considerably increases the orifice of the valve, but the temptation to push Hegar dilators down through it should be avoided as this is likely to cause regurgitation.

17

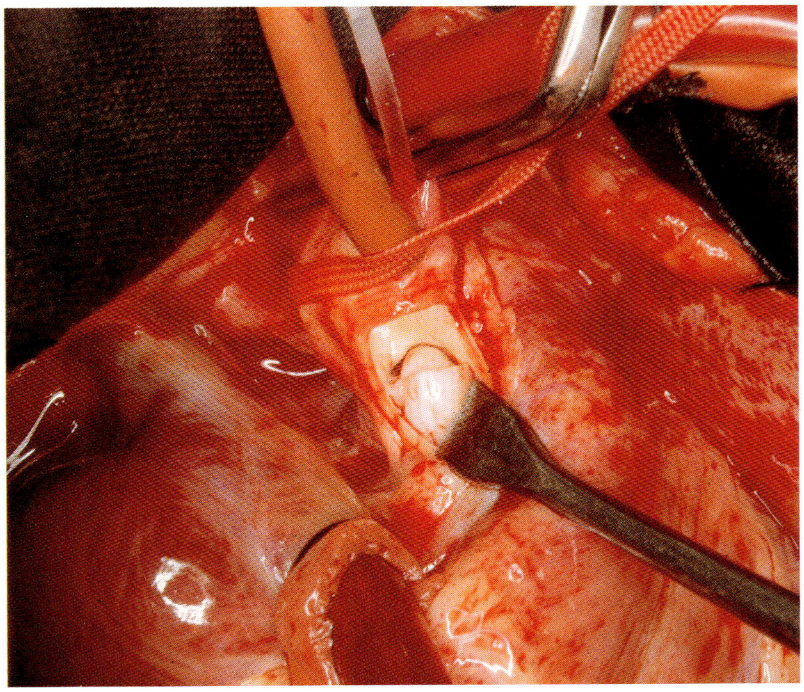

17 The final result looks rather disappointing because of the bicuspid nature of the valve. Although considerable relief of stenosis has been achieved, there is still likely to be a gradient across the valve and the patient will have a murmur. However, the patient should do well for many years but will inevitably need further surgery, probably valve replacement at some time in the future.

18

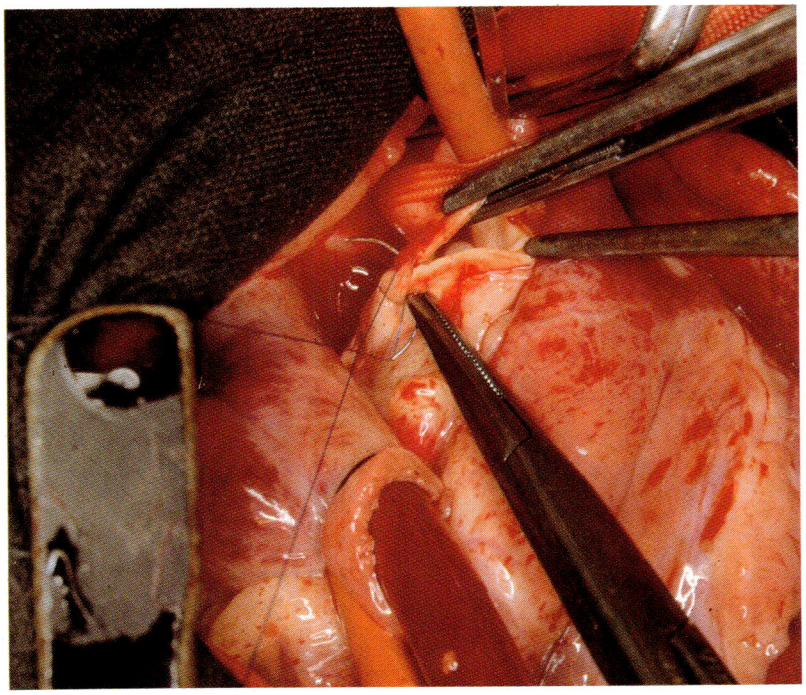

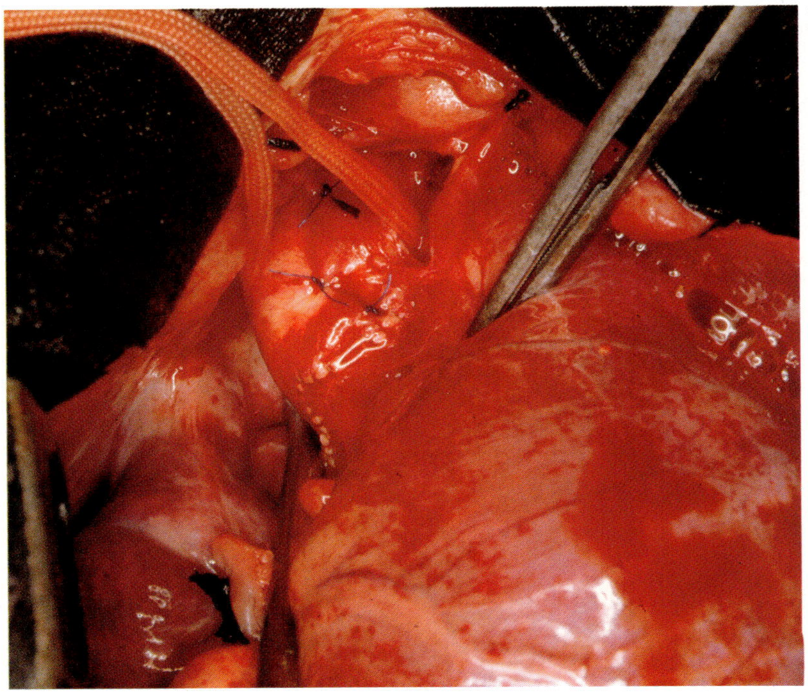

19

18 and 19 The aorta is closed with continuous Prolene, air removed from the heart and the aortic clamp released.

Sub-valvar stenosis

20

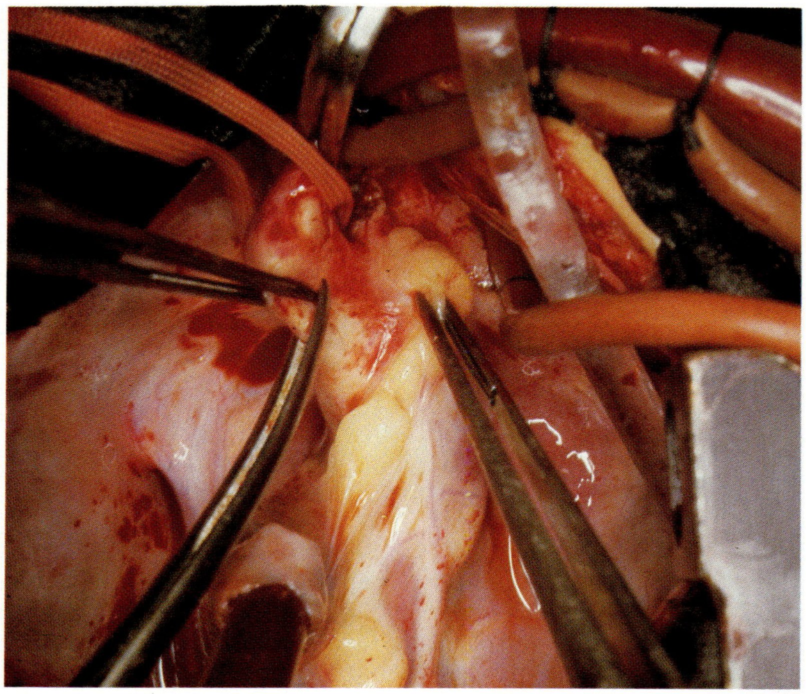

21

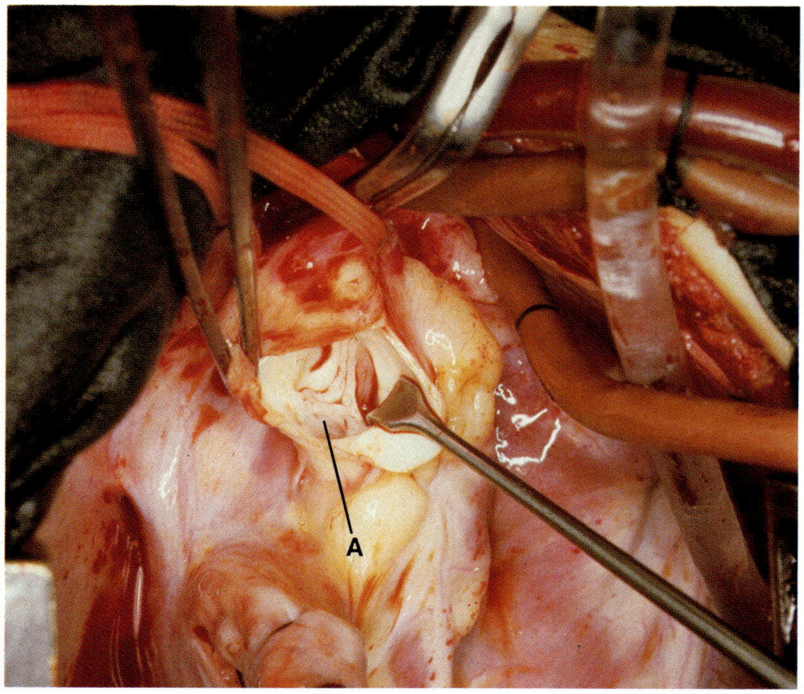

20 and 21 After the institution of cardiopulmonary bypass, the aorta is incised and retracted to reveal a normal aortic valve (**A**).

22

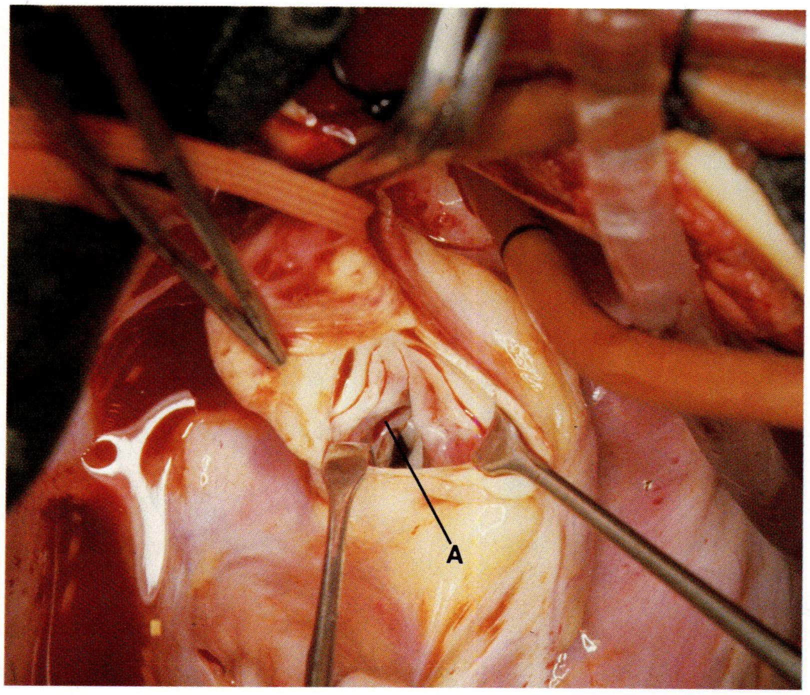

22 With further retraction and allowing the valve cusps to fall back against the aortic wall, the subvalvar obstruction (**A**) is revealed. This obstructing ring is composed of muscle and fibrous tissue.

23

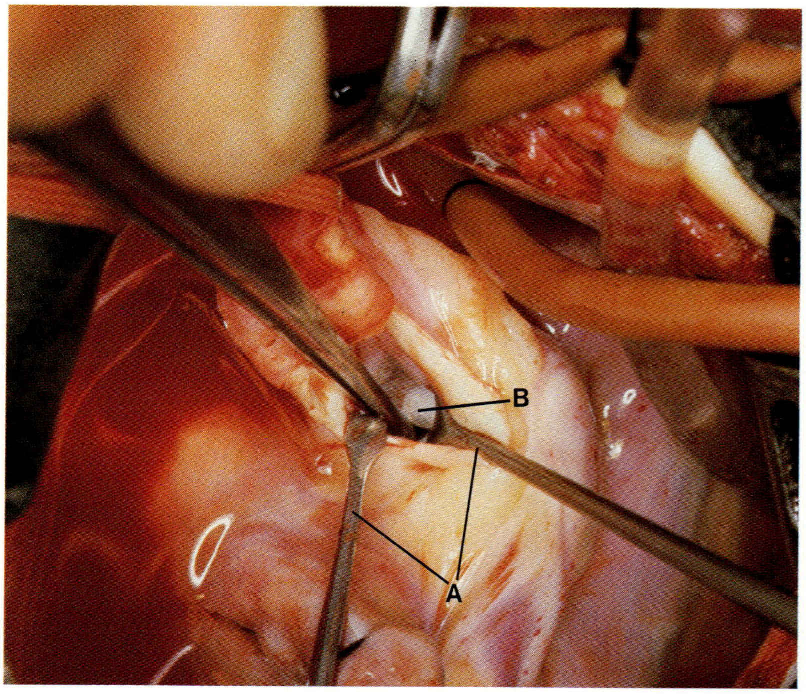

23 The retractors (**A**) have now been placed carefully through the valve so as to retract the cusps better. However, great care must be taken not to damage the cusps or to pull too hard causing pressure on the conduction mechanism and possible heart-block. The fibromuscular shelf (**B**), which is particularly prominent below the commissure between the left and right cusps, is seen clearly.

24

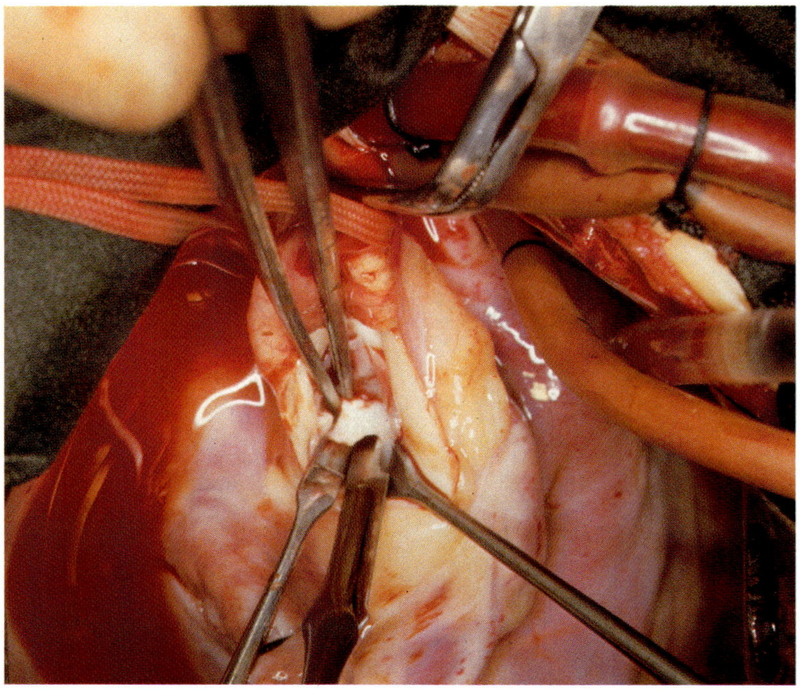

25

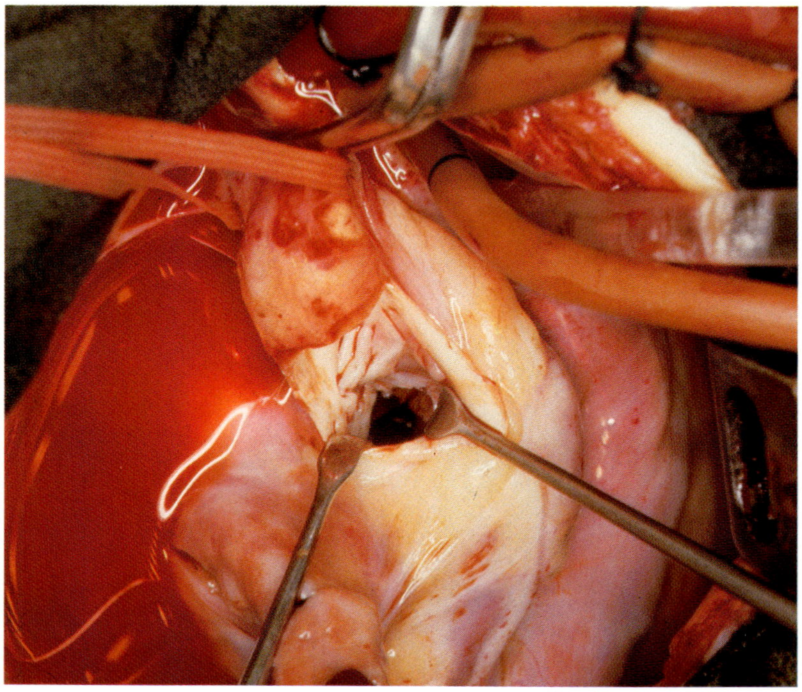

24 and 25 The fibromuscular shelf is cut out with a knife; it is in this region that the incision can be carried into the muscle below the commissure between the left and right cusps without fear of damage to the conduction mechanism or mitral valve and, as in this case, giving good relief of obstruction. The obstructing membrane or shelf usually continues onto the mitral valve and anteriorly onto the membranous septum, but care must be taken when excising it in these regions not to cause damage to underlying structures.

26

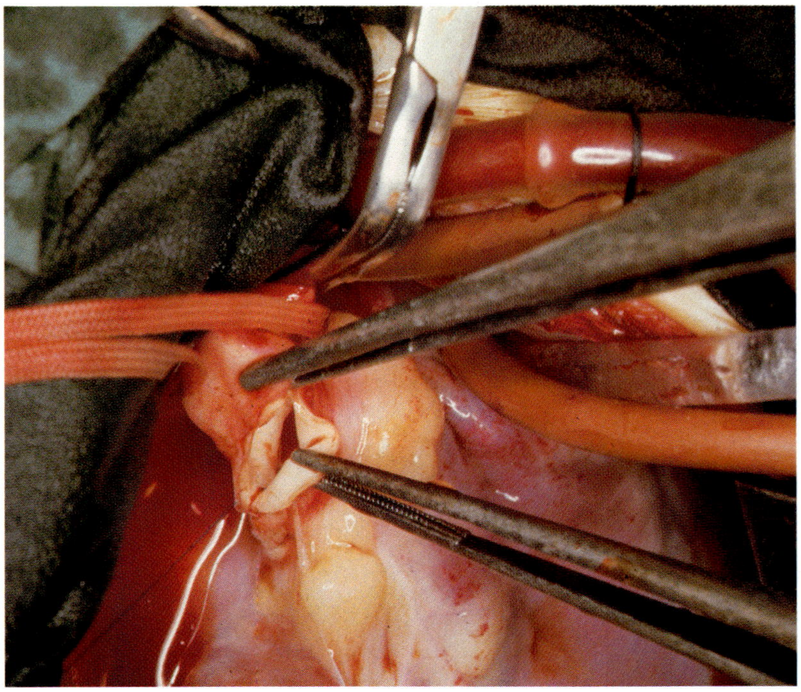

27

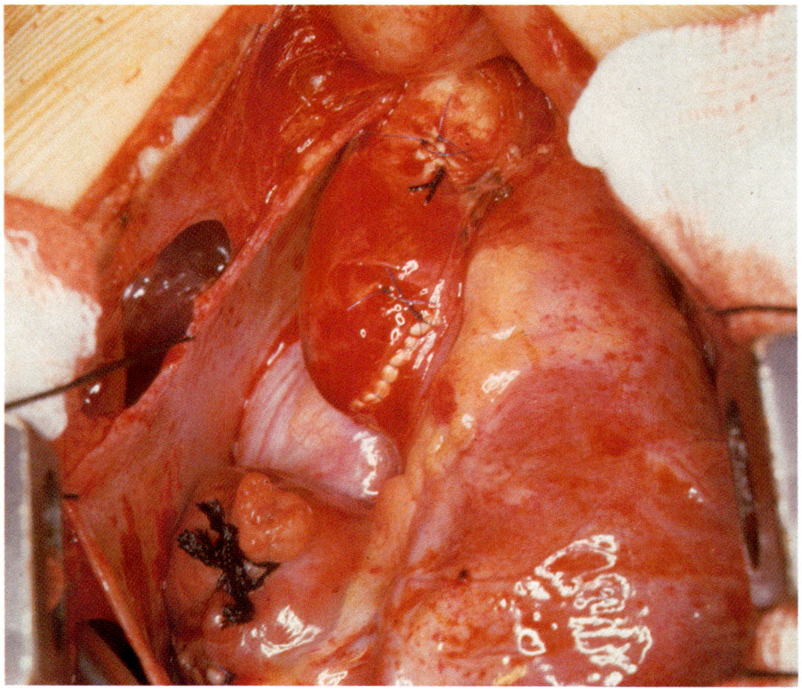

26 and 27 The aorta is then closed with continuous Prolene and the aortic clamp is released.

References

Chapter 1

1 Gross R. E. and Hubbard J. P. (1939) Surgical ligation of a patent ductus arteriosus. *Journal of the American Medical Association* **112,** 729.
2 Crafoord C. and Nylin G. (1945) Congenital coarctation of the aorta and its surgical treatment. *Journal of Thoracic Surgery* **14**, 347.
3 Blalock A. and Taussig H. (1945) The surgical treatment of malformations of the heart. *Journal of the American Medical Association* **128**, 189.
4 Brock R. S. (1948) Pulmonary valvulotomy for the relief of congenital pulmonary stenosis. *British Medical Journal* **1**, 1121.
5 Sellors T. H. (1948) Surgery of pulmonic stenosis. A case in which the pulmonary valve was successfully divided. *Lancet* **1**, 988.
6 Muller W. H. and Damman J. F. (1952) The treatment of certain congenital malformations of the heart by the creation of pulmonary stenosis to reduce pulmonary hypertension and excessive pulmonary blood flow. *Surgery, Gynaecology and Obstetrics* **95**, 213.
7 Swan H. (1954) Techniques of intracardiac surgery under direct vision. *Annals of Surgery* **139**, 385.
8 Lewis F. J., Shumway N. E., Niazi S. A. and Benjamin R. B., (1956) Aortic valvulotomy under direct vision during hypothermia. *Journal of Thoracic Surgery* **32**, 481.
9 Lillehei C. W., Cohen M., Warden H. E., Read R. C., Aust J. B. De Wall R. A. and Varco R. L. (1955) Direct vision intracardiac surgical correction of the tetralogy of Fallot, pentalogy of Fallot and pulmonary atresia defects. Report of first ten cases. *Annals of Surgery* **142,** 418.
10 Gibbon J. H. (1954) Application of a mechanical heart and lung apparatus to cardiac surgery. *Minnesota Med.* **37**, 171.
11 Malm J. R., Bowman F. D., Jesse M. J. and Blumenthal S. (1970) Open-heart surgery in the infant. *American Journal of Surgery* **119**, 613.
12 Hisaka Y., Shirotani H. and Mori C. (1967) Open-heart surgery in infants with the aid of hypothermic anaesthesia. *Arch. Jap. Chir.* **36**, 495.
13 Barratt-Boyes B. G., Simpson M. and Neutze J. M. (1971) Intracardiac surgery in neonates and infants using deep hypothermia with surface cooling and limited cardiopulmonary bypass. *Circulation* **43** and **44,** Supp 1-25.
14 Manners J. M. (1980) Anaesthesia for cardiac surgery. In *Topical Reviews in Anaesthesia.* Ed: J. Norman & J. Whitwam, Vol. **1**, pp. 179-260. Wright, Bristol.
15 Ionescu M. I. (1981) *Techniques in Extracorporeal Circulation.* Butterworths, Sevenoaks.
16 Roe B. B., Hutchinson J. C., Fishman N. H., Ullyot D. J. and Smith D. L. (1977) Myocardial protection with cold, ischaemic, potassium-induced cardioplegia. *Journal of Thoracic and Cardiovascular Surgery* **73**, 366.
17 Manners J. M., Monro J. L. and Edwards J. C. (1980) Corrective cardiac surgery in infants. *Anaesthesia* **35**, 1149.

Chapter 4

1 Gross R. E. and Hubbard J. P. (1939) Surgical ligation of a patent ductus arteriosus. *Journal of the American Medical Association* **112**, 729.

Chapter 5

1 Craafoord C. and Nylin G. (1945) Congenital coarctation of the aorta and its surgical treatment. *Journal of Thoracic Surgery* **14**, 347.
2 Waldhausen A. J. and Nahrwold D. L. (1966) Repair of coarctation of the aorta with subclavian flap. *Journal of Thoracic and Cardiovascular Surgery* **51,** 532.
3 Hamilton D. I., Di Eusanio G., Sandrasagra F. A. and Donelly R. J. (1978) Early and late results of aortoplasty with a left subclavian flap for coarctation of the aorta in infancy. *Journal of Thoracic and Cardiovascular Surgery* **75,** 699.

Chapter 6

1 Blalock A. and Taussig H. (1945) The surgical treatment of malformations of the heart. *Journal of the American Medical Association* **128,** 189.

Chapter 7

1 Waterston D. J. (1962) The treatment of Fallot's tetralogy in infants under the age of one year (In Czech.) *RozhL. Chir.* **41**, 183.
2 Cooley D. A. and Hallman G. L. (1966) Intrapericardial aortic-right pulmonary arterial anastomosis. *Surgery, Gynaecology and Obstetrics* **122**, 1084.

Chapter 8

1 Muller W. H. and Damman J. F. (1952) The treatment of certain congenital malformations of the heart by the creation of pulmonary stenosis to reduce pulmonary hypertension and excessive pulmonary blood flow. *Surgery, Gynaecology and Obstetrics* **95**, 213.

Chapter 9

1 Lewis F. J. (1955) The surgical anatomy of atrial septal defects. Experiences with repair under direct vision. *Annals of Surgery* **142**, 401.
2 Gibbon J. H. (1954) Application of a mechanical heart and lung apparatus to cardiac surgery. *Minnesota Medicine* **37**, 171.

Chapter 10

1 Rastelli G. C., Kirklin J. W. and Titus J. L. (1966) Anatomic observations on complete form of persistent common atrioventricular canal with special reference to atrioventricular valves. *Mayo Clinic Proceedings* **41**, 296.
2 Carpentier A. (1977) Surgical anatomy and management of the mitral component of atrioventricular canal defects. In *Paediatric Cardiology*. Ed: R. H. Anderson and E. A. Shinebourne. Churchill-Livingstone, p. 477.

Chapter 12

1 Fallot A. (1888) Contribution à l'anatomie pathologique de la maladie bleu (cyanose cardiaque). *Marseille Med.* **25**, 77.
2 Lillehei C. W., Cohen M., Warden H. E., Read R. C., Aust J. B., De Wall R. A. and Varco R. L. (1955) Direct vision intracardiac surgical correction of the tetralogy of Fallot, pentalogy of Fallot and pulmonary atresia defects. Report of first ten cases. *Annals of Surgery* **142**, 418.
3 Monro J. L. (1978) Fallot's Tetralogy – necessity for outflow patch. In *Paediatric Cardiology* 1977. Ed: R. H. Anderson and E. A. Shinebourne, Churchill-Livingstone. Edinburgh.
4 Pacifico A. D., Kirklin J. W. and Blackstone E. H. (1977) Surgical management of pulmonary stenosis in tetralogy of Fallot. *Journal of Thoracic and Cardiovascular Surgery* **74**, 382.
5 Kirklin J. W. and Karp R. B. (1970) *The Tetralogy of Fallot from a surgical viewpoint.* Philadelphia, W. B. Saunders Company. Ch. 6.

Chapter 13

1 Rashkind W. J. and Miller W. W. (1966) Creation of an atrial septal defect without thoracotomy. *Journal of the American Medical Association* **196**, 991.
2 Blalock A. and Hanlon C. R. (1950) The surgical treatment of complete transposition of the aorta and pulmonary artery. *Surgery, Gynaecology and Obstetrics* **90**, 1.
3 Mustard W. T. (1964) Successful two-stage correction of transposition of the great vessels. *Surgery* **55**, 469.
4 Senning A. (1959) Surgical correction of transposition of the great vessels. *Surgery* **45**, 966.
5 Jatene A. D., Fontes V. F., Paulista P. P., Souza L. C. B., Neger B., Galantier N. and Sousa J. E. M. R. (1976) Anatomic correction of transposition of the great vessels. *Journal of Thoracic and Cardiovascular Surgery* **72**, 364.
6 Yacoub M. H. (1979) The case for anatomic correction of transposition of the great arteries. *Journal of Thoracic and Cardiovascular Surgery* **78**, 3.

Chapter 14

1 McGoon D. C., Rastelli G. C. and Ongley P. A. (1968) An operation for the correction of truncus arteriosus. *Journal of the American Medical Association* **205**, 69.

Chapter 16

1 Fontan F. and Baudet E. (1971) Surgical repair of tricuspid atresia. *Thorax* **25**, 240.
2 Yacoub M. H. and Radley-Smith R. (1975) Use of a valved conduit from right atrium to pulmonary artery for correction of a single ventricle. *Circulation* **51**, 52. Supplement 2, 101.
3 Kreutzer G., Galindez E. and Bono H. (1973) An operation for the total correction of tricuspid atresia. *Journal of Cardiovascular Surgery* **66**, 613.
4 Bjork V. O., Olin C. L. Bjarke B. B. and Thoren C. A. (1979) Right atrial – right ventricular anastomosis for correction of tricuspid atresia. *Journal of Thoracic and Cardiovascular Surgery* **77**, 452.
5 Fontan F., Deville C., Quaegebeur J., Ottenkamp J., Sourdille N., Choussat A. and Brom G. A. (1983) Repair of tricuspid atresia in 100 patients. *Journal of Thoracic and Cardiovascular Surgery* **85**, 647.

Chapter 17

1 Ross D. N. and Somerville J. (1966) Correction of pulmonary atresia with a homograft aortic valve. *Lancet* **2**, 1446.

Index